Inderbir Singh's

Textbook of
HUMAN HISTOLOGY

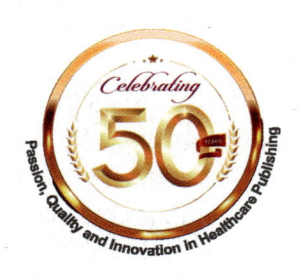

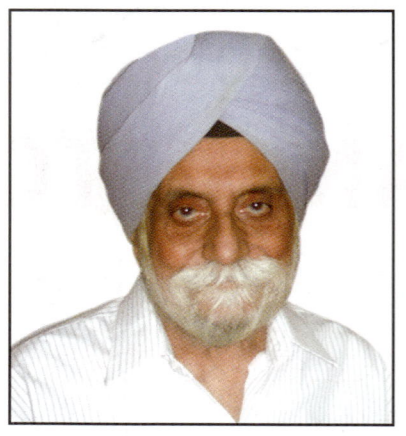

Late **Professor Inderbir Singh**
(1930–2014)

Tribute to a Legend

Professor Inderbir Singh, a legendary anatomist, is renowned for being a pillar in the education of generations of medical graduates across the globe. He was one of the greatest teachers of his times. He was a passionate writer who poured his soul into his work. His eagle's eye for details and meticulous way of writing made his books immensely popular amongst students. He managed to become enmeshed in millions of hearts in his lifetime. He was conferred the title of Professor Emeritus by Maharishi Dayanand University, Rohtak.

On 12th May, 2014, he was awarded posthumously with* Emeritus Teacher Award *by* National Board of Examination *for making invaluable contribution in teaching of Anatomy. This award is given to honour legends who have made tremendous contribution in the field of medical graduate. He was a visionary for his times, and the legacies he left behind are his various textbooks on *Gross Anatomy*, *Histology*, *Neuroanatomy* and *Embryology*. Although his mortal frame is not present amongst us, his genius will live on forever.

Inderbir Singh's

Textbook of
HUMAN HISTOLOGY

With Color Atlas and Practical Guide

NINTH EDITION

Revised and Edited by

Pushpalatha K
MBBS MD (PhD)
Professor and Head
Department of Anatomy
Jagadguru Sri Shivarathreeshwara (JSS) Medical College
Mysuru, Karnataka, India

Deepa Bhat
MBBS MD (PhD)
Associate Professor
Department of Anatomy
Jagadguru Sri Shivarathreeshwara (JSS) Medical College
Mysuru, Karnataka, India

Pushpa NB
MBBS MD
Assistant Professor
Department of Anatomy
Jagadguru Sri Shivarathreeshwara (JSS) Medical College
Mysuru, Karnataka, India

Foreword
Nachiket Shankar

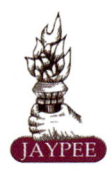

JAYPEE BROTHERS MEDICAL PUBLISHERS
The Health Sciences Publisher
New Delhi | London

Jaypee Brothers Medical Publishers (P) Ltd

Headquarters
Jaypee Brothers Medical Publishers (P) Ltd
4838/24, Ansari Road, Daryaganj
New Delhi 110 002, India
Phone: +91-11-43574357
Fax: +91-11-43574314
Email: jaypee@jaypeebrothers.com

Overseas Office
J.P. Medical Ltd
83 Victoria Street, London
SW1H 0HW (UK)
Phone: +44 20 3170 8910
Fax: +44 (0)20 3008 6180
Email: info@jpmedpub.com

Website: www.jaypeebrothers.com
Website: www.jaypeedigital.com

© 2020, Jaypee Brothers Medical Publishers

The views and opinions expressed in this book are solely those of the original contributor(s)/author(s) and do not necessarily represent those of editor(s) of the book.

All rights reserved. No part of this publication may be reproduced, stored or transmitted in any form or by any means, electronic, mechanical, photocopying, recording or otherwise, without the prior permission in writing of the publishers.

All brand names and product names used in this book are trade names, service marks, trademarks or registered trademarks of their respective owners. The publisher is not associated with any product or vendor mentioned in this book.

Medical knowledge and practice change constantly. This book is designed to provide accurate, authoritative information about the subject matter in question. However, readers are advised to check the most current information available on procedures included and check information from the manufacturer of each product to be administered, to verify the recommended dose, formula, method and duration of administration, adverse effects and contraindications. It is the responsibility of the practitioner to take all appropriate safety precautions. Neither the publisher nor the author(s)/editor(s) assume any liability for any injury and/or damage to persons or property arising from or related to use of material in this book.

This book is sold on the understanding that the publisher is not engaged in providing professional medical services. If such advice or services are required, the services of a competent medical professional should be sought.

Every effort has been made where necessary to contact holders of copyright to obtain permission to reproduce copyright material. If any have been inadvertently overlooked, the publisher will be pleased to make the necessary arrangements at the first opportunity. The **CD/DVD-ROM** (if any) provided in the sealed envelope with this book is complimentary and free of cost. **Not meant for sale.**

Inquiries for bulk sales may be solicited at: jaypee@jaypeebrothers.com

Inderbir Singh's Textbook of Human Histology

First Edition : 1987
Second Edition : 1992
Third Edition : 1992
Fourth Edition : 2002
Reprint : 2005
Fifth Edition : 2006
Reprint : 2008
Reprint : 2009
Sixth Edition : 2011
Seventh Edition : 2014
Eighth Edition : 2016
Ninth Edition : May 2019
Revised Reprint : Sep **2019**

ISBN: 978-93-89034-97-4

Printed at Sanat Printers

Dedicated to

*The Almighty, family, colleagues and friends
for their support and for kindling the fire
within that has led to fulfil the passion to write a book*

FOREWORD

It gives me great pleasure to write the foreword for the latest edition of this well-known textbook of histology. For a number of years, this textbook was the preferred learning resource for health professional students. More recently a number of other textbooks in histology have become available. It is therefore appropriate that this edition has emerged, incorporating the changes that are required for the current generation of students, yet retaining the strengths of the older editions. Each chapter begins with the learning objectives and identification points of the related slides. The text has been presented in a concise, bulleted format that makes for easy readability. Schematic diagrams are presented alongside pictures from actual slides, making it simple for students to identify and draw the key features. The applied histology section provides a relevant clinical context for learning. Each chapter ends with multiple choice questions, which provide an opportunity for students to evaluate their learning. This edition will be ideally suited for the first batch of MBBS students undergoing the recently rolled out competency-based curriculum.

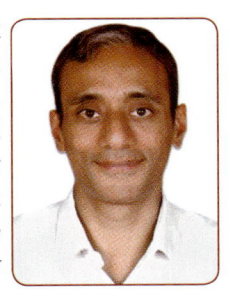

Nachiket Shankar
Professor
Department of Anatomy and Medical Education
St John's Medical College
Bengaluru, Karnataka, India

JSS MEDICAL COLLEGE
(Constituent College)
JSS Academy of Higher Education & Research
(Deemed to be University)
Accredited 'A+' Grade by NAAC

PREFACE

Inderbir Singh's Textbook of Human Histology is widely used by students and faculty of health profession. Ninth edition of this book has been improvised as per current student requirements. The chapters have been revised with simplified representation. The contents are updated incorporating the recent advances that the students must be aware off.

Well-defined learning objectives assist focussed student learning, help to choose appropriate teaching learning methods and assessment strategies. The content has been stratified to must know, good to know and nice to know categories. This intends to progressively take student from basic understanding to in-depth knowledge as per their needs. The content is modified and revised according to the new competency-based curriculum. Optic nerve and umbilical cord is added as per Medical Council of India (MCI) requirements.

The point-wise representation will make the reading easier and understandable.

The histology slides that students' observe during practical classes are similar with newly-added color plates of the textbook. Core highlight of this edition is addition of easily reproducible hand written diagrams of histology slides that student witnesses in the practical class. This will help in practical record writing and during examination.

The clinical features are retained, modified and added keeping in mind their applicability in pathology. Thus the learning carries forward in next phase of MBBS which forms the core vision of competency-based medical education that is being rolled out this academic year.

Identification points are added in the beginning of every chapter that helps the students to identify the slide, for last minute revision and during spotters.

The Multiple Choice Questions (MCQs) added will help the students in preparing for examinations. This book offers a one-stop solution for all histology-related needs.

Effort was made keeping in mind student friendliness yet maintaining the quality. Utmost care has been taken to avoid any errors or omissions. The suggestions, from learned and expertise would always be welcomed wholeheartedly to improve the efficacy of the manuscript. Scope for amendment always remains, and is invited from teachers and students.

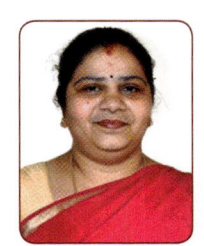

Pushpalatha K

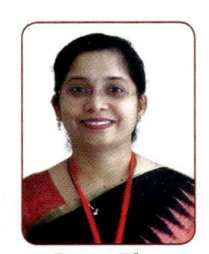

Deepa Bhat

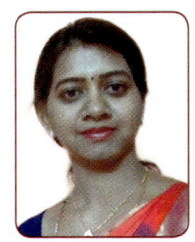

Pushpa NB

ACKNOWLEDGMENTS

We would like to thank all the people for the help and support they provided in the preparation of this book. Thanks to Principal and the staff of JSS Medical College, Mysuru, Karnataka, India, for this opportunity.

Special thanks to Molecular Biology Laboratory, Department of Biochemistry, JSS Medical College, Mysuru, for permitting to capture the photomicrographs that is the salient highlight of this manuscript. Thank those who have directly and indirectly assisted in completion of this task.

Finally our thanks to Shri Jitendar P Vij (Group Chairman), Mr Ankit Vij (Managing Director), Mr MS Mani (Group President), Dr Madhu Choudhary (Publishing Head–Education), Ms Pooja Bhandari (Production Head) and Ms Sunita Katla (Executive Assistant to Group Chairman and Publishing Manager) of M/s Jaypee Brothers Medical Publishers (P) Ltd, New Delhi, India, for this opportunity.

NATIONAL ADVISORY BOARD

Akhilandeswari B
Professor
Department of Anatomy
Bangalore Medical College and Research Institute
Bengaluru, Karnataka, India

Anirban Sadhu
Associate Professor
Department of Anatomy
RG Kar Medical College
Kolkata, West Bengal, India

Anjali Jain
Professor and Head
Department of Anatomy
Christian Medical College
Ludhiana, Punjab, India

Anjoo Yadav
Associate Professor
Department of Anatomy
Lady Hardinge Medical College
New Delhi, India

Anju Partap Kaundal
Professor and Head
Department of Anatomy
Indira Gandhi Medial College
Shimla, Himachal Pradesh, India

Arun Sharma
Head, Department of Anatomy
MLB Medical College
Jhansi, Uttar Pradesh, India

Ashwini C Appaji
Associate Professor
MS Ramaiah Medical College
Bengaluru, Karnataka, India

Avinash Thakur
Assistant Professor
Department of Anatomy
ESIC Medical College and Hospital
Faridabad, Haryana, India

Debabani Bora
Associate Professor
Department of Anatomy
Jorhat Medical College
Jorhat, Assam, India

Dilip Gohil
Associate Professor
Department of Anatomy
MP Shah Medical College
Jamnagar, Gujarat, India

Doris George Yohannan
Assistant Professor
Department of Anatomy
Government Medical College
Thiruvananthapuram, Kerala, India

J Thilagavathi
Professor and Head
Department of Anatomy
Government Medical College
Chennai, Tamil Nadu, India

K Aparna Vedapriya
Professor and Head
Department of Anatomy
Osmania Medical College
Hyderabad, Telangana, India

Kanchan Kapoor
Professor
Department of Anatomy
Government Medical College
Chandigarh, Punjab, India

KK Agarwal
Professor and Head
Department of Anatomy
VCS Government Medical College
Srinagar, Uttarakhand, India

Kunal Chawla
Assistant Professor
Department of Anatomy
Indira Gandhi Medial College
Shimla, Himachal Pradesh, India

Merlin Rachel Thomas
Assistant Professor
Department of Anatomy
Armed Forces Medical College
Pune, Maharashtra, India

Namita Malhotra
Professor and Head
Department of Anatomy
Government Medical College
Mewat, Nalhar, Haryana, India

Navita Aggarwal
Professor and Head
Department of Anatomy
Adesh Institute of Medical Sciences and Research
Bathinda, Punjab, India

Prakash BS
Professor and Head
Department of Anatomy
Hassan, Institute of Medical Sciences
Hassan, Karnataka, India

Pratheepa Sivasankari N
Professor
Department of Anatomy
SRM Institute of Science and Technology
Chennai, Tamil Nadu, India

Preeti Dnyandeo Sonje
Associate Professor
Department of Anatomy
Dr DY Patil Medical College
Pune, Maharashtra, India

Pritha S Bhuiyan
Professor and Head
Department of Anatomy
Seth GS Medical College and KEM Hospital
Mumbai, Maharashtra, India

Purushottam Rao Manvikar
Professor and Head
Department of Anatomy
Dr DY Patil Medical College
Pune, Maharashtra, India

Rakesh Kumar Verma
Associate Professor
Department of Anatomy
King George's Medical College
Lucknow, Uttar Pradesh, India

Renu Mishra
Professor and Head
Department of Anatomy
Saraswati Institute of Medical Sciences
Hapur, Uttar Pradesh, India

Ritesh K Shah
Professor
Department of Anatomy
GCS Medical College
Ahmedabad, Gujarat, India

Ritu Agarwal
Associate Professor
Department of Anatomy
Government Medical College
Pali, Rajasthan, India

Sheetal Joshi
Associate Professor
Department of Anatomy
Lady Hardinge Medical College
New Delhi, India

SK Aggarwal
Professor and Head
Department of Anatomy
Doon Medical College
Dehradun, Uttarakhand, India

Sneh Agarwal
Director, Professor and Head
Department of Anatomy
Lady Hardinge Medical College
New Delhi, India

Sumedh G Sonavane
Associate Professor
Department of Anatomy
TN Medical College and BYL Nair Charitable Hospital
Mumbai, Maharashtra, India

Vanita Gupta
Professor and Head
Department of Anatomy
Rama Medical College
Hapur, Uttar Pradesh, India

Color Atlas — A1–A45

Chapter 1: Light Microscopy and Tissue Preparation — 1
- History — 1
- Parts of a light microscope — 1
- Principle of microscopy — 2
- Practical tips in using a bright-field microscope — 2
- Types of microscopes — 3
- Tissue processing — 3

Chapter 2: Cell Structure — 5
- Components of a cell — 5
- Staining of a cell — 21
- Applied histology — 21

Chapter 3: Epithelia and Glands — 23

Epithelia — 23
- Definition — 23
- General features of epithelial tissue — 23
- Functions — 23
- Classification of epithelia — 23
- Simple epithelium — 23
- Basement membrane — 32
- Projections from the cell surface — 33
- Applied histology — 36

Glands — 37
- Characteristic features — 37
- Classification of glands — 37
- Classification of exocrine glands — 37
- Structural organization — 39
- Development of glands — 40
- Structure of acini — 41
- Applied histology — 42

Chapter 4: General Connective Tissue — 44
- General features — 44
- Classification of connective tissue — 44
- Components of connective tissue — 44
- Fibers of connective tissue — 49
- Intercellular ground substance of connective tissue — 51
- Different forms of connective tissue — 52
- Functions of connective tissue — 56
- Connective tissue with special properties — 57
- Applied histology — 59

Chapter 5: Cartilage — 60
- General features of cartilage — 60
- Perichondrium — 60
- Components of cartilage — 60
- Types of cartilage — 61
- Applied histology — 65

Chapter 6: Bone — 67
- General features — 67
- Composition of bone tissue — 67
- Bone membranes — 69
- Classification and structure of bone — 71
- Formation of bone—ossification — 75
- How bones grow? — 78
- Applied histology — 81

Chapter 7: Muscular Tissue — 83
- Types of muscular tissue — 83
- Skeletal muscle — 84
- Cardiac muscle — 91
- Smooth muscle — 93
- Myoepithelial cells — 96
- Applied histology — 96

Chapter 8: Lymphatics and Lymphoid Tissue — 98
- Classification — 98
- Other classification — 98
- Lymph — 99
- Lymphatic vessels — 99
- Lymphocytes — 100
- Lymph nodes — 100
- Spleen — 103
- Thymus — 106

Mucosa-associated lymphoid tissue	108
Tonsils	109
Further reading	109
Applied histology	111

Chapter 9: Nervous Tissue — 113

Structure of a neuron	113
Neuroglia	116
Types of neurons	120
Peripheral nerves	120
Ganglia	124
Applied histology	126

Chapter 10: Cardiovascular System — 129

Basic structure of a blood vessel	129
Structure of arteries	130
Arterioles	132
Capillaries	133
Veins	134
Venules	135
Nutrition and innervation of blood vessels	135
Heart	137
Further reading	137
Applied histology	138

Chapter 11: Skin and its Appendages — 139

Functions	139
Types of skin	139
Structure of skin	142
Blood supply of the skin	145
Nerve supply of the skin	145
Appendages of the skin	145
Applied histology	150

Chapter 12: Salivary Glands — 152

Salivary glands	152
Applied histology	159

Chapter 13: Placenta and Umbilical Cord — 160

Placenta	**160**
Functions	160
Components	160
Formation of placenta	161
Microscopic structure	162
Placental circulation and barrier	162
Applied histology	164
Umbilical Cord	**164**

Chapter 14: Respiratory System — 166

Common features of air passages	166
Nasal cavities	166
Pharynx	167
Larynx	167
Trachea and principal bronchi	168
Lungs	171
Applied histology	176

Chapter 15: Digestive System: Oral Cavity and Related Structures — 177

Oral cavity	177
Lips	177
Teeth	179
Tongue	180
Applied histology	185
Further reading	185

Chapter 16: Digestive System: General Plan of Gastrointestinal Tract, Stomach and Intestines — 188

General structure of GIT	189
Esophagus	191
Stomach	191
Small intestine	197
Large intestine	204
Applied histology	208

Chapter 17: Hepatobiliary System and Pancreas — 211

Liver	211
Extrahepatic biliary apparatus	217
Pancreas	219
Differences between serous salivary gland and pancreas	222
Applied histology	222

Chapter 18: Urinary System — 224

Functions	224
Kidneys	224
Ureters	234

Urinary bladder	235
Urethra	238
Applied histology	238

Chapter 19: Central Nervous System: Spinal Cord, Cerebellar Cortex and Cerebral Cortex — 240

Spinal cord	240
Cerebral cortex	243
Cerebellar cortex	247
Applied histology	251

Chapter 20: Male Reproductive System — 252

Testis	252
Spermatogenesis	257
Epididymis	260
Ductus deferens	262
Seminal vesicle	262
Prostate	265
Penis	265
Applied histology	268

Chapter 21: Female Reproductive System — 269

Ovary	269
Uterine tubes	276
Uterus	276
Cervix	281
Vagina	282
Female external genitalia	282
Mammary gland	284
Applied histology	287

Chapter 22: Endocrine System — 289

Hormones	289
Distribution of endocrine cells	290
Hypophysis cerebri	290
Thyroid gland	295
Parathyroid glands	298
Suprarenal glands/adrenal glands	300
Pineal gland	302
Some other organs having endocrine functions	303
Applied histology	305

Chapter 23: Special Senses: Eye — 307

Structure of eyeball	307
Outer fibrous coat	307
Lens	317
Accessory visual organs	319
Applied histology	323

Chapter 24: Special Senses: Ear — 325

External ear	325
Middle ear	327
Internal ear	327
Some elementary facts about the mechanism of hearing	336
Applied histology	336

Index — *339*

COMPETENCY TABLE

Number	Competency The student should be able to	Core (Y/N)	Teaching-Learning Methods	Assessment Methods	Ch. No.	Pg. No.
AN 65.1	Identify epithelium under the microscope and describe the various types that correlate to its function		Lecture, Practical	Written/skill assessment	03	23–36
AN 65.2	Describe the ultrastructure of epithelium		Lecture, Practical	Written	03	
Topic: Connective tissue histology	**Number of competencies (2)**		**Number of procedures for certification (NIL)**			
AN 66.1	Describe and identify various types of connective tissue with functional correlation	Y	Lecture, Practical	Written/skill assessment	04	44–59
AN 66.2	Describe the ultrastructure of connective tissue	N	Lecture, Practical	Written	04	
Topic: Muscle histology	**Number of competencies (3)**		**Number of procedures for certification (NIL)**			
AN 67.1	Describe and identify various types of muscle under the microscope	Y	Lecture, Practical	Written/skill assessment	07	83–96
AN 67.2	Classify muscle and describe the structure-function correlation of the same	Y	Lecture, Practical	Written	07	
AN 67.3	Describe the ultrastructure of muscular tissue	N	Lecture, Practical	Written	07	
Topic: Nervous tissue histology	**Number of competencies (3)**		**Number of procedures for certification (NIL)**			
AN 68.1	Describe and identify multipolar and unipolar neuron, ganglia, peripheral nerve	Y	Lecture, Practical	Written/skill assessment	09	113–126
AN 68.2	Describe the structure-function correlation of neuron	Y	Lecture, Practical	Written		
AN 68.3	Describe the ultrastructure of nervous tissue	N	Lecture, Practical	Written		
Topic: Blood vessels	**Number of competencies (3)**		**Number of procedures for certification (NIL)**			
AN 69.1	Identify elastic and muscular blood vessels, capillaries under the microscope	Y	Lecture, Practical	Skill assessment	10	129–138
AN 69.2	Describe the various types and structure-function correlation of blood vessel	Y	Lecture, Practical	Written		
AN 69.3	Describe the ultrastructure of blood vessels	Y	Lecture, Practical	Written		
Topic: Glands and lymphoid tissue	**Number of competencies (2)**		**Number of procedures for certification (NIL)**			
AN 70.1	Identify exocrine gland under the microscope and distinguish between serous, mucous and mixed acini	Y	Lecture, Practical	Written/skill assessment	12	152–159
AN 70.2	Identify the lymphoid tissue under the microscope and describe microanatomy of lymph node, spleen, thymus, tonsil and correlate the structure with function	Y	Lecture, Practical	Written/skill assessment	08	98–111
Topic: Bone and cartilage	**Number of competencies (2)**		**Number of procedures for certification (NIL)**			
AN 71.1	Identify bone under the microscope; classify various types and describe the structure-function correlation of the same	Y	Lecture, Practical	Written/skill assessment	06	67–81
AN 71.2	Identify cartilage under the microscope and describe various types and structure-function correlation of the same	Y	Lecture, Practical	Written/skill assessment	05	60–65

Contd...

Contd...

Number	Competency The student should be able to	Core (Y/N)	Teaching-Learning Methods	Assessment Methods	Ch. No.	Pg. No.
Topic:	Integumentary system	Number of competencies (1)		Number of procedures for certification (NIL)		
AN 72.1	Identify the skin and its appendages under the microscope and correlate the structure with function	Y	Lecture, Practical	Written/skill assessment	11	139–150
AN 9.2	**Breast:** Describe the location, extent, deep relations, structure, age changes, blood supply, lymphatic drainage, microanatomy and applied anatomy of breast				21	284–287
AN 25.1	Identify, draw and label a slide of trachea and lung				14	168–174
AN 43.2	Identify, describe and draw the microanatomy of pituitary gland, thyroid, parathyroid gland, suprarenal				22	289–305
	Tongue				15	181–185
	Salivary glands				12	152–159
	Tonsil				08	109–112
	Epiglottis				14	168–169
	Cornea				23	308–310
	Retina				23	312–317
AN 43.3	Identify, describe and draw microanatomy of olfactory epithelium				14	167
	Eyelid				23	319–320
	Lip				15	177–178
	Sclero-corneal junction				23	308
	Optic nerve				09	121–123
	Cochlea—organ of Corti				24	330–335
	Pineal gland				22	302–303
AN 52.2	Describe and identify the microanatomical features of: Urinary system: Kidney, Ureter and urinary bladder				18	224–239
	Male reproductive system: Testis, epididymis, vas deferens, prostate and penis				20	252–268
	Female reproductive system: Ovary, uterus, uterine tube, cervix				21	269–288
	Placenta and umbilical cord				13	160–165
AN 52.3a	Describe and identify the microanatomical features of: Esophagus, stomach, small intestine, large intestine				16	191–210
	Liver, pancreas				17	211–223
AN 64.1	Describe and identify the microanatomical features of spinal cord, cerebellum and cerebrum				19	240–251

Color Atlas

HISTOLOGY AND ITS STUDY

The study of histology is very important for the understanding of the normal functioning of the human body. It also forms the essential basis for the study of the changes in various tissues and organs in disease (This is the science of pathology). From these points of view the study of histology is best done taking one organ system at a time. That is the approach most teachers prefer to take in practical classes of histology. It is also the basis on which the chapters of this book have been organized.

However, in practical examinations, the emphasis is on the ability of the student to recognize a tissue or organ that is being viewed through a microscope. Here it becomes necessary to know how to distinguish between similar looking tissues or organs belonging to different systems. This atlas has been organized to serve this objective. Tissues and organs that have a similar appearance are considered in one lot. For example, if a slide presents something that looks like a tube, whether it be an artery or the ureter or the ductus deferens, these are considered together. This makes the grouping unusual, but this is exactly what the student needs at the time of an examination.

At the same time it is true that an organ can be composed of several tissues (or layers), and the ability to recognize them can go a long way in arriving at a correct diagnosis of the organ being seen. We will, therefore, first try to study and identify the various tissues that make up different organs. We will then have a good basis for identifying any organ that we are required to recognize.

BASIC TISSUES THAT CAN BE RECOGNIZED IN HISTOLOGICAL SECTIONS

Epithelia

The outer surface of the body, and the luminal surfaces of cavities (big or small) lying within the body are lined by one or more layers of cells that completely cover them. Such layers of cells are called epithelia. Epithelial tissue forms the lining of the general body surfaces, passages and cavities within the body. Basement membrane connects the epithelium to the underline subepithelial tissues.

Classification of epithelial tissue is based on shape of the cells, number of cell layers and special modifications seen on the cells. Epithelia may be **simple**, when they consist of only one layer of cells, or **stratified** when there are several layers of cells. Epithelial cells may be flat (or squamous), cuboidal, or columnar.

Several types of epithelia can be recognized. Learning to identify an epithelium can be of considerable help in finding out what organ you are seeing.

EPITHELIA AND GLANDS

Simple Squamous Epithelium

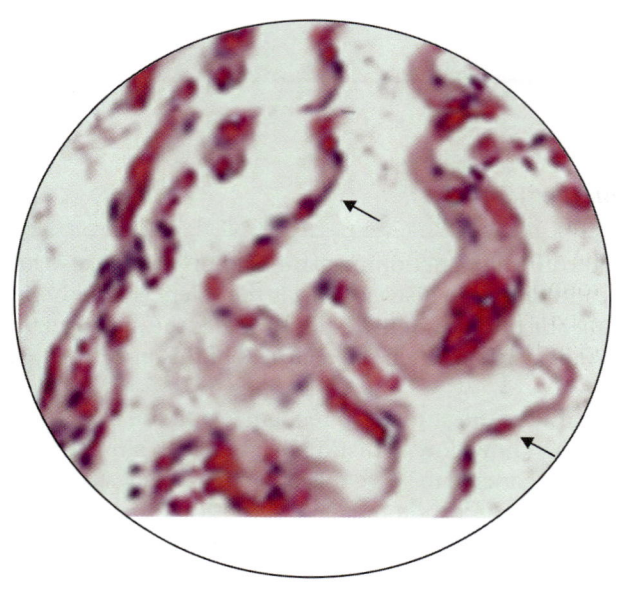

Fig. A1.1: An alveolus of the lung showing a lining of simple squamous epithelium (*see* arrows).

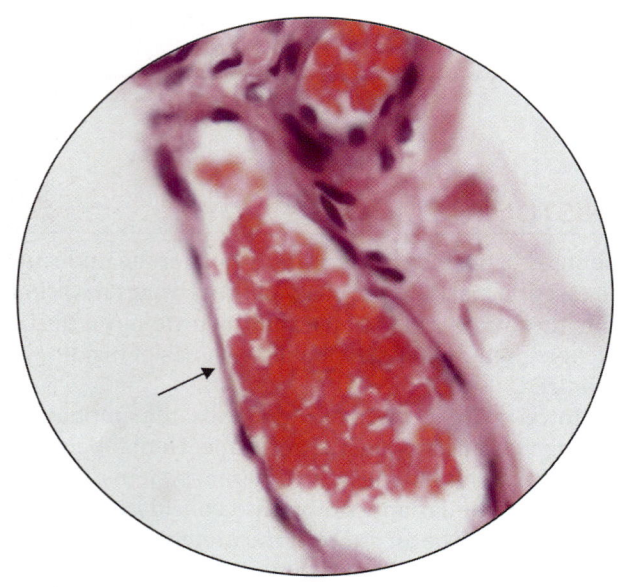

Fig. A1.2: A capillary lined by endothelium (*see* arrow).

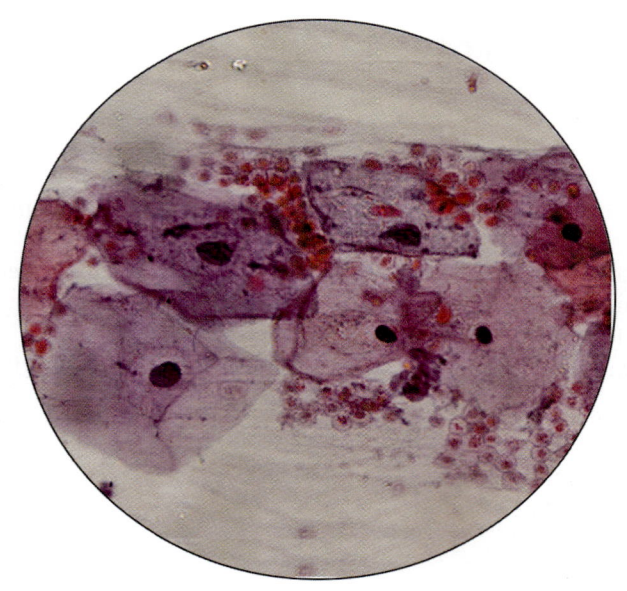

Fig. A1.3: Surface view as seen in buccal smear.

Points of identification
- The cells of this epithelium are flattened in sections. They appear so thin that bulgings are produced on the surface by their nuclei
- In surface view the cells have polygonal outlines that interlock with those of adjoining cells.

Simple Cuboidal Epithelium

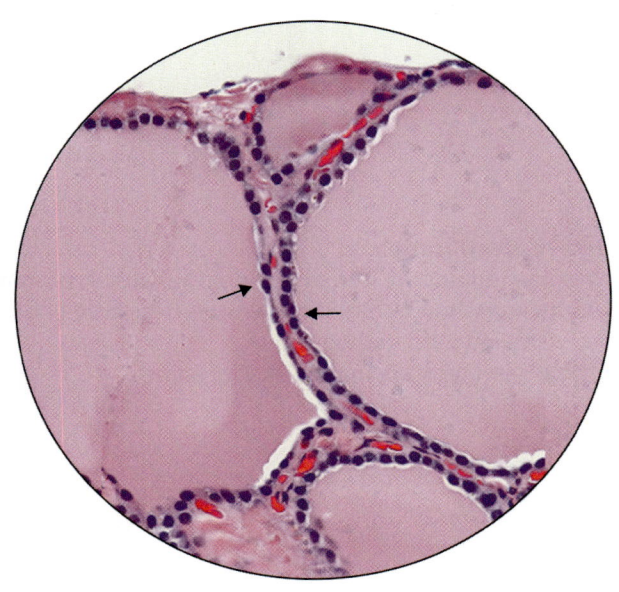

Fig. A1.4: Thyroid follicle lined by simple cuboidal epithelium (*see* arrows).

Points of identification
- This epithelium is made up of cells that look like squares (in which the length and breadth are equal). Nuclei are rounded
- A typical cuboidal epithelium lines follicles of the thyroid gland, ducts of salivary gland, and tubules of kidney.

Simple Columnar Epithelium

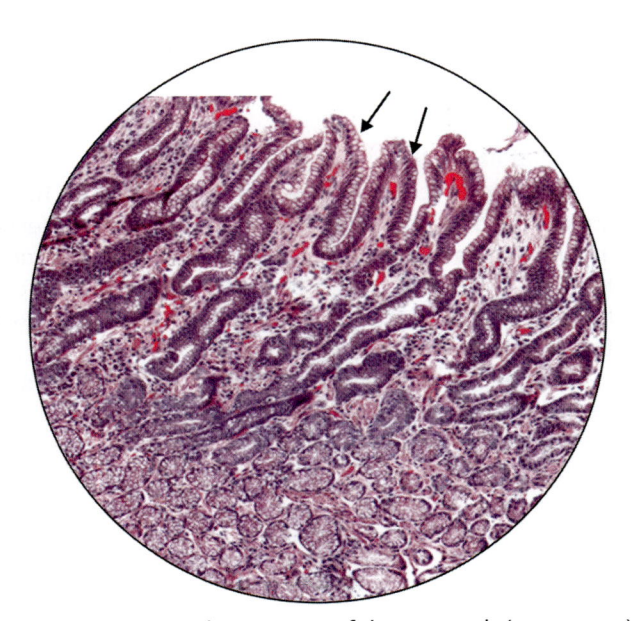

Fig. A1.5: Lining the mucosa of the stomach (*see* arrows).

Points of identification
- The height of the cells in this epithelium is much greater than their width. The nuclei are oval being elongated in the same direction as the cells. They lie near the bases of the cells. Because of this we see a zone of clear cytoplasm above the nuclei
- A simple columnar epithelium (non-ciliated) lines the mucous membrane of the stomach and of the large intestine.

Columnar Epithelium Showing Striated Border

Points of identification
- In some regions the free surfaces of the cells of columnar epithelium show a thickening with vertical striations in it, this is called a striated border
- This is seen typically in the small intestine.

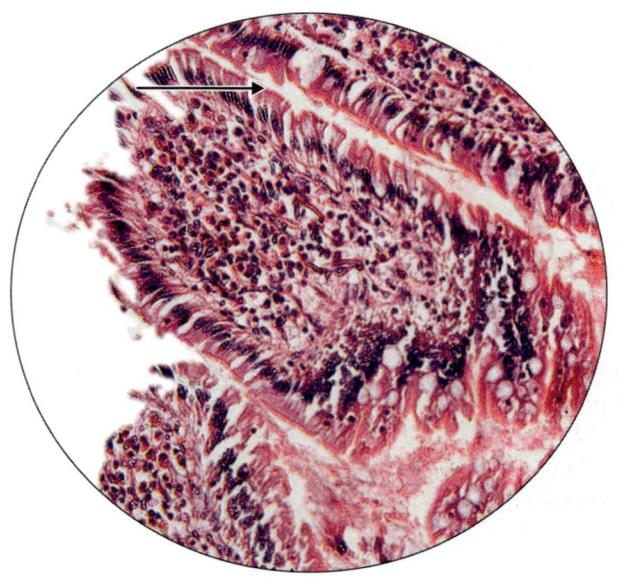

Fig. A1.6: Columnar epithelium with a striated border in the small intestine (*see* arrow).

Pseudostratified Ciliated Columnar Epithelium

Points of identification
- It is not a true stratified epithelium but appears to be stratified. Normally, in columnar epithelium the nuclei lie in a row, toward the basal part of the cells. Sometimes, however, the nuclei appear to be arranged in two or more layers giving the impression that the epithelium is more than one cell thick
- In some situations, pseudostratified columnar epithelium bears hair-like projections called cilia
- Pseudostratified ciliated columnar epithelium is seen in trachea and in large bronchi.

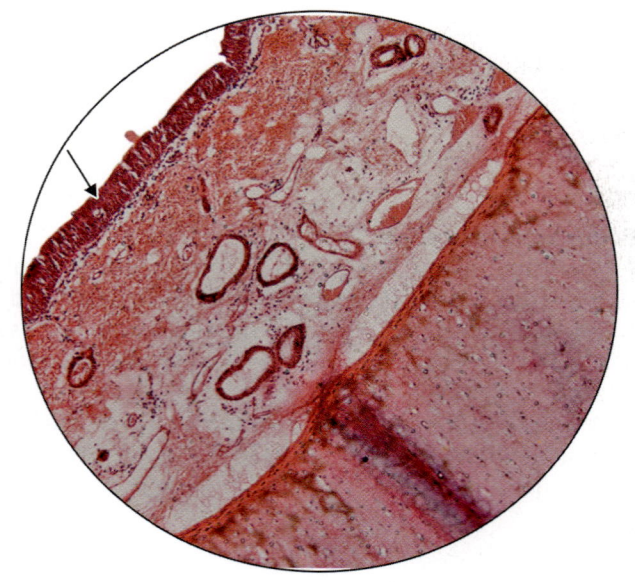

Fig. A1.7: Pseudostratified ciliated columnar epithelium in trachea (*see* arrow).

Color Atlas

Stratified Squamous Epithelium

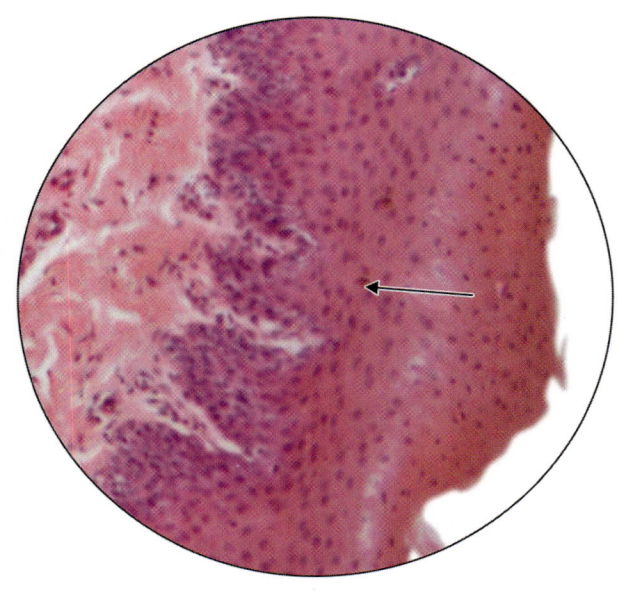

Fig. A1.8: Nonkeratinized stratified squamous epithelium: As seen in esophagus (*see* arrow).

Points of identification
- Although this is called stratified squamous epithelium, only the most superficial cells are squamous (flattened)
- The cells in the deepest (or basal) layer are columnar. In the middle layers, they are polyhedral, while the more superficial layers show increasing degrees of flattening
- The nuclei are oval in the basal layer, rounded in the middle layer, and transversely elongated in the superficial layers
- The surface layer shows squamous cells with flattened nuclei
- This kind of epithelium is seen lining some internal organs, like the esophagus or the vagina
- Here the deeper layers are covered by additional layers that represent stages in the conversion of cells into nonliving fibers. This process is called keratinization (or cornification).

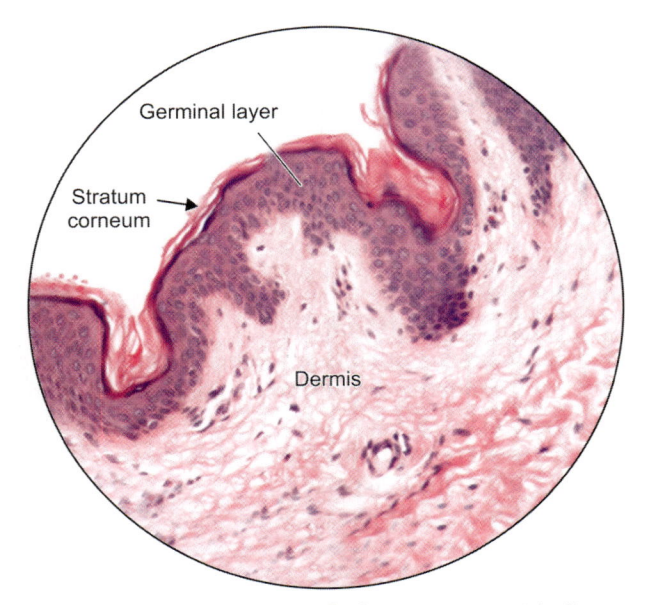

Fig. A1.9: Keratinized stratified squamous epithelium.

Points of identification
- The surface layer is made up of keratin which appears as fibers. No cellular outline or nuclei can be seen
- It is seen typically in epidermis of the skin.

Transitional Epithelium

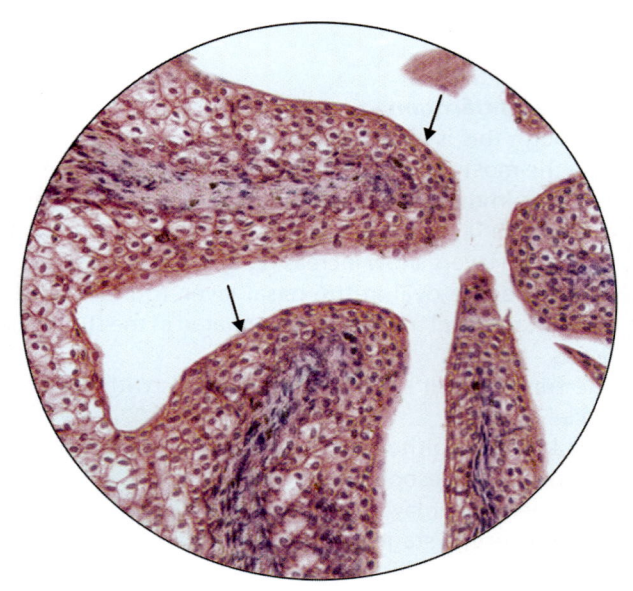

Fig. A1.10: Transitional epithelium seen at high magnification in ureter (*see* arrows).

Points of identification
- In this type of epithelium, several layers of round nuclei are seen
- The superficial cells are not flattened but are umbrella shaped
- Their nuclei appear rounded and may show mitotic figures
- This epithelium lines many parts of the urinary tract.

GENERAL CONNECTIVE TISSUE

Dense Regular Connective Tissue

Nuclei of fibroblast

Collagen fibers

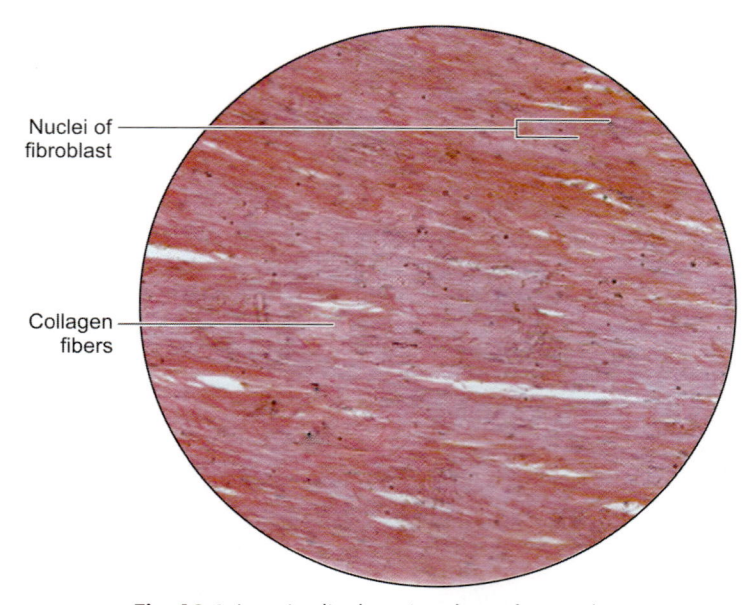

Fig. A2.1: Longitudinal section through a tendon.

Points of identification
- Presence of collagen fibers (or fiber bundles) arranged in orderly fashion parallel to each other
- Nuclei of some cells (mainly fibroblasts) are seen between the bundles of collagen. They are elongated (elliptical)
- Ground substance is less in amount.

Color Atlas | A7

Dense Irregular Connective Tissue (Dermis of Skin)

Collagen fibers

Nuclei of fibroblast

Points of identification
- Irregularly arranged bundles of collagen fibers that stain pink. In stretch preparation they are seen in wavy bundles. Other fibers present (elastic, reticular) can be seen only with special stains
- Few cells (fibroblast) and less ground substance.

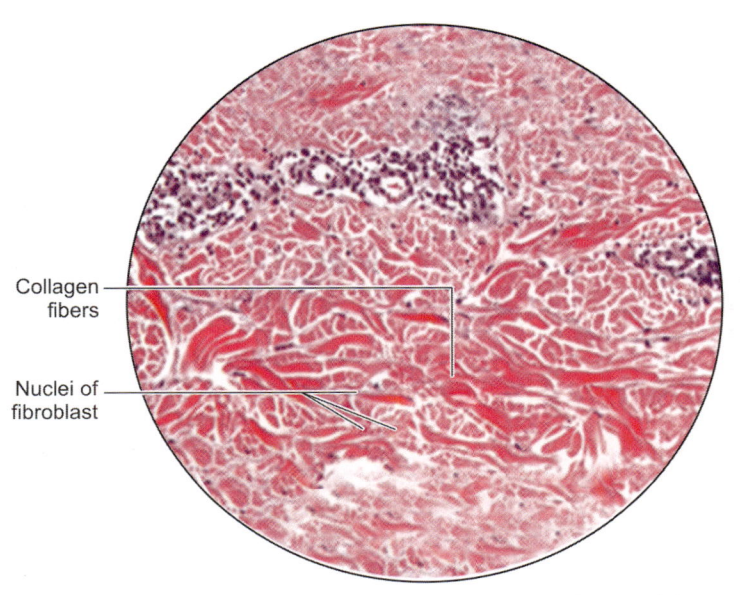

Fig. A2.2: Dense irregular connective tissue as seen in dermis of skin.

Adipose Tissue

Adipocyte

Blood vessel

Points of identification
- Presence of fat cells. In routine sections the cells appear empty as the fat in them gets dissolved during preparation of the section giving it a honeycomb appearance
- The cytoplasm of each cell is seen as a pink rim
- The nucleus is flat and lies to one side (eccentric).

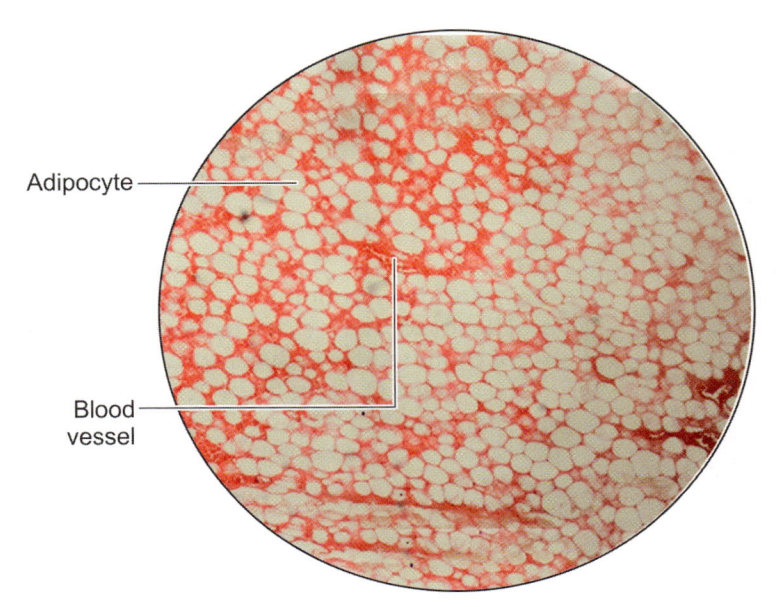

Fig. A2.3: Adipose tissue.

CARTILAGE

Hyaline Cartilage

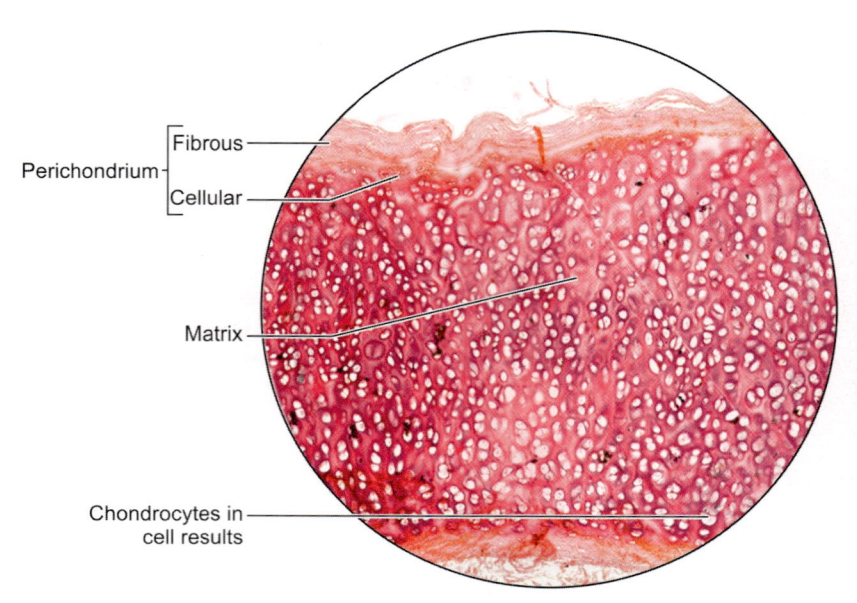

Fig. A3.1: Hyaline cartilage.
Courtesy: Balakrishna Shetty, Sweekritha H Poonja. HISTOLOGY Practical Manual, 4th edition. New Delhi: Jaypee Brothers Medical Publishers (P) Ltd; 2019. p. 18.

Points of identification
- Hyaline cartilage is characterized by isogenous groups of chondrocytes called as cell nest
- Chondrocytes are surrounded by a homogeneous basophilic matrix which separates the cells widely
- Chondrocytes increase in size from periphery to center
- Near the surface of the cartilage the cells are flattened and merge with the cells of the overlying connective tissue. This connective tissue forms the perichondrium
- Perichondrium displays an outer fibrous and inner cellular layer.

Elastic Cartilage

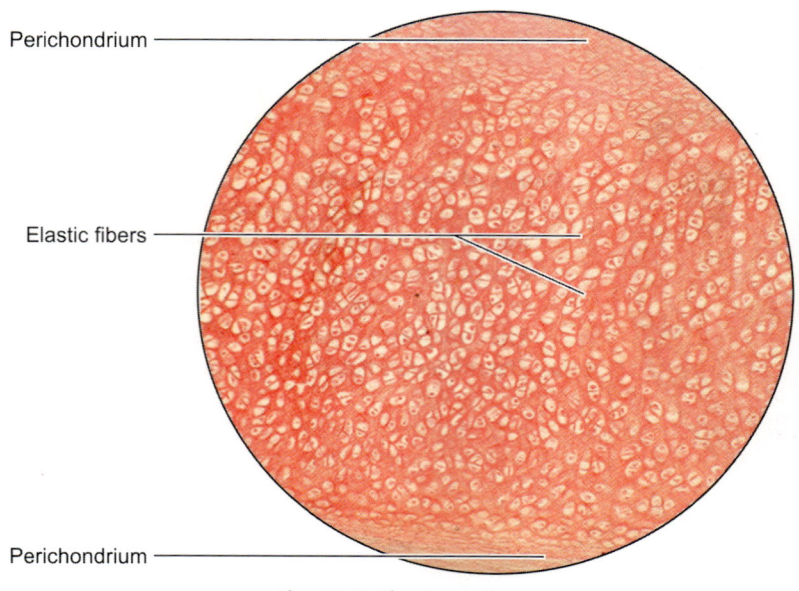

Fig. A3.2: Elastic cartilage.

Points of identification
- Elastic cartilage is characterized by presence of chondrocytes within lacuna surrounded by bundles of elastic fibers
- Perichondrium is present showing an outer fibrous and inner cellular layer.

Fibrocartilage

Points of identification
- Presence of prominent collagen fibers arranged in bundles with rows of chondrocytes intervening between the bundles
- Perichondrium is absent
- This kind of cartilage can be confused with the appearance of a tendon. However, the chondrocytes in fibrocartilage are rounded but in a tendon, fibrocytes are flattended and elongated.

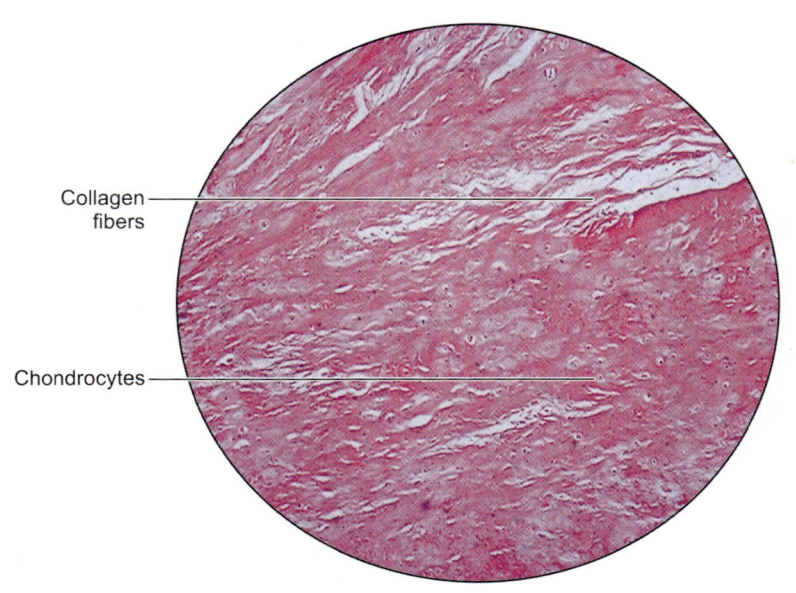

Fig. A3.3: Fibrocartilage.

BONE

Compact Bone (Transverse Section)

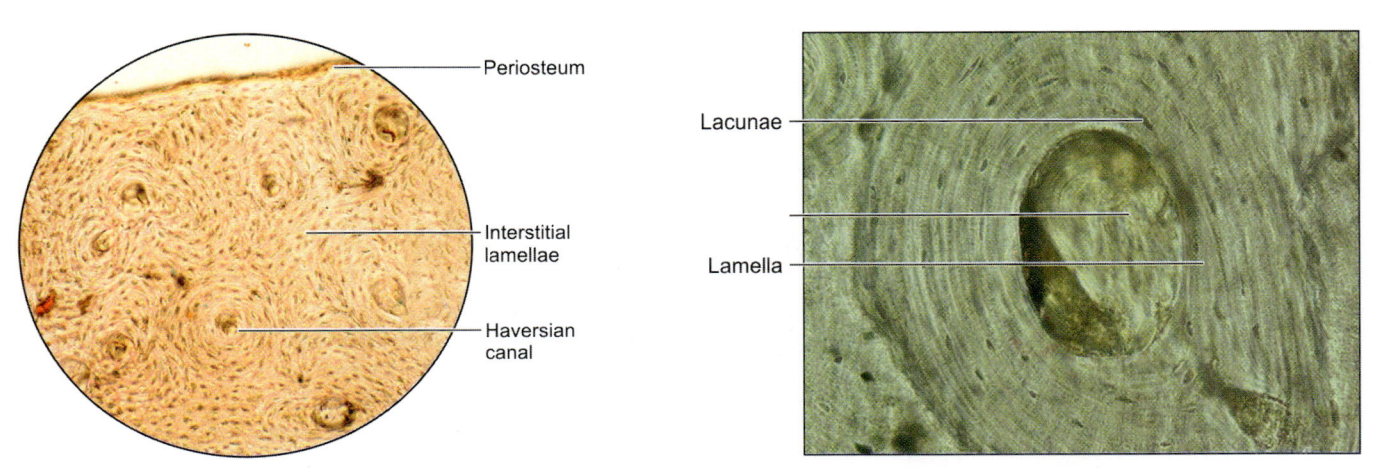

Fig. A4.1: Ground section.

Fig. A4.2: Haversian system.

Points of identification
- Haversian system made up of concentric lamellae, lacunae with osteocytes, Haversian (central) canal containing blood vessels and nerves are seen
- Three types of lamellae are seen—(1) circumferential, (2) concentric, and (3) interstitial
- Canaliculi radiate from lacunae.

Compact Bone (Longitudinal Section)

Labels: Lamella; Lacunae with osteocytes

Points of identification
- Volkmann's canal interconnecting Haversian systems is seen
- Lacunae with osteocytes.

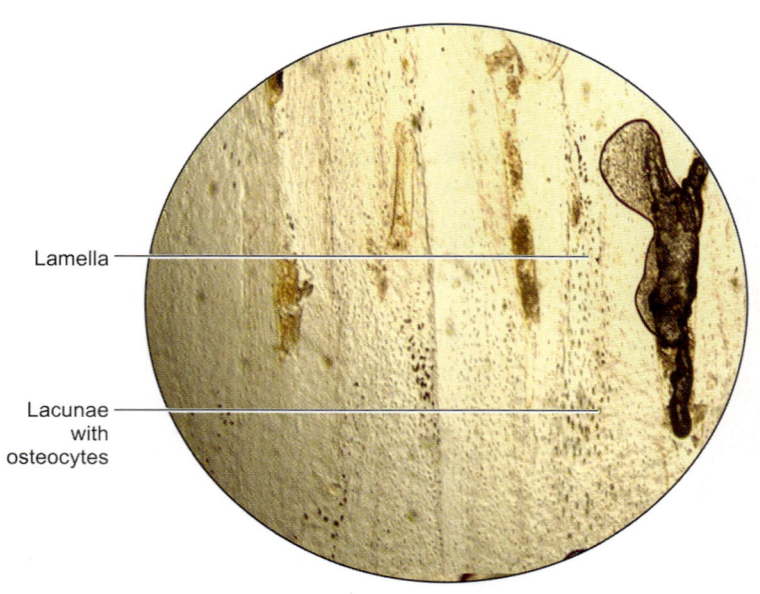

Fig. A4.3: Compact bone: Transverse section.

MUSCULAR TISSUE

Longitudinal Section Through Skeletal Muscle

Labels: Peripherally placed nuclei; Muscle fibers with transverse striations

Points of identification
- In a longitudinal section through skeletal muscle, the fibers are easily distinguished as they show characteristic transverse striations
- The fibers are long and parallel without branching
- Many flat nuclei are placed at the periphery
- The muscle fibers are separated by some connective tissue.

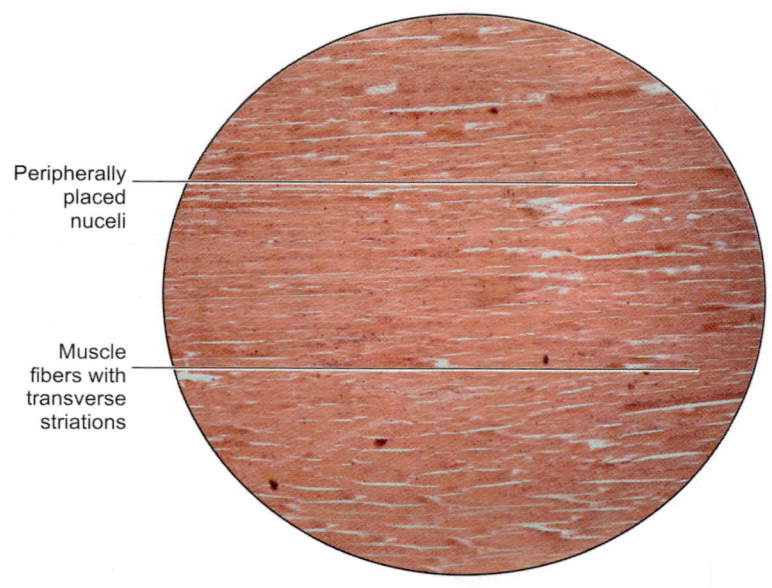

Fig. A5.1: Longitudinal section through skeletal muscle (low power).

Transverse Section Through Skeletal Muscle

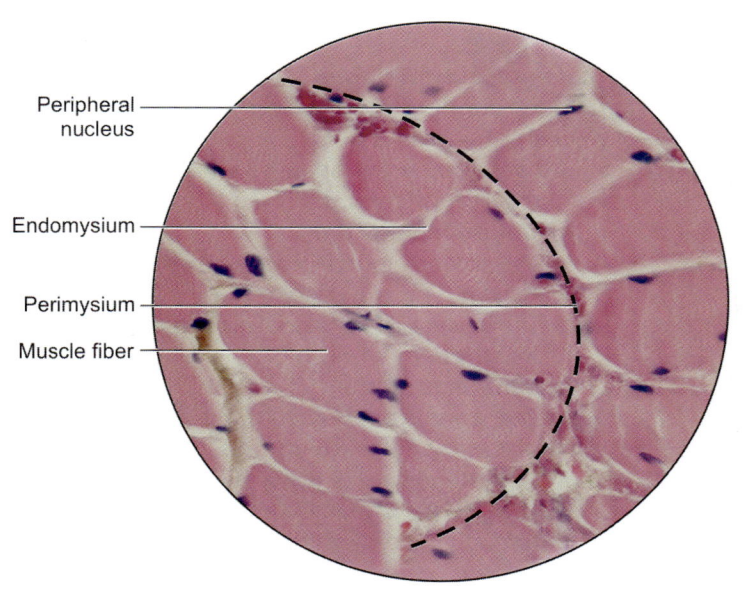

Fig. A5.2: Transverse section through skeletal muscle.

Labels: Peripheral nucleus, Endomysium, Perimysium, Muscle fiber

Points of identification
The transverse section of a skeletal muscle fiber is characterized by:
- Fibers seen as irregularly round structures with peripheral nuclei
- Muscle fibers grouped into numerous fasciculi
- Dots within the fibers are myofibrils which are seen at higher magnification.

The connective tissue of the muscle consists of:
- **Epimysium**: Connective tissue sheath of muscle (not seen in photomicrograph)
- **Perimysium**: Connective tissue covering of each fascicle
- **Endomysium**: Loose connective tissue surrounding each muscle fiber.

Cardiac Muscle

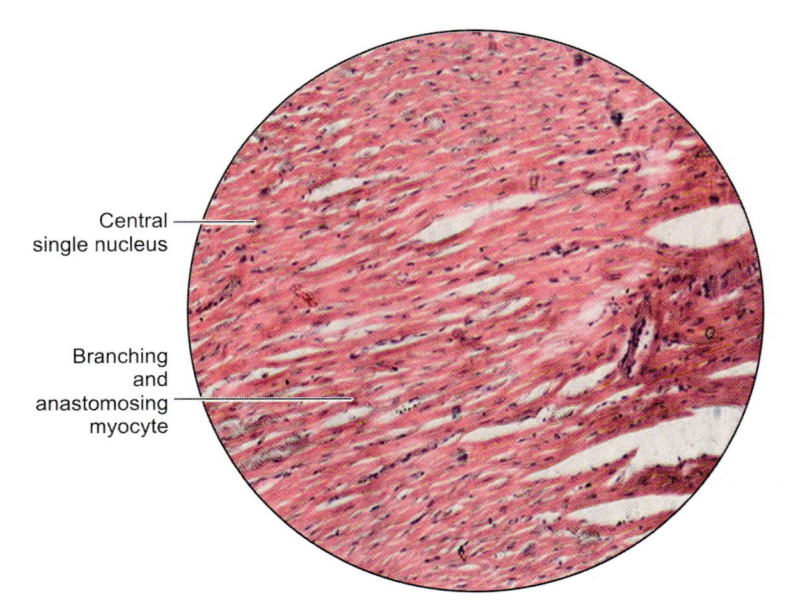

Fig. A5.3: Cardiac muscle.

Labels: Central single nucleus, Branching and anastomosing myocyte

Points of identification
- The fibers are made up of "cells" each of which has a centrally placed nucleus and transverse striations
- A clear space called perinuclear halo is seen around the nucleus
- Adjacent cells are separated from one another by transverse lines called intercalated discs
- Fibers show branching
- Blood vessels are also seen.

Smooth Muscle

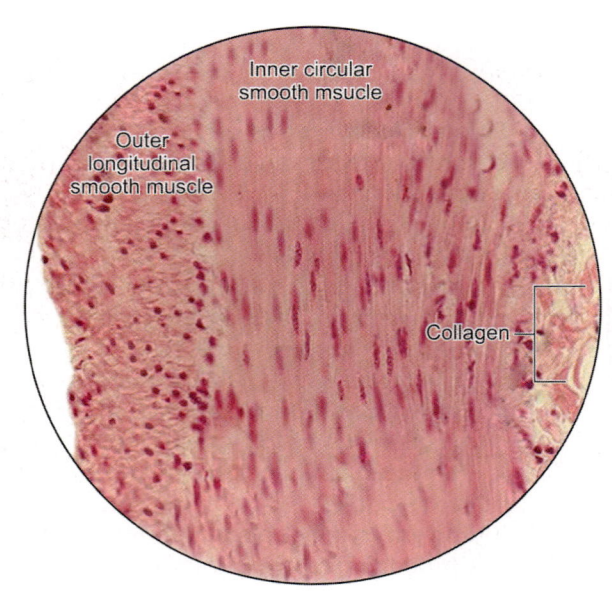

Fig. A5.4: Smooth muscle.

Points of identification

In the drawing, muscle is seen cut longitudinally as well as transversely.
- Loose connective tissue is seen above and below the layers of muscle.

In longitudinal section:
- The smooth muscle fibers are **spindle-shaped** cells with tapering ends
- The nucleus is elongated and centrally placed
- *No striations* are seen.

In transverse section:
- The spindle-shaped cells are cut at different places along the length resulting in various shapes and sizes of the cells
- The nucleus is seen in those cells which are cut through the center. Others do not show nuclei.

LYMPHATICS AND LYMPHOID TISSUE

Lymph Node

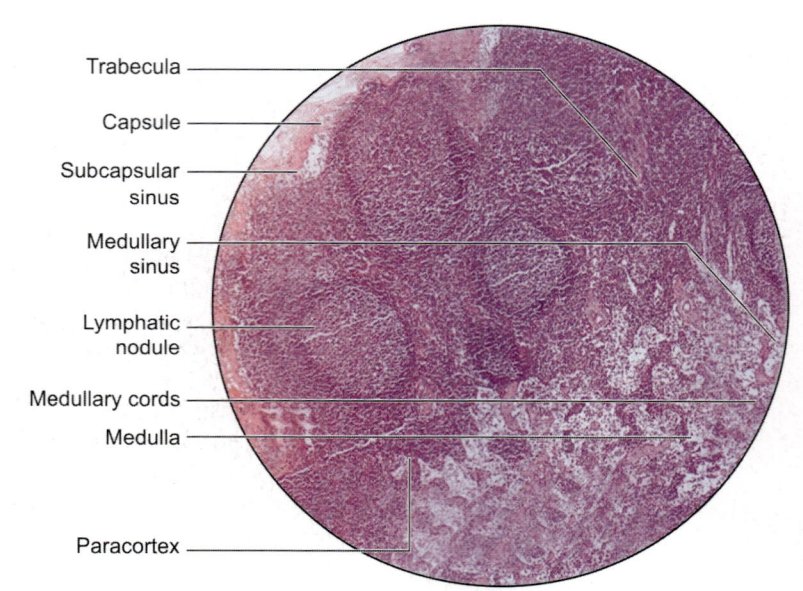

Fig. A6.1: Lymph node.

Points of identification
- A thin capsule surrounds the lymph node and sends in trabeculae
- Just beneath the capsule a clear space is seen. This is the subcapsular sinus
- A lymph node has an outer cortex and an inner medulla
- The cortex is packed with lymphocytes. A number of rounded lymphatic follicles (or nodules) are present. Each nodule has a pale staining germinal center surrounded by a zone of densely packed lymphocytes
- Within the medulla the lymphocytes are arranged in the form of anastomosing cords. Several blood vessels can be seen in the medulla.

Note: All lymphoid tissue are easily recognized due to presence of aggregation of dark staining nuclei. The nuclei belong to lymphocytes.

Spleen

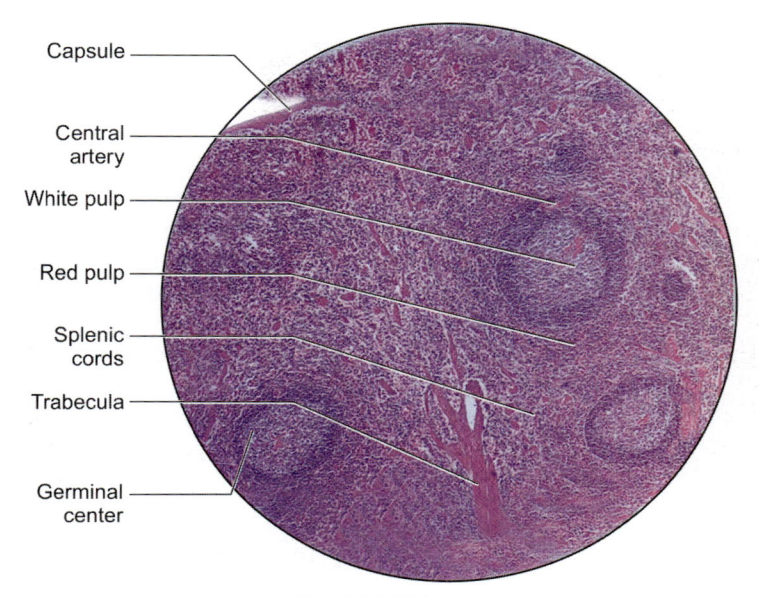

Labels (Fig. A6.2):
- Capsule
- Central artery
- White pulp
- Red pulp
- Splenic cords
- Trabecula
- Germinal center

Fig. A6.2: Spleen.

Points of identification
- The spleen is characterized by a thick capsule with trabeculae extending from it into the organ (not shown in photomicrograph)
- The substance of the organ is divisible into the red pulp in which there are diffusely distributed lymphocytes and numerous sinusoids; and the white pulp in which dense aggregations of lymphocytes are present. The latter are in the form of cords surrounding arterioles
- When cut transversely the cords resemble the lymphatic nodules of lymph nodes, and like them they have germinal centers surrounded by rings of densely packed lymphocytes. However, the nodules of the spleen are easily distinguished from those of lymph nodes because of the presence of an arteriole in each nodule
- This arteriole occupies an eccentric position in the nodule.

Thymus

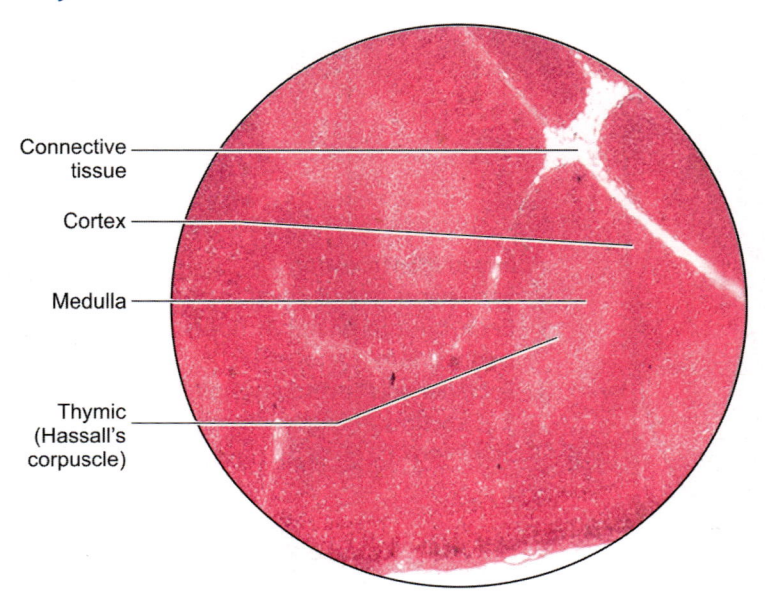

Labels (Fig. A6.3):
- Connective tissue
- Cortex
- Medulla
- Thymic (Hassall's corpuscle)

Fig. A6.3: Thymus.

Points of identification
- The thymus is made up of lymphoid tissue arranged in the form of distinct lobules. The presence of this lobulation enables easy distinction of the thymus from all other lymphoid organs
- The lobules are partially separated from each other by connective tissue septae
- In each lobule an outer darkly stained cortex (in which lymphocytes are densely packed); and an inner lightly stained medulla (in which the cells are diffuse) are present
- Whereas the cortex is confined to one lobule, the medulla is continuous from one lobule to another
- The medulla contains pink staining rounded masses called the corpuscles of Hassall.

Palatine Tonsil

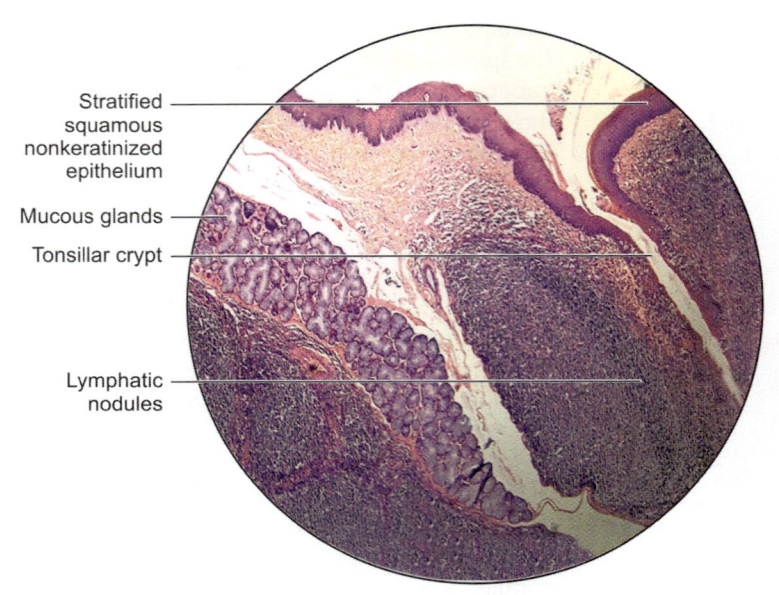

Labels: Stratified squamous nonkeratinized epithelium; Mucous glands; Tonsillar crypt; Lymphatic nodules

Fig. A6.4: Palatine tonsil.

Points of identification
- Palatine tonsil is an aggregation of lymphoid tissue that is readily recognized by the fact that it is covered by a stratified squamous epithelium
- At places the epithelium dips into the tonsil in the form of deep crypts
- Deep to the epithelium there is diffuse lymphoid tissue in which typical lymphatic nodules can be seen.

NERVOUS TISSUE

Peripheral Nerve

Labels: Nerve fibers; Perineurium

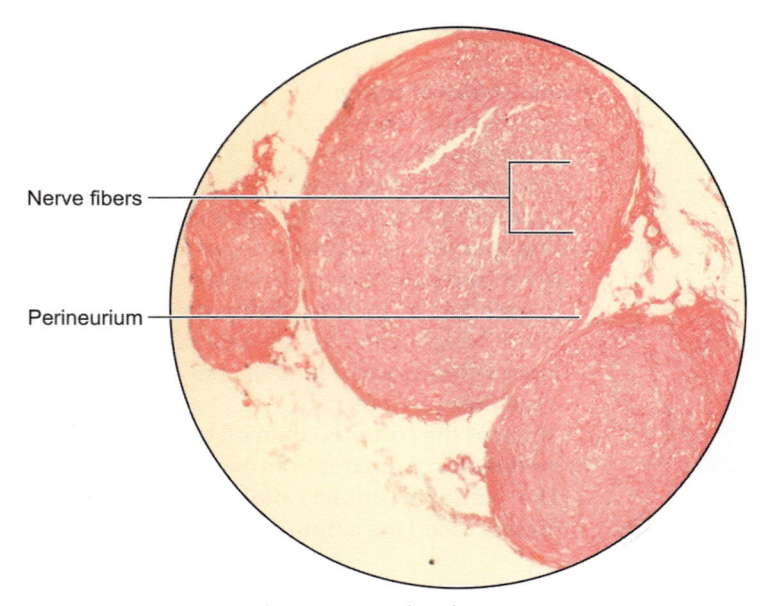

Fig. A7.1: Preipheral nerve.

Points of identification
- Each nerve fiber is covered by endoneurium
- Each bundle of nerve fibers is covered by perineurium
- Each nerve is covered by epineurium
- Cut section of axon with myelin sheath and Schwann cell nucleus.

Optic Nerve

Labels: Optic nerve fibers; Central retinal artery and vein; Pial septa

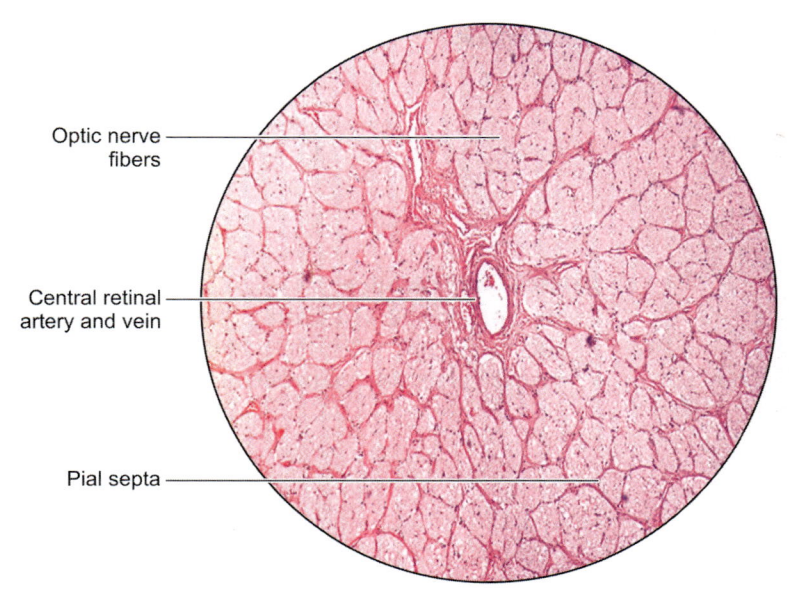

Fig. A7.2: Optic nerve.

Points of identification
- Covered by meninges—dura mater, arachnoid mater, and pia mater
- Central retinal artery and vein are seen
- Pial septa divides the nerve into bundles.

Sensory Ganglia

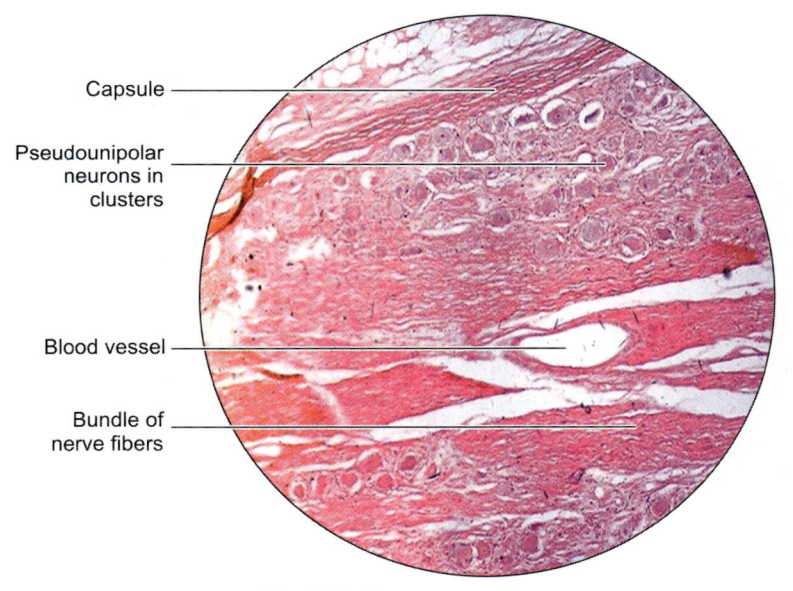

Labels: Capsule; Pseudounipolar neurons in clusters; Blood vessel; Bundle of nerve fibers

Fig. A7.3: Sensory ganglia.

Points of identification
- Unipolar neurons with centrally placed nucleus
- Neurons are presented in a group between the group of nerve fibers
- Prominent satellite cells are seen.

Autonomic Ganglia

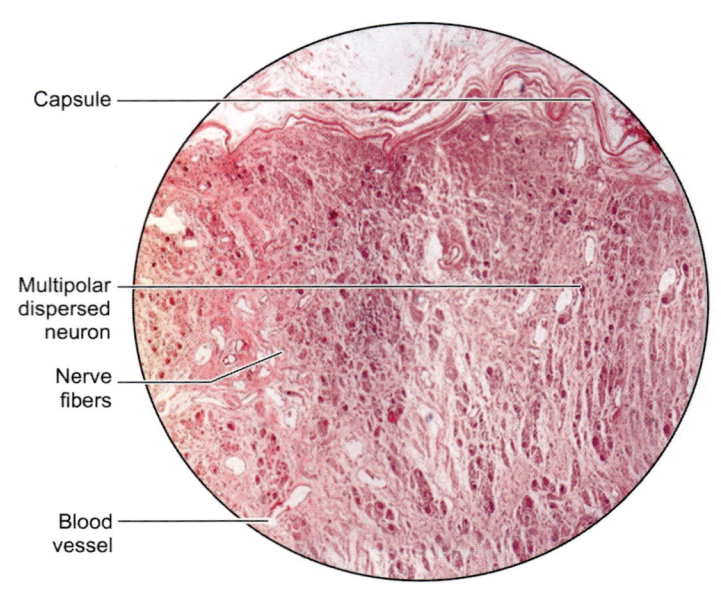

Fig. A7.4: Autonomic ganglia.

Labels: Capsule; Multipolar dispersed neuron; Nerve fibers; Blood vessel

Points of identification
- Multipolar neurons with eccentrically placed nucleus
- Neurons are scattered between the nerve fibers.

CARDIOVASCULAR SYSTEM

Elastic Artery

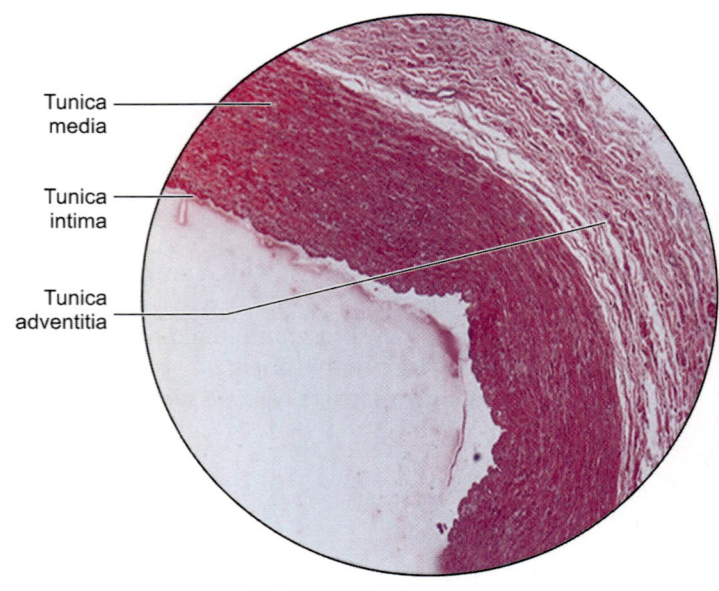

Fig. A8.1: Elastic artery.

Labels: Tunica media; Tunica intima; Tunica adventitia

Points of identification
Elastic artery is characterized by presence of:
- Tunica intima consisting of endothelium, subendothelial connective tissue, and internal elastic lamina
- The first layer of elastic fibers is called the internal elastic lamina. The internal elastic lamina is not distinct from the elastic fibers of media
- Well developed subendothelial layer in tunica intima
- Thick tunica media with many elastic fibers and some smooth muscle fibers
- Tunica adventitia containing collagen fibers with several elastic fibers
- Vasa vasorum in the tunica adventitia (Not seen in this slide).

Color Atlas

Muscular (Medium Size) Artery

Tunica adventitia
Tunica media
Tunica intima

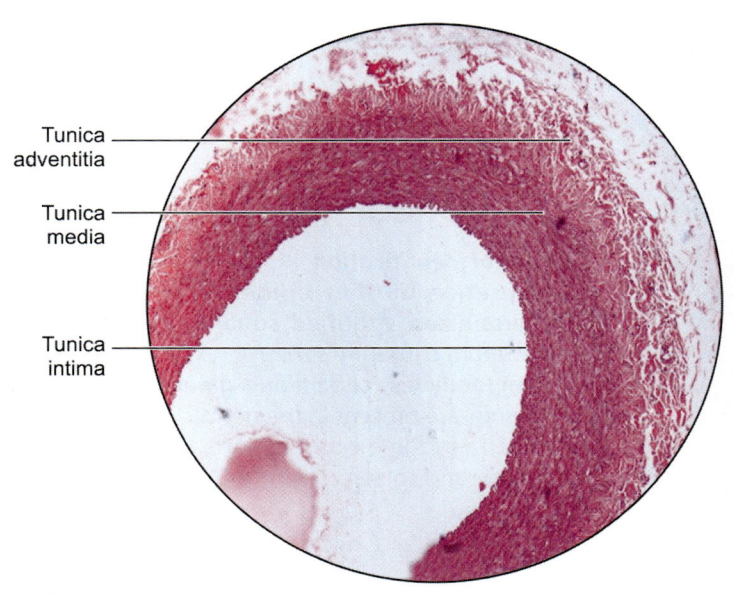

Fig. A8.2: Muscular (medium size) artery.

Points of identification
- In muscular arteries, the tunica intima is made up of endothelium and internal elastic lamina, which is thrown into wavy folds due to contraction of smooth muscle in the media
- Tunica media is composed mainly of smooth muscle fibers arranged circularly
- Tunica adventitia contains collagen fibers and few elastic fibers.

Large-sized Vein

Tunica intima
Tunica media
Tunica adventitia

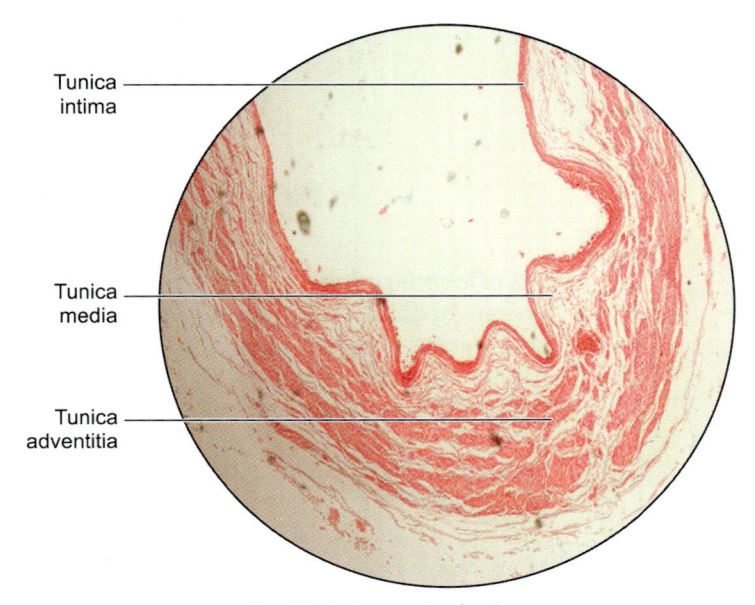

Fig. A8.3: Large-sized vein.

Points of identification
- The vein has a thinner wall and a larger lumen than the artery
- The tunica intitma, media, and adventitia can be made out, but they are not sharply demarcated
- The media is thin and contains a much larger quantity of collagen fibers than arteries. The amount of elastic tissue or of muscle is much less
- The adventitia is relatively thick and contains considerable amount of elastic and muscle fibers.

Note: The luminal surface appears as a dark line, with an occasional nucleus along it.

SKIN AND ITS APPENDAGES

Thin Skin or Hairy Skin

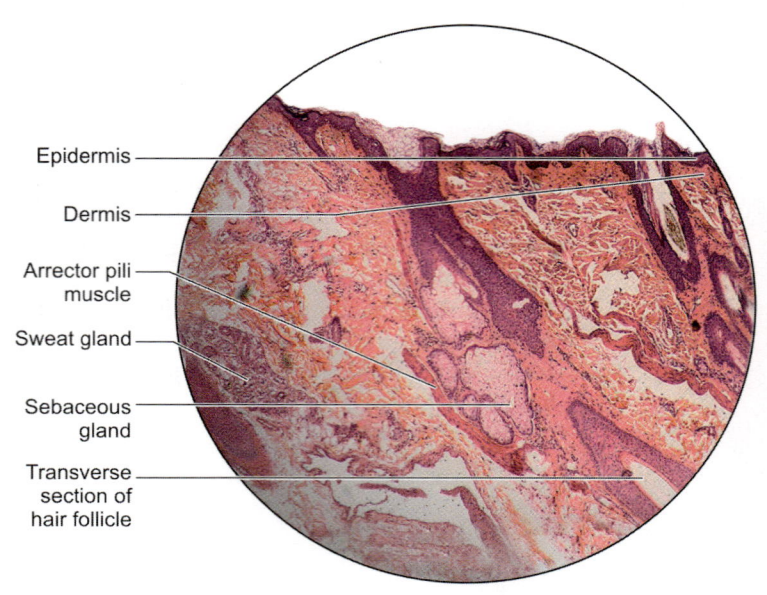

Fig. A9.1: Thin skin or hairy skin (low magnification).

Labels: Epidermis, Dermis, Arrector pili muscle, Sweat gland, Sebaceous gland, Transverse section of hair follicle

Points of identification
- Presence of thin epidermis made up of keratinized stratified squamous epithelium (stratum corneum is thin)
- Hair follicles, sebaceous glands and sweat glands are present in the dermis
- It is found in all others parts of body except palms and soles.

Thick Skin

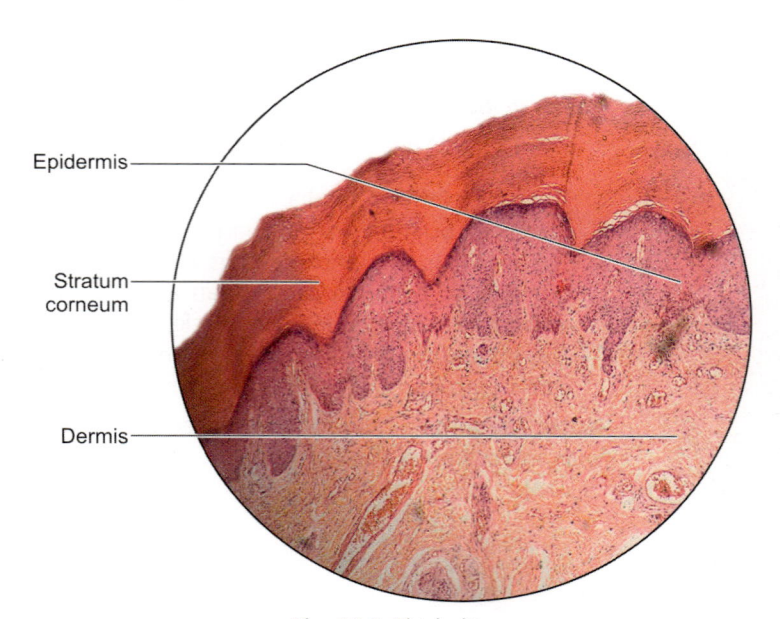

Fig. A9.2: Thick skin.

Labels: Epidermis, Stratum corneum, Dermis

Points of identification
- Presence of thick epidermis made up of keratinized stratified squamous epithelium (stratum corneum is very thick)
- Hair follicles and sebaceous glands are absent in dermis
- Sweat glands are present in the dermis
- It is found in palms of hands and soles of feet.

Color Atlas

Hair Follicle and Sebaceous Gland

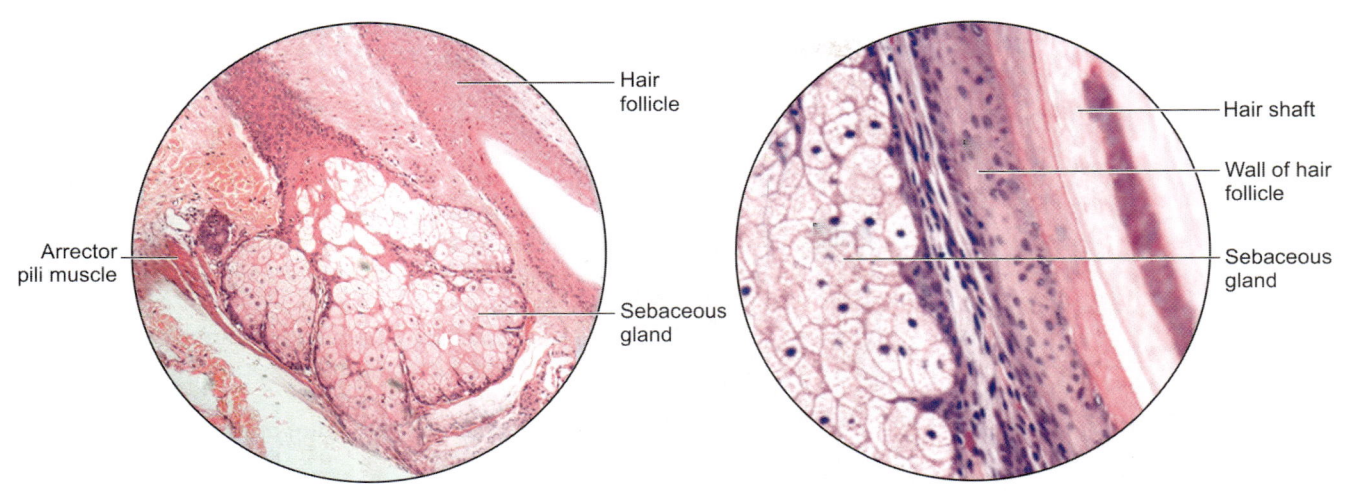

Fig. A9.3: Hair follicle and sebaceous gland (Low magnification).

Fig. A9.4: Hair follicle and sebaceous gland (High magnification).

Points of identification
- In figures small areas of skin at higher magnification are shown
- The parts of a sebaceous gland and hair follicle containing a hair root can be seen
- Each sebaceous gland consists of a number of alveoli that open into a hair follicle
- Each alveolus is pear shaped. It consists mainly of a solid mass of polyhedral cells.

SALIVARY GLANDS

Parotid Gland

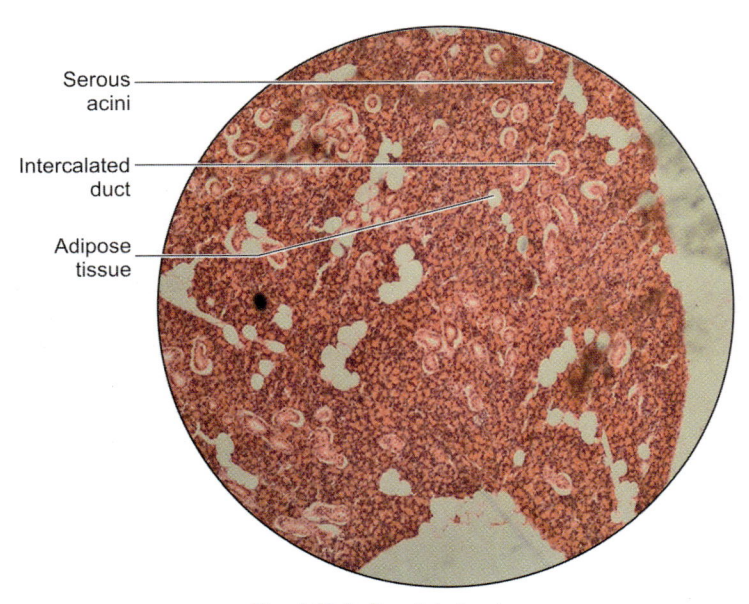

Fig. A10.1: Parotid gland.

Points of identification
The parotid gland is a serous salivary gland. The characteristic features are:
- Only serous acini are present which contain basophilic zymogen granules and are darkly stained
- Intercalated and striated (intralobular) ducts are seen
- Interlobular duct can be seen
- It also contains adipocytes.

Submandibular Gland (Low Magnification)

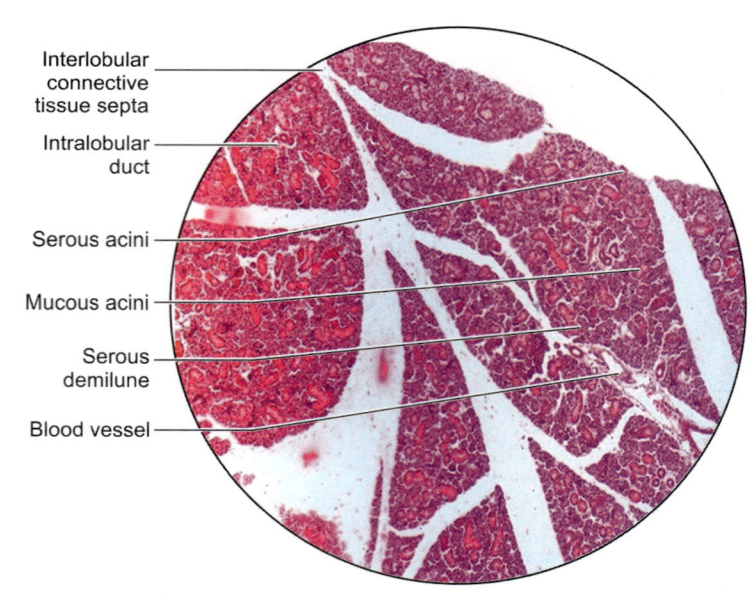

Fig. A10.2: Submandibular gland (Low magnification).

Labels: Interlobular connective tissue septa, Intralobular duct, Serous acini, Mucous acini, Serous demilune, Blood vessel

Points of identification
- The submandibular gland is a mixed salivary gland, predominantly serous with a few mucous acini
- Serous cells are frequently located at the periphery of mucous acini in the form of a crescent and called as demilunes
- Striated ducts are more prominent than those in parotid gland.

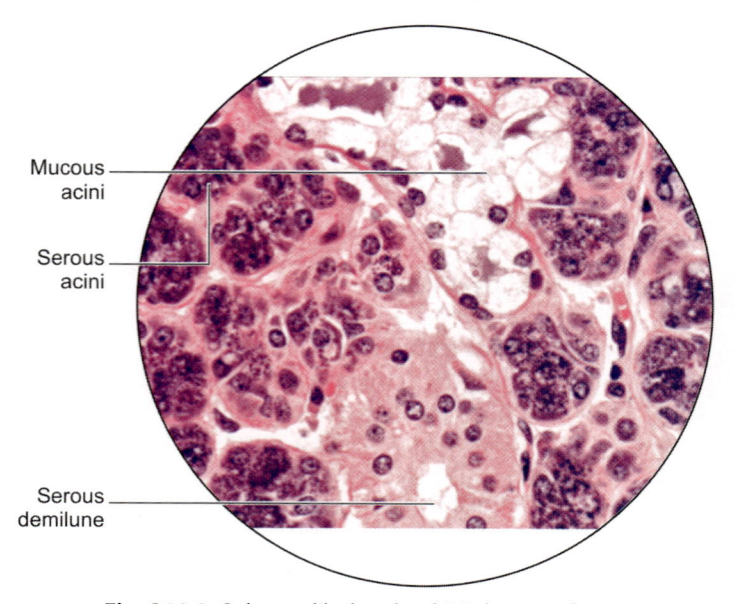

Submandibular Gland (High Magnification)

Fig. A10.3: Submandibular gland (High magnification).

Labels: Mucous acini, Serous acini, Serous demilune

Points of identification
- In the high power view the serous and mucous acini can be identified by their staining reaction, and shape and position of nucleus
- The serous acini are darkly stained and have rounded nucleus placed near the center of the cell
- The mucous acini are lightly stained with flat nucleus placed toward the basement membrane
- The mucous acini are often associated with darkly stained crescentic patch of serous cells called serous demilune.

Sublingual Salivary Gland

Labels: Intercalated duct, Interlobular connective tissue septa, Mucous acini, Blood vessels

Points of identification
- The sublingual gland is predominantly a mucous gland but few serous acini may also be seen
- Serous demilunes may be present.

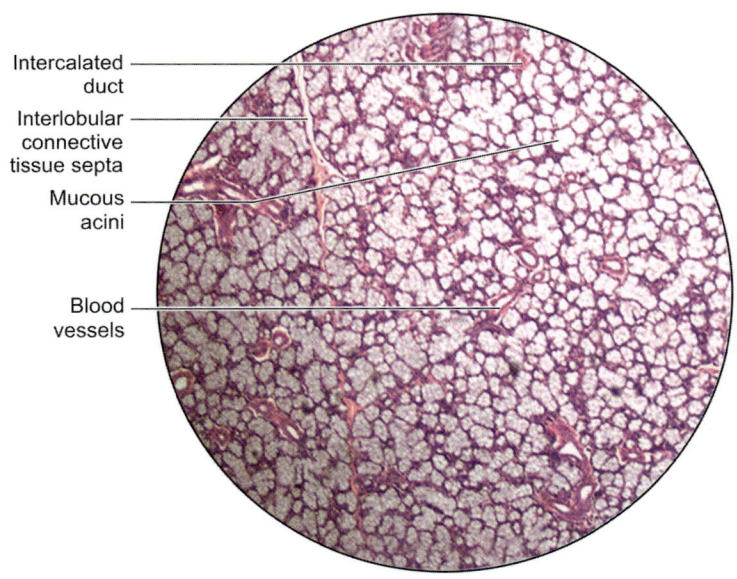

Fig. A10.4: Sublingual salivary gland.

PLACENTA

Placenta (Low Magnification)

Labels: Anchoring villi, Intervillous space with maternal blood, Floating villi

Points of identification
- Tertiary villi of various size and shapes seen
- Inter villous space containing maternal blood
- Truncus chorii, ramus chorii, ramuli chorii and floating villi in intervillous space seen
- Section of tertiary villi has core of mesoderm surrounded by cyto- and syncytiotrophoblast.

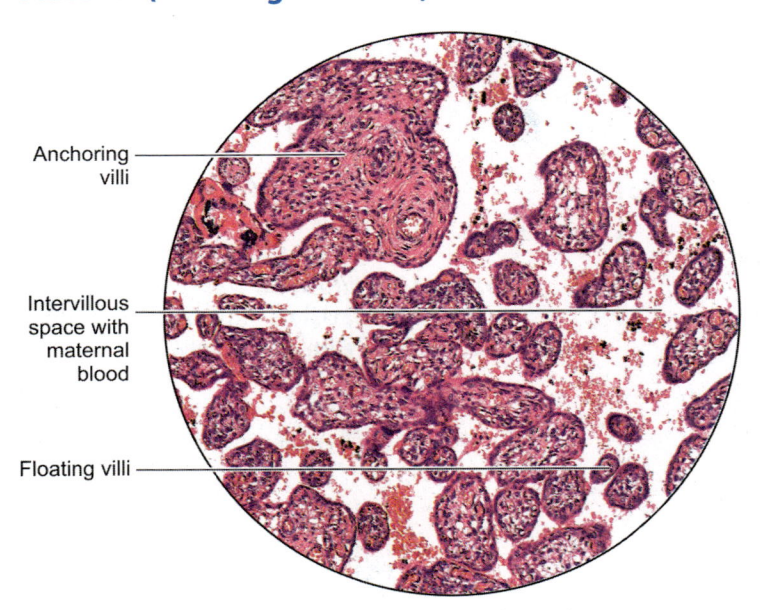

Fig. A11.1: Placenta (Low magnification).

RESPIRATORY SYSTEM

Epiglottis

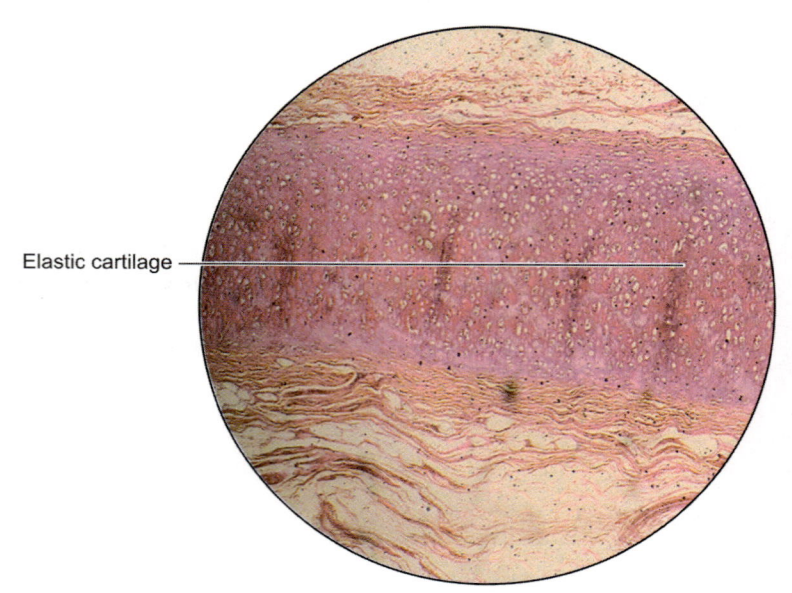

Elastic cartilage

Fig. A12.1: Epiglottis.

Points of identification
- Lined by pseudostratified ciliated columnar epithelium
- Lamina propria with serous and mucous glands
- Central core of elastic tissue.

Trachea

Hyaline cartilage
Adventitia
Perichondrium
Lamina propria
Pseudostratified ciliated columnar epithelium
Blood vessels

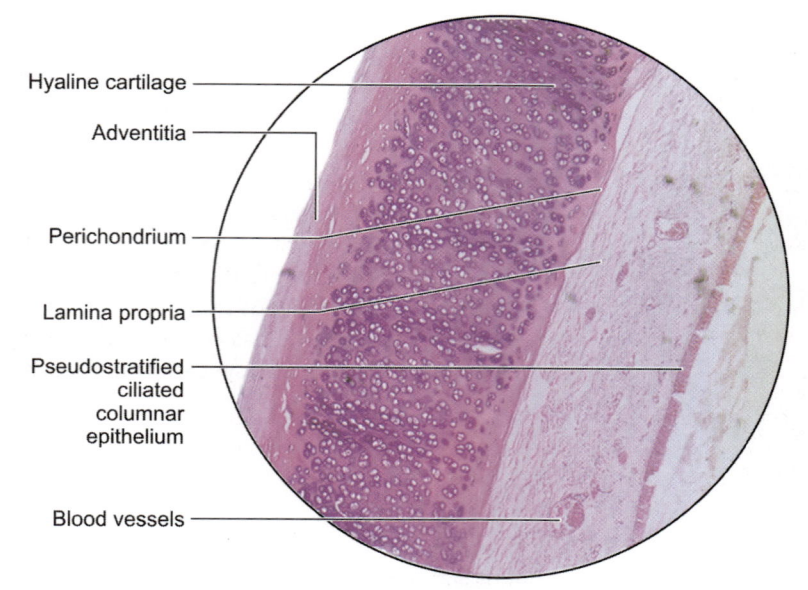

Fig. A12.2: Trachea.

Points of identification
- Pseudostratified ciliated columnar epithelium with goblet cells
- Lamina propria
- Submucosa with serous and mucous glands
- Presence of hyaline cartilage and trachealis muscle.

Lung

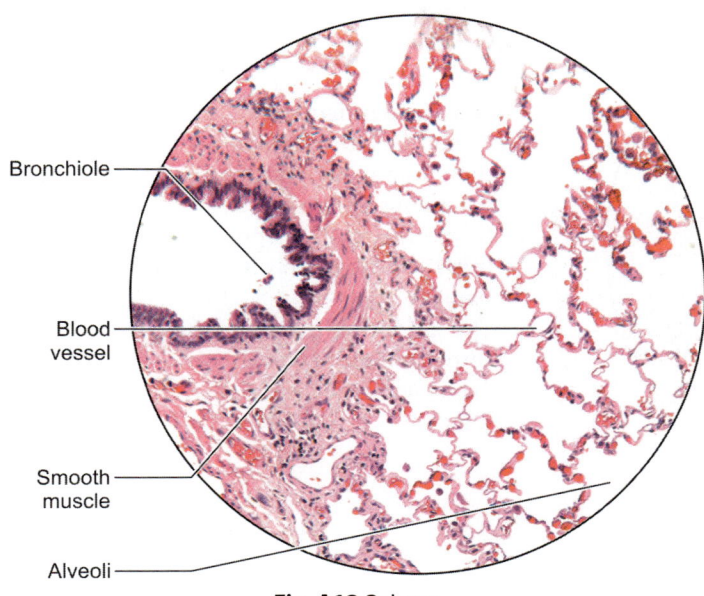

Fig. A12.3: Lung.

Labels: Bronchiole, Blood vessel, Smooth muscle, Alveoli

Courtesy: Ivan Damjanov. Atlas of Histopathology, 1st edition. New Delhi: Jaypee Brothers Medical Publishers (P) Ltd; 2012. p. 37.

Points of identification
- Presence of alveolar ducts
- Alveolar sac lined by simple squamous epithelium
- Presence of intrapulmonary bronchus with varying amount of islands cartilage and smooth muscles
- Respiratory bronchioles with simple cuboidal epithelial lining lacking cilia and goblet cells.

DIGESTIVE SYSTEM: ORAL CAVITY AND RELATED STRUCTURES

Tongue (Anterior Part)

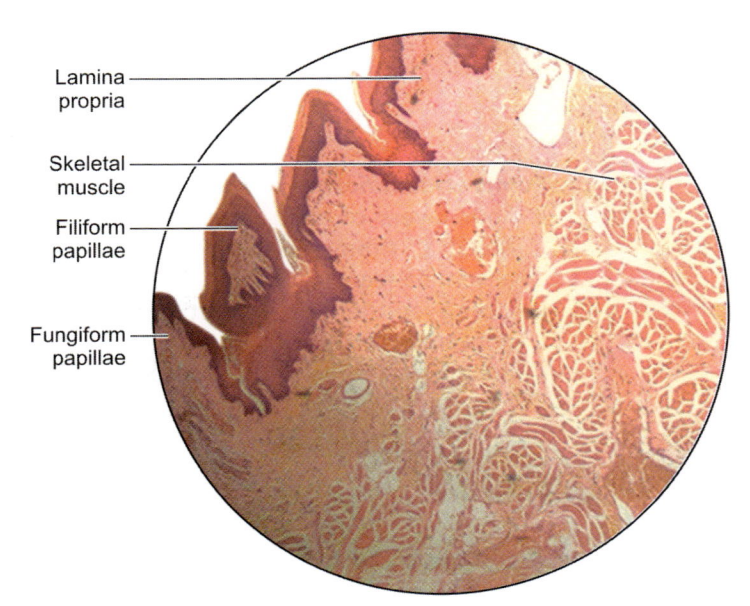

Fig. A13.1: Tongue (Anterior part).

Labels: Lamina propria, Skeletal muscle, Filiform papillae, Fungiform papillae

Points of identification
- The tongue is covered on both surfaces by stratified squamous epithelium (nonkeratinized)
- The ventral surface of the tongue is smooth, but on the dorsum the surface shows numerous projections or papillae
- Each papilla has a core of connective tissue covered by epithelium. Some papillae are pointed (filiform), while others are broad at the top (fungiform). A third type of papilla is circumvallate, the top of this papilla is broad and lies at the same level as the surrounding mucosa
- The main mass of the tongue is formed by skeletal muscle seen below the lamina propria. Muscle fibers run in various directions so that some are cut longitudinally and some transversely
- Numerous serous and mucous glands are present amongst the muscle fibers.

Vallate Papilla

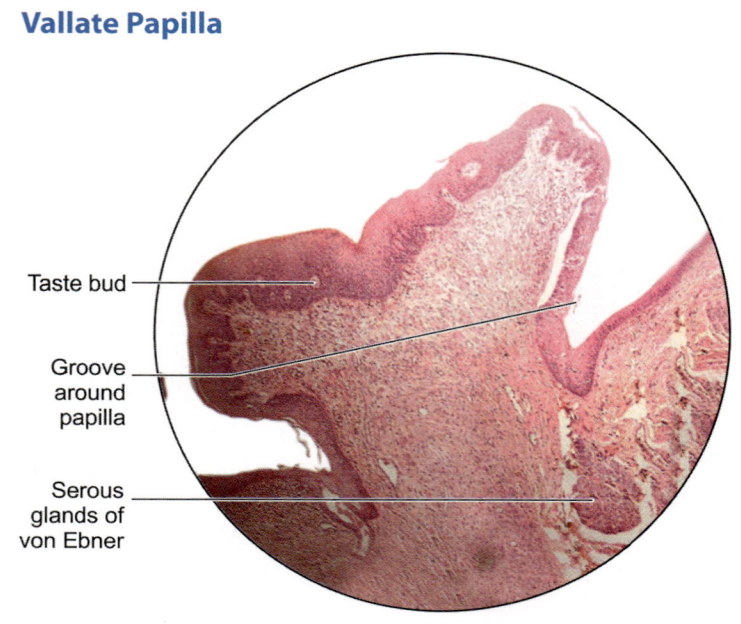

Fig. A13.2: Vallate papilla.

Labels: Taste bud; Groove around papilla; Serous glands of von Ebner

Points of identification
- Circumvallate papillae are characterized by their dome-shaped structure lined by stratified squamous epithelium
- Numerous oval-shaped lightly stained taste buds can be seen on the lateral wall of the papillae
- The underlying connective tissue contains serous glands of von Ebner
- Skeletal muscle can be seen extending into the papillae.

DIGESTIVE SYSTEM: GENERAL PLAN OF GASTROINTESTINAL TRACT, STOMACH AND INTESTINES

Esophagus

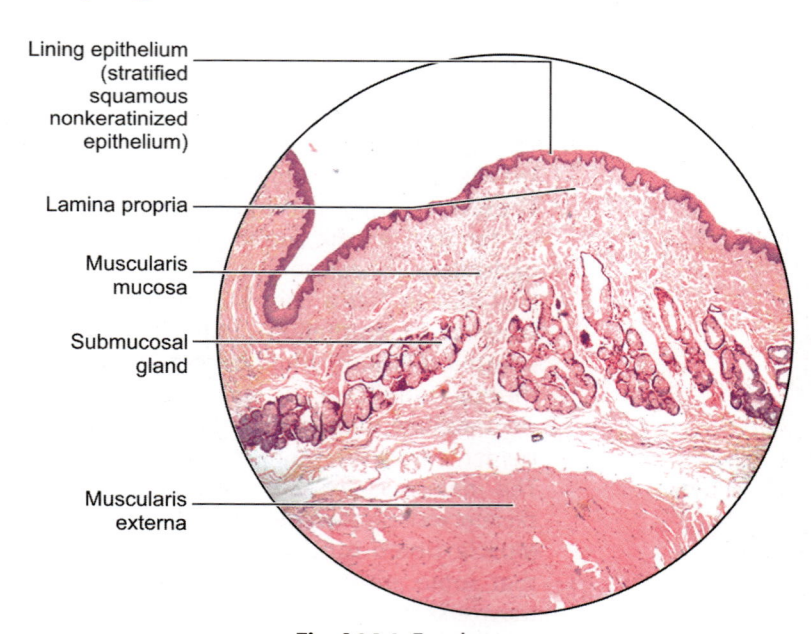

Fig. A14.1: Esophagus.

Labels: Lining epithelium (stratified squamous nonkeratinized epithelium); Lamina propria; Muscularis mucosa; Submucosal gland; Muscularis externa

Points of identification
- Four layers of gastrointestinal tract (GIT): Mucosa, submucosa, muscularis externa, adventitia seen
- Lining epithelium is stratified squamous nonkeratinized epithelium
- Submucosa is studded with mucus-secreting esophageal glands.

Stomach (Fundus)

Fig. A14.2: Stomach (Fundus): Low power.

Fig. A14.3: Stomach (Fundus): High power.

Points of identification
- Presence of four layers—mucosa, submucosa, muscularis externa, and serosa
- Shallow gastric pits occupying superficial one-fourth or less of the mucosa
- Presence of gastric glands in the mucosa
- Gastric glands with numerous oxyntic cells which give beaded appearance.

Stomach (Pylorus)

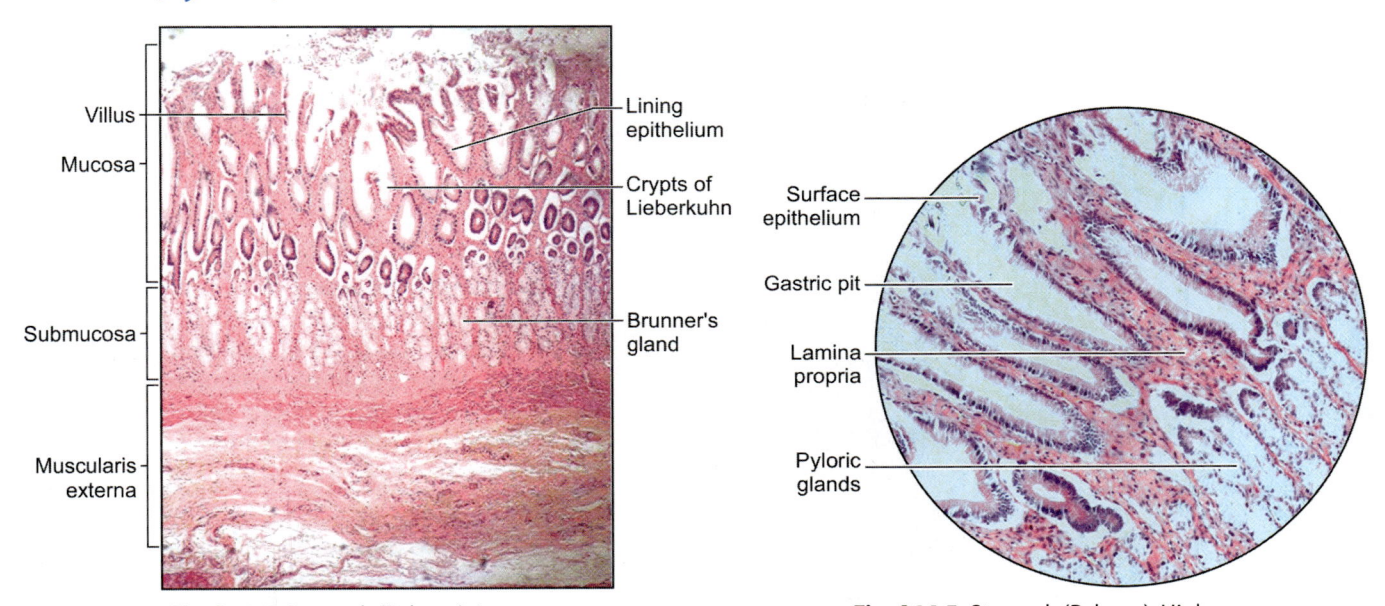

Fig. A14.4: Stomach (Pylorus): Low power.

Fig. A14.5: Stomach (Pylorus): High power.

Points of identification
- Presence of four layers—mucosa, submucosa, muscularis externa, and serosa
- Deep gastric pits occupying two-thirds of the depth of the mucosa
- Presence of pyloric glands (mucous glands) in the mucosa that are simple/branched tubular glands which are coiled.

Duodenum

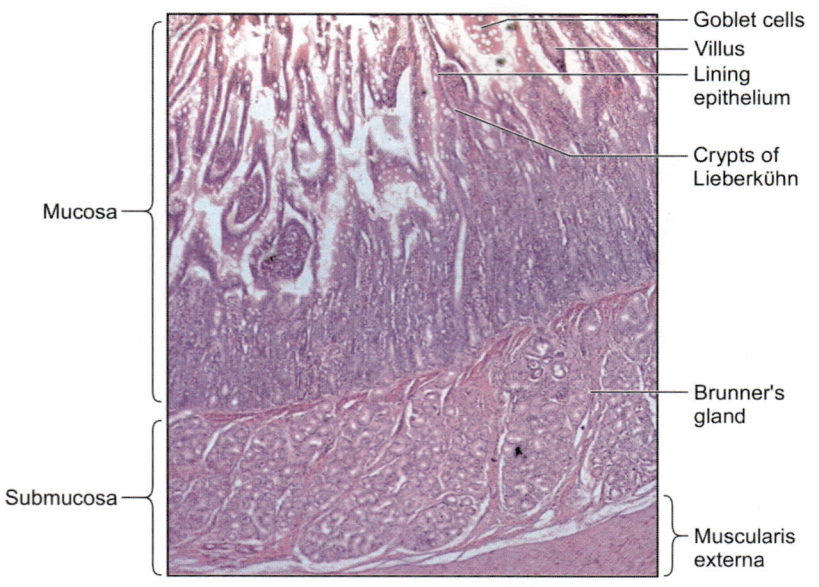

Fig. A14.6: Duodenum.

Points of identification
- Wall made up of four layers
- Mucosa—presence of numerous broad villi, lined by simple columnar epithelium with microvilli and goblet cells
- Presence of submucous Brunner's gland.

Jejunum

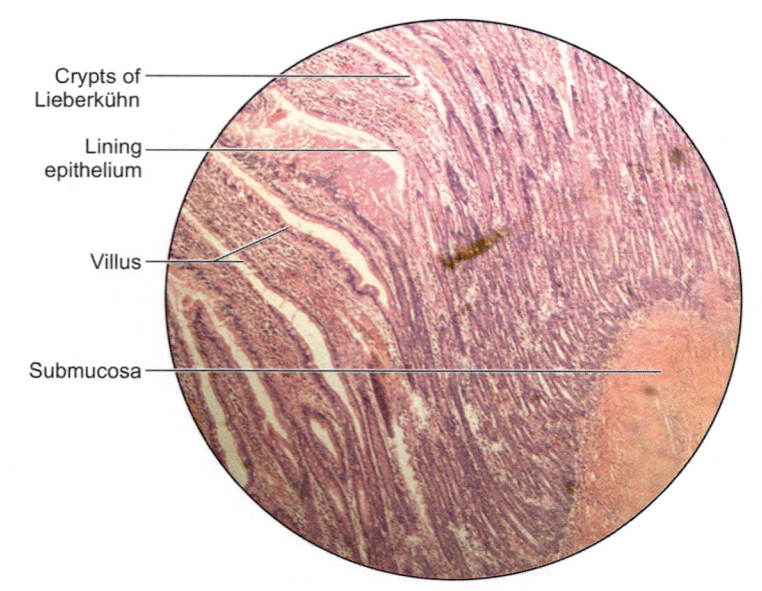

Fig. A14.7: Jejunum.

Points of identification
- Wall made up of four layers
- Mucosa—presence of numerous tall slender villi, lined by simple columnar epithelium with microvilli and goblet cells
- Absence of submucous Brunner's gland.

Ileum

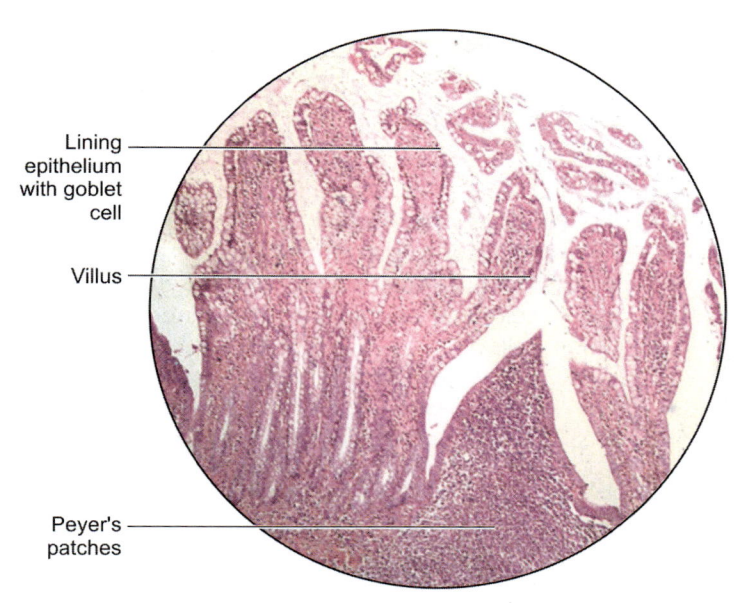

Fig. A14.8: Ileum.

Labels: Lining epithelium with goblet cell; Villus; Peyer's patches

Points of identification
- Wall made up of four layers
- Mucosa—presence of short, small fewer villi, lined by simple columnar epithelium with microvilli and numerous goblet cells
- Absence of submucous Brunner's gland.

Colon

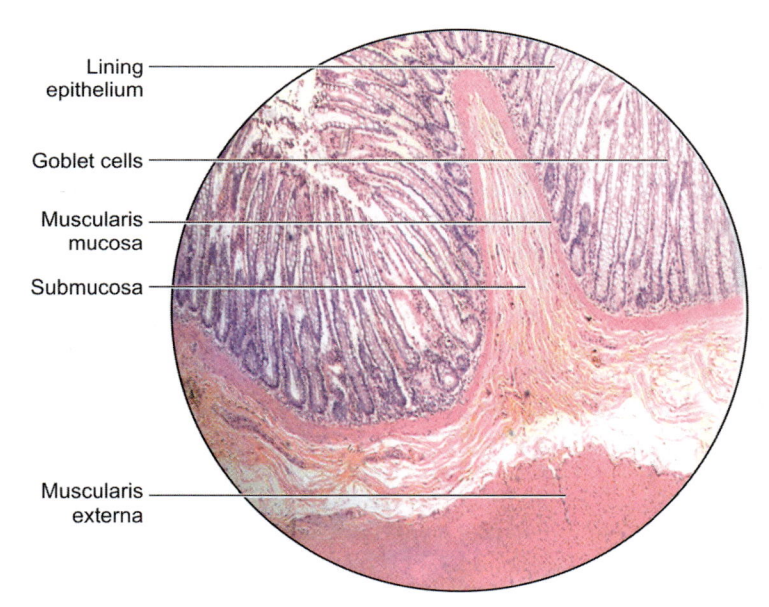

Fig. A14.9: Colon.

Labels: Lining epithelium; Goblet cells; Muscularis mucosa; Submucosa; Muscularis externa

Points of identification
- Wall made up of four layers
- Mucosa—absence of villi, lined by simple columnar epithelium with numerous goblet cells
- Lymphatic follicles dispersed in the lamina propria
- Presence of taenia coli, appendices epiploicae.

Vermiform Appendix

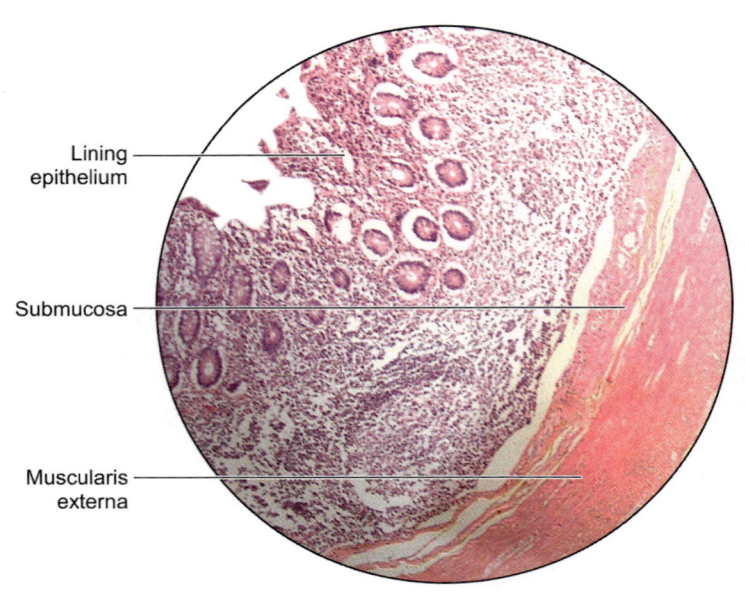

Fig. A14.10: Vermiform appendix.

Labels: Lining epithelium, Submucosa, Muscularis externa

Points of identification
- Wall made up of four layers
- Mucosa—absence of villi, lined by simple columnar epithelium with numerous goblet cells
- Submucosa packed with numerous lymphatic follicles, extending into lamina propria
- Absence of taenia coli, appendices epiploicae.

HEPATOBILIARY SYSTEM AND PANCREAS

Liver (Panoramic View)

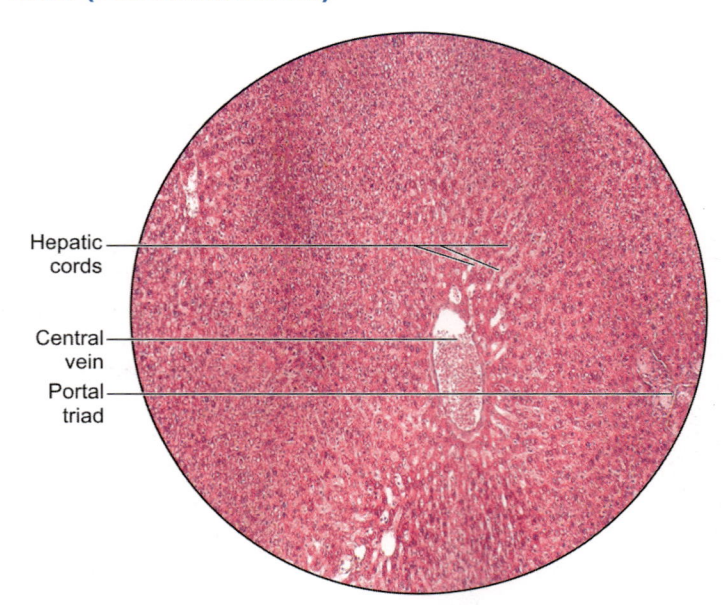

Fig. A15.1: Liver (Panoramic view).

Labels: Hepatic cords, Central vein, Portal triad

Points of identification
- The panoramic view of liver shows many hexagonal areas called hepatic lobules. The lobules are partially separated by connective tissue
- Each lobule has a small round space in the center. This is the central vein
- A number of broad irregular cords of cells seem to pass from this vein to the periphery of the lobule. These cords are made up of polygonal liver cells—hepatocytes
- Along the periphery of the lobules, there are angular intervals filled by connective tissue
- Each such area contains a branch of the portal vein, a branch of the hepatic artery, and an interlobular bile duct
- These three constitute a portal triad.

Color Atlas

Liver (High Magnification)

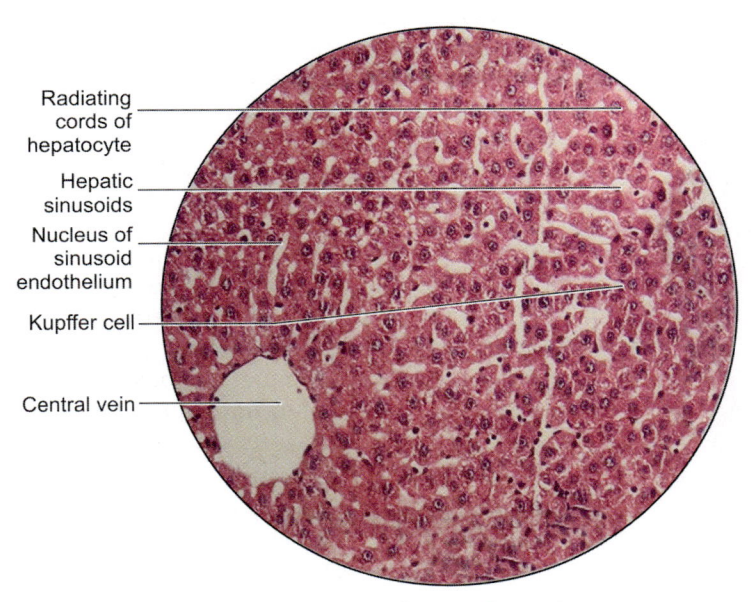

Labels on figure:
- Radiating cords of hepatocyte
- Hepatic sinusoids
- Nucleus of sinusoid endothelium
- Kupffer cell
- Central vein

Fig. A15.2: Liver (High magnification).

Points of identification
On high magnification:
- The lobule is made up of polygonal liver cells arranged in the form of radiating cords
- The central round nucleus of hepatocyte is surrounded by abundant pink cytoplasm
- The cords are separated from each other by spaces called sinusoids
- The sinusoids are lined by endothelial cells and Kupffer cells (macrophage cells)
- Each portal tract contains a hepatic arteriole, portal venule, and one or two interlobular bile ducts. Normally, these structures are surrounded by fibroconnective tissue and a few lymphocytes.

Gallbladder

Labels on figure:
- Lamina propria
- Simple columnar epithelium with brush border
- Mucosal folds
- Fibromuscular layer

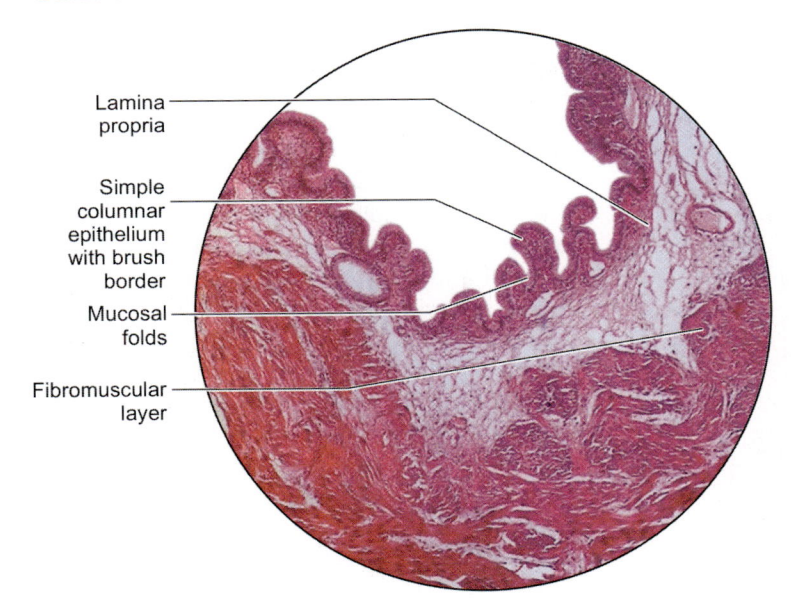

Fig. A15.3: Gallbladder.

Points of identification
- The mucous membrane is lined by tall columnar cells with striated border
- The mucosa is highly folded and some of the folds might look-like villi
- Crypts may be found in lamina propria
- Submucosa is absent
- The muscle coat is poorly developed with numerous connective tissue fibers interspersed among muscle. This is called as fibromuscular coat
- A serous covering lined by flattened mesothelium is seen.

Note: Gallbladder can be differentiated from small intestine by absence of villi, goblet cells, submucosa, and proper muscularis externa.

Pancreas

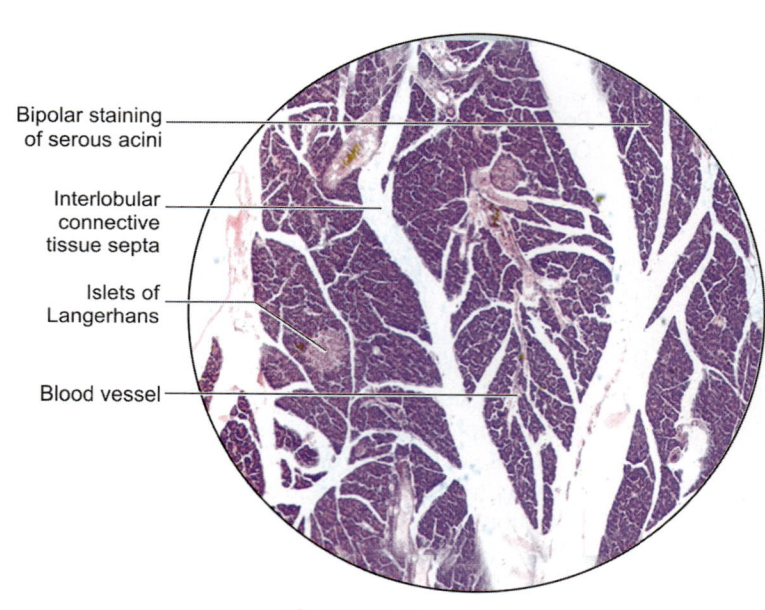

Fig. A15.4: Pancreas.

Labels: Bipolar staining of serous acini; Interlobular connective tissue septa; Islets of Langerhans; Blood vessel

Points of identification
- Made up of serous acini
- The cells forming the acini of the pancreas are highly basophilic (bluish staining). The lumen of the acinus is very small
- Some acini may show pale staining (centroacinar cell) in the center
- Among the acini, some ducts are seen
- The ducts have a distinct lumen, lined by cuboidal epithelium
- At some places, the acini are separated by areas where we see aggregations of cells quite different from those of the acini
- These aggregations form the pancreatic islets: pale staining cells arranged as groups, surrounded by blood vessels
- In the photomicrograph, an interlobular duct lined by cuboidal epithelium is surrounded by lobules of acinar cells which have small basal nuclei and granular eosinophilic or slightly basophilic cytoplasm. Islets of Langerhans appear as groups of small cells with lightly stained cytoplasm.

URINARY SYSTEM

Kidney (Low Magnification)

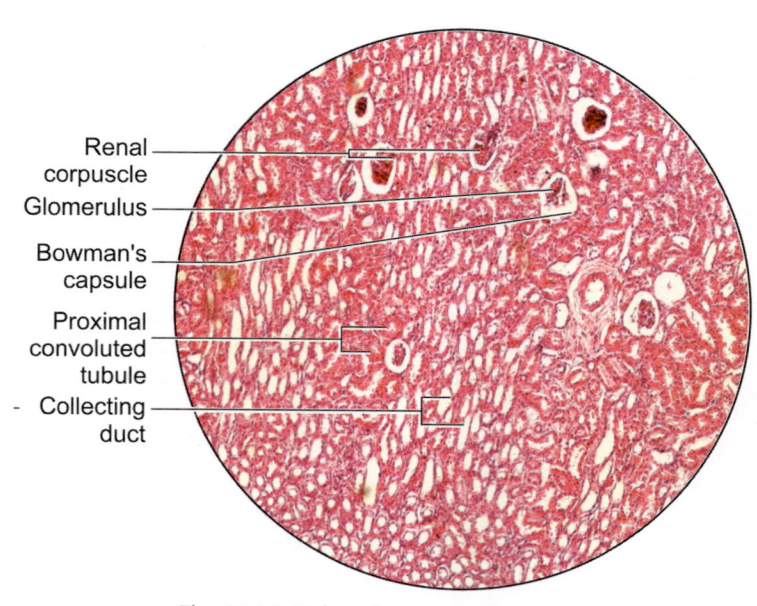

Fig. A16.1: Kidney (Low magnification).
Courtesy: Balakrishna Shetty, Sweekritha H Poonja. HISTOLOGY Practical Manual, 4th edition. New Delhi: Jaypee Brothers Medical Publishers (P) Ltd; 2019. p. 108.

Labels: Renal corpuscle; Glomerulus; Bowman's capsule; Proximal convoluted tubule; Collecting duct

Points of identification
- The kidney is covered by a capsule, deep to which is the cortex
- Deep to the cortex there is the medulla
- In the cortex we see circular structures called renal corpuscles surrounding which there are tubules cut in various shapes
- The dark pink stained tubules are parts of the proximal convoluted tubules (PCT): their lumen is small and indistinct. It is lined by cuboidal epithelium with brush border
- Lighter staining tubules, each with a distinct lumen, are the distal convoluted tubules (DCT). They are lined by simple cuboidal epithelium
- PCT are more in number than DCT
- In the medulla we see very light staining, elongated, parallel running tubules. These are collecting ducts and loop of Henle. Some of them extend into the cortex forming a medullary ray. The collecting ducts are lined by simple cuboidal epithelium and loop of Henle (thin segments) are lined by simple squamous epithelium
- Cut sections of blood vessels are seen both in the cortex and medulla.

Renal Cortex (High Magnification)

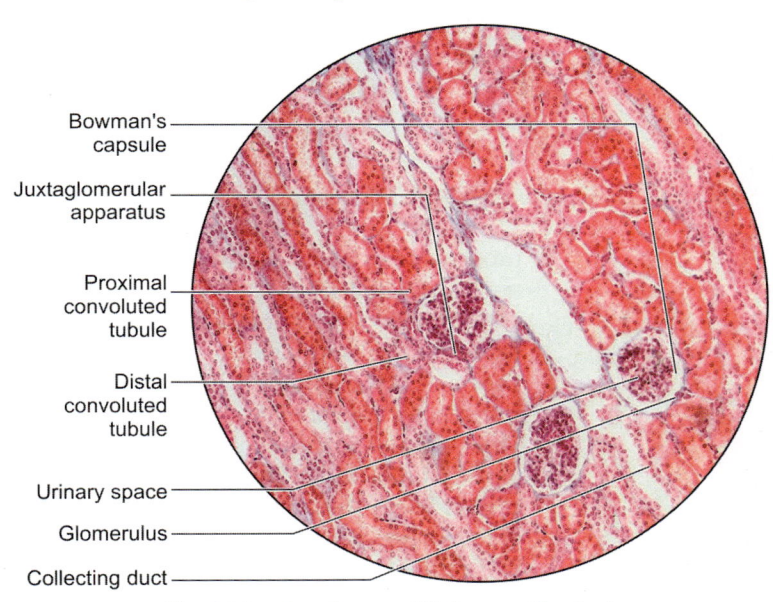

Fig. A16.2: Renal cortex (High magnification).

Labels: Bowman's capsule, Juxtaglomerular apparatus, Proximal convoluted tubule, Distal convoluted tubule, Urinary space, Glomerulus, Collecting duct

Points of identification
- In the high power view of renal cortex large renal corpuscles can be identified
- The renal corpuscle consists of a tuft of capillaries that form a rounded glomerulus, and an outer wall, the glomerular capsule (Bowman's capsule)
- A urinary space between the glomerulus and the capsule is seen
- Proximal convoluted tubules are dark staining. They are lined by cuboidal cells with a prominent brush border. Their lumen is indistinct
- Distal convoluted tubules are lighter staining. The cuboidal cells lining them do not have a brush border. Their lumen is distinct.

Renal Medulla (High Magnification)

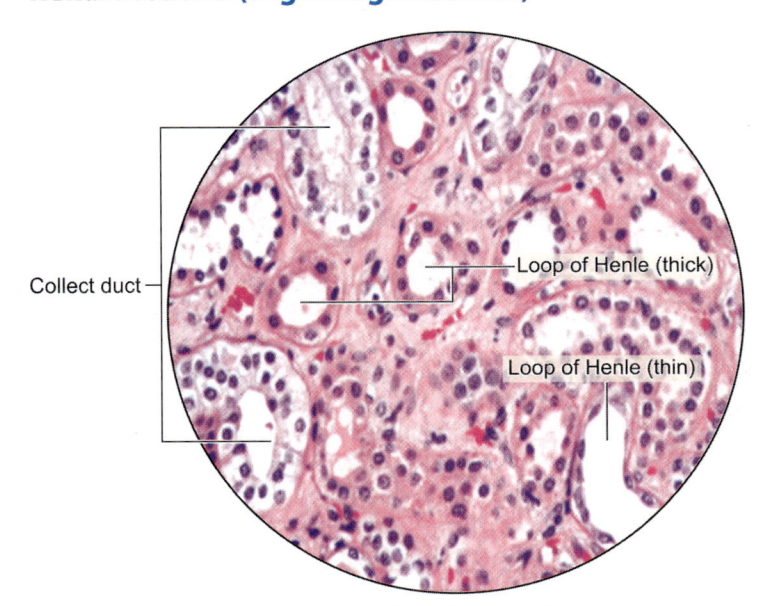

Fig. A16.3: Renal medulla (High magnification).

Labels: Collect duct, Loop of Henle (thick), Loop of Henle (thin)

Points of identification
- A high power view of a part of the renal medulla shows a number of collecting ducts cut longitudinally or transversely
- They are lined by a cuboidal epithelium, the cells of which stain lightly. Cell boundaries are usually distinct. The lumen of the tubule is also distinct
- Sections of the thin segment of the loop of Henle are seen. They are lined by flattened cells, the walls being very similar in appearance to those of blood capillaries
- Sections through the thick segments of loops of Henle are seen. They are lined by cuboidal epithelium.

Ureter

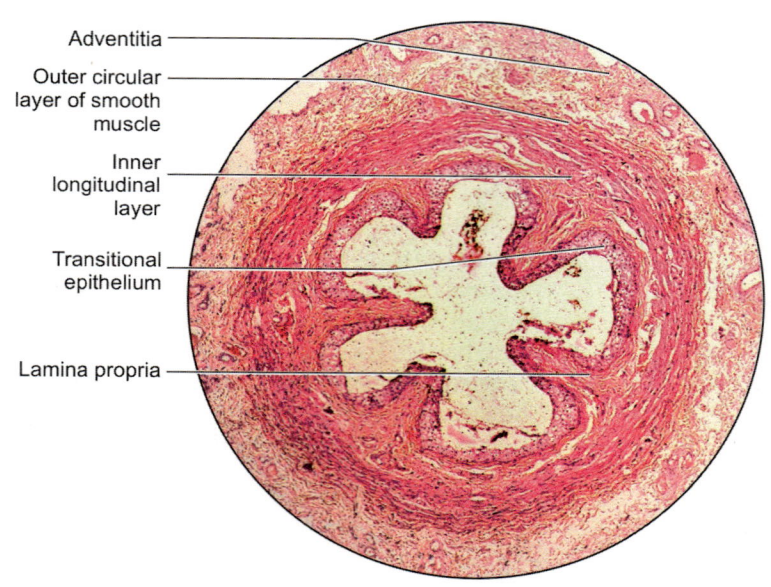

Fig. A16.4: Ureter (Low magnification).

Points of identification
- The ureter can be recognized because it is tubular and its mucous membrane is lined by transitional epithelium
- The epithelium rests on a layer of connective tissue (lamina propria)
- The mucosa shows folds that give the lumen a star-shaped appearance
- The muscle coat has an inner layer of longitudinal fibers and an outer layer of circular fibers. This arrangement is the reverse of that in the gut
- The muscle coat is surrounded by connective tissue—adventitia in which blood vessels and fat cells are present.

Urinary Bladder

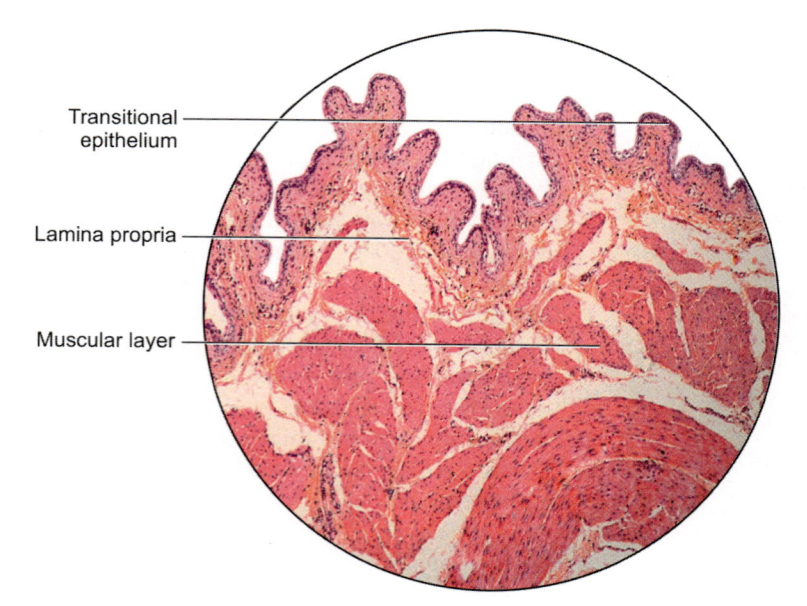

Fig. A16.5: Urinary bladder.

Points of identification
- The urinary bladder is easily recognized because the mucous membrane is lined by transitional epithelium
- The epithelium rests on lamina propria
- The muscle layer is thick. It has inner and outer longitudinal layers between which there is a layer of circular or oblique fibers. The distinct muscle layers may not be distinguishable
- The outer surface is lined in parts by peritoneum (serosa) (not seen in the photomicrograph).

CENTRAL NERVOUS SYSTEM: SPINAL CORD, CEREBELLAR CORTEX AND CEREBRAL CORTEX

Spinal Cord

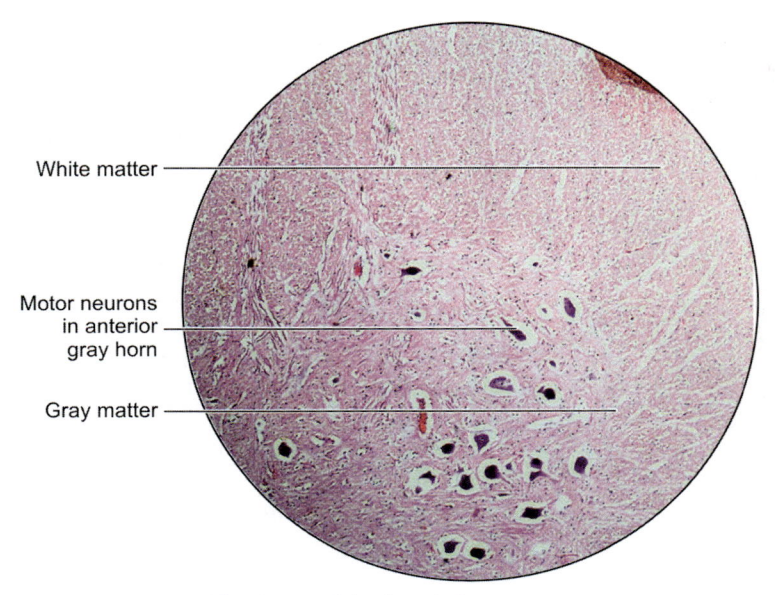

Fig. A17.1: Spinal cord: Gray matter.

Points of identification
- The spinal cord has a characteristic oval shape
- It is made up of white matter (containing mainly of myelinated fibers), and gray matter (containing neurons and unmyelinated fibers)
- The gray matter lies toward the center and is surrounded all round by white matter
- The gray matter consists of a centrally placed mass and projections (horns) that pass forwards and backwards.

Cerebral Cortex

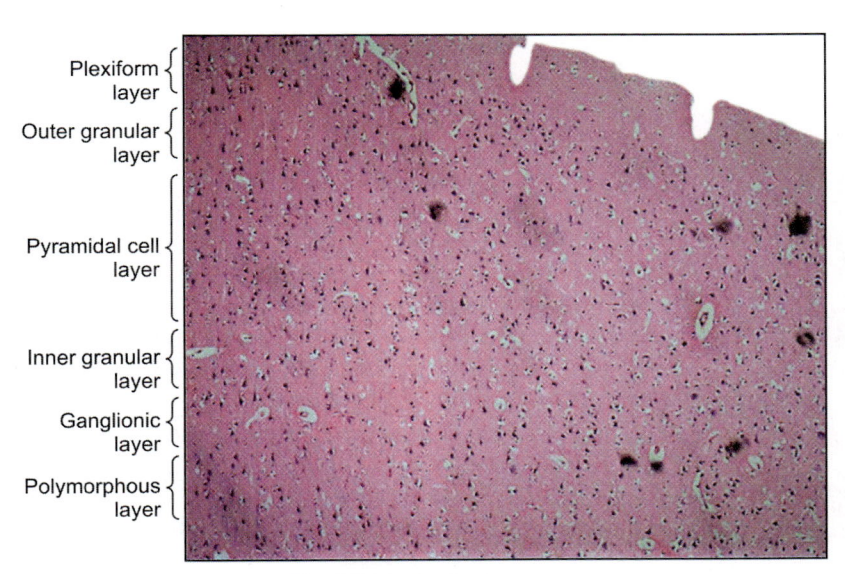

Fig. A17.2: Cerebral cortex.

Points of identification
- A slide of cerebral cortex shows outer gray and inner white matter
- Multipolar neurons of various shapes are arranged in six layers in the gray matter
- Axons of these neurons are present in the white matter
- Neuroglia and blood vessels are present in gray and white matter.

Cerebellar Cortex

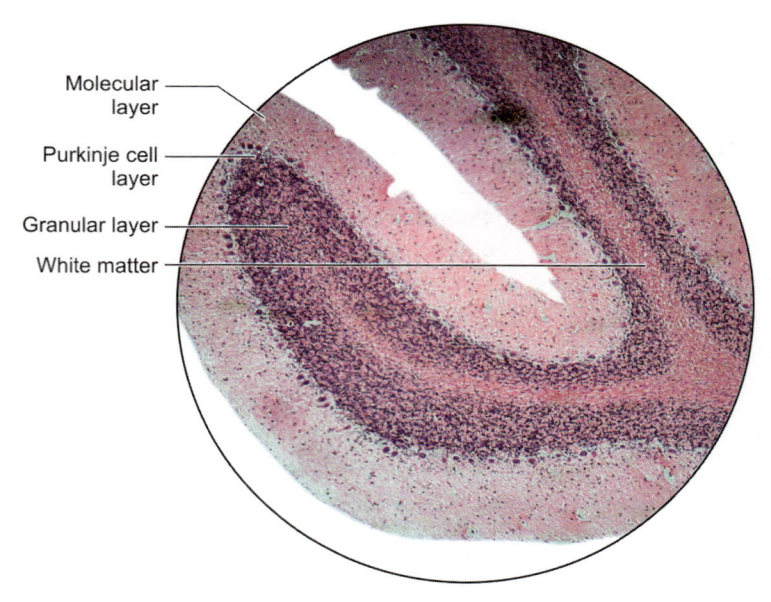

Fig. A17.3: Cerebellar cortex.

Points of identification
- The section of cerebellum shows leaf-like folia
- The cortex is covered by pia mater which appears as a thin layer of collagen fibers. Blood vessels may be seen just beneath the pia mater
- Outer gray matter is arranged in three layers from without inwards:
  1. *Molecular layer*: Very few nuclei of neurons seen. Many cell processes present. Appears pale
  2. *Purkinje cell layer*: Single layer of big flask-shaped pink neurons
  3. *Granular cell layer*: Appears very dark blue because of presence of abundant nuclei of neurons
- Inner white matter shows axons which appear as pink fibers
- Nuclei of neuroglia are present both in gray and white matter.

MALE REPRODUCTIVE SYSTEM

Testis (Low Magnification)

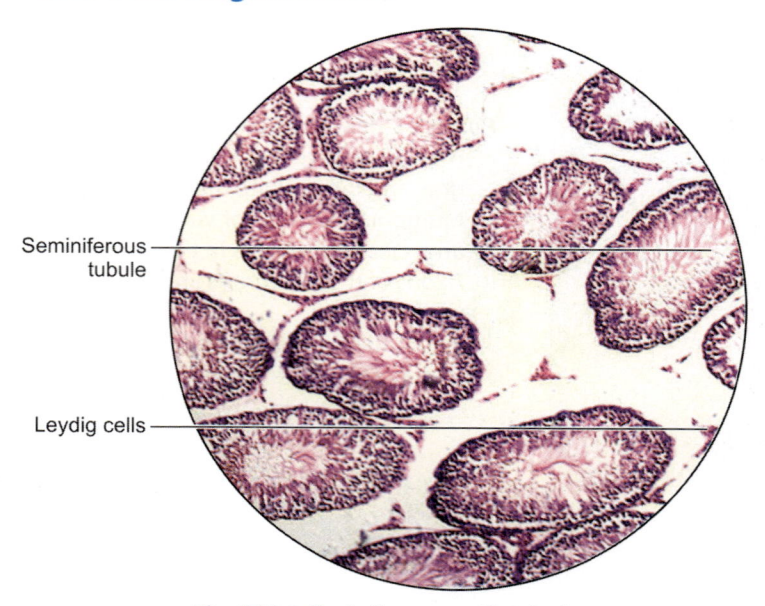

Fig. A18.1: Testis (Low magnification).

Points of identification
The testis has an outer fibrous layer, the tunica albuginea deep to which:
- A number of seminiferous tubules cut in various directions are seen
- The tubules are separated by connective tissue, containing blood vessels and groups of interstitial cells of Leydig
- Each seminiferous tubule is lined by several layers of cells
- Cells are of two types:
  1. Spermatogenic cells which produce spermatozoa
  2. Sustentacular (Sertoli) cells which have a supportive function.

Testis (High Magnification)

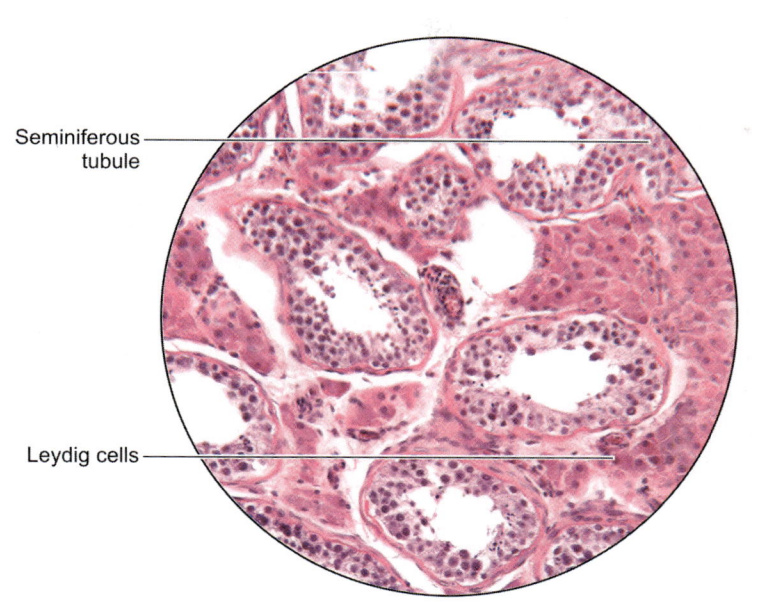

Fig. A18.2: Testis (High magnification).
Courtesy: Ivan Damjanov. Atlas of Histopathology, 1st edition. New Delhi: Jaypee Brothers Medical Publishers (P) Ltd; 2012. p. 203.

Labels: Seminiferous tubule; Leydig cells

Points of identification
- The outermost row of nuclei belongs to sustentacular cells (Sertoli) and to spermatogonia, some of which are undergoing mitosis (note very dense nucleus of irregular shape)
- Passing inwards toward the center of the tubule we have large darkly staining nuclei of spermatocytes, and many smaller nuclei of spermatids
- Toward the center of the tubule a number of developing spermatozoa are seen. The sperms are often found in clusters embedded in the cytoplasm of Sertoli cells
- In the adult testis, sustentacular cells are less prominent than germ cells. They are more prominent than germ cells before puberty and in old age.

Epididymis

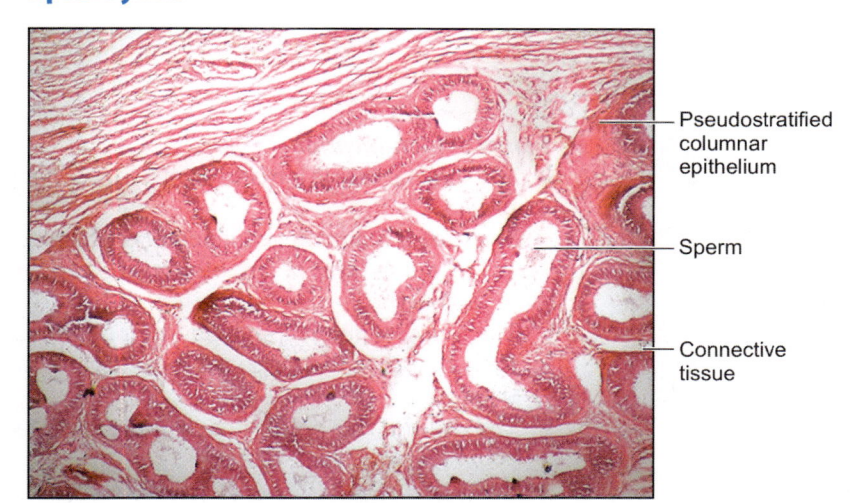

Fig. A18.3: Epididymis.

Labels: Pseudostratified columnar epithelium; Sperm; Connective tissue

Points of identification
- The body of the epididymis is a long convoluted duct
- A section shows number of tubules lined by pseudostratified columnar epithelium in which there are tall columnar cells and shorter basal cells that do not reach the lumen. The columnar cells bear stereocilia
- Smooth muscles are present in the wall of the duct
- Clumps of spermatozoa are present in the lumen of the duct.

Ductus Deferens

Pseudostratified Columnar epithelium
Layer of smooth muscles

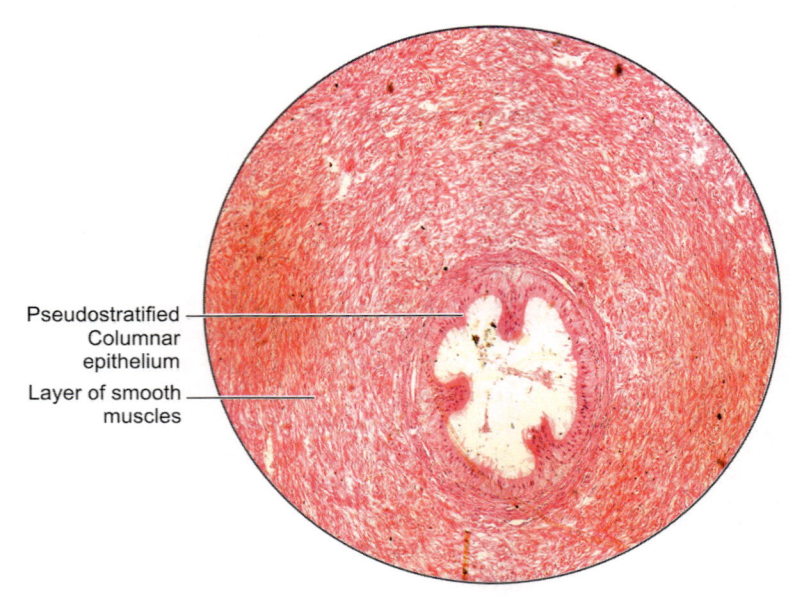

Fig. A18.4: Ductus deferens.
Courtesy: Balakrishna Shetty, Sweekritha H Poonja. HISTOLOGY Practical Manual, 4th edition. New Delhi: Jaypee Brothers Medical Publishers (P) Ltd; 2019. p. 120.

Points of identification
This tubular structure displays:
- A small irregular lumen
- Mucous membrane lined by pseudostratified columnar epithelium with underlying lamina propria
- The muscle coat is very thick. Three layers, inner longitudinal, middle circular, and outer longitudinal are seen
- Outer most layer is adventitia composed of collagen fibers and containing blood vessels.

Seminal Vesicle (Low Magnification)

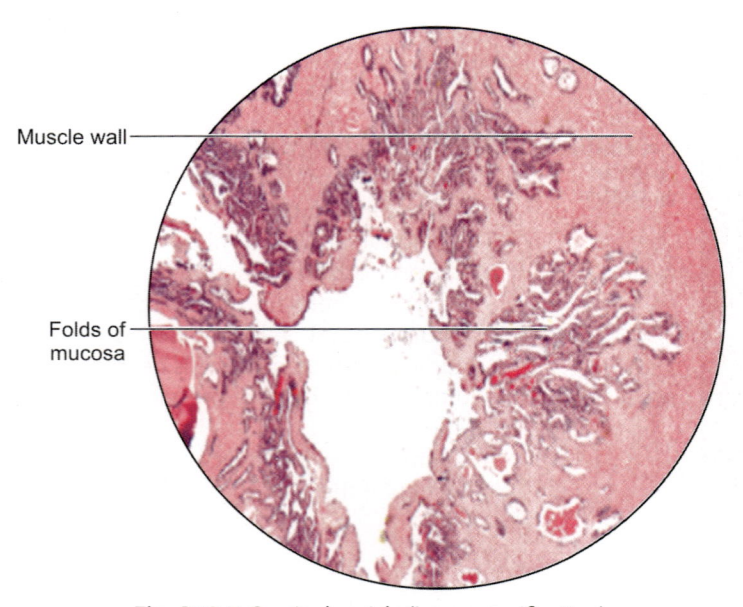

Muscle wall
Folds of mucosa

Fig. A18.5: Seminal vesicle (Low magnification).

Points of identification
- The seminal vesicle is made up of a convoluted tubule
- The tube has an outer covering of connective tissue, a thin layer of smooth muscle and an inner mucosa
- The mucosal lining is thrown into numerous folds that branch and anastomose to form a network
- The lining epithelium is usually simple columnar or pseudostratified.

Prostate (Low Magnification)

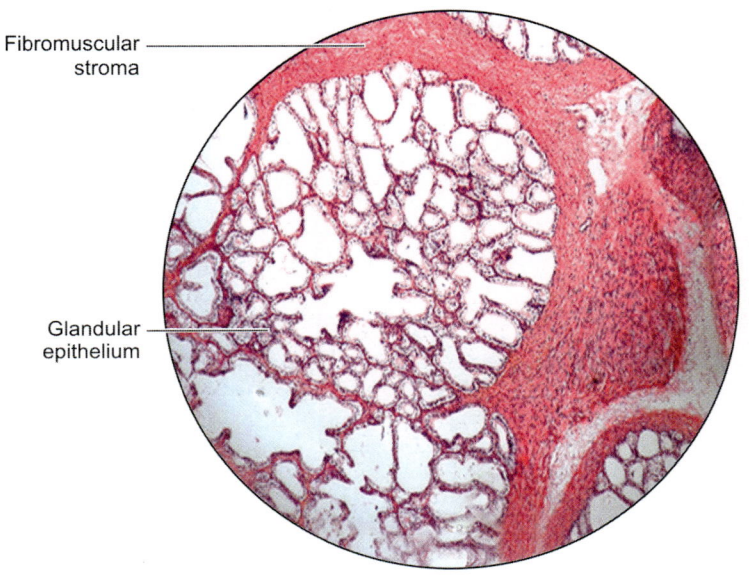

Fig. A18.6: Prostate (Low magnification).

Labels: Fibromuscular stroma; Glandular epithelium

Points of identification
- The prostate consists of glandular tissue embedded in prominent fibromuscular stroma
- The glandular tissue is in the form of follicles with serrated edges. They are lined by columnar epithelium. The lumen may contain amyloid bodies
- The follicles are separated by broad bands of fibromuscular tissue.

FEMALE REPRODUCTIVE SYSTEM

Ovary

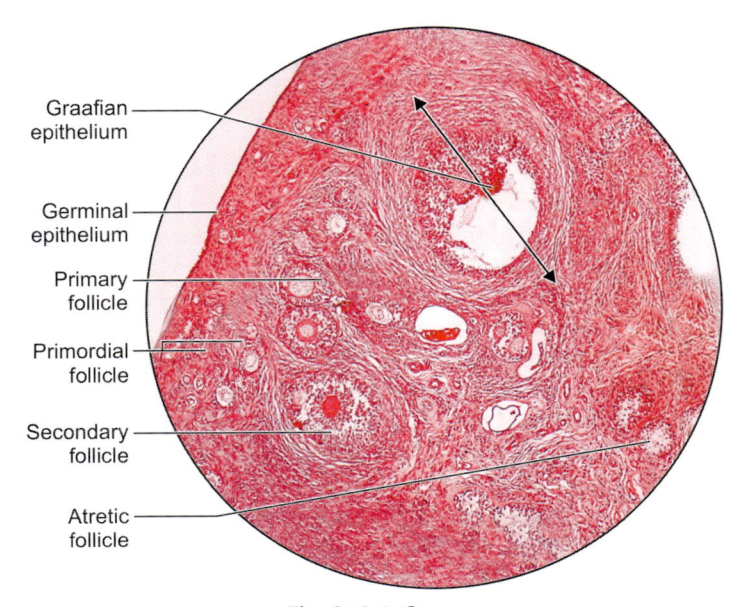

Fig. A19.1: Ovary.

Courtesy: Balakrishna Shetty, Sweekritha H Poonja. HISTOLOGY Practical Manual, 4th edition. New Delhi: Jaypee Brothers Medical Publishers (P) Ltd; 2019. p. 126.

Labels: Graafian epithelium; Germinal epithelium; Primary follicle; Primordial follicle; Secondary follicle; Atretic follicle

Points of identification
- The surface is covered by a cuboidal epithelium. Deep to the epithelium, there is a layer of connective tissue that constitutes the tunica albuginea
- The substance of the ovary has an outer cortex in which follicles of various sizes are present, and an inner medulla consisting of connective tissue containing numerous blood vessels
- Just deep to the tunica albuginea, many primordial follicles each of which contains a developing ovum surrounded by flattened follicular cells are present
- Large follicles have a follicular cavity surrounded by several layers of follicular cells
- The cells surrounding the ovum constitute the cumulus oophorus
- The follicle is surrounded by a condensation of connective tissue which forms a capsule for it
- The capsule consists of an inner cellular part (the theca interna), and an outer fibrous part (the theca externa) collectively called as theca folliculi. The follicle is surrounded by a stroma made up of reticular fibers and fusiform cells.

Fallopian Tube

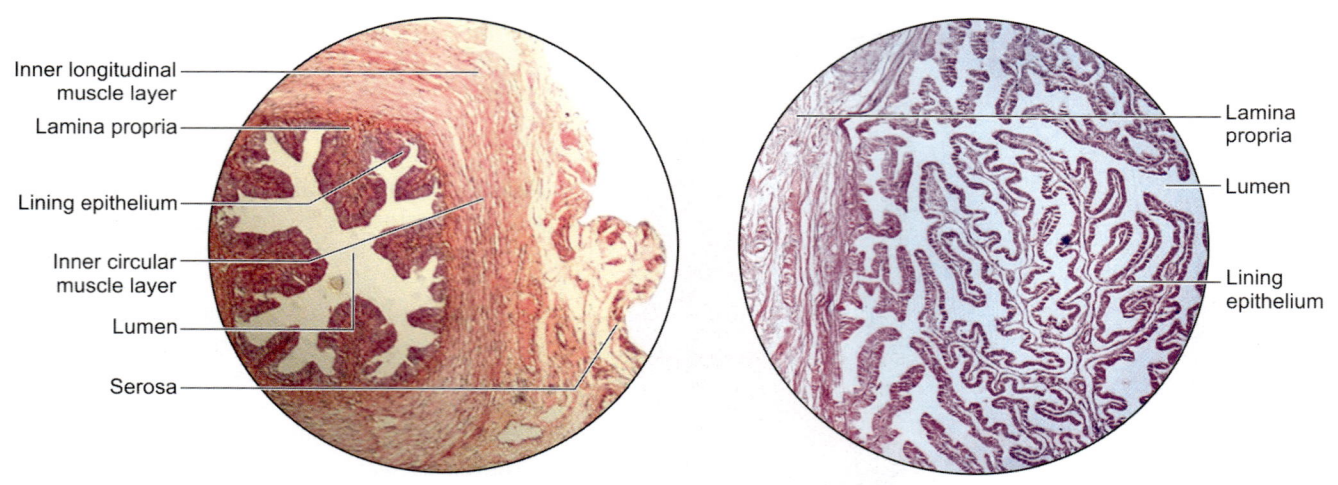

Fig. A19.2: Fallopian tube (Low magnification).

Fig. A19.3: Fallopian tube (High magnification).

Points of identification
- The uterine tube is characterized by the presence of numerous branching mucosal folds that almost fill the lumen of the tube
- The mucosa is lined by ciliated columnar epithelium
- The uterine tube has a muscular wall with an inner circular and outer longitudinal muscle layer.

Uterus (Proliferative Phase)

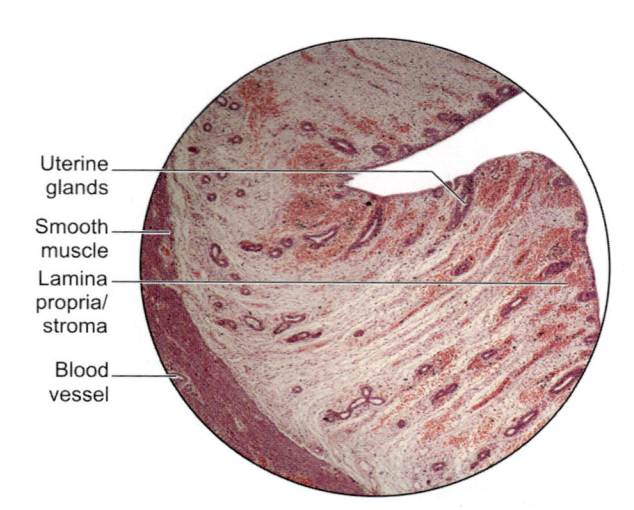

Fig. A19.4: Uterus (Proliferative phase).

Points of identification
- The wall of the uterus consists of a mucous membrane (called the endometrium) and a very thick layer of muscle (the myometrium). The thickness of the muscle layer helps to identify the uterus easily
- The endometrium has a lining of columnar epithelium that rests on a stroma of connective tissue
- Numerous tubular uterine glands dip into the stroma
- The appearance of the endometrium varies considerably depending upon the phase of the menstrual cycle. The endometrium is thin and progressively increases in thickness. The uterine glands are straight and tubular in this phase.

Uterus (Secretory Phase)

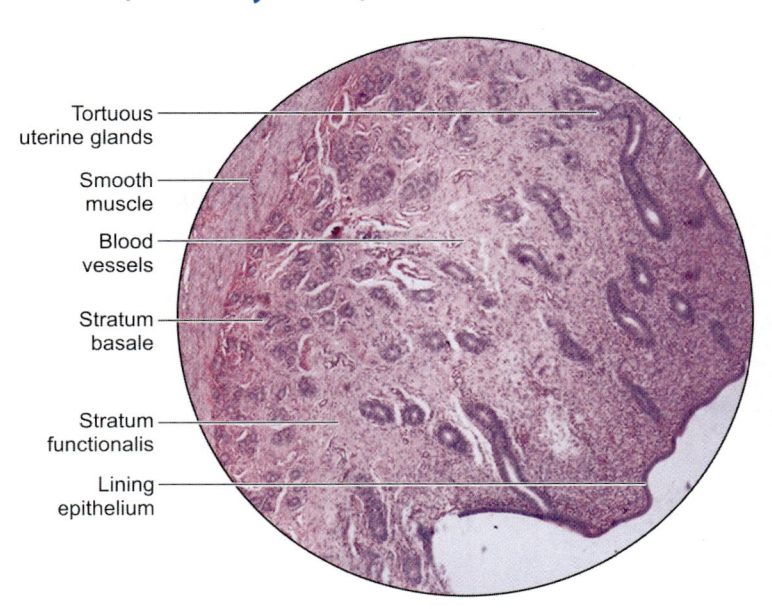

Labels: Tortuous uterine glands, Smooth muscle, Blood vessels, Stratum basale, Stratum functionalis, Lining epithelium

Fig. A19.5: Uterus (Secretory phase).

Points of identification
In the secretory phase:
- The thickness of the endometrium is much increased
- The uterine glands elongate, become dilated, and tortuous as a result of which they have saw-toothed margins in sections
- Blood vessels extend in the upper portion of endometrium.

Vagina

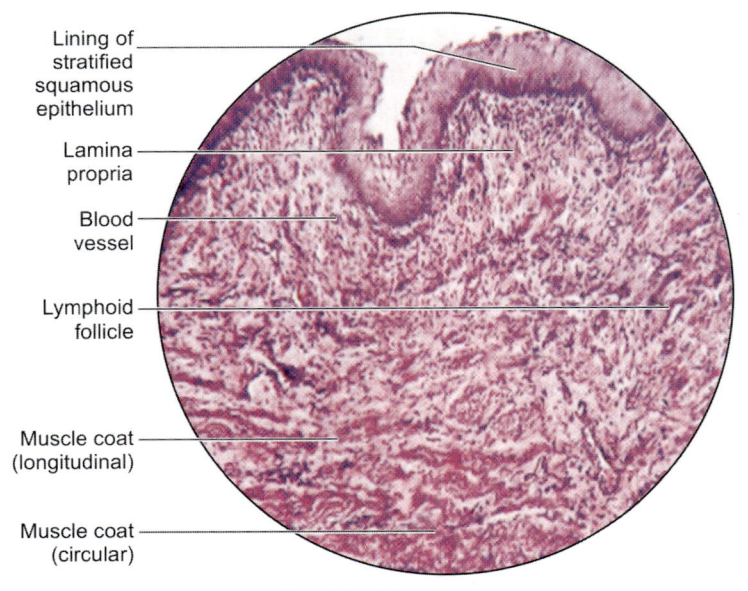

Labels: Lining of stratified squamous epithelium, Lamina propria, Blood vessel, Lymphoid follicle, Muscle coat (longitudinal), Muscle coat (circular)

Fig. A19.6: Vagina.

Points of identification
- The vagina is a fibromuscular structure consisting of an inner mucosa, a middle muscular layer, and an outer adventitia
- The mucosa consists of stratified squamous nonkeratinized epithelium and loose fibroelastic connective tissue lamina propria with many blood vessels and no glands
- The mucosa of vagina is rich in glycogen and hence, the cells are pale stained which distinguishes it from esophagus
- Muscular layer consists of smooth muscle fibers.

Mammary Gland (Resting)

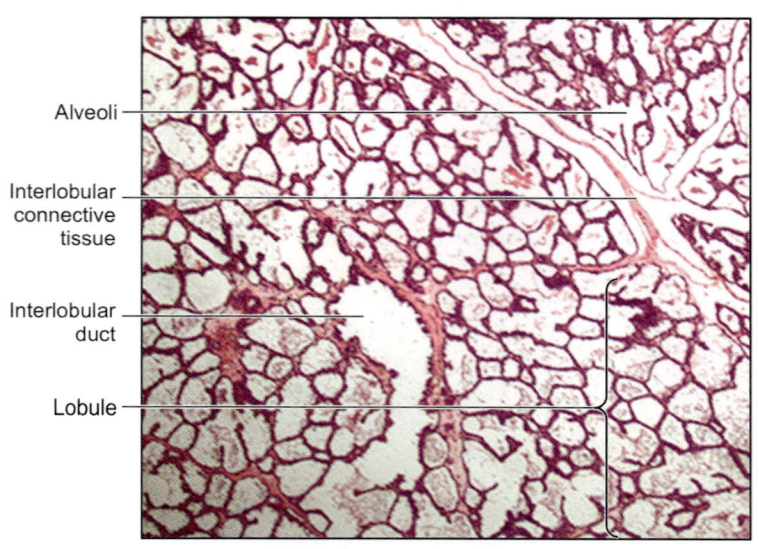

Fig. A19.7: Mammary gland (Resting).

Labels: Alveoli, Interlobular connective tissue, Interlobular duct, Lobule

Points of identification
- Mammary gland consists of lobules of glandular tissue separated by considerable quantity of connective tissue and fat
- Nonlactating mammary glands contain more connective tissue and less glandular tissue
- The glandular elements or alveoli are distinctly tubular. They are lined by cuboidal epithelium and have a large lumen so that they look like ducts. Some of them may be in form of solid cords of cells
- Extensive branching of duct system seen.

Mammary Gland (Lactating)

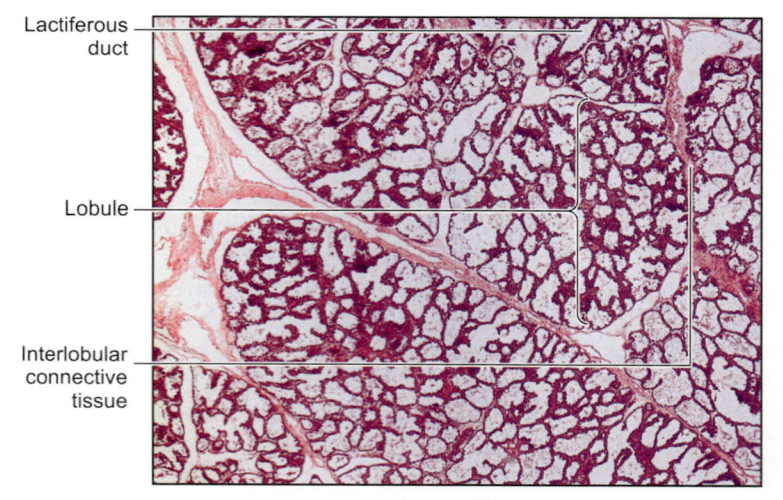

Fig. A19.8: Mammary gland (Lactating).

Labels: Lactiferous duct, Lobule, Interlobular connective tissue

Points of identification
- In lactating mammary gland, the glandular elements proliferate so that they become relatively more prominent than the connective tissue
- The interlobular connective tissue septum is very thin
- The lobules are formed by compactly arranged alveoli
- The alveoli are lined by simple cuboidal secretory epithelium and associated myoepithelial cells. Their lumen contains eosinophilic secretory material which appears vacuolated due to the presence of fat droplets.

Color Atlas

ENDOCRINE SYSTEM

Hypophysis Cerebri

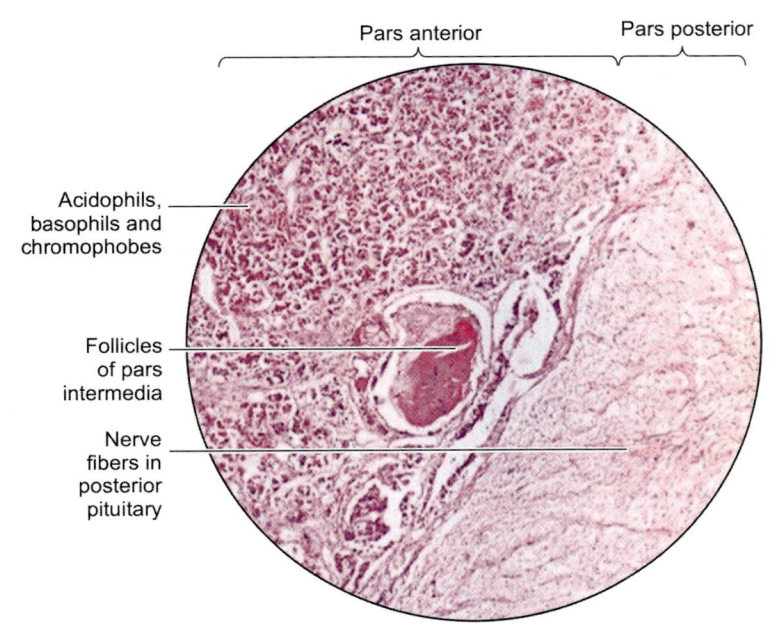

Fig. A20.1: Hypophysis cerebri.

Points of identification
The hypophysis cerebri consists of three main parts:
- Pars anterior is cellular
- Pars intermedia is variable in structure
- Pars posterior consists of fibers, and is lightly stained.

Pars Anterior

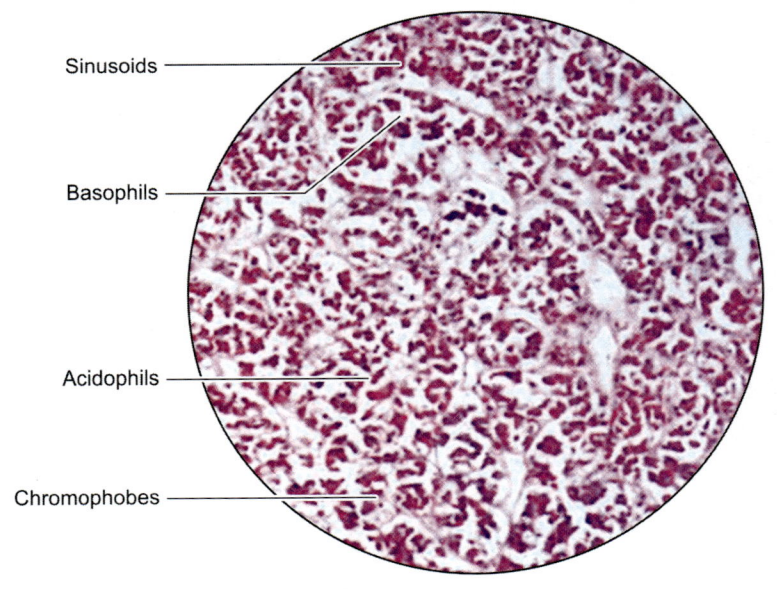

Fig. A20.2: Pars anterior.

Points of identification
- It consists of groups or cords of cells.
- The cells are of three types:
  1. The pink staining cells are alpha cells or acidophils
  2. The cells with bluish cytoplasm are beta cells or basophils
  3. Cells in which the cytoplasm is not conspicuous, and the nuclei are closely packed, are chromophobe cells
- Numerous sinusoids are present between the groups of cells.

Thyroid Gland

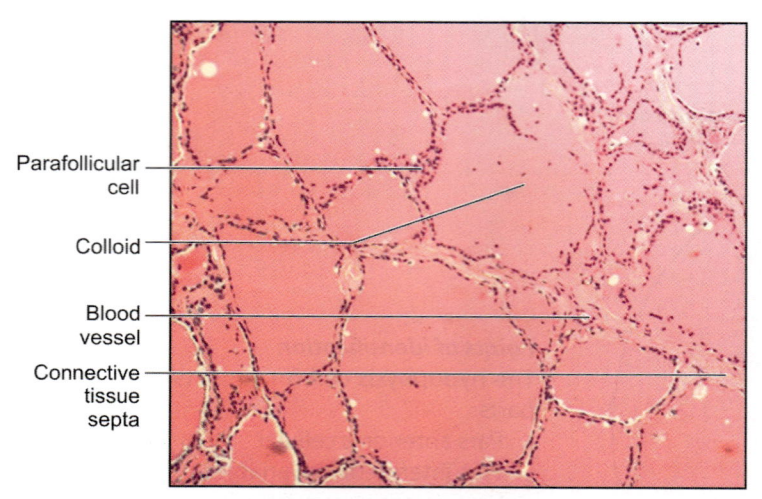

Fig. A20.3: Thyroid gland (Low magnification).

Points of identification
- The thyroid gland is made up of follicles lined by cuboidal epithelium
- In photomicrograph, in low magnification, it can be seen that follicles vary in shape and size
- Each follicle is filled with a homogenous pink colloid proteinaceous material composed primarily of thyroglobulin that has been produced by the follicular epithelial cells
- Parafollicular cells are present in relation to the follicles and also as groups in the connective tissue
- In the intervals between the follicles, there is some connective tissue and blood vessels between follicles.

Parathyroid Gland

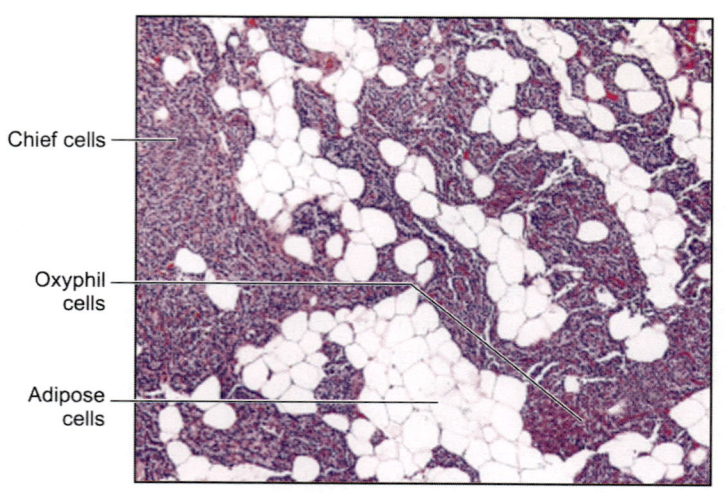

Fig. A20.4: Parathyroid gland.
Courtesy: Damjanov I. Atlas of Histopathology, 1st edition. New Delhi: Jaypee Brothers Medical Publishers (P) Ltd; 2012. p. 290.

Points of identification
- These glands are made up of masses of cells with numerous capillaries in between
- Most of the cells (of which only nuclei are seen) are the chief cells which appear as small basophilic cells
- Oxyphil cells appear as large as eosinophilic (pink) cells
- Oxyphil cells are few in number
- Adipose cells are also seen.

Suprarenal Gland

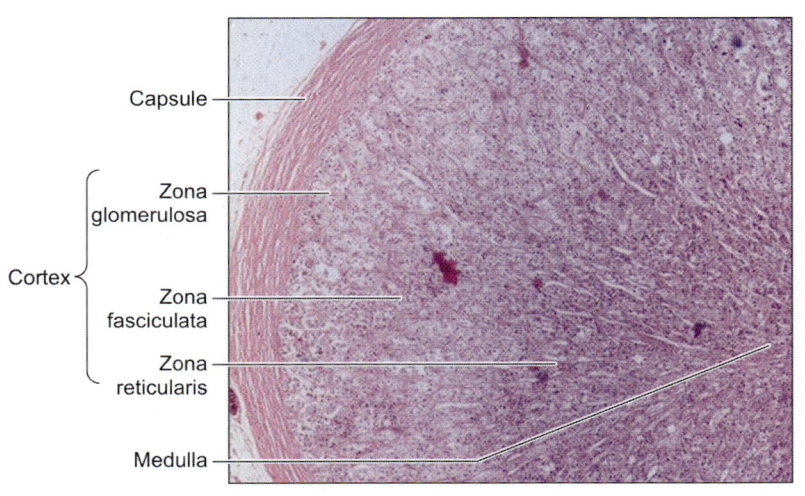

Fig. A20.5: Suprarenal gland.

Labels: Capsule, Zona glomerulosa, Zona fasciculata, Zona reticularis (Cortex), Medulla

Points of identification
- The suprarenal gland is made up of a large number of cells arranged in layers. It consists of an outer cortex and an inner medulla
- The cortex is divisible into three zones
- The zona glomerulosa is most superficial. Here, the cells are arranged in the form of inverted U-shaped structures or acinus-like groups
- In the zona fasciculata, the cells are arranged in straight columns (typically two-cell thick). Sinusoids intervene between the columns
- The zona reticularis is made up of cords of cells that branch and form a network
- The medulla is made up of groups of cells separated by wide sinusoids. Some sympathetic neurons are also present.

SPECIAL SENSES: EYE

Cornea

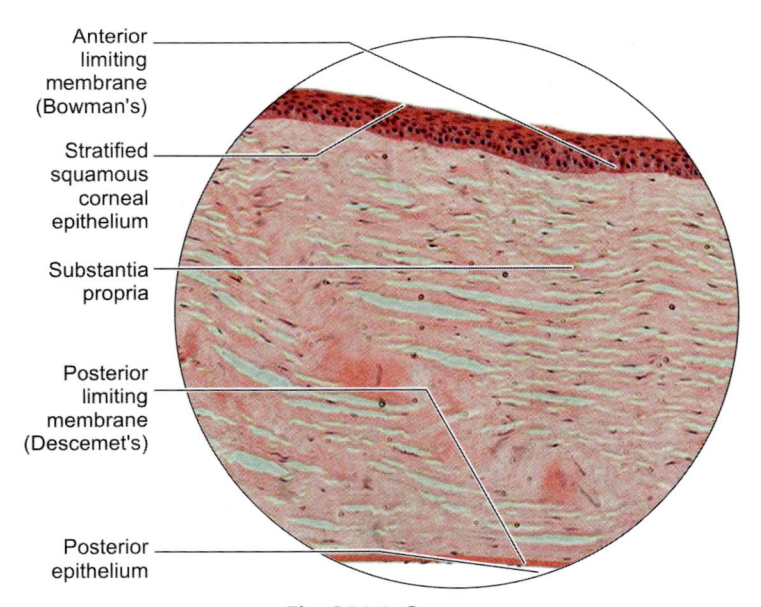

Fig. A21.1: Cornea.

Labels: Anterior limiting membrane (Bowman's), Stratified squamous corneal epithelium, Substantia propria, Posterior limiting membrane (Descemet's), Posterior epithelium

Points of identification
- The cornea is made up of five layers: corneal epithelium, anterior limiting membrane, or Bowman's membrane, corneal stroma, posterior limiting lamina, and endothelium
- The corneal epithelium is nonkeratinized stratified squamous epithelium
- The substantia propria is made up of collagen fibers embedded in a ground substance
- Endothelium is lined by a single layer of flattened or cuboidal cells.

Retina

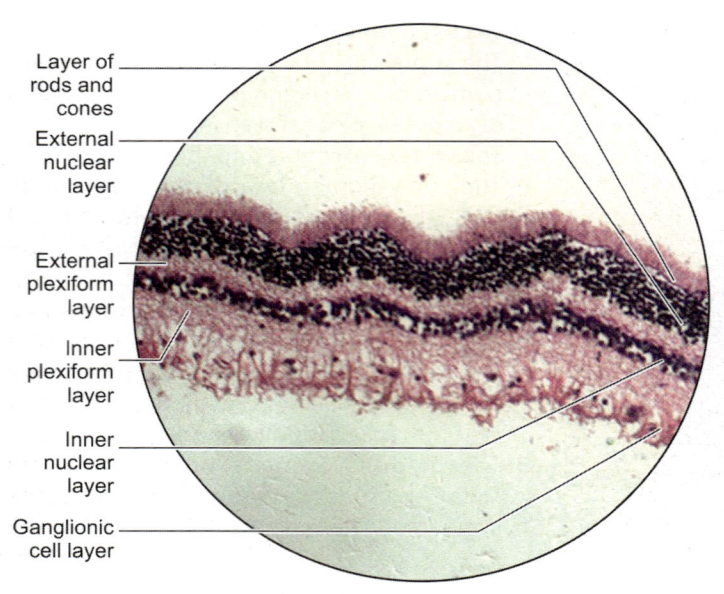

Fig. A21.2: Retina.

Labels: Layer of rods and cones; External nuclear layer; External plexiform layer; Inner plexiform layer; Inner nuclear layer; Ganglionic cell layer

Points of identification
- Made up of ten layers: pigment epithelium, layer of rods and cones, external limiting membrane, outer nuclear layer, outer plexiform layer, inner nuclear layer, inner plexiform layer, ganglionic cell layer, nerve fiber layer, and internal limiting membrane
- Outer pigment epithelium is made up of simple cuboidal epithelium
- The outer nuclear layer is thicker with densely packed nuclei than in the inner nuclear layer
- Ganglion cell layer is made up of a single row of cells of varying size.

SPECIAL SENSES: EAR

Pinna

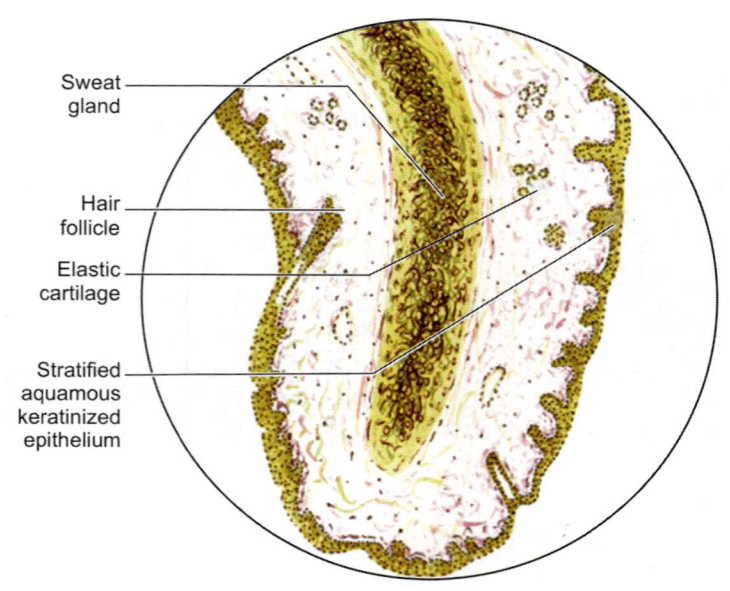

Fig. A22.1: Pinna.

Labels: Sweat gland; Hair follicle; Elastic cartilage; Stratified aquamous keratinized epithelium

Point of identification
The pinna has a core of elastic cartilage covered on both sides by true skin in which hair follicles and sweat glands are seen.

Cochlea

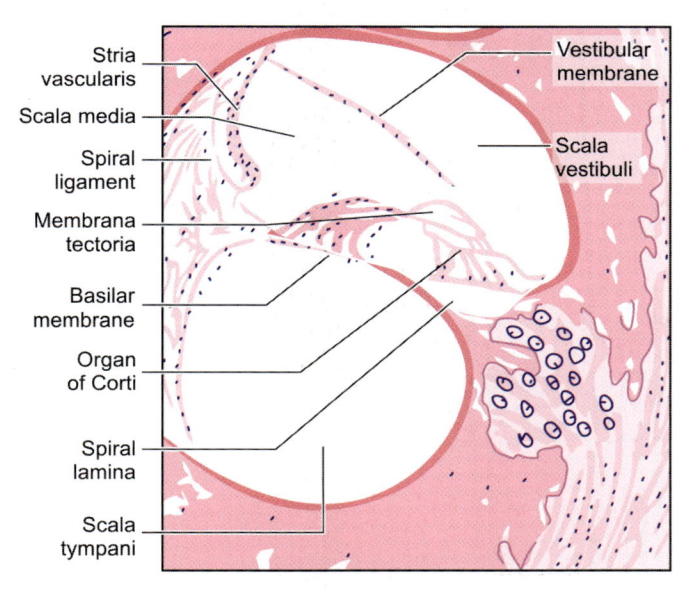

Fig. A22.2: Cochlea.

Points of identification

- The cochlea is embedded in the petrous temporal bone
- It is in the form of a spiral canal and is, therefore, cut up six times
- The cone-shaped mass of bone surrounded by these turns of the cochlea is called the modiolus which contains a canal through which fibers of the cochlear nerve pass
- A mass of neurons belonging to the spiral ganglion lies to the inner side of each turn of the cochlea
- The parts to be identified in each turn of the cochlea are the scala vestibuli, scala media, the scala tympani, the vestibular membrane, the basilar membrane, the membrana tectoria, and the organ of Corti, and the spiral lamina
- Outer wall of the cochlear turn is the spiral ligament and it is lined by avascularized epithelium (stria vascularis).

CHAPTER 1

Light Microscopy and Tissue Preparation

Learning objectives

To study the:
- Components of a light microscope
- Principles of a conventional bright-field microscope
- Practical tips in using a bright-field microscope
- Types of microscopes
- Tissue processing

INTRODUCTION

Microscope is an instrument used to see the structures that are very small to be visualized by naked eyes. Microscopy is the science which deals with the study of small objects using microscope.

HISTORY

Use of hand lens to observe small object dates back to 13th century, but it was Robert Hooke who first used the microscope which could provide magnification up to 42 times. Improved version with magnification of up to 300 times was developed by Antony van Leeuwenhoek (Father of Microscopy). Bonnannus added source of light, condenser, rack, and pinion for better focusing.

PARTS OF A LIGHT MICROSCOPE

In the histology laboratory, students use light microscope. It is also called as compound microscope or bright-field microscope (Fig. 1.1). It is mandatory to have the proper knowledge of parts of the light microscope for optimal focusing and proper handling of the microscope. Following are the essential parts of light microscope (Fig. 1.2):
- Stand
- Eyepiece
- Revolving nose piece with objective lenses
- Focus knob
- Stage
- Light source—mirror
- Diaphragm and condenser
- Mechanical stage.

Stand or base: It supports the microscope. It bears arm or limb. At the upper end of the arm, their lies body tube.

Body tube: It bears eyepiece at one end and objective lenses at the other end.

Eye piece: Eye piece or ocular lens is used to bring the image into the focus of eye. It enlarges the image produced by particular objective lens.

Objective lenses: These lenses are usually fitted into the revolving nose piece/objective turret, which allow the user to switch between objective lenses. They are powerful magnifying lenses which produces best possible image of an object. Compound microscopes nowadays have more than one objective lenses with magnification ranging from

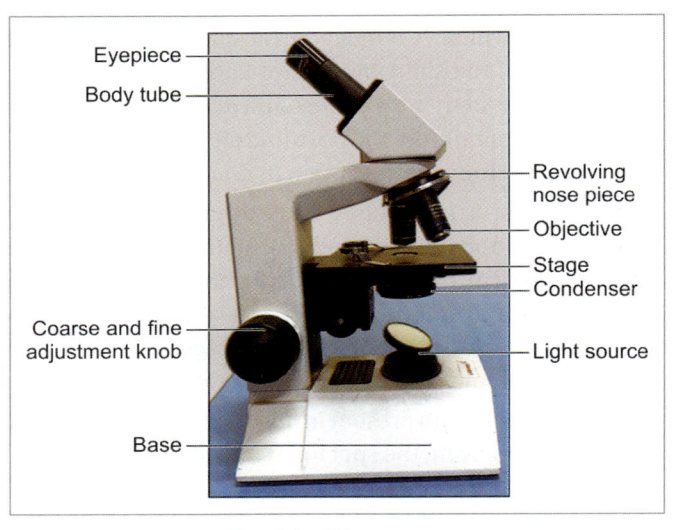

Fig. 1.1: Microscope.

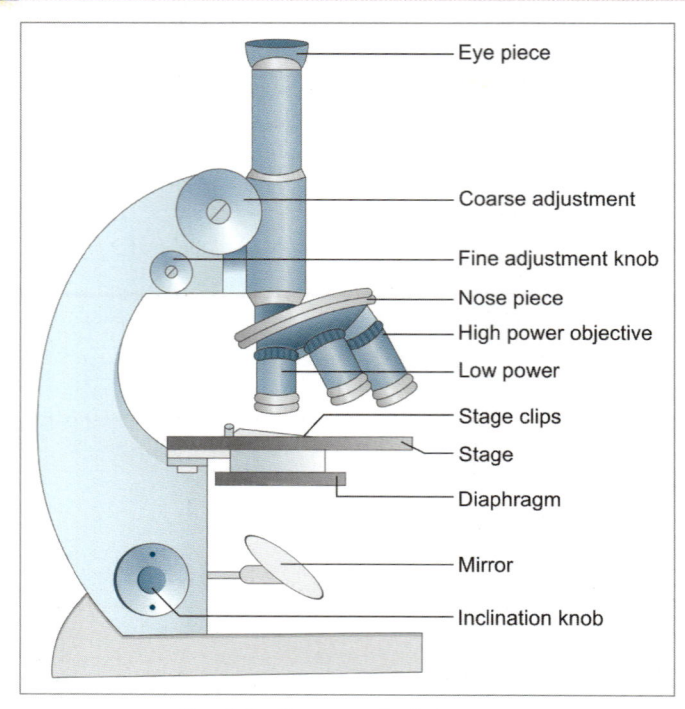

Fig. 1.2: Compound microscope.

5X to 100X and numerical aperture varying from 0.14 to 0.7, respectively. Objective lenses with very low power objective (3X, 4X, or 5X magnification) are used to scan the field, low power objective produces 10X magnification (10 times), high power objective produces 40X, and oil immersion gives 100X magnification. Objective lenses will have color coding for easy identification.

Stage: The stage is a platform below the objective which supports the slide being viewed. Center of the stage has aperture through which light passes to illuminate the specimen. The stage usually has arms to hold slides. Recent microscopes will have a mechanical stage that allows tiny movements of the slide via control knobs that reposition the slide as desired. With a mechanical stage, slides move on two horizontal axes for positioning the slide, thereby facilitating to study the specimen in detail.

Focus knobs: It includes coarse adjustment and fine adjustment knobs. Coarse adjustment knob moves the stage in vertical direction to bring the specimen into focus. Slight movement of the coarse adjustment brings about large vertical movement of the stage. Hence, coarse adjustment should only be used with low power objective.

Fine adjustment knob present inside the coarse adjustment knob is used to bring the specimen into sharp focus.

Light source: Natural or artificial sources of light can be used. Daylight is directed via a mirror. Most microscopes have their own adjustable and controllable light source, most often it is a halogen bulb. Other options being illumination using laser and LEDs.

Condenser: The condenser is a lens designed to focus light from the illumination source onto the slide. Most of the times, condenser also include other features, such as a diaphragm/or filters, to manage the quality and intensity of the illumination. Thus, condenser controls the quality of image formed by the objective. With the condenser, it is always advisable to use only plane mirror to focus the light. Condenser can be moved up and down using rack and pinion. Condenser should be at optimal height for proper lighting, hence for better resolution.

Mirror: Microscopes without integral light sources are provided with mirror. Mirror will have two surfaces—plane and concave. Concave surface converts beam of light into cone of light. Hence, it is ideal to use concave mirror with low power objective. While focussing with natural light it is ideal to use plane mirror.

PRINCIPLE OF MICROSCOPY

Objective lens of the microscope forms enlarged image of the object under observation, this image is called as primary image (I1) and the magnification caused is called primary or initial magnification which is engraved on the objective. The primary image acts as object for the eyepiece and a secondary image (I2) is formed within the barrel by first lens (field lens). The eye lens, which is above the field lens, forms a smaller image (of millimeter diameter) of the secondary image called Ramsden's disk (I3). The lens of observer's eye converts this image into actual image (I4) that is formed on the retina of the observer.

PRACTICAL TIPS IN USING A BRIGHT-FIELD MICROSCOPE

1. Microscope should be placed on the level surface.
2. Switch on the power supply for light source. If there is no inbuilt light source, then natural light has to be focused, so that light strikes the center of mirror and directed toward the condenser.
3. Adjust the condenser at optimal position. Remember only plane mirror has to be used with condenser. Open the aperture of the iris diaphragm fully.
4. Focusing starts at lower magnification in order to center the specimen by the user on the stage. Place the slide on

CHAPTER 1: Light Microscopy and Tissue Preparation

the center of the stage just below the objective, ensure that the coverslip faces upward.

5. Move the stage using coarse adjustment until the slide comes close to the objective and focus the section sharp. Care should be taken not to strike the objective on the slide. So, it is always better to keep the objective as near as possible to the slide and then moving it away until the specimen is focused.
6. Finally use fine adjustment for optimal focusing and better view.

TYPES OF MICROSCOPES

Microscopes are mainly classified based on the source of light they use. Following are some varieties of microscopes other than bright-field microscope:

1. **Dark-field microscope:** In this microscope, only the objects are illuminated by strong oblique peripheral light, whereas the central beam of light is prevented from entering the objective lens by central patch stop fitted into condenser. It is used to study extremely tiny particles (colloid suspension) and transparent objects like crystals, protozoa, etc.
2. **Phase-contrast microscope:** It mainly works on the difference in the refractive indices of different media and object. With difference in the refractive indices, there occurs phase difference and image will be formed due to interference between direct light (not passed through object) and diffracted light (passed through the object). The phase differences are converted into differences of amplitude, hence objects which causes more difference in the phase leads to more difference in amplitude, thus results in brighter image without staining.
3. **Interference microscope:** In this microscope, beam of light from single source is split and passed through the object and outside. Later, they are recombined by beam recombiner at image plane. After recombination, difference in retardation caused by interference is used to measure the refractive index, thereby measuring the thickness of the object under observation.
4. **Polarization microscope:** It is a conventional microscope having rotating stage with 2 polarizing elements and balsam. Polarizer is interfered below the condenser and analyzer is placed above the objective lens. Polarizing microscope is mainly used to distinguish between amorphous and crystalline biological specimens like bones, lipid droplets, etc.
5. **Fluorescence microscope:** In this microscope, ultraviolet light is incident on object and made to emit the visible light. Tissues treated with fluorescent dye are examined with ultraviolet light, by emitting light of longer wavelength. They are seen as bright objects against dark background.
6. **Ultraviolet microscope:** In this microscope, ultraviolet light is used as source. Amount of light absorbed is recorded photographically and the molecules in the specimen are detected. Mainly, nucleic acids, purine, and pyrimidine are detected by this kind of microscope.
7. **Electron microscope:** Is a refracting microscope where a stream of high-velocity electrons is used instead of light. Since it provides resolution around 3–5 Å, finer details of structure can studied. As electrons are used, the image is focused by the magnetic coils on fluorescent screen. There are two types of electron microscopes—transmission electron microscope and scanning electron microscope.

TISSUE PROCESSING

1. Always carry the microscope in both hands. Hold the arm in one hand and support the base of the microscope with other hand.
2. After tissue is procured, it has to be properly fixed in ideal fixative. Fixation is done in order to enable the tissue to withstand further steps of tissue processing. An ideal fixative acts rapidly, causes immediate death of the tissue and preserves life-like appearance. It also prevents autolysis, putrefaction neither shrinks nor swells the tissue, cheap, nontoxic, and provides wide range of staining options. Commonly used are alcohol, acetone, formalin, Zenker's fluid, etc.
3. Once the tissue is properly "fixed", it is later dehydrated using increasing strengths of alcohol ending with absolute alcohol.
4. After tissue is dehydrated, excess of alcohol is removed by a process called "dealcoholization" or "clearing". Clearing agents raises the refractive index of the tissue and makes it transparent. Commonly used are xylene, cedar wood oil, chloroform, etc.
5. Cleared tissue is impregnated both externally and internally by embedding media (paraffin), hence blocks are prepared. Embedded tissue is sectioned with microtome into very thin slices without distortion and attached to glass slide.
6. Mounted paraffin sections are deparaffinized before staining. In routine histology laboratory, thin sections are stained using hematoxylin and eosin stains. Hematoxylin

is a basic dye, hence it combines with acid components of the cell like DNA, RNA, and renders them purple/blue color. Hematoxylin usually stains cell nuclei, myelin, elastic fibers, fibrin, neuroglia, and muscle striations. Whereas eosin is acidic dye, hence it combines with basic components of cytoplasm like proteins (amino acids) and stains it pink.

7. After hematoxylin and eosin (H & E) staining, slide is cleared, mounted using DPX, and covered with coverslip for future use.

8. Special stains are used when particular components have to be studied. For example, collagen is stained by Van Gieson method, elastic fibers by Verhoeff's method, and so on.

Note: Bipolar staining—in this, basal portion of the cell stained blue because of extensive rough endoplasmic reticulum and apical part stained pink because of eosinophilic zymogen granules. Bipolar staining is exhibited by pancreatic acini, serous acini of salivary gland.

CHAPTER 2

Cell Structure

Learning objectives

To study the:
- Introduction and types of cell
- Components of a cell—plasma membrane, cell organelles, nucleus, and cytoskeleton
- Cell junctions
- Staining of a cell
- Applied histology

INTRODUCTION

Cells are the structural and functional units of all the tissues. There are two types of cells—(1) Cells which lack membrane-bound nucleus and membrane-bound organelles are called prokaryotic cells (e.g. bacteria) and (2) Cells with membrane-bound nucleus and membrane-bound organelles are called eukaryotic cells. In this chapter, we will discuss about the eukaryotic cells.

COMPONENTS OF A CELL (FIG. 2.1)

- A cell is bounded by a ***cell membrane/plasma membrane*** within which is enclosed by a complex material called ***protoplasm***.
- The protoplasm consists of a central, denser part called the ***nucleus***, and an outer less dense part called the ***cytoplasm***. The nucleus is separated from the cytoplasm by a nuclear membrane.
- The cytoplasm has a fluid base (matrix) which is referred to as the ***cytosol*** or ***hyaloplasm***. The cytosol contains a number of ***organelles*** which have distinctive structure and functions. Many of them are in the form of membranes that enclose spaces. These spaces are collectively referred to as the ***vacuoplasm***.

Cell Membrane/Plasma Membrane

- The membrane which separates the interior of the cell from surrounding structure is called plasma membrane. It has high permeability property and regulates the cellular metabolism.
- *Structure of plasma membrane*: The structure of cell membrane is called as **fluid mosaic model**. In electron microscopy (EM), the average cell membrane is seen to be about 7.5 nm thick. It consists of two densely stained layers separated by a lighter zone, thus creating a trilaminar appearance (Fig. 2.2).
- Cell membranes are mainly made up of lipids, proteins, and carbohydrates.

Fluid Mosaic Model

Lipids in Cell Membranes

- It is now known that the trilaminar structure of membranes is produced by the arrangement of lipid molecules (predominantly phospholipids) that constitute the basic framework of the membrane (Fig. 2.2).
- Each phospholipid molecule consists of an enlarged head in which the phosphate portion is located, and of two thin tails (Fig. 2.3). The head end is also called the ***polar end*** while the tail end is the ***nonpolar end***. The head end is soluble in water and is said to be **hydrophilic**. The tail end is insoluble and is said to be **hydrophobic**.
- When such molecules are suspended in an aqueous medium, they arrange themselves so that the hydrophilic ends are in contact with the medium but not the hydrophobic ends thus, forming a bilayer.
- The dark staining parts of the membrane are formed by the heads of the molecules, while the light staining intermediate zone is occupied by the tails, thus giving the membrane its trilaminar appearance.

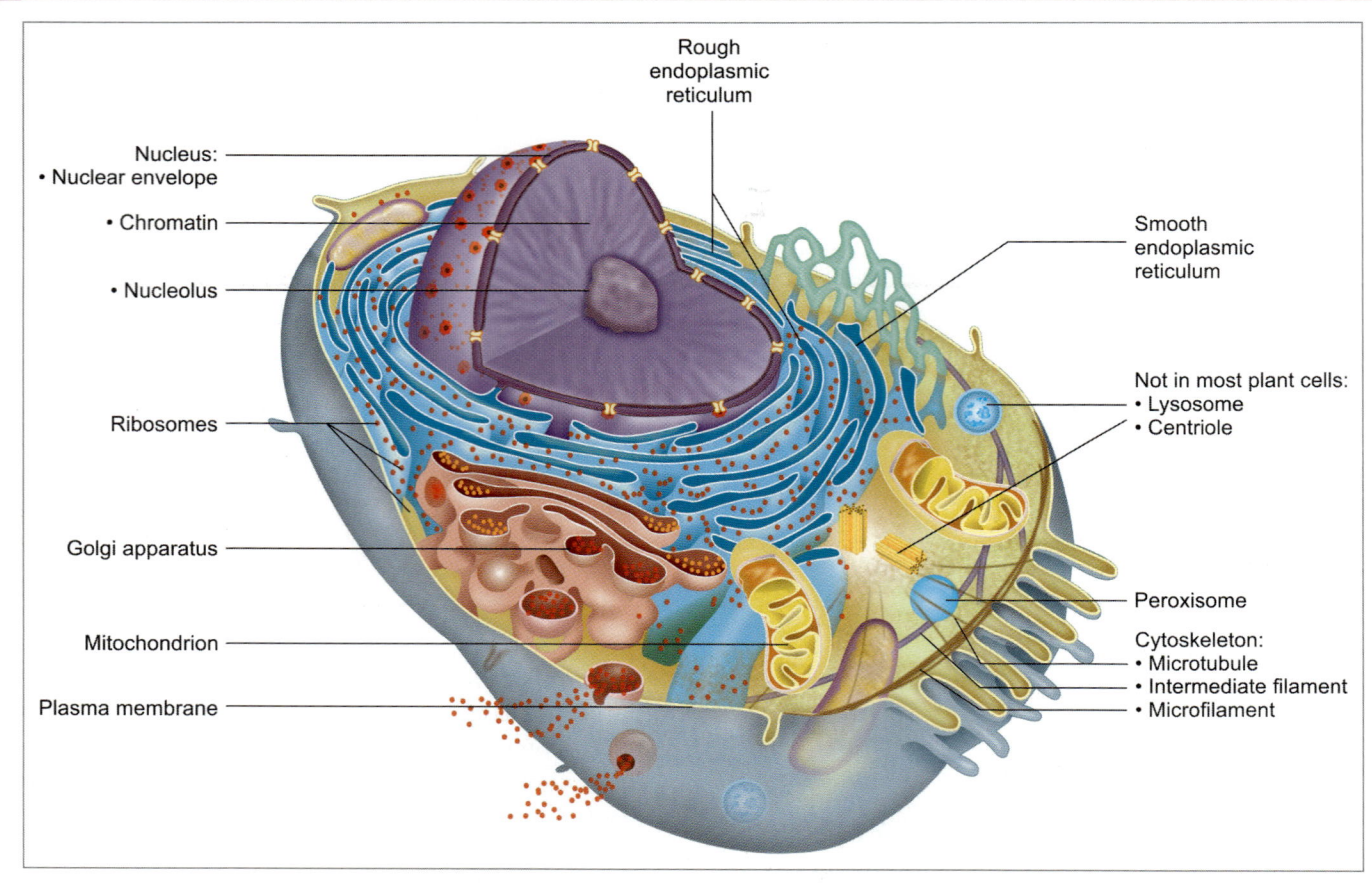

Fig. 2.1: Schematic representation of eukaryotic cell and its components.

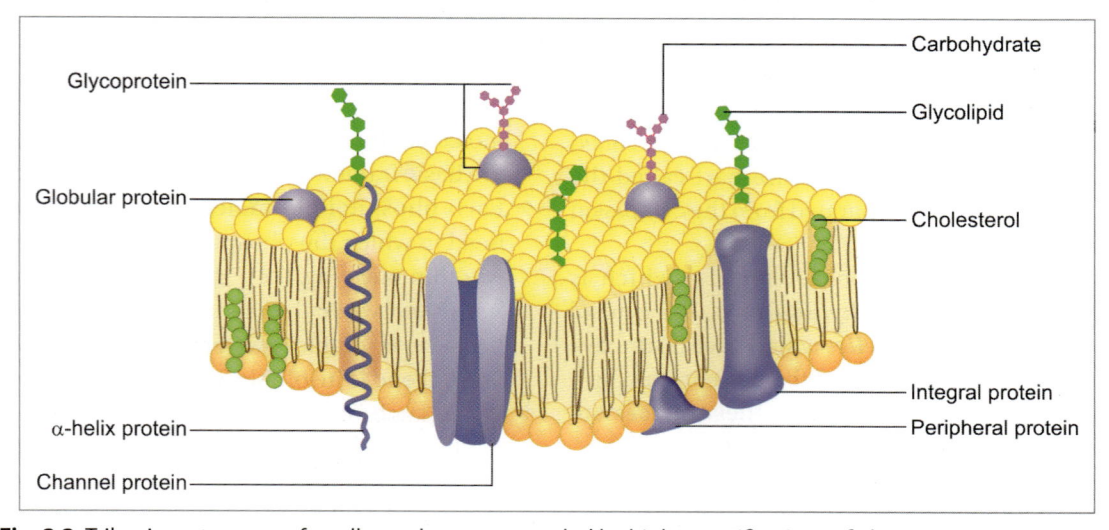

Fig. 2.2: Trilaminar structure of a cell membrane as revealed by high magnifications of electron microscopy (EM).

CHAPTER 2: Cell Structure

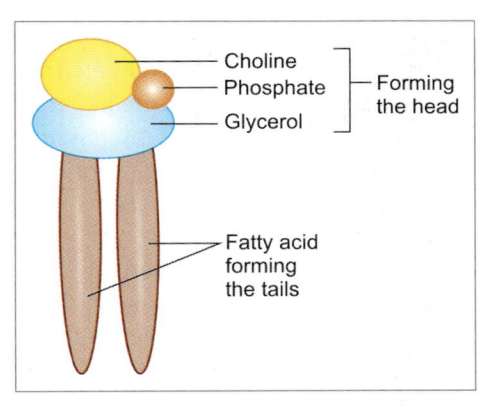

Fig. 2.3: Diagram showing the structure of a phospholipid molecule (phosphatidylcholine) seen in a cell membrane.

❖ Because of the manner of its formation, the membrane is to be regarded as a fluid structure that can readily reform when its continuity is disturbed. For the same reasons, proteins present within the membrane can move freely within the membrane.

Proteins in Cell Membranes

❖ The proteins are present in the form of irregularly rounded masses. Most of them are embedded within the thickness of the membrane and partly project on either outer or inner surface. Some proteins occupy the entire thickness of the membrane and may project out of both its surfaces and are called as transmembrane proteins (Fig. 2.4).
❖ *Significance of proteins of the cell membrane*:
  - They form an essential part of the structure of the membrane
  - Play a vital role in transport across the membrane and act as pumps. Ions get attached to the protein on one surface and move with the protein to the other surface
  - Some proteins form passive channels through which substances can diffuse through the membrane
  - Some proteins act as receptors for specific hormones or neurotransmitters
  - Some proteins act as enzymes.

Carbohydrates of Cell Membranes

❖ In addition to the phospholipids and proteins, carbohydrates are present at the surface of the membrane. They are attached either to the proteins forming glycoproteins or to the lipids forming glycolipids (Fig. 2.5).
❖ The carbohydrate layer is especially well developed on the external surface of the plasma membrane forming the cell boundary. This layer is referred to as the cell coat or *glycocalyx*.

> **Added Information**
>
> The glycocalyx is made up of the carbohydrate portions or glycoproteins and glycolipids present in the cell membrane. Some functions attributed to the glycocalyx are as follows:
> ➢ Special adhesion molecules present in the layer enable the cell to adhere to specific types of cells, or to specific extracellular molecules.
> ➢ The layer contains antigens. These include major histocompatibility complex (MHC). In erythrocytes, the glycocalyx contains blood group antigens.
> ➢ Most molecules in the glycocalyx are negatively charged causing adjoining cells to repel one another. This force of repulsion maintains the 20 nm interval between cells. However, some molecules that are positively charged adhere to negatively-charged molecules of adjoining cells, holding the cells together at these sites.

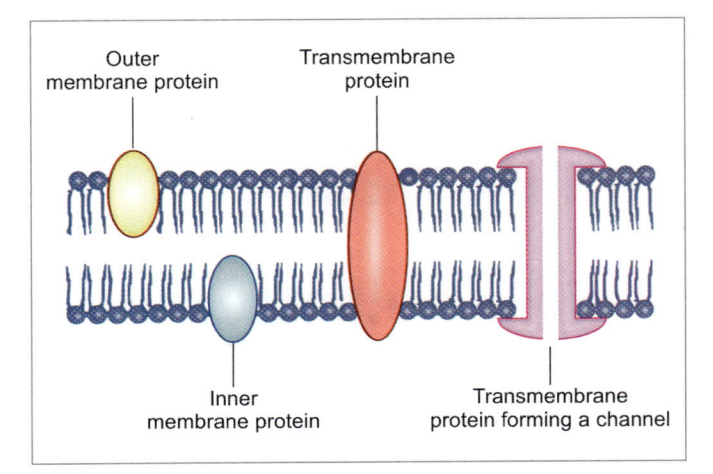

Fig. 2.4: Some varieties of membrane proteins.

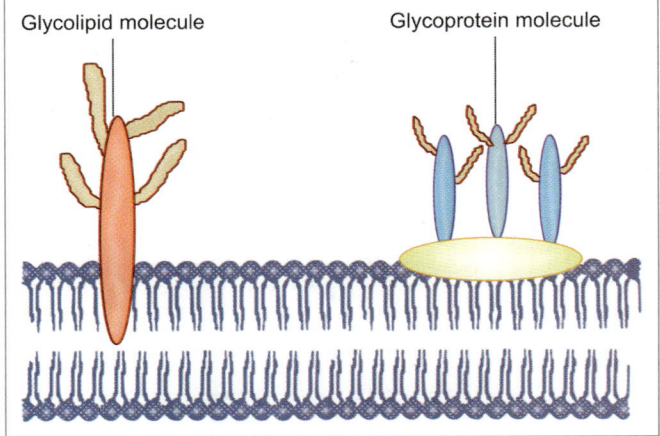

Fig. 2.5: Glycolipid and glycoprotein molecules attached to the outer aspect of cell membrane.

Functions of the Cell Membrane

i. It maintains the shape of the cell.
ii. It controls the passage of all substances into or out of the cell.
iii. The cell membrane forms a sensory surface. This function is most developed in nerve and muscle cells.
iv. The surface of the cell membrane bears *receptors* for hormones and enzymes. Stimulation of these receptors (e.g. by the specific hormone) can produce profound effects on the activity of the cell. Receptors also play an important role in absorption of specific molecules into the cell.
v. Membrane proteins help to maintain the structural integrity of the cell by giving attachment to cytoskeletal filaments. They also help to provide adhesion between cells and extracellular materials.
vi. Cell membranes of some cells may show a high degree of specialization in some cells. For example, the membranes of rod and cone cells of retina bear proteins that are sensitive to light.

Transport of Material Across the Cell Membrane

- Transport across the plasma membrane can be either **active transport** which requires energy or **passive transport** which does not require any energy.
- Passive transport can be either by simple diffusion (e.g. water, oxygen, glycerol, carbon dioxide, etc.) or facilitated diffusion (e.g. ions, urea, glucose, etc.).
- Some molecules can enter cells by passing through passive channels in the cell membrane and large molecules enter the cell by the process of **endocytosis** (Fig. 2.6A).
- Endocytosis is the process of actively transporting molecules into the cell by engulfing it with its membrane. In endocytosis, the molecule invaginates a part of the cell membrane and gets surrounded by it and then separates from the rest of the cell membrane to form an **endocytic vesicle**. This vesicle can move through the cytosol to other parts of the cell. Some cells use the process of endocytosis to engulf foreign matter (e.g. bacteria) and it is then referred to as *phagocytosis (cell eating)*.
- *Pinocytosis (cell drinking)* is a process similar to endocytosis where the vesicles formed are used for absorption of fluids or other small molecules into the cell.
- **Exocytosis** is a form of active transport in which a cell transports molecules out of the cell. Molecules produced within the cytoplasm (e.g. secretions) are enclosed in membranes to form vesicles (**exocytic vesicles**) that approach the cell membrane and fuse with its internal surface. The vesicle then ruptures releasing the molecule to the exterior (Fig. 2.6B).

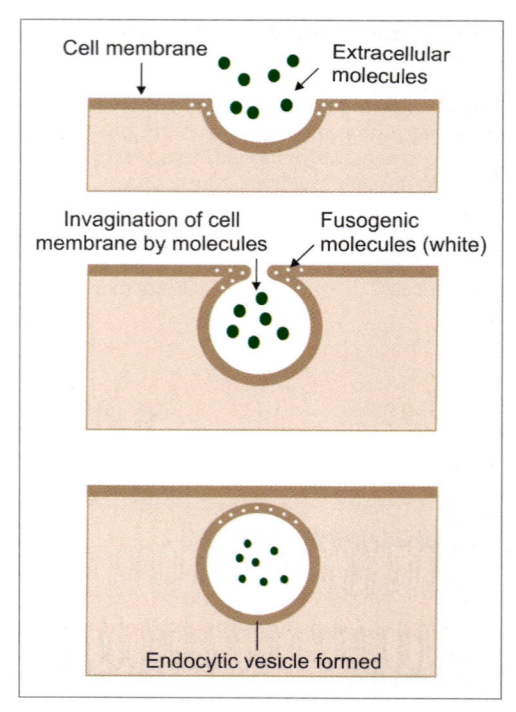

Fig. 2.6A: Three stages in the absorption of extracellular molecules by endocytosis.

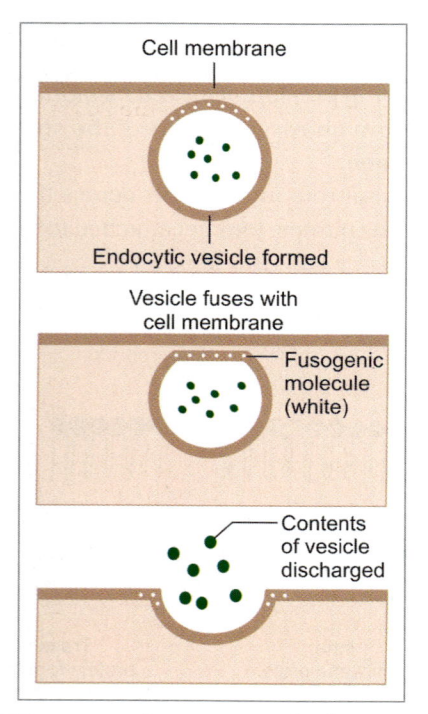

Fig. 2.6B: Three stages in exocytosis. The fusogenic proteins facilitate adhesion of the vesicle to the cell membrane.

CHAPTER 2: Cell Structure

Cell Junctions

Cell junctions are intercellular connections between the plasma membranes of adjacent cells of animal tissues. Intercellular connections between adjacent cells resulting in varying degrees of fusion and specialized functions of animal tissues. They are formed by multiprotein complexes. These junctions can be recognized by electron microscope.

Classification of Cell Junctions

There are three major types of cell junctions:
1. *Anchoring junctions or adhesive junctions*: Bind cells together.
2. *Occluding junctions/tight junctions*.
3. *Communicating junctions/gap junctions*: Direct transport of some substances from cell to cell.

Unspecialized Contacts

- These are contacts that do not show any specialized features on EM examination. At such sites, adjoining cell membranes are held together as follows.
- Some glycoprotein molecules, present in the cell membrane, are called **cell adhesion molecules** (CAMs). These molecules occupy the entire thickness of the cell membrane (i.e. they are transmembrane proteins). At its cytosolic end, each CAM is in contact with **an intermediate protein/link protein**.
- Fibrous elements of the cytoskeleton are attached to this intermediate protein (and thus, indirectly, to CAMs). The other end of the CAM juts into the 20 nm intercellular space, and comes in contact with a similar molecule from the opposite cell membrane. In this way, a path is established through which forces can be transmitted from the cytoskeleton of one cell to another (Fig. 2.7).
- Cell adhesion molecules and intermediate proteins are of various types. Contacts between cells can be classified on the basis of the type of CAMs proteins present. The adhesion of some CAMs is dependent on the presence of calcium ions, while some others are not dependent

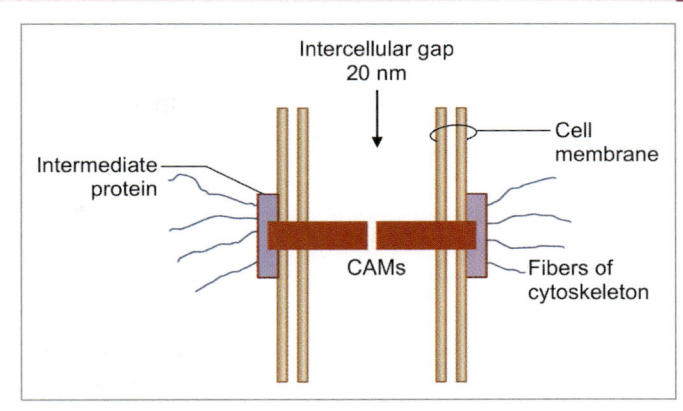

Fig. 2.7: Scheme to show the basic structure of an unspecialized contact between two cells. (CAMs: cell adhesion molecules).

on them (Table 2.1). Intermediate proteins are also of various types (catenins, vinculin, and α-actinin).

Anchoring Junctions

- Anchoring junctions are cell junctions that are attached to one another and with the components of the extracellular matrix. They are commonly found in tissues that are prone to constant mechanical stress, e.g. skin and heart.
- Anchoring junctions are of the following types:
  - Adhesive spots/desmosomes/macula adherens
  - Adhesive belts/zonula adherens
  - Adhesive strips/fascia adherens.

Adhesion spots (desmosomes, macula adherens) (Figs. 2.8 and 2.10)

- These are the most common type of junctions between adjoining cells. Desmosomes are present where strong anchorage between cells is needed, e.g. between cells of the epidermis.
- At the site of a desmosome, the plasma membrane is thickened due to presence of a dense layer of proteins on its inner surface. The thickened areas of the two sides are separated by a gap of 25 nm. The region of the gap is rich in glycoproteins. The thickened areas of the two membranes are held together by fibrils that appear to

Table 2.1: Types of cell adhesion molecules (CAM).

Type of CAM	Subtypes	Present in
Calcium dependent	Cadherins (of various types)	Most cells including epithelia
	Selectins	Migrating cells, e.g. leukocytes
	Integrins	Between cells and intercellular substances. About 20 types of integrins, each attaching to a special extracellular molecule
Calcium independent	Neural cell adhesion molecule (NCAM)	Nerve cells
	Intercellular adhesion molecule (ICAM)	Leukocytes

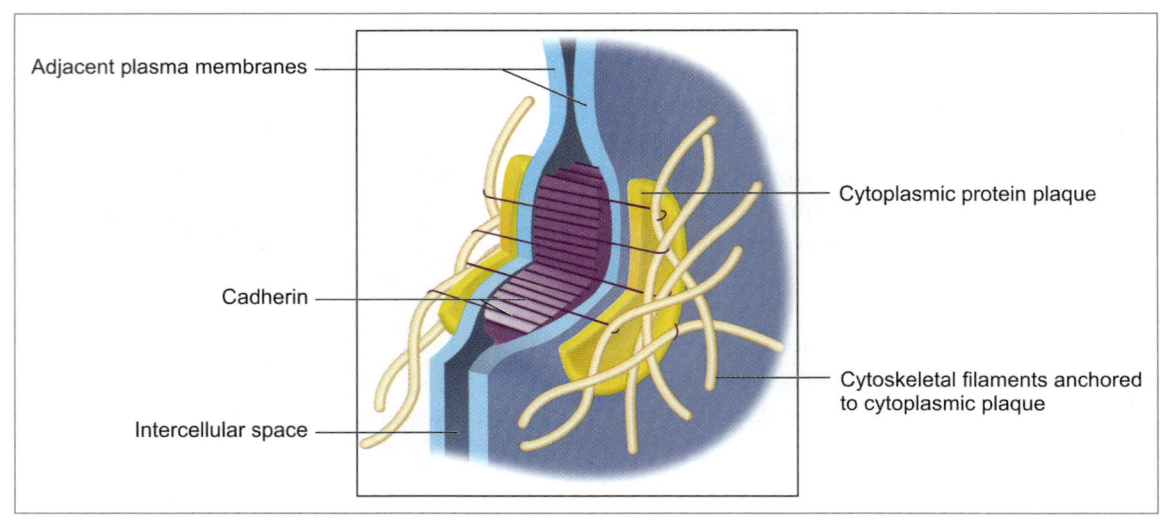

Fig. 2.8: Electron microscopy (EM) appearance of a desmosome.

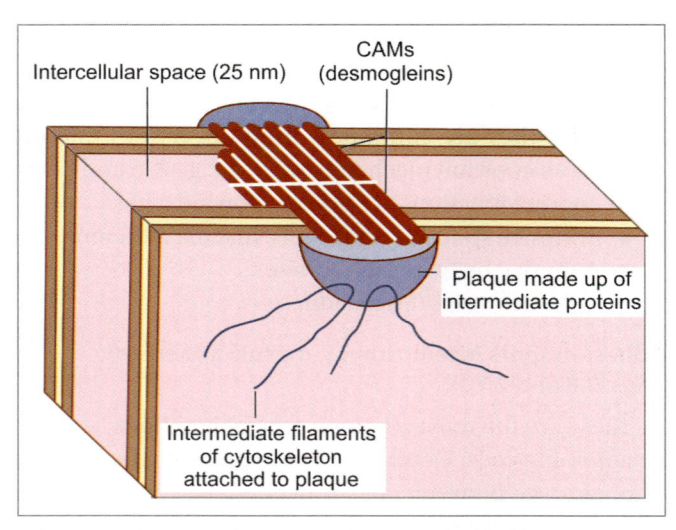

Fig. 2.9: Schematic diagram to show the detailed structure of a desmosome (in the epidermis). (CAMs: cell adhesion molecules).

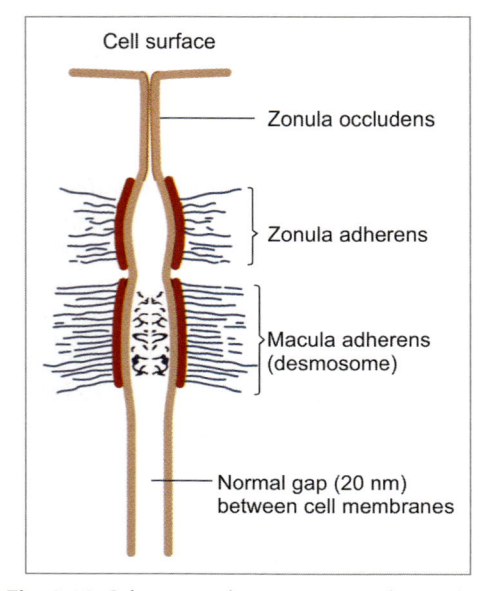

Fig. 2.10: Scheme to show a junctional complex.

pass from one membrane to the other across the gap (Fig. 2.9).

Adhesive belts (zonula adherens)

It is usually seen near the apices of epithelial cells. This is similar to a desmosome in being marked by thickenings of the two plasma membranes, to the cytoplasmic aspects of which fibrils are attached. However, the gap between the thickenings of the plasma membranes of the two cells is not traversed by filaments (Fig. 2.10).

Adhesive strips (fascia adherens)

- ❖ These are similar to adhesive belts. They differ from the latter in that the areas of attachment are in the form of short strips and do not go all round the cell. These are seen in relation to smooth muscle, intercalated discs of cardiac muscle, and in junctions between glial cells and nerves. Modified anchoring junctions attach cells to extracellular material. Such junctions are seen as *hemidesmosomes*, or as *focal spots*.
- ❖ *Hemidesmosomes* are similar to desmosomes, but the thickening of cell membrane is seen only on one side. Hemidesmosomes are common where basal epidermal cells lie against connective tissue.
- ❖ *Focal spots* are also called *focal adhesion plaques*, or *focal contacts*. They represent areas of local adhesion of a cell to extracellular matrix. Such junctions are of a

transient nature (e.g. between a leukocyte and a vessel wall). Such contacts may send signals to the cell and initiate cytoskeletal formation.

Occluding Junctions/Tight Junctions/ Zonula Occludens

- Like the zonula adherens, the zonula occludens are seen most typically near the apices of epithelial cells. At such a junction, the two plasma membranes are in actual contact (Figs. 2.11A and B).
- These junctions act as barriers that prevent the movement of molecules into the intercellular spaces. For example, intestinal contents are prevented by them from permeating into the intercellular spaces between the lining cells (Fig. 2.12).

Functions of tight junctions

- These junctions separate areas of cell membrane that are specialized for absorption or secretion from the rest of the cell membrane.
- In cells involved in active transport against a concentration gradient, occluding junctions prevent back diffusion of transported substances.

Apart from epithelial cells, zonula occludens are also present between endothelial cells.

In some situations, occlusion of the gaps between the adjoining cells may be incomplete and the junction may allow slow diffusion of molecules across it. These are referred to as *leaky tight junctions*.

Communicating Junctions (Gap Junctions)

- At these junctions, the plasma membranes are not in actual contact, but lie very close to each other, the

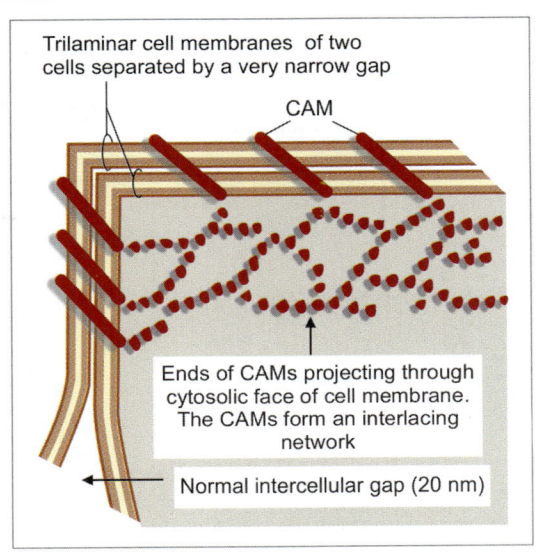

Fig. 2.12: Schematic diagram to show the detailed structure of part of an occluding junction. (CAMs: cell adhesion molecules).

gap being reduced from the normal 20 nm to 3 nm. In transmission electron micrographs, this gap is seen to contain bead-like structures (Fig. 2.11B).

- A minute canaliculus passing through each "bead" connects the cytoplasm of the two cells thus, allowing the free passage of some substances (sodium, potassium, calcium, and metabolites) from one cell to the other (also see here). Gap junctions are, therefore, also called *macula communicans*. They are widely distributed in the body.
- Changes in pH or in calcium ion concentration can close the channels of gap junctions. By allowing passing of ions, they lower transcellular electrical resistance. Gap junctions form electrical synapses between some neurons.
- The wall of each channel is made up of six protein elements (called *nexins*, or *connexons*). The "inner" ends of these elements are attached to the cytosolic side of the cell membrane while the "outer" ends project into the gap between the two cell membranes (Fig. 2.13). Here, they come in contact with (and align perfectly with) similar nexins projecting into the space from the cell membrane of the opposite cell, to complete the channel.

Cell Organelles

- The cytoplasm of a typical cell contains various structures that are referred to as organelles. They include the endoplasmic reticulum (ER), ribosomes,

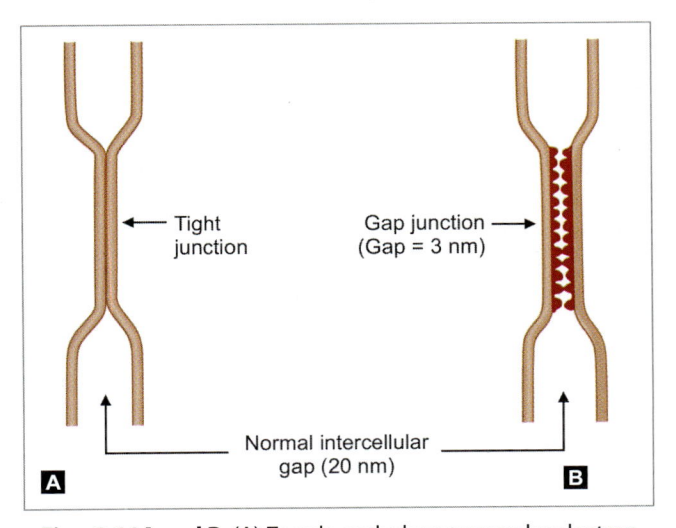

Figs. 2.11A and B: (A) Zonula occludens as seen by electron microscopy (EM); (B) Gap junction as seen by EM.

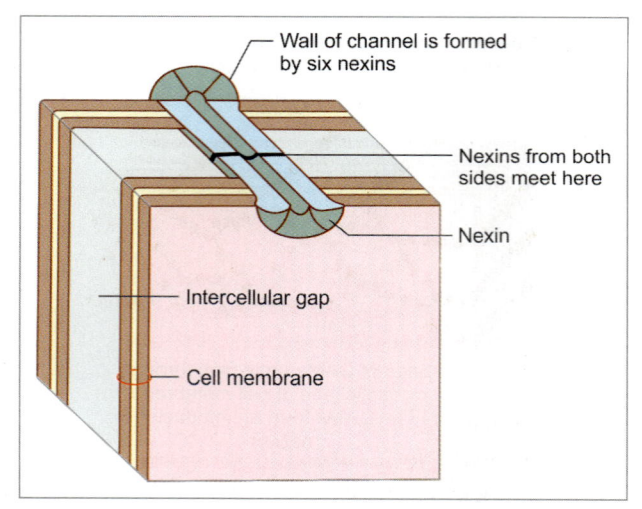

Fig. 2.13: Diagram to show the constitution of one channel of a communicating junction.

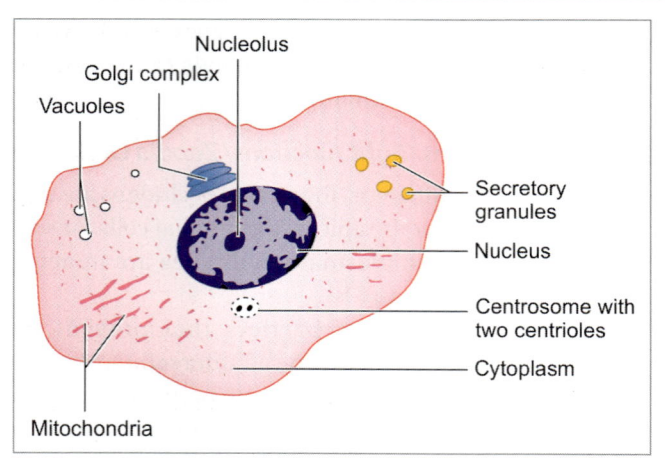

Fig. 2.14: Some features of a cell that can be seen with a light microscope.

mitochondria, the Golgi complex, and various types of vesicles (Fig. 2.14).

❖ The cytosol also contains a cytoskeleton made up of microtubules, microfilaments, and intermediate filaments. Centrioles are closely connected with microtubules.

Endoplasmic Reticulum

❖ It is a network of membranous tubules within the cytoplasm of a cell and it is continuous with the nuclear membrane. It is involved in protein and lipid synthesis.
❖ The membranes form the boundaries of channels that may be arranged in the form of flattened sacs (or cisternae) or of tubules. Ribosomes and enzymes are present on the "outer" surfaces of the membranes of the reticulum.
❖ Because of the presence of the ER, the cytoplasm is divided into two components, one within the channels and one outside them (Fig. 2.15). The cytoplasm within the channels is called the ***vacuoplasm***, and that outside the channels is the ***hyaloplasm*** or ***cytosol***.
❖ There are two types of ER within each cell: (1) Smooth endoplasmic reticulum (SER) and (2) Rough endoplasmic reticulum (RER).
❖ In most places, the membranes forming the ER are studded with minute particles of ribonucleic acid (RNA) called ***ribosomes***. The presence of these ribosomes gives the membrane a rough appearance and they are called RER.

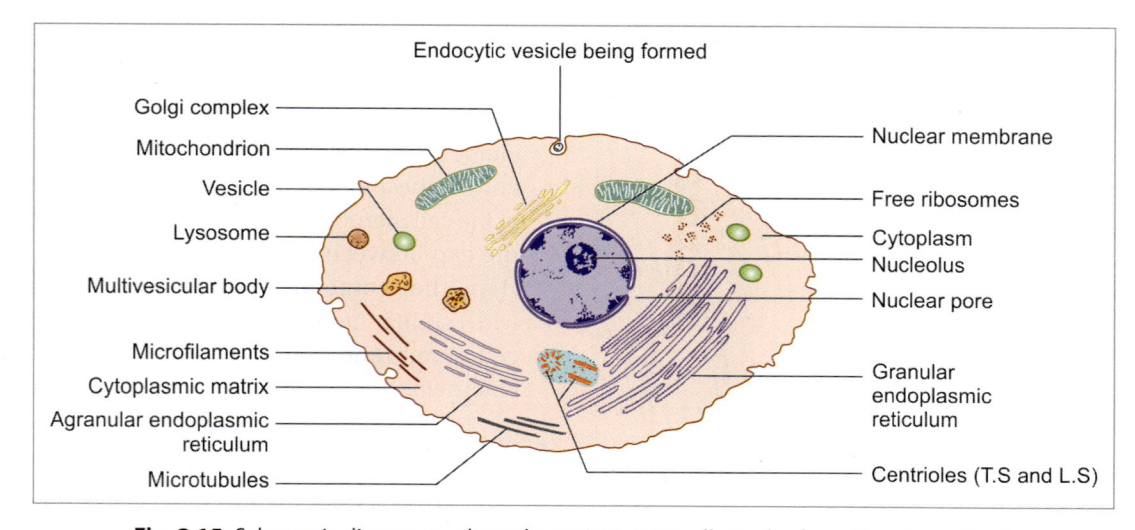

Fig. 2.15: Schematic diagram to show the various organelles to be found in a typical cell. (*Various structures shown are not drawn to scale*).

CHAPTER 2: Cell Structure

- Rough endoplasmic reticulum represents the site at which proteins are synthesized. The attached ribosomes play an important role in this process. The lumen of RER is continuous with the perinuclear space. It is also continuous with the lumen of SER.
- Smooth endoplasmic reticulum is involved in lipid metabolism and acts as the calcium store for the cell. It is involved in the synthesis of lipids, especially that of membrane phospholipids. It is often located near the periphery of the cell. SER is responsible for further processing of proteins synthesized in RER.
- Products synthesized by the ER are stored in the channels within the reticulum.

Ribosomes

- We have seen earlier that ribosomes are present in relation to RER. They may also lie free in the cytoplasm.
- They may be present singly in which case they are called **monosomes or** in groups which are referred to as **polyribosomes** or **polysomes**. Each ribosome consists of proteins and RNA and is about 15 nm in diameter. Ribosomes play an essential role in protein synthesis.

Mitochondria

- The mitochondrion is a double membrane-bound organelle and can be seen with the light microscope in specially stained preparations. They are so called because they appear either as granules or as rods (mitos = granule; chondrium = rod).
- The number of mitochondria varies from cell to cell being greatest in cells with high metabolic activity (e.g. in secretory cells). Mitochondria vary in size, most of them being 0.5–2 μm in length. Mitochondria are large in cells with a high oxidative metabolism.
- The mitochondrion is bounded by a smooth **outer membrane** within which there is an inner membrane, the two being separated by an **intermembranous space**. The inner membrane is highly folded on itself forming incomplete partitions called **cristae**. The space bounded by the inner membrane is filled by a granular material called the **matrix** (Fig. 2.16).
- The matrix contains numerous enzymes. It also contains some RNA and deoxyribonucleic acid (DNA): These are believed to carry information that enables mitochondria to duplicate themselves during cell division. All mitochondria are derived from those in the fertilized ovum, and are entirely of maternal origin.
- The most prominent roles of mitochondria are to produce the energy of the cell (**power house of the cell**). Primary function of mitochondria is to generate large quantities of energy in the form of adenosine triphosphate (ATP). They contain many enzymes including some that play an important part in Krebs cycle (TCA cycle). In addition to producing energy, mitochondria store calcium for cell signaling activities, generate heat, and mediate cell growth and death.

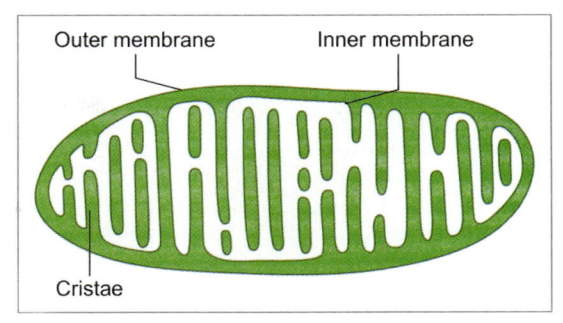

Fig. 2.16: Structure of a mitochondrion.

- Adenosine triphosphate and guanosine triphosphate (GTP) are formed in mitochondria and from there they pass to other parts of the cell and provide energy for various cellular functions. These facts can be correlated with the observation that within the cell mitochondria tend to concentrate in regions where energy requirements are greatest.

Golgi Complex

- Golgi apparatus, also called Golgi complex or Golgi body, is a membrane-bound organelle of cells that is made up of a series of flattened, stacked pouches called cisternae. It is involved in secretion and intracellular transport.
- In light microscopic preparations, suitably treated with silver salts, the Golgi complex can be seen as a small structure of irregular shape, usually present near the nucleus (*see* Fig. 2.14).
- When examined with the EM, the complex is seen to be made up of membranes similar to those of SER. The membranes form the walls of a number of flattened sacs that are stacked over one another. Toward their margins, the sacs are continuous with small rounded vesicles (Fig. 2.17). The cisternae of the Golgi complex form an independent system. Their lumen is not in communication with that of ER. Material from ER reaches the Golgi complex through vesicles.
- The Golgi apparatus is made up of approximately four to eight cisternae, although in some single-celled organisms, it may consist of as many as 60 cisternae. The cisternae are held together by matrix proteins, and the

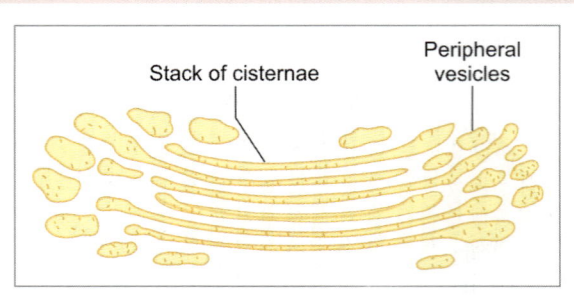

Fig. 2.17: Structure of the Golgi complex.

whole of the Golgi apparatus is supported by cytoplasmic microtubules. The apparatus has three regions known generally as: (1) "Cis" (cisternae nearest the endoplasmic reticulum), (2) "Medial" (central layers of cisternae), and (3) "Trans" (cisternae farthest from the ER).

- Material synthesized in RER travels through the ER lumen into SER. Vesicles budding off from SER transport this material to the cis face of the Golgi complex. Some proteins are phosphorylated here. From the cis face, all these materials pass into the medial Golgi. Here, sugar residues are added to proteins to form protein-carbohydrate complexes.
- Finally, all material passes to the trans face, which performs the following functions (Fig. 2.18):
  a. Proteolysis of some proteins converts them from inactive to active forms
  b. Like the medial Golgi, the trans face is also concerned in adding sugar residues to proteins
  c. In the trans face, various substances are sorted out and packed in appropriate vesicles. The latter may be secretory vesicles, lysosomes, or vesicles meant for transport of membrane to the cell surface.

Other Storage Vesicles

Materials such as lipids, or carbohydrates, may also be stored within the cytoplasm in the form of membrane-bound vesicles.

Lysosomes

- These vesicles contain enzymes that can destroy unwanted material present within a cell. Such material may have been taken into the cell from outside (e.g. bacteria), or may represent organelles that are no longer of use to the cell. The enzymes present in lysosomes include proteases, lipases, carbohydrases, and acid phosphatase (as many as 40 different lysosomal enzymes have been identified).
- The stages in the formation of a lysosome are as follows:
  - Acid hydrolase enzymes synthesized in ER reach the Golgi complex where they are packed into vesicles (Fig. 2.19). The enzymes in these vesicles are inactive because of the lack of an acid medium (these are

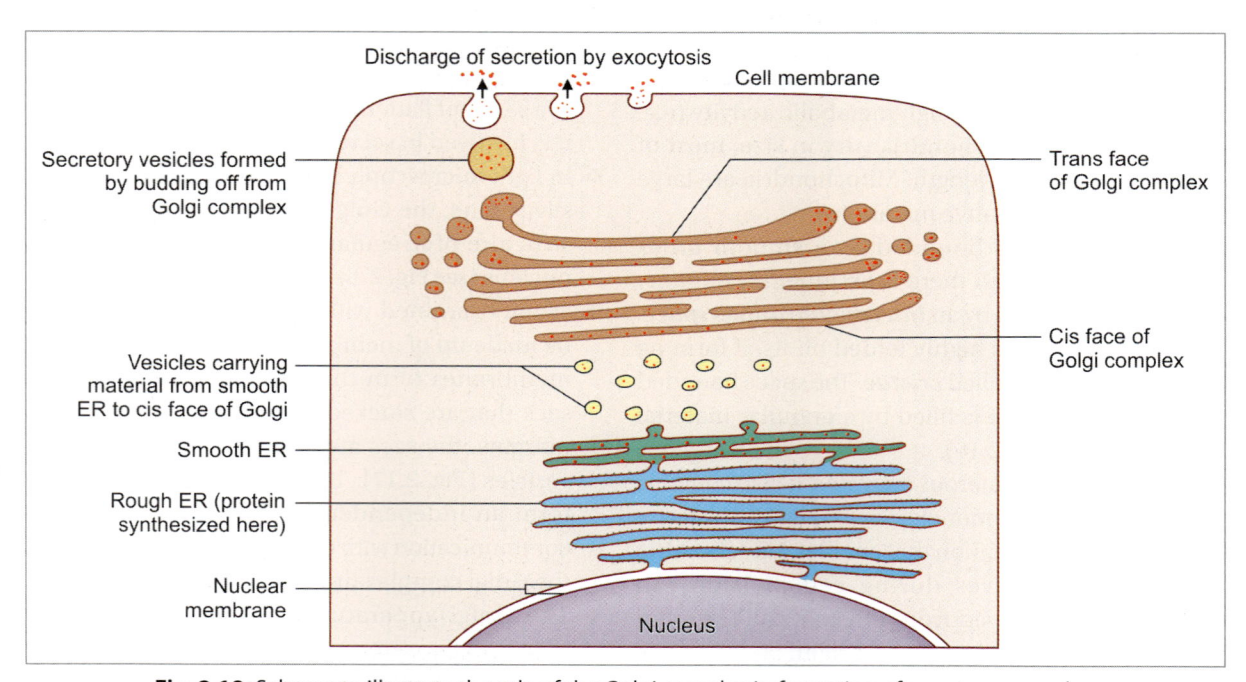

Fig. 2.18: Scheme to illustrate the role of the Golgi complex in formation of secretory vacuoles.

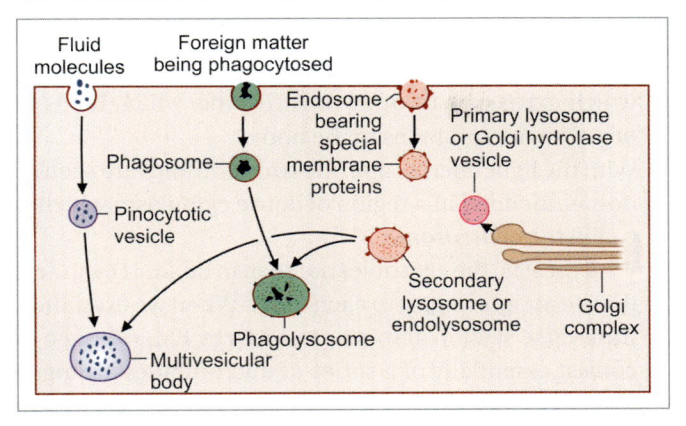

CHAPTER 2: Cell Structure

Fig. 2.19: Scheme to show how lysosomes, phagolysosomes, and multivesicular bodies are formed.

called ***primary lysosomes*** or ***Golgi hydrolase vesicles***) (Flowchart 2.1).

- These vesicles fuse with other vesicles derived from cell membrane (***endosomes***). These endosomes possess the membrane proteins necessary for producing an acid medium. The product formed by fusion of the two vesicles is an ***endolysosome*** or ***secondary lysosome*** (Flowchart 2.1).
- H^+ ions are pumped into the vesicle to create an acid environment. This activates the enzymes and a mature lysosome is formed.

❖ Lysosomes help in "digesting" the material within phagosomes. A lysosome, containing appropriate enzymes, fuses with the phagosome so that the enzymes of the former can act on the material within the phagosome. These bodies consisting of fused phagosomes and lysosomes are referred to as ***phagolysosomes*** (Fig. 2.19).

❖ In a similar manner, lysosomes may also fuse with pinocytotic vesicles. The structures formed by such fusion often appear to have numerous small vesicles within them and are, therefore, called ***multivesicular bodies***.

❖ Lysosomes are present in all cells except mature erythrocytes. They are a prominent feature in neutrophil leukocytes.

Flowchart 2.1: Types of lysosomes.

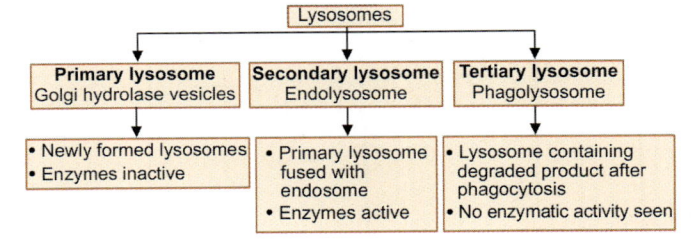

```
                    Lysosomes
        ┌───────────────┼───────────────┐
   Primary lysosome  Secondary lysosome  Tertiary lysosome
   Golgi hydrolase     Endolysosome      Phagolysosome
   vesicles
  ─────────────────  ─────────────────  ─────────────────
  • Newly formed    • Primary lysosome  • Lysosome containing
    lysosomes         fused with          degraded product after
  • Enzymes inactive  endosome            phagocytosis
                    • Enzymes active    • No enzymatic activity seen
```

Peroxisomes

❖ These are similar to lysosomes in that they are membrane-bound vesicles containing enzymes.

❖ The enzymes in most of them react with other substances to form hydrogen peroxide which is used to detoxify various substances by oxidizing them. The enzymes are involved in oxidation of very long chain fatty acids. Hydrogen peroxide resulting from the reactions is toxic to the cell. Other peroxisomes contain the enzyme catalase which destroys hydrogen peroxide, thus preventing the latter from accumulating in the cell. Peroxisomes are most prominent in cells of the liver and in cells of renal tubules.

Cytoskeleton

❖ The cytoskeleton is a network of filaments and tubules that extends throughout a cell, through the cytoplasm, except for the nucleus.

❖ The cytoskeleton supports the cell, gives it shape, organizes and tethers the organelles, and has role in molecule transport, cell division, and cell signaling.

❖ The elements that constitute the cytoskeleton consist of the following:
- Microfilaments
- Microtubules
- Intermediate filaments.

Microfilaments

❖ Microfilaments are made up of actin filaments so they are also called actin filaments. Their structure is two strands of actin wound in a spiral. They are about 7 nm thick, making them the thinnest filaments in the cytoskeleton.

❖ They facilitate in cytokinesis, cell motility, and allow single-celled organisms like amebas to move. They are also involved in cytoplasmic streaming, which is the flowing of cytosol throughout the cell. Cytoplasmic streaming transports nutrients and cell organelles.

❖ Microfilaments are also part of muscle cells and allow these cells to contract, along with myosin.

Microtubules

❖ Microtubules are the largest cytoskeletal filaments in cells, with a diameter of 25 nm.

❖ The basic constituent of microtubules is the ***protein tubulin***. Chains of tubulin form ***protofilaments***. The wall of a microtubule is made up of 13 protofilaments that run longitudinally (Fig. 2.20). The tubulin protofilaments are stabilized by ***microtubule-associated proteins*** (MAPs).

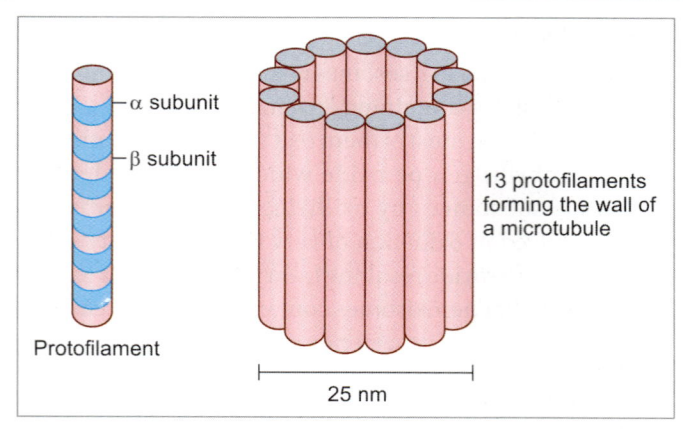

Fig. 2.20: Scheme to show how a microtubule is constituted.

- Microtubules are formed in centrioles which constitute a microtubule organizing center.

Functions of microtubules

- They have role in cell movement, cell division, and transporting materials within cells.
- As part of the cytoskeleton, they provide stability to the cell. They prevent tubules of ER from collapsing.
- They facilitate transport within the cell. As part of the cytoskeleton, microtubules help to move organelles inside a cell's cytoplasm.
- In dividing cells, microtubules form the mitotic spindle.
- Cilia and flagella are made up of microtubules.

Intermediate Filaments

- These are so called as their diameter (10 nm) is intermediate between that of microfilaments (5 nm) and of microtubules (25 nm). The proteins constituting these filaments vary in different types of cells.
- They include *cytokeratin* (in epithelial cells), *neurofilament protein* (in neurons), *desmin* (in muscle), *glial fibrillary acidic protein* (in astrocytes), *lamin* (in the nuclear lamina of cells), and *vimentin* (in many types of cells).

Functions of intermediate filaments

- Intermediate filaments link cells together. The filaments also facilitate cell attachment to extracellular elements at hemidesmosomes.
- In the epithelium of the skin, the filaments undergo modification to form keratin. They also form the main constituent of hair and of nails.
- The neurofilaments of neurons are intermediate filaments. Neurofibrils help to maintain the cylindrical shape of axons.
- The nuclear lamina consists of intermediate filaments.

Centrioles

- A centriole is a small structure made up of microtubules which exists as part of the centrosome, which helps to organize microtubules in the body.
- With the light microscope, the two centrioles are seen as dots embedded in a region of dense cytoplasm which is called the **centrosome**.
- With the EM, the centrioles are seen to be short cylinders that lie at right angles to each other. When we examine a transverse section across a centriole by EM, it is seen to consist essentially of a series of microtubules arranged in a circle. There are nine groups of tubules, each group consisting of three tubules (Fig. 2.21).
- Centrioles play an important role in the formation of various cellular structures that are made up of microtubules. These include the mitotic spindles of dividing cells, cilia, flagella, and some projections of specialized cells (e.g. the axial filaments of spermatozoa). It is of interest to note that cilia, flagella, and the tails of spermatozoa all have the 9 + 2 configuration of microtubules that are seen in a centriole.

Nucleus

- The nucleus constitutes the central and denser parts of the cell. It is usually rounded or ellipsoid. Occasionally, it may be elongated, indented, or lobed. It is usually 4–10 µm in diameter.
- It is a highly specialized organelle that serves as the information processing and administrative center of the cell. It has two major functions: (1) It stores the cell's hereditary material, or DNA, and (2) It coordinates the cell's activities, which include growth, intermediary metabolism, protein synthesis, and cell division.
- In usual classroom slides stained with hematoxylin and eosin, the nucleus stains dark purple or blue while the

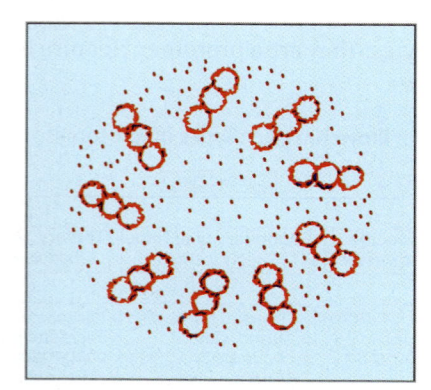

Fig. 2.21: Transverse section across a centriole (near its base). Note nine groups of tubules, each group having three microtubules.

cytoplasm is usually stained pink. In some cells, the nuclei are relatively large and light staining.
- Nuclei appear to be made up of a delicate network of fibers: The material making up the fibers of the network is called **chromatin** (because of its affinity for dyes). At some places in the nucleus, the chromatin is seen in the form of irregular dark masses that are called **heterochromatin**. At other places, the network is loose and stains lightly: The chromatin of such areas is referred to as **euchromatin**.
- Nuclei which are large and in which relatively large areas of euchromatin can be seen are referred to as **open-face nuclei**. Nuclei that are made up mainly of heterochromatin are referred to as **closed-face nuclei** (Figs. 2.22A and B).
- In addition to the masses of heterochromatin, the nucleus shows one or more rounded, dark staining bodies called **nucleoli**. The nucleolus is a membraneless organelle within the nucleus that manufactures ribosomes, the cell's protein-producing structures.
- Through the microscope, the nucleolus looks like a large dark spot within the nucleus. A nucleus may contain up to four nucleoli.
- After a cell divides, a nucleolus is formed when chromosomes are brought together into nucleolar organizing regions and during cell division, the nucleolus disappears.
- The nucleus also contains various small granules, fibers, and vesicles. The spaces between the various constituents of the nucleus described earlier are filled by a base called the **nucleoplasm**.
- With the EM, the nucleus is seen to be surrounded by a double-layered **nuclear membrane** or **nuclear envelope**. The outer nuclear membrane is continuous with ER. The space between the inner and outer membranes is the **perinuclear space**. This is continuous with the lumen of RER.
- The inner layer of the nuclear membrane provides attachment to the ends of chromosomes. Deep to the inner membrane, there is a layer containing proteins and a network of filaments: This layer is called the **nuclear lamina**. Specific proteins present in the inner nuclear membrane give attachment to filamentous proteins of the nuclear lamina.
- At several points, the inner and outer layers of the nuclear membrane fuse leaving gaps called **nuclear pores**. Each pore is surrounded by dense protein arranged in the form of eight complexes. These proteins and the pore together form the **pore complex**.
- Nuclear pores represent sites at which substances can pass from the nucleus to the cytoplasm and vice versa (*see* Fig. 2.15). The nuclear pore is about 80 nm across. It is partly covered by a diaphragm that allows passage only to particles less than 9 nm in diameter. A typical nucleus has 3,000–4,000 pores.
- It is believed that pore complexes actively transport some proteins into the nucleus, and ribosomes out of the nucleus.
- Building blocks for building DNA and RNA are allowed into the nucleus as well as molecules that provide the energy for constructing genetic material.

Nature and Significance of Chromatin
- Chromatin is made up of a substance called **deoxyribonucleic acid** (usually abbreviated to DNA), and of proteins. It is in the form of a long chain of nucleotides.
- Most of the proteins in chromatin are **histones**. Some nonhistone proteins are also present. Filaments of DNA form coils around histone complexes.
- The structure formed by a histone complex and the DNA fiber coiled around it is called a **nucleosome**. Nucleosomes are attached to one another forming long chains (Fig. 2.23). These chains are coiled on themselves (in a helical manner) to form filaments having 30 nm in diameter. These filaments constitute chromatin.
- The DNA fibril makes two turns around a complex formed by histones to form a nucleosome. Nucleosomes give the chromatin fiber the appearance of a beaded string. The portion of the DNA fiber between the nucleosomes is called linkerDNA.
- Filaments of chromatin are again coiled on themselves (**supercoiling**), and this coiling is repeated several times. Each coiling produces a thicker filament. In this way, a

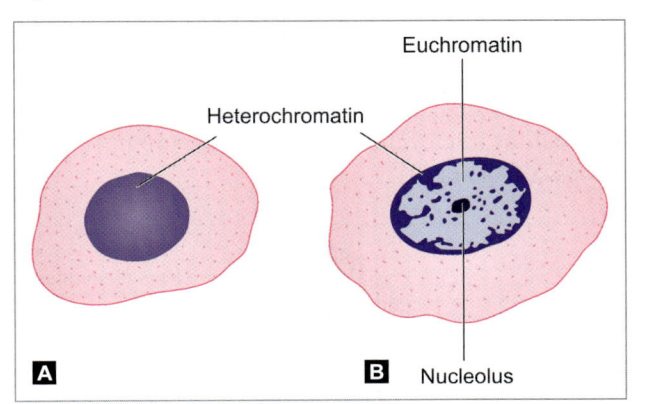

Figs. 2.22A and B: Comparison of a heterochromatic nucleus (A), and a euchromatic nucleus (B).

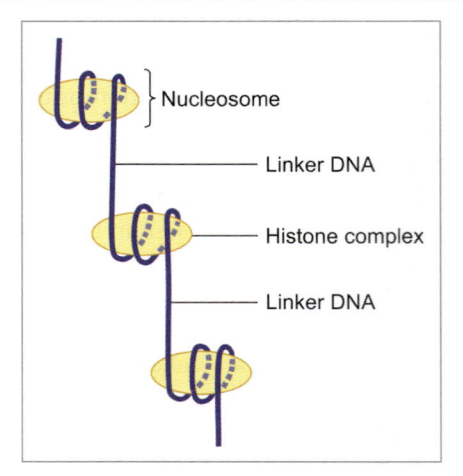

Fig. 2.23: Scheme to show the structure of a chromatin fiber. (DNA: deoxyribonucleic acid)

filament of DNA that is originally 50 mm long can be reduced to a chromosome by only 5 µm in length.

- Five types of histones are recognized. These are H1, H2A, H2B, H3, and H4 (Fig. 2.24). Two molecules each of H2A, H2B, H3, and H4 join to form a granular mass, the *nucleosome core.* The DNA filament is wound *twice* around this core, the whole complex forming a nucleosome. The length of the DNA filament in one nucleosome contains 146 nucleotide pairs. One nucleosome is connected to the next by a short length of *linker DNA*. Linker DNA is made up of about 50 nucleotide pairs.
- Heterochromatin represents areas where chromatin fibers are tightly coiled on themselves forming "solid" masses. In contrast, euchromatin represents areas where coiling is not so marked. During cell division, the entire chromatin within the nucleus becomes very tightly coiled and takes on the appearance of a number of short, thick, and rod-like structures called *chromosomes*. Chromosomes are made up of DNA and proteins. Proteins stabilize the structure of chromosomes.

Nucleoli

- Nuclei contain one or more nucleoli and are spherical and about 1–3 µm in diameter. They stain intensely both with hematoxylin and eosin, the latter giving them a slight reddish tinge. Nucleoli are larger and more distinct in cells that are metabolically active.
- Using histochemical procedures that distinguish between DNA and RNA, it is seen that the nucleoli have a high RNA content. With the EM, nucleoli are seen to have a central filamentous zone (*pars filamentosa*) and an outer granular zone (*pars granulosa*) both of which are embedded in an amorphous material (*pars amorpha*) (Fig. 2.25).
- Parts of the chromosomes located within nucleoli constitute the *pars chromosoma* of nucleoli.
- Nucleoli are sites where ribosomal RNA is synthesized.

Projections from the Cell Surface

Many cells show projections from the cell surface. The various types of projections are described here.

Cilia

- These can be seen, with the light microscope, as minute hair-like projections from the free surfaces of some epithelial cells (Fig. 2.26). In the living animal, cilia can be seen to be motile.
- The free part of each cilium is called the *shaft*. The region of attachment of the shaft to the cell surface is called the *base*. The free end of the shaft tapers to a tip.
- Each cilium is 0.25 µm in diameter. It consists of: (a) an outer covering that is formed by an extension of the cell membrane; and (b) an inner core (*axoneme*) that is formed by microtubules arranged in a definite manner (Figs. 2.27A and B).

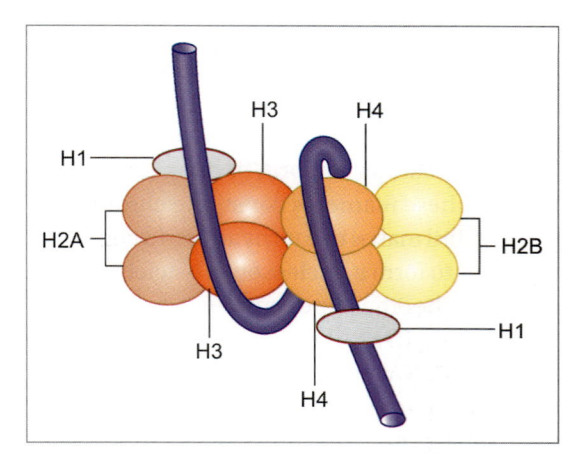

Fig. 2.24: Diagram showing detailed composition of a histone complex forming the nucleosome core.

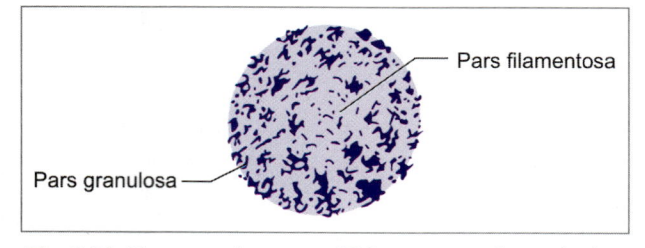

Fig. 2.25: Electron microscopy (EM) structure of a nucleolus.

CHAPTER 2: Cell Structure

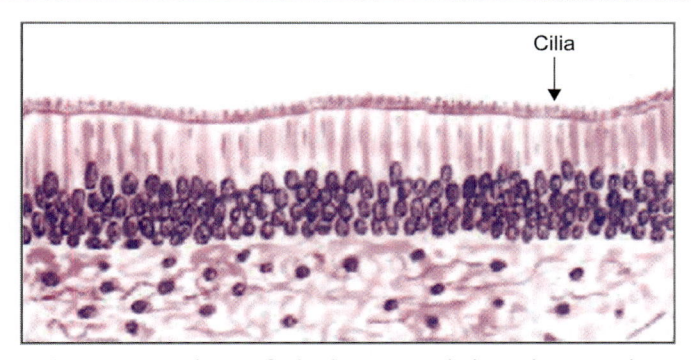

Fig. 2.26: Pseudostratified columnar epithelium showing cilia.

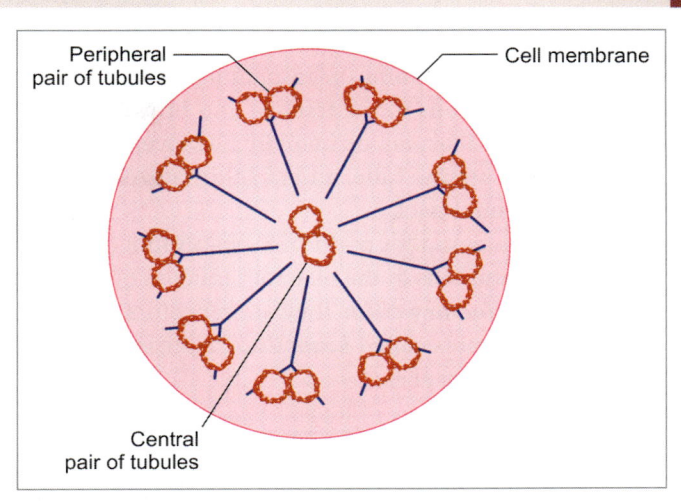

Fig. 2.28: Transverse section across a cilium.

is represented by one tubule only. Just near the tip, only the central pair of tubules is seen (Fig. 2.29).
- At the base of the cilium, one additional tubule is added to each outer pair so that here the nine outer groups of tubules have three tubules each, exactly as in the centriole.
- Microtubules in cilia are bound with proteins (dynein and nexin). Nexin holds the microtubules together. Dynein molecules are responsible for bending of tubules, and thereby for movements of cilia.

Functions of cilia
- The cilia lining an epithelial surface move in coordination with one another, the total effect being that like a wave. As a result, fluid, mucous, or small solid objects lying on the

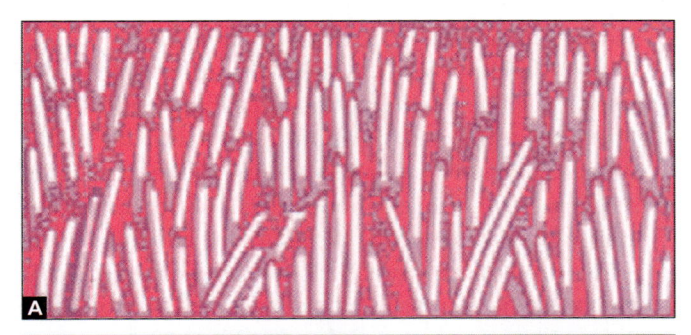

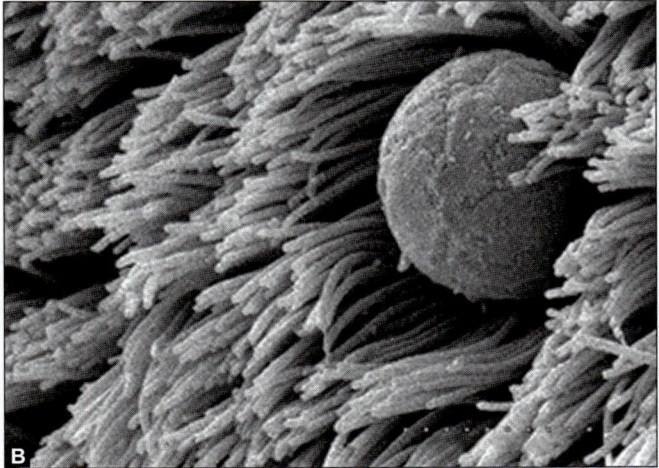

Figs. 2.27A and B: Drawing of cilia as seen by scanning electron microscopy.

- It has a striking similarity to the structure of a centriole. There is a central pair of tubules that is surrounded by nine pairs of tubules. The outer tubules are connected to the inner pair by radial structures like the spokes of a wheel. Other projections pass outward from the outer tubules (Fig. 2.28).
- As the tubules of the shaft are traced toward the tip of the cilium, it is seen that one tubule of each outer pair ends short of the tip so that near the tip each outer pair

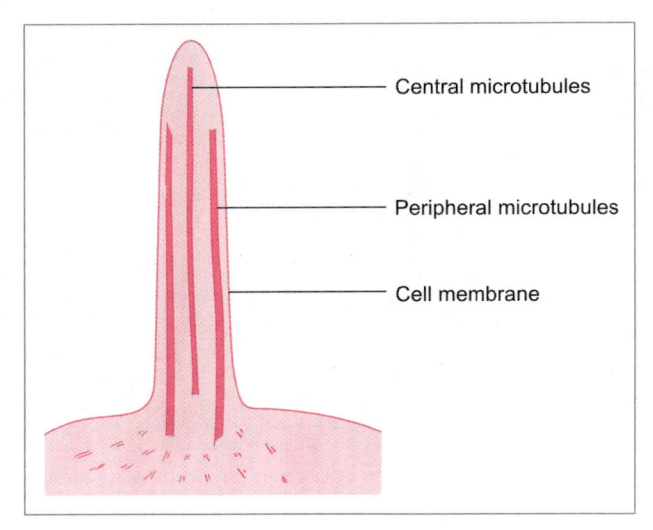

Fig. 2.29: Longitudinal section through a cilium.

epithelium can be caused to move in a specific direction. Movements of cilia lining the respiratory epithelium help to move secretions in the trachea and bronchi toward the pharynx. Ciliary action helps in the movement of ova through the uterine tube, and of spermatozoa through the male genital tract.

❖ In some situations, they perform a sensory function. Cilia present on the cells in the olfactory mucosa of the nose are called **olfactory cilia**: They are receptors for smell. Similar structures called **kinociliaare** present in some parts of the internal ear.

Flagella

❖ These are somewhat larger processes having the same basic structure as cilia. In the human body, the best example of a flagellum is the tail of the spermatozoon.

❖ In a flagellum, movement starts at its base. The segment nearest the base bends in one direction. This is followed by bending of succeeding segments in opposite directions, so that a wave-like motion passes down the flagellum. When a spermatozoon is suspended in a fluid medium, this wave of movement propels the spermatozoon forward.

Microvilli and Basolateral Folds

❖ Microvilli are finger-like projections from the cell surface that can be seen by EM (Figs. 2.30A and B).

❖ Each microvillus consists of an outer covering of plasma membrane and a cytoplasmic core in which there are numerous microfilaments (actin filaments). The filaments are continuous with actin filaments of the cell cortex.

❖ Numerous enzymes and glycoproteins concerned with absorption have been located in microvilli.

❖ With the light microscope, the free borders of epithelial cells lining the small intestine appear to be thickened: The thickening has striations perpendicular to the surface. This **striated border** of light microscopy (Figs. 2.31A and B) has been shown by EM to be made up of long microvilli arranged parallel to one another.

❖ In some cells, the microvilli are not arranged so regularly. With the light microscope, the microvilli of such cells give the appearance of a **brush border** (Fig. 2.32).

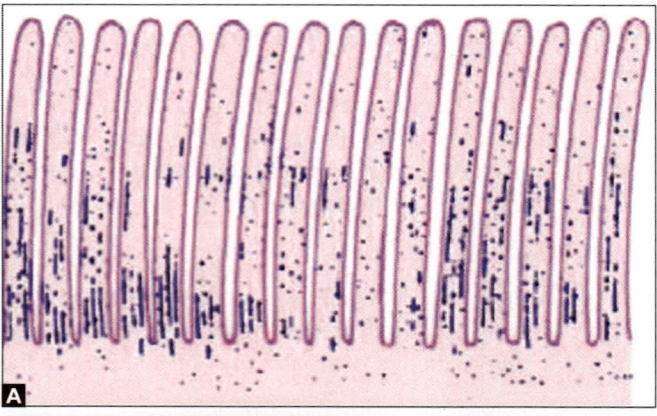

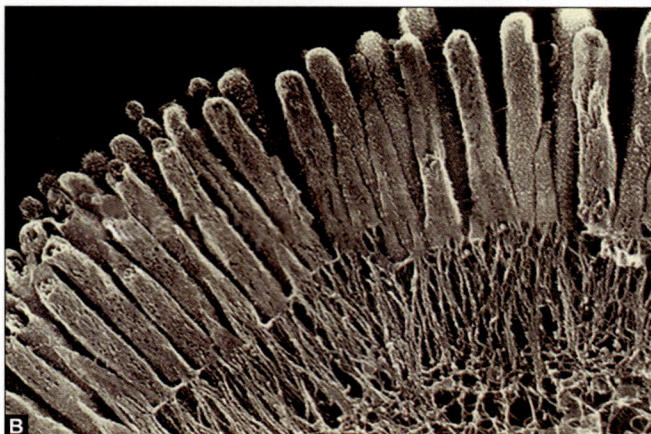

Figs. 2.30A and B: Microvilli as seen in longitudinal section. The regular arrangement of microvilli is characteristic of the striated border of intestinal absorptive cells.

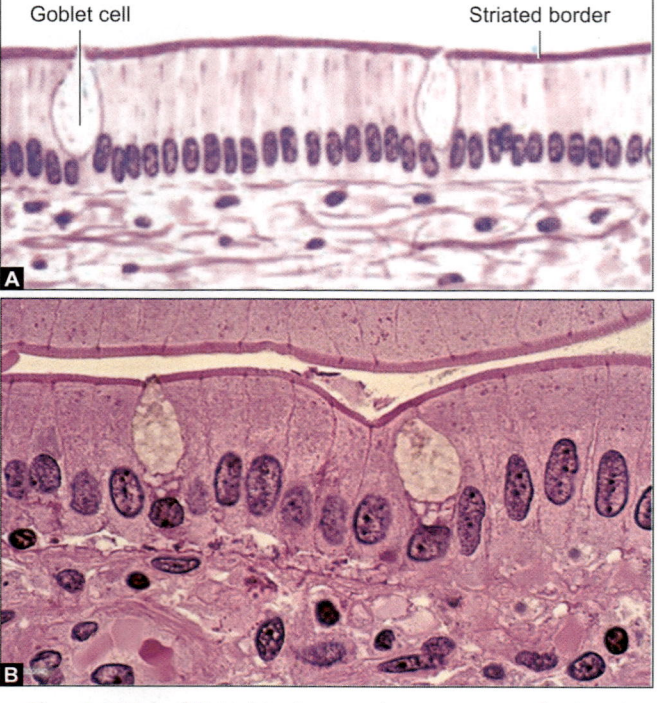

Figs. 2.31A and B: Light microscopic appearance of striated border formed by microvilli.

CHAPTER 2: Cell Structure

Fig. 2.32: Light microscopic appearance of a brush border in epithelium lining renal tubules.

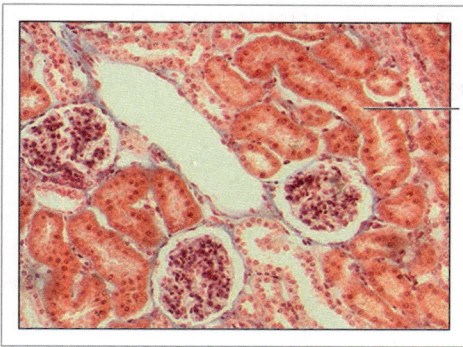

- Microvilli greatly increase the surface area of the cell and are, therefore, seen most typically at sites of active absorption, e.g. the intestine, and the proximal and distal convoluted tubules of the kidneys.
- Modified microvilli called *stereocilia* are seen on receptor cells in the internal ear, and on the epithelium of the epididymis.
- In some cells, the cell membrane over the basal or lateral aspects of the cell shows deep folds (basolateral folds). Like microvilli, basolateral folds are an adaptation to increase cell surface area.
- Basal folds are seen in renal tubular cells, and in cells lining the ducts of some glands. Lateral folds are seen in absorptive cells lining the gut (Fig. 2.32).

STAINING OF A CELL

Nuclei are stained blue, whereas the cytoplasm and extracellular matrix have varying degrees of pink staining.

- **Structures that are stained purple** (basophilic): DNA (heterochromatin and the nucleolus) in the nucleus, and RNA in ribosomes and in the RER are both acidic, and so hematoxylin binds to them and stains them purple. Some extracellular materials (i.e. carbohydrates in cartilage) are also basophilic.
- **Structures that are stained pink** (eosinophilic or acidophilic): Most proteins in the cytoplasm are basic, and so eosin binds to these proteins and stains them pink. This includes cytoplasm, cell membrane, cytoplasmic filaments in muscle cells, intracellular membranes, and extracellular fibers.

Mucous cells like goblet cell produce **mucus**, which does not stain very darkly, so the **mucous cells** look almost clear. Mucous cells stain very poorly because they contain little RER and their mucin granules tend to react poorly with most stains.

Serous cells produce a watery secretion that contains a lot of proteins and stain fairly well due to the presence of RER and secretory granules in the cytoplasm.

APPLIED HISTOLOGY

- Mitochondrial DNA can be abnormal. This interferes with mitochondrial and cell functions, resulting in disorders referred to as *mitochondrial cytopathy syndromes*. The features (which differ in intensity from patient to patient) include muscle weakness, degenerative lesions in the brain, and high levels of lactic acid. The condition can be diagnosed by EM examination of muscle biopsies. The mitochondria show characteristic paracrystalline inclusions.
- Genetic defects can lead to absence of specific acid hydrolases that are normally present in lysosomes. As a result, some molecules cannot be degraded, and accumulate in lysosomes. Examples of such disorders are *lysosomal glycogen storage disease* in which there is abnormal accumulation of glycogen, and *Tay-Sachs disease* in which lipids accumulate in lysosomes and lead to neuronal degeneration.
- Defects in enzymes of peroxisomes can result in metabolic disorders associated with storage of abnormal lipids in some cells (brain and adrenal).
- Cilia can be abnormal in persons with genetic defects that interfere with synthesis of ciliary proteins. This leads to the *immotile cilia syndrome*. As secretions are not removed from respiratory passages, the patient has repeated and severe chest infections. Women affected by the syndrome may be sterile as movement of ova along the uterine tube is affected. Ciliary proteins are present in the tails of spermatozoa, and an affected male may be sterile because of interference with the motility of spermatozoa.

MULTIPLE CHOICE QUESTIONS

1. A structure that is continuous with rough endoplasmic reticulum (RER) is the:
   a. Golgi apparatus
   b. Nucleolus
   c. Outer nuclear membrane
   d. Euchromatin
2. Which of the following is not a membranous organelle?
   a. Centrioles
   b. Mitochondria
   c. Lysosomes
   d. Endoplasmic reticulum
3. "Cell drinking" is also called as:
   a. Endocytosis
   b. Exocytosis
   c. Pinocytosis
   d. Phagocytosis
4. Protein synthesis occurs at:
   a. Ribosomes
   b. Microfilaments
   c. Centrioles
   d. Nucleoli
5. Junction that segregates two cell compartments from mixing is:
   a. Gap junction
   b. Desmosomes
   c. Tight junction
   d. Cell junction
6. A type of junctions that has protein extending from one cell to another:
   a. Gap junction
   b. Desmosomes
   c. Tight junction
   d. Cell junction

Answers
1. c
2. a
3. c
4. a.
5. c.
6. d

CHAPTER 3

Epithelia and Glands

Learning objectives

To study the:

Epithelia
- Definition, general features and functions of epithelial tissue
- Classification of the epithelial tissue with example
- Basement membrane
- Cell surface projections
- Applied histology

Glands
- Definition of glands
- Classification with example
- Structure of serous and mucous salivary glands
- Applied histology

EPITHELIA

DEFINITION

One or more layers of cells that cover the outer surface (of the body) or line the luminal surface of tubular structures and cavities of the body are called **epithelia** (singular = epithelium).

GENERAL FEATURES OF EPITHELIAL TISSUE

- Very little intercellular space (20 nm)
- Usually avascular and nourishment is by diffusion from the adjacent supporting tissue
- Cells rest on a basement membrane
- Cells show polarity
- Cells show surface modifications
- Good regenerative capacity
- Metaplasia (changes from one type to another) can take place
- Derived from all three germ layers.

FUNCTIONS

- **Protection** from abrasion and injury
- **Absorption** of the material from lumen
- **Secretion** of mucus, hormones, enzymes, etc.
- **Exchange**/transcellular transport across the epithelial layers.

CLASSIFICATION OF EPITHELIA

Epithelial tissue is classified depending on the **cell arrangements and morphology** (Flowchart 3.1).

An epithelium may consist of only one layer of cells when it is called a ***unilayered*** or ***simple*** epithelium. Alternatively, it may be ***multilayered*** (***stratified***) or it can be ***pseudostratified***.

- ***Unilayered (simple) epithelia***: Single layer of cells resting on a basement membrane. It may be further classified according to the shape of the cells constituting them.
- ***Multilayered (stratified) epithelia***: Epithelia which consist of multiple layers with the basal layer resting on the basement membrane. The epithelium is named according to the shape of cells of the most superficial layer.
- ***Pseudostratified epithelia***: Single-layered cells but giving a false appearance of stratification.

SIMPLE EPITHELIUM

Based on the shape of the cells constituting them, simple epithelia can be classified as squamous, cuboidal, and columnar.

Flowchart 3.1: Classification of epithelia.

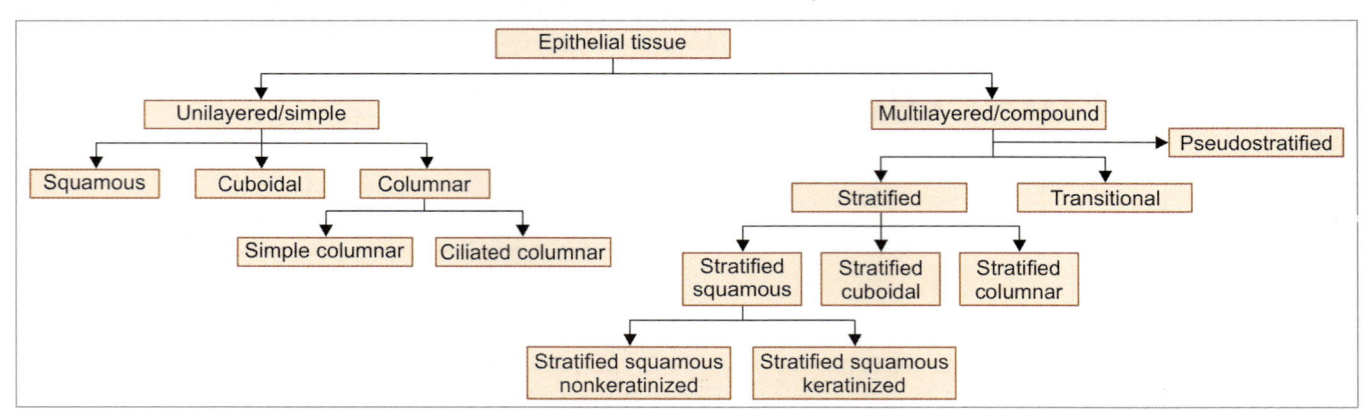

Simple Squamous Epithelium

- It is composed of single layer of flattened cells, their height being very little as compared to their width. Such an epithelium is called a **squamous epithelium**. The cytoplasm of cells forms only a thin layer. The nuclei produce bulging of the cell surface (Plate 3.1).
- In surface view, the cells have polygonal outlines that interlock with those of adjoining cells (Plate 3.1D). In a section, the cells appear flattened and their height being much less as compared to their width (Fig. 3.1).
- *Functions*: It helps in rapid transport of substances, diffusion of gases, and filtration of fluids.
- With the electron microscope (EM) the junctions between cells are marked by occluding junctions. The junctions are, thus, tightly sealed, and any substance passing through the epithelium has to pass through the cells, and not between them.

Examples

- Alveoli of the lungs.
- Free surface of the serous pericardium, the pleura, and the peritoneum; here it is called **mesothelium**.
- Inside the heart, where it is called **endocardium** and inside the blood vessels and lymphatics, where it is called **endothelium**.

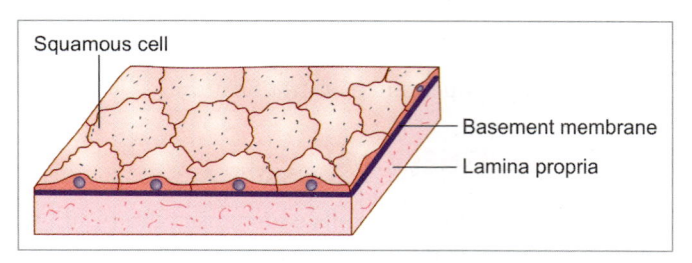

Fig. 3.1: Simple squamous epithelium (schematic representation).

- Squamous epithelium is also found lining some parts of the renal tubules, and in some parts of the internal ear.

Simple Cuboidal Epithelium

- When the height and width of the cells of the epithelium are more or less equal (i.e. they look like squares in section), it is described as a **cuboidal epithelium**.
- The nuclei are usually rounded and centrally placed (Plate 3.2).
- In sectional view, cells appear cuboidal in shape. When viewed from surface, cells are hexagonal in shape (Fig. 3.2).
- *Function*: It is mainly concerned with secretory, absorptive, and excretory functions.

Examples

- It is seen in the follicles of the thyroid gland, in the ducts of many glands, and on the surface of the ovary, the choroid plexuses, the inner surface of the lens, and the pigment cell layer of the retina.
- A cuboidal epithelium with a prominent brush border is seen in the proximal convoluted tubules (PCTs) of the kidneys.

Simple Columnar Epithelium

- When the height of the cells of the epithelium is distinctly greater than their width, it is described as a **columnar epithelium**.
- Nuclei are elongated and located in the lower half of the cells. Nuclei of all cells are placed at the same level (Fig. 3.3 and Plate 3.3).
- In vertical section, the cells of this epithelium are rectangular. On surface view (or in transverse section), the cells are polygonal (Fig. 3.3).

CHAPTER 3: Epithelia and Glands

Plate 3.1: Simple squamous epithelium

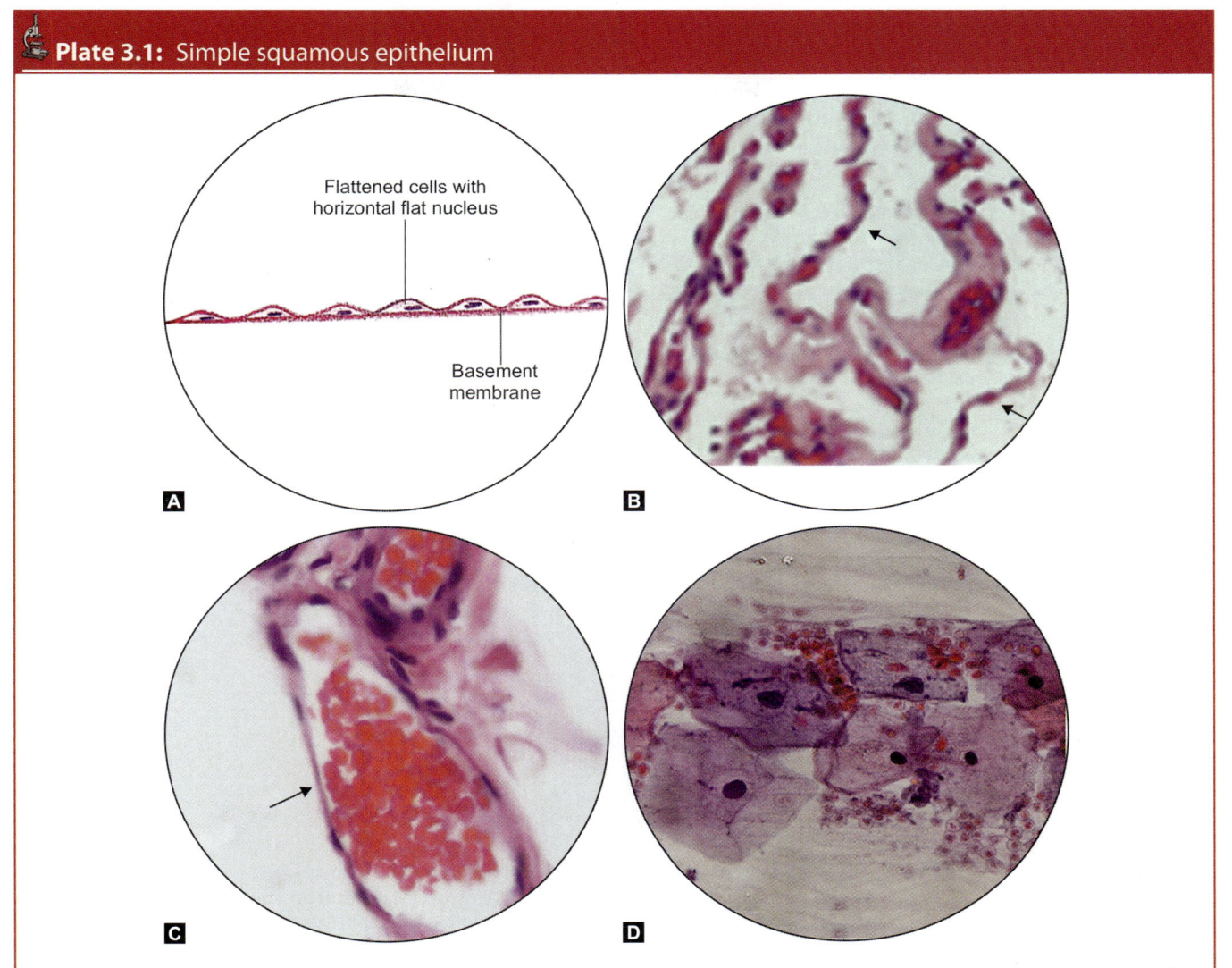

A — Flattened cells with horizontal flat nucleus; Basement membrane

B

C

D

Simple squamous epithelium: (A) As seen in drawing; (B) An alveolus of the lung showing a lining of simple squamous epithelium (photomicrograph) (*see* arrows); (C) A capillary lined by endothelium (photomicrograph) (*see* arrow); (D) Surface view as seen in buccal smear (photomicrograph).

Points of identification
- The cells of this epithelium are flattened in sections. They appear so thin that bulgings are produced on the surface by their nuclei
- In surface view the cells have polygonal outlines that interlock with those of adjoining cells.

Columnar epithelium can be further classified according to the nature of the free surfaces of the cells as follows:
1. **Simple columnar epithelium**: In some situations, the cell surface has no particular specialization. A simple columnar epithelium (nonciliated) lines the mucous membrane of the stomach and of the large intestine. They may even contain goblet cells.

Goblet cells are glandular simple columnar epithelial cells which perform the major function of secreting mucus. The name **goblet** is derived due to the special shape of these cells (Fig. 3.4). It has a narrow base and expanded apical portion. Since the mucus gets washed away during routine hematoxylin and eosin (H & E) staining, the upper expanded portions appear empty.

26   **Textbook of Human Histology**

Plate 3.2: Simple cuboidal epithelium

Simple cuboidal epithelium: (A) As seen in a section (drawing); (B) Thyroid follicle lined by simple cuboidal epithelium (photomicrograph) (*see* arrows); (C) Duct of salivary gland (photomicrograph) (*see* arrow).

Points of identification
- This epithelium is made up of cells that look like squares (in which the length and breadth are equal). Nuclei are rounded
- A typical cuboidal epithelium lines follicles of the thyroid gland, ducts of salivary gland, and tubules of kidney.

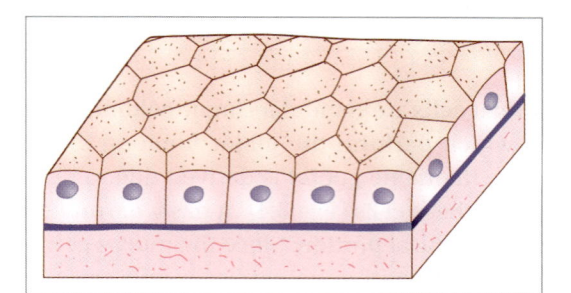

Fig. 3.2: Simple cuboidal epithelium. Note that the cells appear cuboidal in section and hexagonal in surface view (schematic representation).

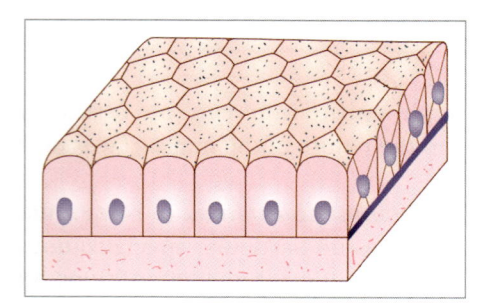

Fig. 3.3: Simple columnar epithelium. Note the basally placed oval nuclei. The cells appear hexagonal in surface view (schematic representation).

CHAPTER 3: Epithelia and Glands

Plate 3.3: Simple columnar epithelium

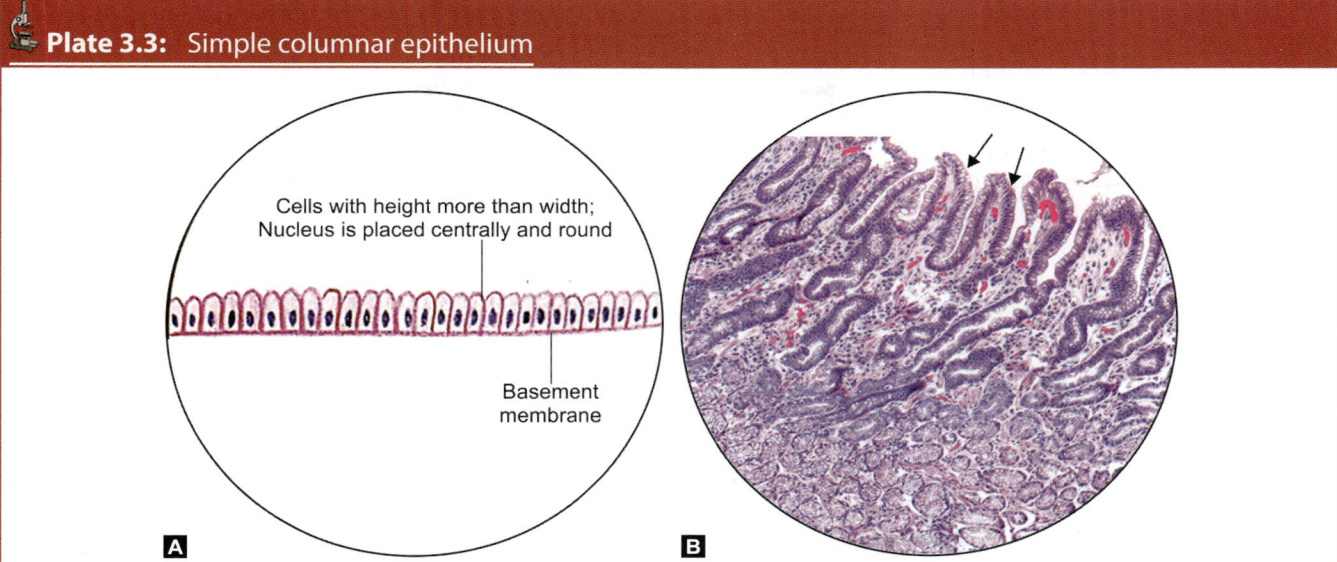

Simple columnar epithelium: (A) As seen in a section (drawing); (B) Lining the mucosa of the stomach (photomicrograph) (*see* arrows)

Points of identification
- The height of the cells in this epithelium is much greater than their width. The nuclei are oval being elongated in the same direction as the cells. They lie near the bases of the cells. Because of this we see a zone of clear cytoplasm above the nuclei
- A simple columnar epithelium (non-ciliated) lines the mucous membrane of the stomach and of the large intestine.

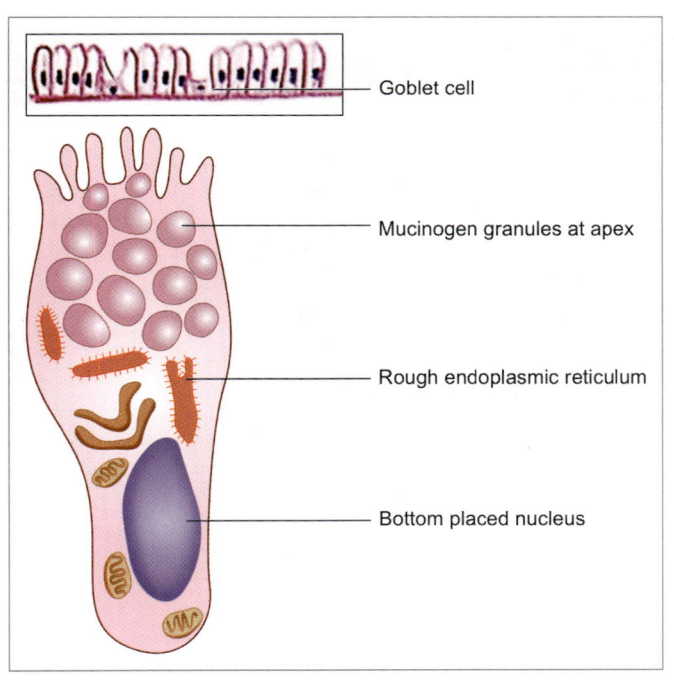

Fig. 3.4: Goblet cells.

The nucleus is round and pushed to the bottom due to accumulated mucinogen.

2. ***Ciliated columnar epithelium***: In some situations, the cell surface bears cilia, e.g. lining epithelium of fallopian tube.

3. At some places, the surface is covered with **microvilli**. Although the microvilli are visible only with the EM, they are seen as a ***striated border*** with the light microscope (when the microvilli are arranged regularly) or as a ***brush border*** (when the microvilli are irregularly placed) (Figs. 3.5A and B).

Functions

❖ Mainly columnar cells have a secretory and absorption function.
❖ In the intestines, many of them secrete mucous that accumulates in the apical part of the cell making it very

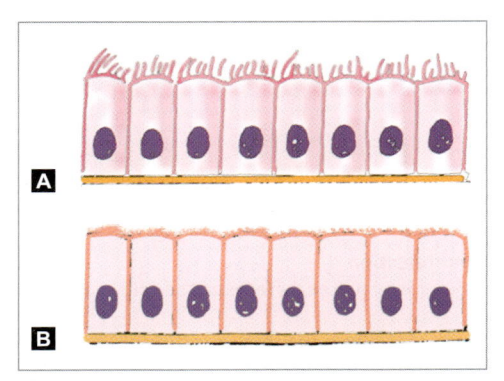

Figs. 3.5A and B: (A) Columnar epithelium showing cilia; (B) Columnar epithelium showing a striated border made up of microvilli (schematic representation).

light staining. These cells acquire a characteristic shape and are called **goblet cells**.
- Columnar epithelial cells can be found in the linings of the ears, nose, and on the taste buds of the tongue. These cells are designed to respond to stimuli.
- Ciliated columnar epithelium can be found in the lining of some organs, such as the fallopian tubes and in the lungs. Cilia are specialized bundles of protein which can move together to help propel material in one direction.
- Columnar epithelial cells are rather thick, which allows them to withstand mild amounts of damage.
- Microvilli increase the surface area for absorption.

Examples

- Simple columnar epithelium is present over the mucous membrane of the stomach and the large intestine.
- Columnar epithelium with a striated border is seen most typically in the small intestine, and with a brush border in the gallbladder (Plate 3.4).
- Ciliated columnar epithelium lines most of the respiratory tract, the uterus, and the uterine tubes. It is also seen in the efferent ductules of the testis, parts of the middle ear and auditory tube, and the ependyma lining the central canal of the spinal cord and the ventricles of the brain.
- In the respiratory tract, the cilia move mucous accumulating in the bronchi (and containing trapped dust particles) toward the larynx and pharynx. When excessive, this mucous is brought out as sputum during coughing. In the uterine tubes, the movements of the cilia help in the passage of ova toward the uterus.

Pseudostratified Epithelium

- It is not a true stratified epithelium but appears to be stratified. All the cells are in contact with basal lamina, but only few cells reach the surface. Tall cells have narrow base and broad apical part, but short cells have broad base and narrow apical part, and nuclei are located at the broad end of the cells, which gives appearance as many layers (Fig. 3.6 and Plate 3.5). However, the nuclei appear to be arranged in two or more layers giving the impression that the epithelium is more than one cell thick.
- The epithelium may bear cilia (ciliated epithelium) and may contain goblet cells. The cilia are capable of

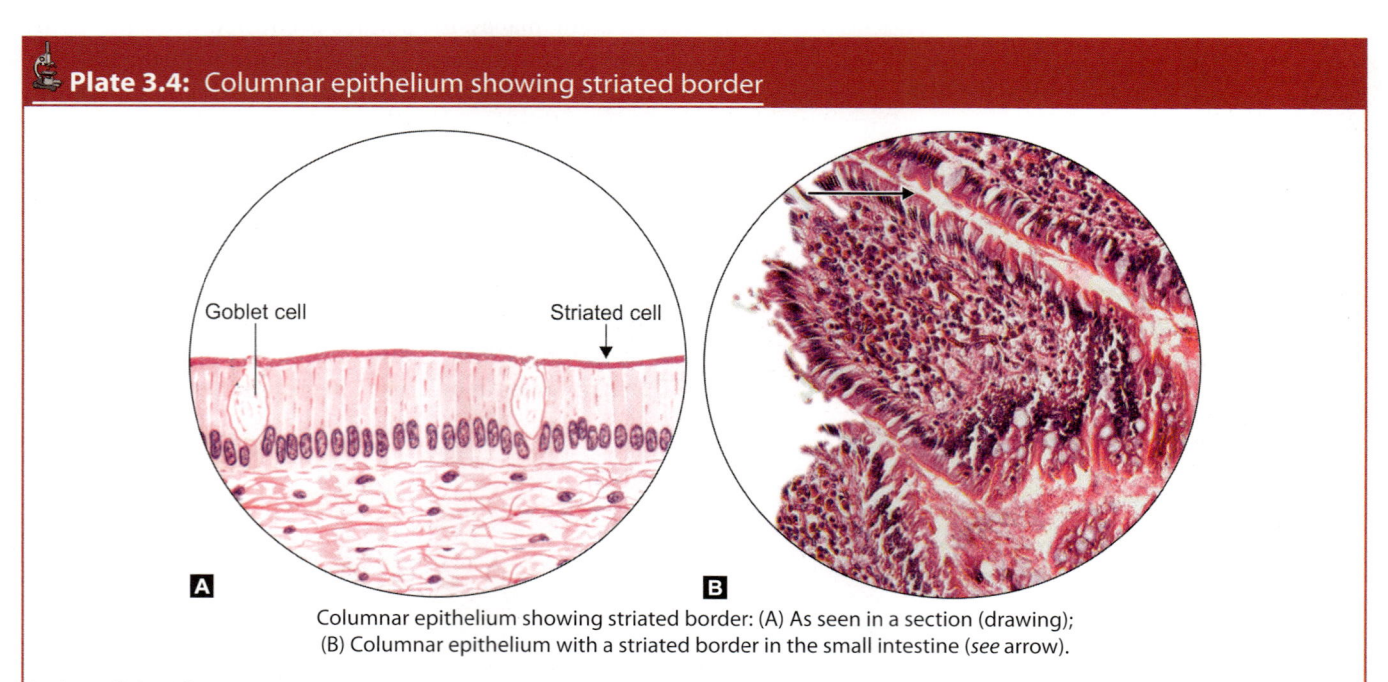

Plate 3.4: Columnar epithelium showing striated border

Columnar epithelium showing striated border: (A) As seen in a section (drawing); (B) Columnar epithelium with a striated border in the small intestine (*see* arrow).

Points of identification
- In some regions the free surfaces of the cells of columnar epithelium show a thickening with vertical striations in it, this is called a striated border
- This is seen typically in the small intestine.

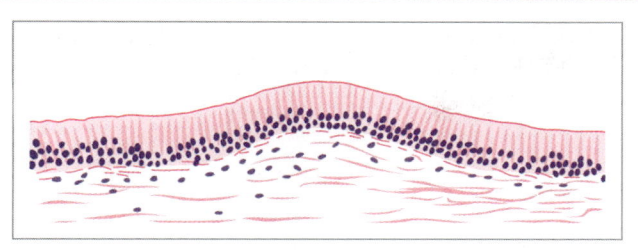

CHAPTER 3: Epithelia and Glands

Fig. 3.6: Pseudostratified columnar epithelium as seen in a section.

movement. At some sites, this epithelium may display stereocilia.

Function

The tall columnar cells are secretory in nature, while the short, basal cells are stem cells which constantly replace the tall cells. The cilia help in clearance of the mucous. The stereocilia help in absorption.

Examples

- Nonciliated pseudostratified columnar epithelium is found in some parts of the auditory tube, the ductus deferens, and the male urethra (membranous and penile parts).
- Ciliated pseudostratified columnar epithelium is seen in the trachea and in large bronchi.
- Pseudostratified columnar epithelium with stereocilia (long microvilli) is seen in epididymis.

Stratified Epithelium

It is stratified more than one layer of cells. It is classified according to the cell shape of the superficial layer as squamous, cuboidal, and columnar.

Stratified Squamous Epithelium

- This type of epithelium is thick and made up of several layers of cells (Plate 3.6 and Fig. 3.7).
- The cells of the deepest (or basal) layer rest on the basement membrane, they are usually columnar in shape. Lying over the columnar cells, there are polyhedral or cuboidal cells. As we pass toward the surface of the epithelium, these cells become progressively more flat, so that the most superficial cells consist of flattened squamous cells.
- Stratified squamous epithelium is found over those surfaces of the body that are subject to friction. As a result

---

Plate 3.5: Pseudostratified ciliated columnar epithelium

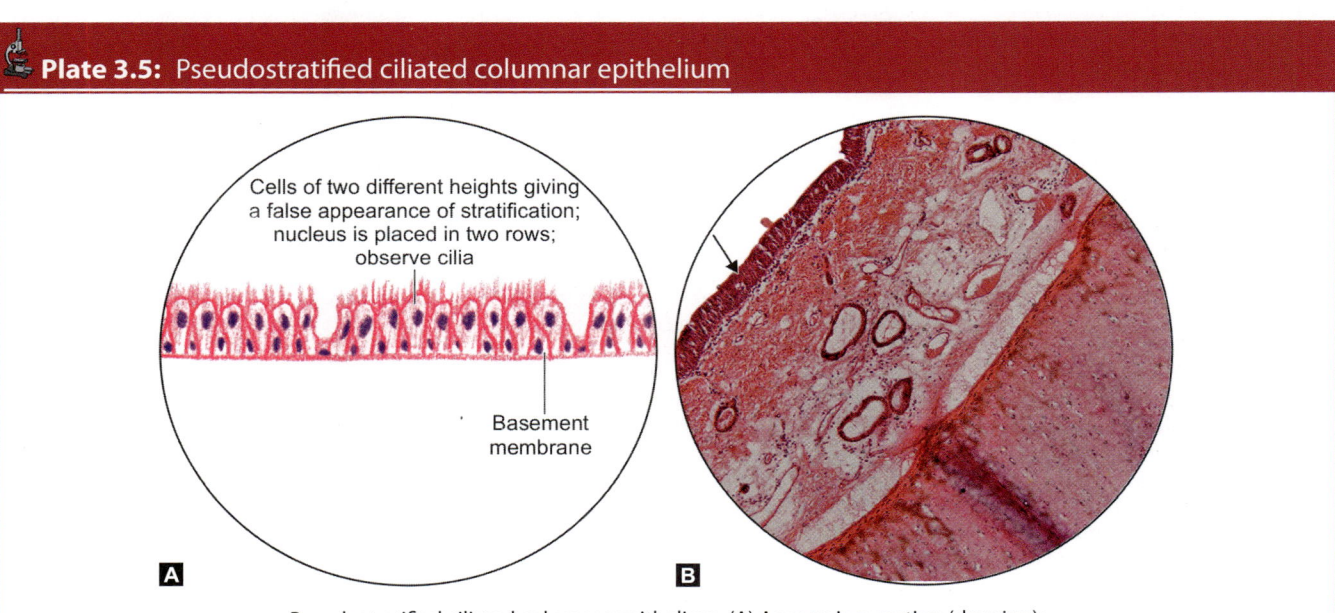

Pseudostratified ciliated columnar epithelium: (A) As seen in a section (drawing); (B) Pseudostratified ciliated columnar epithelium in trachea (photomicrograph) (*see* arrow).

Points of identification
- It is not a true stratified epithelium but appears to be stratified. Normally, in columnar epithelium the nuclei lie in a row, toward the basal part of the cells. Sometimes, however, the nuclei appear to be arranged in two or more layers giving the impression that the epithelium is more than one cell thick
- In some situations, pseudostratified columnar epithelium bears hair-like projections called cilia
- Pseudostratified ciliated columnar epithelium is seen in trachea and in large bronchi.

Plate 3.6: Stratified squamous epithelium

A — Uppermost layer of flattened nucleated cells; Polygonal cells; Basement membrane with columnar cells

B

C — Keratinized layer; Flat nucleated cells; Polygonal cells; Basement membrane with columnar cells

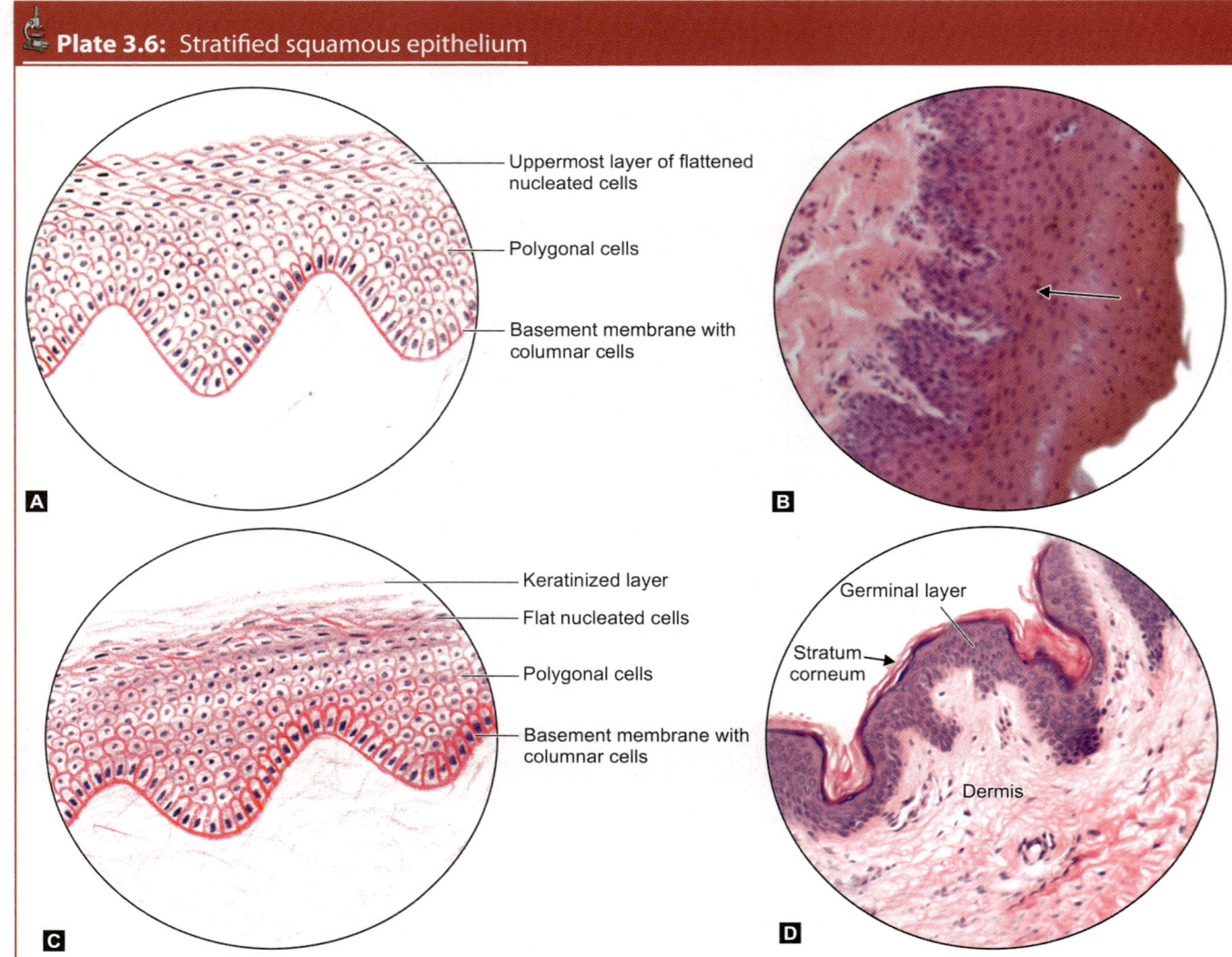

D — Germinal layer; Stratum corneum; Dermis

Stratified squamous epithelium: (A) As seen in a section (drawing); (B) As seen in esophagus (photomicrograph) (see arrow); (C) Keratinized stratified squamous epithelium as seen in skin (drawing); (D) Photomicrograph.

Points of identification
- Although this is called stratified squamous epithelium, only the most superficial cells are squamous (flattened)
- The cells in the deepest (or basal) layer are columnar. In the middle layers, they are polyhedral, while the more superficial layers show increasing degrees of flattening
- The nuclei are oval in the basal layer, rounded in the middle layer, and transversely elongated in the superficial layers
- The surface layer shows squamous cells with flattened nuclei
- This kind of epithelium is seen lining some internal organs, like the esophagus or the vagina.
- Here the deeper layers are covered by additional layers that represent stages in the conversion of cells into nonliving fibers. This process is called keratinization (or cornification)
- The surface layer is made up of keratin which appears as fibers. No cellular outline or nuclei can be seen
- It is seen typically in epidermis of the skin.

CHAPTER 3: Epithelia and Glands

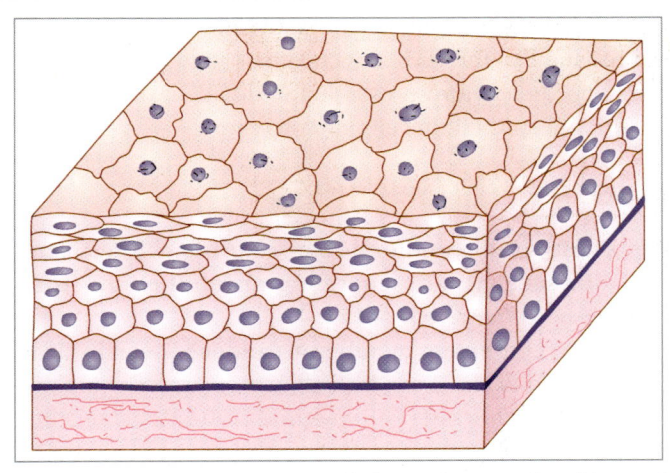

Fig. 3.7: Stratified squamous epithelium. There is a basal layer of columnar cells that rests on the basement membrane. Overlying the columnar cells of this layer, there are a few layers of polygonal cells or rounded cells. Still more superficially, the cells undergo progressive flattening, becoming squamous (schematic representation).

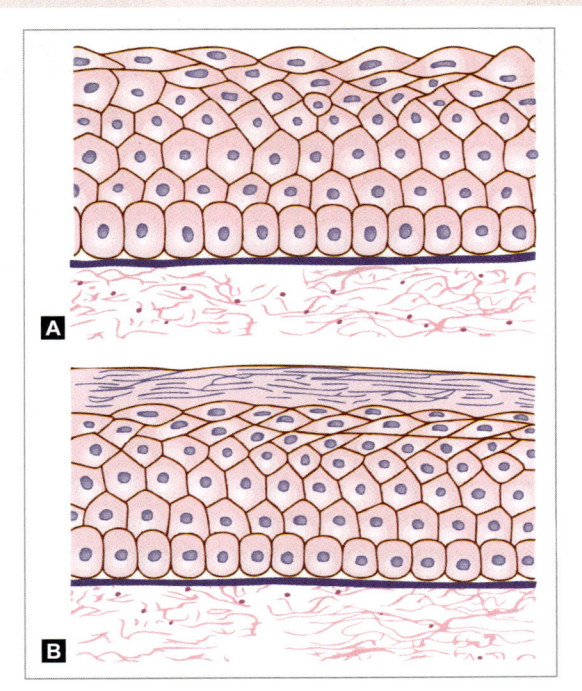

Figs. 3.8A and B: Stratified squamous epithelium. (A) Nonkeratinized; (B) Keratinized (schematic representation).

of friction the most superficial layers are constantly being removed and are replaced by the proliferation of cells from the basal layer. This layer, therefore, shows frequent mitoses.

Stratified squamous epithelium can be divided into two types—(1) *Nonkeratinized* and (2) *Keratinized*.
1. *Nonkeratinized stratified squamous epithelium*: Stratified epithelium, where the surface of the squamous epithelium remains moist, the most superficial cells are living, and nuclei can be seen in them. This kind of epithelium is described as nonkeratinized stratified squamous epithelium (Fig. 3.8A).
   Examples: It is usually wet and is found in lining the mouth, oropharynx, esophagus, true vocal folds, and vagina.
2. *Keratinized stratified squamous epithelium*: *It is similar to nonkeratinized epithelium, except that* epithelial surface is dry, and the most superficial layers of epithelium are composed of dead cells whose nuclei and cytoplasm have been replaced with **keratin**. This kind of epithelium constitutes keratinized stratified squamous epithelium (Fig. 3.8B and Plate 3.6).
   Example: Epithelium covers the skin of whole of the body and forms the epidermis.

Functions
- It is protective in nature
- Keratin prevents dehydration of underlying tissue.

Stratified Cuboidal Epithelium

It consists of only two layers of cuboidal cells. It is found in ducts of sweat glands.

Stratified Columnar Epithelium

It is composed of two layers, polyhedral to cuboidal deeper layer and superficial layer of columnar cells. It is found in conjunctiva of eye, certain large excretory ducts, like pancreas and salivary glands, and regions of male urethra.

Function

Like all stratified epithelia, it is protective in function, and it also helps in conducting the secretion of the glands.

Transitional Epithelium

This is a multilayered epithelium with four to six cells thick and which can contract and expand as needed.
- It is called transitional because it is transitional between stratified squamous and stratified columnar epithelia.
- It differs from stratified squamous epithelium in that the cells at the surface are not squamous. The deepest cells are columnar or cuboidal. The middle layers are made up of polyhedral or pear-shaped cells. The cells

of the surface layer are large and often shaped like an umbrella (Plate 3.7).
- ❖ The superficial cell layer, which lines the lumen, is the only fully differentiated layer of the epithelium.
- ❖ It provides an impenetrable barrier between the lumen and the bloodstream. It is exclusively located in urinary system and named as urothelium.
- ❖ In the urinary bladder, it is seen that cells of transitional epithelium can be stretched considerably without losing their integrity. When stretched, it appears to be thinner, and the cells become flattened (Figs. 3.9A and B).

Example

Transitional epithelium is found in the renal pelvis and calyces, the ureter, the urinary bladder, and part of the urethra. Because of this distribution, it is also called **urothelium**.

Functions

At the surface of the epithelium, the plasma membranes are unusual. Embedded in the lipid layer of the membranes, there are special glycoproteins. It is believed that these glycoproteins make the membrane impervious and resistant to the toxic effects of substances present in urine and thus, afford protection to adjacent tissues. The transitional epithelium cells stretch readily.

▌BASEMENT MEMBRANE

It is a thin, delicate membrane of protein fibers and mucopolysaccharides separating an epithelium from underlying connective tissue.
- ❖ A distinct basement membrane cannot be seen in H&E preparations, but it can be well demonstrated using the periodic acid-Schiff (PAS) method. The latter stains the glycoproteins present in the membrane.
- ❖ Under the EM a basement membrane is seen to have a **basal lamina** (nearest to the epithelial cells) and a **reticular lamina** or **fibroreticular lamina** (consisting of reticular tissue and merging into surrounding connective tissue). The basal lamina is divisible into the **lamina densa** containing fibrils and the **lamina lucida** which appears to be transparent. The lamina lucida lies against the cell membranes of epithelial cells.

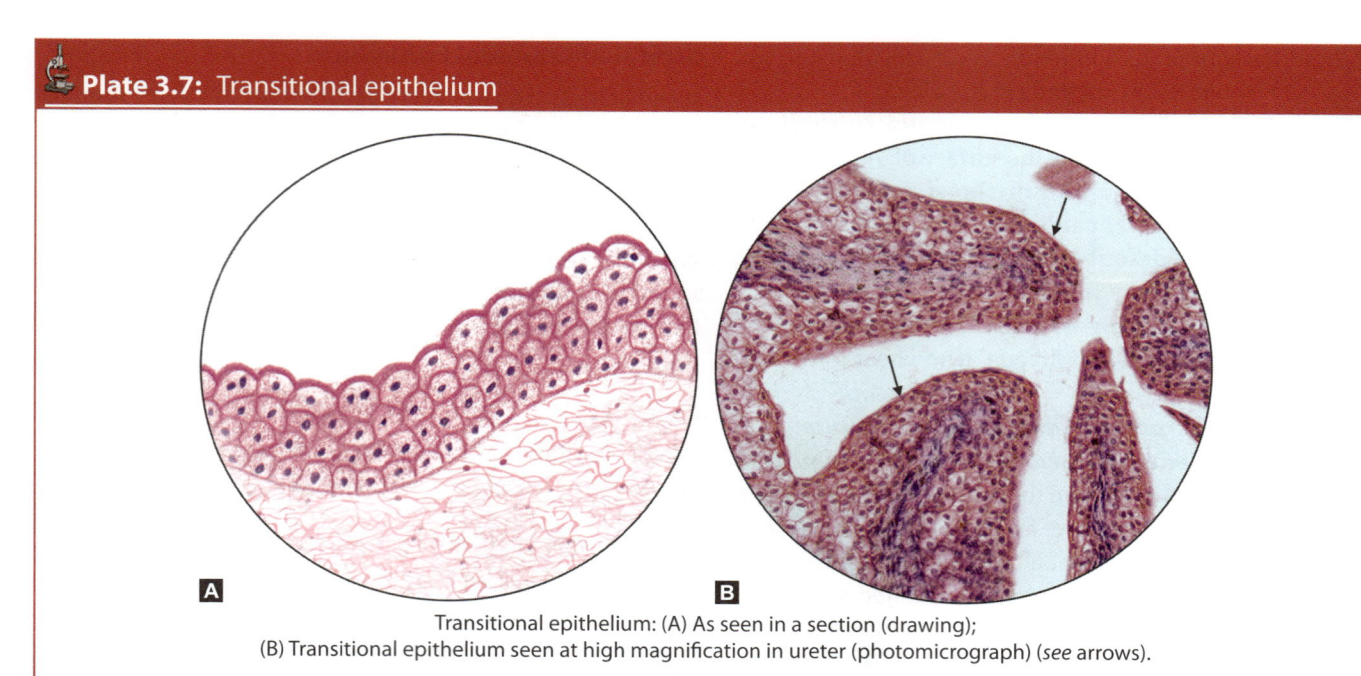

Plate 3.7: Transitional epithelium

Transitional epithelium: (A) As seen in a section (drawing); (B) Transitional epithelium seen at high magnification in ureter (photomicrograph) (*see* arrows).

Points of identification
- ➢ In this type of epithelium, several layers of round nuclei are seen
- ➢ The superficial cells are not flattened but are umbrella shaped
- ➢ Their nuclei appear rounded and may show mitotic figures
- ➢ This epithelium lines many parts of the urinary tract.

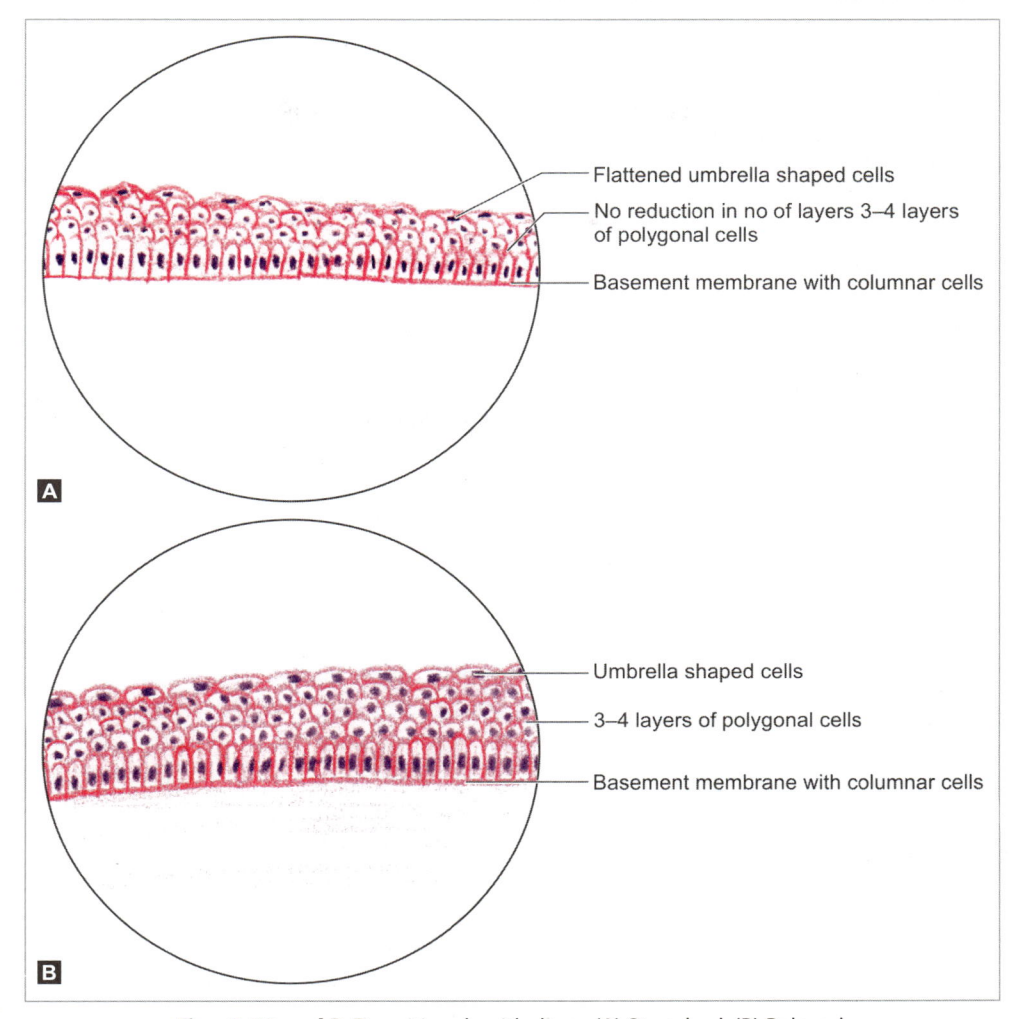

Figs. 3.9A and B: Transitional epithelium: (A) Stretched; (B) Relaxed.

- Basal membrane also present where other cell types come in contact with connective tissues, like muscle, adipose and nervous tissue.
- Main component is type IV collagen fibers, glycoproteins laminin and entactin, and proteoglycans.

Functions of Basement Membrane

- It provides structural support to the cells. It provides adhesion on one side of epithelial cells.
- It acts as a barrier that limits or regulates the exchange of molecules. The barrier function varies with location (because of variations in pore size). Large proteins are prevented from passing out of blood vessels, but (in the lung) diffusion of gases is allowed.
- It influences cell polarity, regulates cell proliferation and differentiation by binding with growth factors, influences cell metabolism, and serves as pathways for cell migration.
- The membranes may influence the regeneration of peripheral nerves after injury and may play a role in re-establishment of the neuromuscular junctions.

PROJECTIONS FROM THE CELL SURFACE

The free or epical surface epithelial cells show projections from the cell surface. The various types of projections are as follows:
- Cilia
- Microvilli
- Stereocilia.

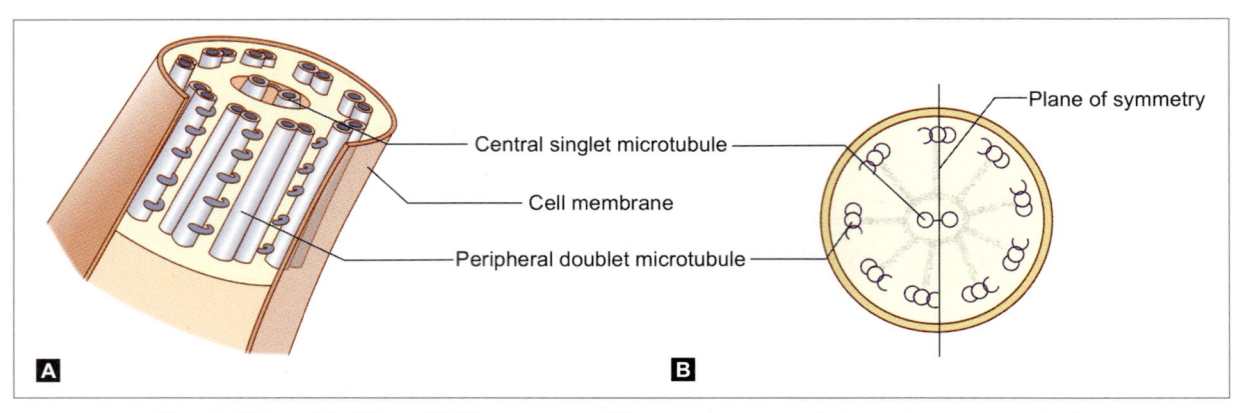

Figs. 3.10A and B: Cilium. (A) Ultrastructure; (B) Internal structure (schematic representation).

Cilia

Cilia are slender, long, motile, microscopic, hair-like structures, or organelles that extend from the epical surface of some epithelial cells. In the living animal, cilia can be seen to be motile.

Structure

- The detailed structure of cilia can only be made out by electron microscopy.
- The free part of each cilium is called the *shaft*. The region of attachment of the shaft to the cell surface is called the *base* (also called the *basal body*, *basal granule*, or *kinetosome*). The free end of the shaft tapers to a tip. Each cilium is 10 μm in length and 0.25 μm in diameter.
- It consists of: (1) an outer covering that is formed by an extension of the cell membrane; and (2) an inner core (*axoneme*) that is formed by microtubules arranged in a definite manner (Figs. 3.10A and B).
- It has a striking similarity to the structure of a centriole. There is a central pair of tubules that is surrounded by nine pairs of tubules. The outer tubules are connected to the inner pair by radial structures (which are like the spokes of a wheel). Other projections pass outward from the outer tubules (Fig. 3.11).
- As the tubules of the shaft are traced toward the tip of the cilium, it is seen that one tubule of each outer pair ends short of the tip so that near the tip each outer pair is represented by one tubule only. Just near the tip, only the central pair of tubules is present.
- At the base of the cilium, one additional tubule is added to each outer pair so that here the nine outer groups of tubules have three tubules each, exactly as in the centriole. Microtubules in cilia are bound with proteins (dynein and nexin). Nexin holds the microtubules together. Dynein molecules are responsible for bending of the tubules, and thereby for the movements of cilia (Fig. 3.11).

Functional Significance

The cilia lining an epithelial surface move in coordination with one another, the total effect being that like a wave. As a result fluid, mucous, or small solid objects lying on the epithelium can be caused to move in a specific direction.

- Movements of cilia lining the respiratory epithelium help to move secretions in the trachea and bronchi toward the pharynx.
- Ciliary action helps in the movement of ova through the uterine tube, and of spermatozoa through the male genital tract.
- In some situations, there are cilia-like structures that perform a sensory function. They may be nonmotile, but can be bent by external influences. Such "cilia" present on the cells in the olfactory mucosa of the nose are called *olfactory cilia*, they are receptors for smell. Similar structures called *kinocilia* are present in some parts of the internal ear.

Note: *Flagella*: These are somewhat larger processes having the same basic structure as cilia. In the human body, the best

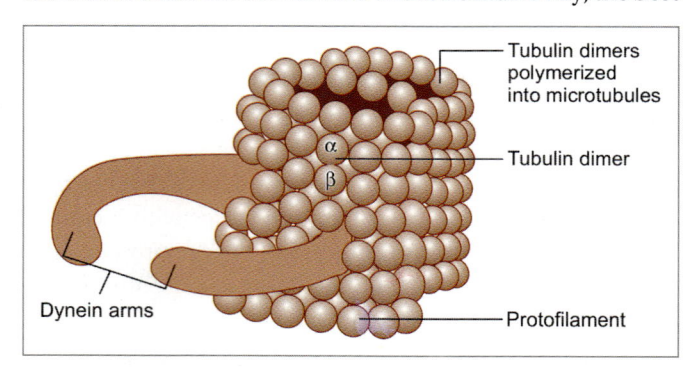

Fig. 3.11: Helical structure of microtubule (schematic representation).

example of a flagellum is the tail of the spermatozoon. The movements of flagella are different from those of cilia. In a flagellum, movement starts at its base. The segment nearest to the base bends in one direction. This is followed by the bending of succeeding segments in opposite directions, so that a wave-like motion passes down the flagellum.

Microvilli

- Microvilli are small finger-like cytoplasmic projections from the free surface of the cell that can be seen by EM measuring 1–2 mm in length and about 75–90 μm in diameter. Microvilli are covered by a polysaccharide surface coat called as **glycocalyx**.
- Each microvillus consists of an outer covering of plasma membrane and a cytoplasmic core in which there are numerous microfilaments (actin filaments). The filaments are continuous with actin filaments of the cell cortex.

Numerous enzymes and glycoproteins, concerned with absorption, have been located in microvilli.

In some places, like epithelial cells lining the small intestine, the microvilli appear to be thickened, the thickening has striations perpendicular to the surface and arranged regularly giving a **striated border appearance.**

In some places, like PCTs of kidney, the microvilli are not arranged so regularly. With the light microscope, the microvilli of such cells give the appearance of a **brush border**.

Functional Significance

Microvilli are nonmotile processes which greatly increase the surface area of the cell and are, therefore, seen most typically at the sites of active absorption, e.g. the intestine, and the PCTs of the kidney (Table 3.1).

Table 3.1: Differences between cilia and microvilli.

Cilia	Microvilli
10 μm in length and 0.25 μm in diameter	1–2 mm in length and about 75–90 μm in diameter
Motile	Nonmotile
Contains 9+2 pattern of microtubules	Contains numerous microfilaments (actin filaments)
Concerned with the movement of ova through uterine tube and movement of secretions in trachea and bronchi toward pharynx	Concerned with absorptive functions
Seen over lining epithelium of respiratory tract and uterine tube.	Seen over intestinal epithelium and proximal convoluted tubule of kidney

Added Information

- *Renewal of epithelial cells*: Epithelial cells have a high turnover rate which is related to their location and function, and the time frame for renewal is constant for a particular cell type. For example, cells of epidermis are constantly being renewed, and it takes about 28 days for complete process from basal layer to keratinization. Small intestine cells are replaced every 4–6 days.
- *Transitional epithelium*:
  ◊ With the EM, the cells of transitional epithelium are seen to be firmly united to one another by numerous desmosomes. Because of these connections, the cells retain their relative position when the epithelium is stretched or relaxed.
  ◊ The cells in the basal layer of transitional epithelium show occasional mitoses, but these are much less frequent than those in stratified squamous epithelium, as there is normally little erosion of the surface. Many cells of the superficial (luminal) layers of the epithelium may contain two nuclei. In some cells, the nucleus is single, but contains multiples of the normal number of chromosomes (i.e. it may be polyploid).
  ◊ According to some workers, all cells of transitional epithelium reach the basal lamina through thin processes. Even though the cells are stratified, they retain a contact with the basement membrane. Hence, this is a transition from unilayered to multilayered epithelium.
- The shape of epithelial cells is related to the amount of contained cytoplasm and organelles. These in turn are related to metabolic activity. Squamous cells are least active. Columnar cells contain abundant mitochondria and endoplasmic reticulum and are highly active.
- Laterally, epithelial cells are in contact with other epithelial cells. The contact between adjoining cells is generally an intimate one because of the presence of desmosomes, zonulae adherens, and zonulae occludens. The intimate contact ensures that materials passing through the epithelium have to pass through the cells, rather than between them.
- Some epithelial cells contain pigment. Such cells are present in the skin, the retina, and the iris.
- Epithelia are generally devoid of blood vessels. Their cells obtain nutrition by diffusion from blood vessels in underlying tissues. In contrast, delicate nerve fibers frequently penetrate into the intervals between epithelial cells.
- Epithelia have considerable capacity for repair after damage. They grow rapidly after injury, to repair the defect.
- It should be remembered that same epithelial cells could have very different functions at different locations. For example, cuboidal cells lining follicles of the thyroid gland have very little in common with cuboidal cells covering the surface of the ovary.
- Epithelial cells in which transport of ions is an important function (e.g. renal tubules) are marked by the presence of basolateral folds, and the presence of large numbers of mitochondria, which provide adenosine triphosphate (ATP) for ion transport. Tight junctions between the cells prevent the passive diffusion of the ions.
- Epithelial cells contain some proteins not present in nonepithelial cells. These include cytokeratin (present in intermediate filaments). Such proteins can be localized using immunohistochemical techniques.

Stereocilia

Stereocilia are very long, nonmotile, and thick microvilli measuring about 5–10 µm in length. They are seen on receptor cells in the internal ear, and on the epithelium of the epididymis. They increase the cells surface area for absorption in epididymis and probably function in signal generation in the hair cells of internal ear.

Note: *Basal folds:* In some cells, the cell membrane over the basal or lateral aspect of the cell shows deep folds (basolateral folds). Like microvilli, basolateral folds are an adaptation to increase cell surface area. Basal folds are seen in renal tubular cells, and in cells lining the ducts of some glands. Lateral folds are seen in absorptive cells lining the gut.

APPLIED HISTOLOGY

- ❖ Each epithelium has its own unique characteristics, location, and morphology which are related to its function. Sometimes, the cell population of an epithelium may undergo metaplasia, transforming it into another epithelial type.
  - *Squamous metaplasia*: Pseudostratified ciliated columnar epithelium of the bronchi in heavy smokers may transform into stratified squamous epithelium.
  - A tumor (or neoplasm) can arise from any tissue if there is uncontrolled growth of cells. Such a tumor may be benign, when it remains localized, or may be malignant. A malignant growth invades surrounding tissues.
  - A malignant tumor arising from an epithelium is called a carcinoma. If it arises from a squamous epithelium, it is a squamous cell carcinoma; and if it arises from glandular epithelium, it is called an adenoma.
  - Quite commonly, cells in tumors resemble those of the tissue from which they are derived, and this is useful in pathological diagnosis. However, in metastases of fast growing tumors, the cells may not show the characteristics of the tissue of origin (undifferentiated tumor), and it may be difficult to find out the location of the primary growth. In such cases, diagnosis can be aided by the localization of proteins that are present only in epithelia. As mentioned earlier, this can be done by using immunohistochemical techniques.
- ❖ *Abnormalities of cilia*:
  - Immotile cilia syndrome (ICS) is an autosomal recessive disease with extensive genetic heterogeneity characterized by abnormal ciliary motion and impaired mucociliary clearance. Ultrastructural and functional defects of cilia result in the lack of effective ciliary motility, causing abnormal mucociliary clearance. As secretions are not removed from respiratory passages, the patient has repeated and severe chest infections. Women affected by the syndrome may be sterile as the movement of ova along the uterine tube is affected. Ciliary proteins are present in the tails of spermatozoa, and an affected male may be sterile because of interference with the motility of spermatozoa.
  - *Kartagener's syndrome*: It is aone type of ICS. It is an autosomal recessive genetic ciliary disorder comprising the triad of situs inversus, chronic sinusitis, and bronchiectasis. The basic problem lies in the defective movement of cilia, leading to recurrent chest infections, ear/nose/throat symptoms, and infertility.
  - Ciliary action is also necessary for normal development of the tissues in embryonic life. Migration of cells during embryogenesis is dependent on ciliary action, and if the cilia are not motile, various congenital abnormalities can result.

SUMMARY

Types	Subtypes	Examples	Main functions
Simple	Squamous	Lung alveoli, blood vessels (endothelium), lining of pericardium, pleura, and peritoneum (mesothelium)	Active transport/exchange
	Cuboidal	Thyroid follicle, covering of ovary	Covering, secretion
	Columnar	Gastrointestinal tract (GIT), gallbladder	Protection, lubrication, absorption, and secretion
Pseudostratified		Trachea, bronchi, nasal cavity	Protection, secretion
Stratified	Stratified squamous keratinized	Skin	Protection
	Stratified squamous nonkeratinized	Oral cavity, esophagus	Protection, secretion
	Stratified cuboidal	Ducts of sweat glands	Absorption, secretion
	Stratified columnar	Conjunctiva, some large excretory ducts, and part of male urethra	Protection, secretion, and absorption
Transitional		Urinary tract from renal calyces to urethra	Protection, distensible

CHAPTER 3: Epithelia and Glands

GLANDS

INTRODUCTION

A gland is a group of cell body that synthesizes substances, like hormones, sweat, saliva, mucus, or acids, for release into the bloodstream or into cavities inside the body or its outer surface.

CHARACTERISTIC FEATURES

- Glands originate from specialized secretory epithelial cells that leave the surface from where they developed and penetrate into the underlying connective tissue and form a basal lamina around them.
- Glandular epithelium is formed by the cells specialized to produce secretion. The secretory molecules are stored in the cells in small membrane-bound vesicle called secretory granules. Glandular cells may synthesize, store, and secrete proteins, lipids, or complexes of carbohydrate and proteins.
- Glands are under hormonal or nervous control through chemical messengers.
- They may be exocrine or endocrine.

CLASSIFICATION OF GLANDS

- **Based on the number of cells**:
  - *Unicellular*: Unicellular glands are interspersed among other (nonsecretory) epithelial cells. They can be found in the epithelium lining the intestines, e.g. goblet cells.
  - *Multicellular*: Most glands are *multicellular*. Such glands develop as diverticula from epithelial surfaces. The "distal" parts of the diverticula develop into secretory elements, while the "proximal" parts form ducts through which secretions reach the epithelial surface, e.g. lacrimal gland, parotid gland, etc.
- **Based on the site of secretion**:
  - *Exocrine glands*: Glands that pour their secretions onto an epithelial surface, directly or through ducts, are called **exocrine glands** (or **externally secreting glands**), e.g. salivary glands.
  - *Endocrine glands*: Some glands lose all contact with the epithelial surface from which they develop, and they pour their secretions into blood. Such glands are called **endocrine glands**, **internally secreting glands**, or **ductless glands**. They secrete the products through the basal lamina onto the blood stream, e.g. thyroid, pituitary, and adrenal.
  - *Paracrine glands*: Glands that secrete a hormone which has effect only in the vicinity of the gland secreting it/hormones that diffuses to short distances to other cells. e.g. enteroendocrine cells of gastrointestinal tract (GIT).

CLASSIFICATION OF EXOCRINE GLANDS (FLOWCHART 3.2)

Unicellular Goblet Cells

It is dispersed individually among the epithelia of the GIT and respiratory tract. They protect the linings. They derive their name from their shape like a goblet. They have thin basal and expanded apical part. Cytoplasm is filled with membrane-bound secretory droplets, which displaces the cytoplasm to the periphery and pushes the nucleus toward base.

Multicellular Exocrine Glands

Multicellular exocrine glands can be further classified as follows:

- **Based on the mode of secretion (Figs. 3.12A to C)**:
  - *Merocrine*: It is a type of exocrine gland. The secretion is released by exocytosis without losing a part of the secretory cell, e.g. salivary glands, some sweat glands, and pancreas.
  - *Apocrine*: Small apical part of the cell is released along with secretory product, e.g. sweat glands in the axillae, areola and nipples of the breast, ear canal, eyelids, wings of the nostril, perianal region, and some parts of the external genitalia.
  - *Holocrine*: As the secretory cell matures, it dies and becomes the secretory product, e.g. sebaceous gland, tarsal gland.
  - *Cytocrine*: In testis, the cells are released as secretion.
- **Based on the nature of secretion**:
  - *Serous gland*: The secretions of serous glands are protein in nature. Cells secrete an enzyme-rich watery fluid. Cells of serous acini are triangular in shape with a rounded nucleus. Their nuclei are centrally placed, e.g. pancreas.
  - *Mucous gland*: In mucous glands, the secretion contains mucopolysaccharides. Cells secrete mucus which is thick, viscous, and jelly-like protective lubricant known as mucin. Cell of mucous acini are tall with flat nuclei at their bases. The lumen of these acini is larger than the serous acini, e.g. goblet cells, minor salivary glands of tongue and palate.

Flowchart 3.2: Classification of glands.

```
                        Glands
          Without ducts    │    With ducts
                ↓                  ↓
           Endocrine           Exocrine
                                  │
                    ┌─────────────┴─────────────┐
                    ↓                           ↓
               Unicellular                 Multicellular
                    │
               Goblet cell
```

- On the basis of number of ducts that drain the gland
  - Simple
  - Compound
- On the basis of shape of the secretory unit
  - Tubular
  - Acinar
  - Alveolar
- On the basis of nature of secretory product
  - Serous
  - Mucous
  - Mixed
- On the basis of secretory mechanism
  - Merocrine
  - Apocrine
  - Holocrine

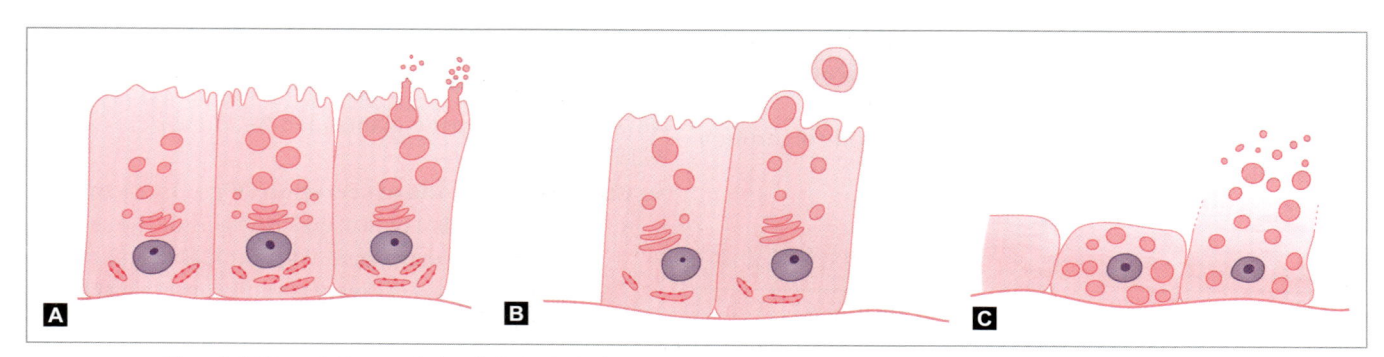

Figs. 3.12A to C: Types of glands based on the manner in which their secretions are poured out of the cells. (A) Merocrine; (B) Apocrine; (C) Holocrine (schematic representation).

- **Mixed gland**: Gland contains acini that secrete both mucus and serous secretions, e.g. submandibular and sublingual glands.
- ❖ **Based on the branching of ducts**:
  - **Simple**: All the secretory cells of an exocrine gland discharge into one duct, e.g. gastric glands, sweat glands, etc.
  - **Compound**: There are a number of groups of secretory cells, and each group discharging into its own duct. These ducts unite to form larger ducts that ultimately drain onto an epithelial surface, e.g. parotid gland, pancreas, etc.
- ❖ **Based on the shape of the secretory unit**: Both in simple and in compound glands, the secretory cells may be arranged in various ways:
  - **Tubular glands**: Glands with secretory unit tubular in shape. The tube may be straight, coiled, or branched, e.g. gastric glands.
  - **Acinar glands**: Glands with secretory unit round or oval in shape, e.g. salivary glands.
  - **Alveolar glands**: Glands with secretory unit flask-shaped. However, it may be noted that the terms acini and alveoli are often used as if they were synonymous. Glands in which the secretory elements are greatly distended are called **saccular glands**.

Note: Combinations of the earlier may be present in a single gland. From what has been said earlier, it will be seen that an exocrine gland may be:

- ❖ Unicellular
- ❖ Simple tubular
- ❖ Simple alveolar (or acinar)
- ❖ Compound tubular
- ❖ Compound alveolar
- ❖ Compound tubuloalveolar (or racemose).

CHAPTER 3: Epithelia and Glands

Some further subdivisions of these are shown in Figures 3.13A to I.

STRUCTURAL ORGANIZATION

Exocrine Glands

All exocrine glands have basically the same structural organization consisting of three components—(1) parenchyma, (2) stroma, and (3) duct system.

- *Parenchyma*: The secretory cells of a gland constitute its *parenchyma*.
- *Stroma*: The connective tissue in which the parenchyma lies is called the *stroma*. The glandular tissue is often divisible into lobules separated by connective tissue septa. Aggregations of lobules may form distinct lobes. The connective tissue covering the entire gland forms a *capsule* for it. Blood vessels and nerves pass along the connective tissue septa to reach the secretory elements. Their activity is under nervous or hormonal control (Fig. 3.14).
- *Duct system*: The ducts convey the secretory product of the gland. When a gland is divided into lobes, the ducts draining it may be *intralobular* (lying within a lobule), *interlobular* (lying in the intervals between lobules), or *interlobar* (lying between adjacent lobes), in increasing order of size (Fig. 3.14).

Endocrine Glands

- They are the sources of many of the body's chemical messengers, known as **hormones** that act at a distance from their origin.
- They are very varied in their size, location, and appearance.
- Many are solid organs, but few are made up of widely distributed single cells.
- Several endocrine glands consist of more than one type of secretory cell and may release more than one hormone product.
- They can be (a) individual cells (unicellular glands), e.g. enteroendocrine cells; (b) endocrine tissue in

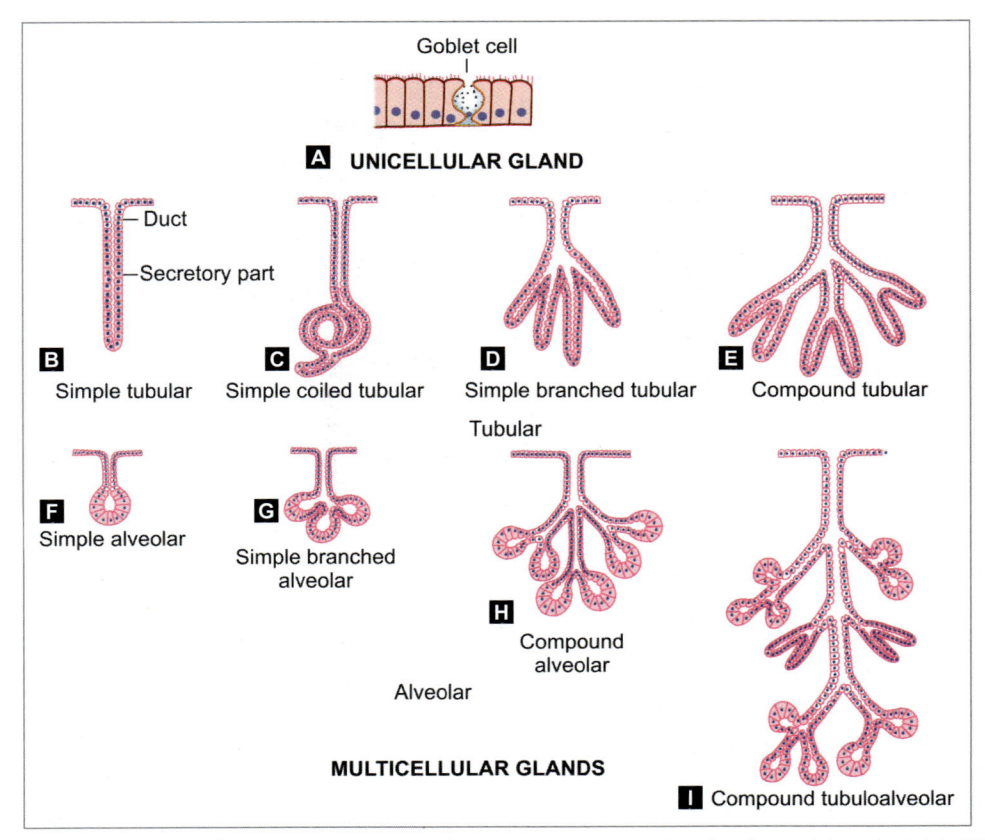

Figs. 3.13A to I: Scheme to show various ways in which the secretory elements of a gland may be organized. (A) Unicellular gland; (B to G) Multicellular glands with a single duct are simple glands; and (H and I) Multicellular glands with branching duct system are compound glands.

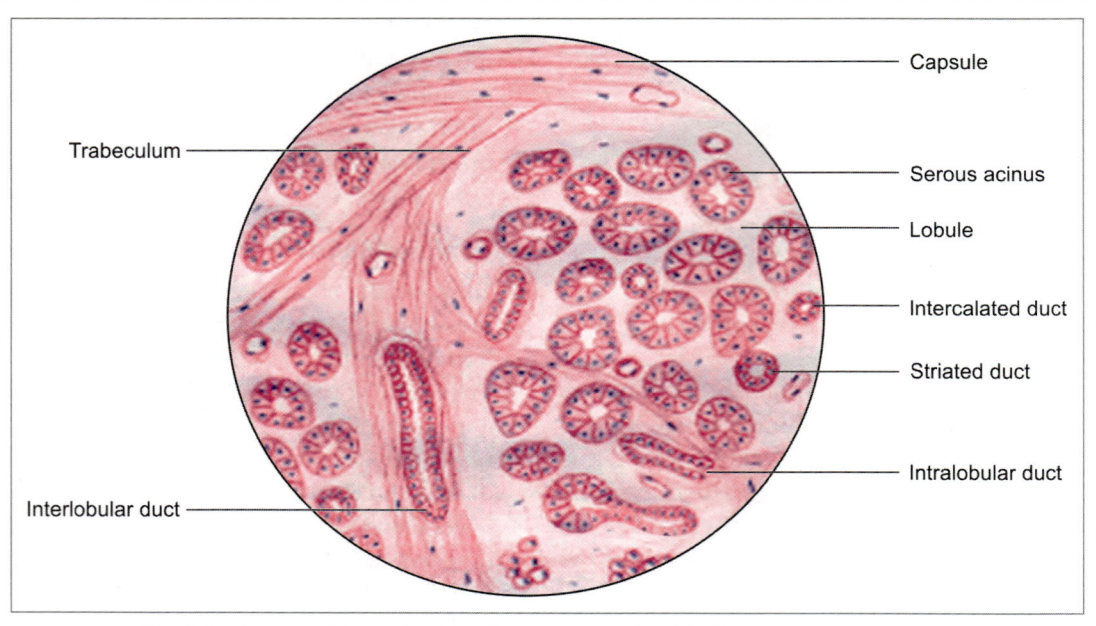

Fig. 3.14: Structural organization of an exocrine gland (schematic representation).

mixed glands (both endocrine and exocrine) as seen in pancreas and male and female reproductive organs; and (c) separate endocrine organs, e.g. pituitary gland, thyroid glands, parathyroid glands, and adrenal glands (Fig. 3.15).

- **Types:**
  a. ***Cord and clump type***: Endocrine glands are usually arranged in cords or in clumps that are intimately related to a rich network of blood capillaries or of sinusoids
  b. ***Follicular type***: In some cases (for example, the thyroid gland), the cells may form rounded follicles.
- Endocrine cells and their blood vessels are supported by delicate connective tissue, and are usually surrounded by a capsule.

Diffuse Neuroendocrine System

The diffuse neuroendocrine system produces paracrine and endocrine hormones. They are widely spread throughout the digestive tract and in the respiratory system, they are interspersed among other secretory cells. Cells are capable of taking up precursors of amines and decarboxylating amino acids, and they are also called amine precursor uptake and decarboxylation (**APUD**) cells. The cells are stained with silver salts so they are also called **argentaffin** and **argyophil** cells.

DEVELOPMENT OF GLANDS

- Glands, both exocrine and endocrine, develop as diverticula of the epithelium (Fig. 3.15).
- The *exocrine* develops as a solid bud from the epithelium into the underlying connective tissue. Soon it elongates, undergoes canalization, and displays a secretory and conducting portion. The conducting part forms the duct and is continuous with the epithelium. Hence, an endocrine gland discharges its secretions through a duct.
- *Endocrine gland* also develops in a similar manner to exocrine gland, but with further development, it breaks the continuity with overlying epithelium. It appears as a

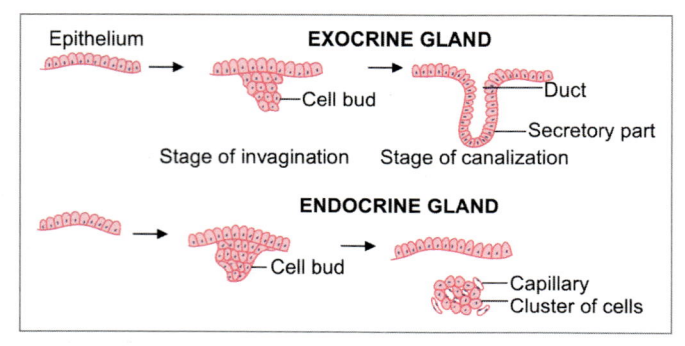

Fig. 3.15: Development of glands (schematic representation).

clump of cells. Soon these groups of cells get surrounded by blood vessels into which they pour their secretions.

Note: In this chapter, we have considered the general features of glands. Further details of the structure of exocrine and endocrine glands will be considered while studying individual glands.

STRUCTURE OF ACINI

Epithelia in secretory portions of glands show specializations of structure depending upon the nature of secretion as follows (Table 3.2):

- Cells that are protein secreting (e.g. hormone-producing cells) have a well-developed rough endoplasmic reticulum (ER), and a supranuclear Golgi complex. Secretory granules often fill the apical portions of the cells. The staining characters of the granules differ in cells producing different secretions (the cells being described as acidophil, basophil, etc.).
- Mucin-secreting cells have a well-developed rough ER (where the protein component of mucin is synthesized) and a very well-developed Golgi complex (where proteins are glycosylated).
- Steroid-producing cells are characterized by the presence of extensive smooth ER and prominent mitochondria.

Serous Cells

- Serous cells are usually arranged in the form of rounded acini. As a result, each cell is roughly pyramidal having a broad base and a narrow apex with a single, round, and basally located nucleus (Figs. 3.16A to C).
- Some microvilli and pinocytotic vesicles are seen at the apex of the cell. The lumen of the acinus often extends for some distance between adjacent cells: these extensions are called *intercellular secretory canaliculi*. Deep to these canaliculi, the cell membranes of adjoining cells are united by tight junctions. Deep to these junctions, the lateral cell margins show folds that interdigitate with those of adjoining cells. The apical cytoplasm contains secretory granules that are small, homogeneous, and electron dense. The cytoplasm also contains a prominent Golgi complex and abundant rough ER, both features indicating considerable synthetic activity. Mitochondria, lysosomes, and microfilaments are also present.

Mucous Cells

- Mucous cells are usually arranged in the form of tubular secretory elements (Figs. 3.16A to C). The cells lining mucous cells tend to be columnar rather than pyramidal with an elongated nucleus at the basal part of the cell.

Table 3.2: Comparison between serous and mucous acini.	
Serous acini	*Mucous acini*
Triangular cells with rounded nucleus at the base. Cell boundaries are indistinct	Tall cells with flat nucleus at the base. Cell boundaries are distinct
Contain zymogen granules	Contain mucoid material
Darkly stained with H & E (because of the presence of zymogen granules, the color varies from pink to dark purple)	Lightly stained and appear empty with hematoxylin and eosin (H & E)
Thin watery secretion	Thick mucoid secretion
Example: Parotid gland	*Example:* Sublingual gland

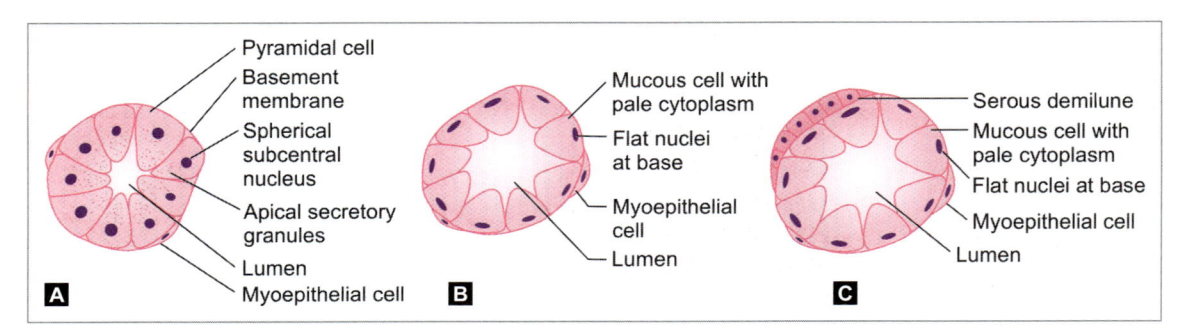

Figs. 3.16A to C: Types of acini. (A) Serous; (B) Mucous; (C) Mucous acini with serous demilune (schematic representation).

- Crescents present in relation to them are located at the ends of the tubules. Their secretory granules are large and ill defined. Rough ER and Golgi complex are similar to those in serous cells, but microvilli, foldings of plasma membrane, and intercellular canaliculi are not usually seen.

Seromucous Cells

From the point of view of ultrastructure, many cells of salivary glands are intermediate between serous and mucous cells. They are referred to as *seromucous cells*. Most of the cells identified as serous with light microscopy in the parotid and submandibular glands are really seromucous. The secretions of all types of salivary secretory cells contain protein–carbohydrate complexes. Their concentration is lowest in the cases of serous cells, very high in mucous cells, and with widely differing concentrations in seromucous cells.

APPLIED HISTOLOGY

- Neoplasms can arise from the epithelium lining a gland. A benign growth arising in a gland is an **adenoma**; and a malignant growth is an **adenocarcinoma**.
- **Sialorrhea (ptyalism)**: Increased flow of saliva is termed sialorrhea or ptyalism.
- **Xerostomia**: Decreased salivary flow is termed xerostomia.
- **Sialadenitis**: Inflammation of salivary glands is called as sialadenitis.
- **Tumors of salivary glands**:
  a. *Pleomorphic adenoma (mixed salivary tumor)*: It is the most common tumor of major and minor salivary glands. It is characterized by pleomorphic or mixed appearance in which there are epithelial elements present in a matrix of mucoid, myxoid, and chondroid tissue;
  b. *Mucoepidermoid carcinoma*: It is the most common malignant salivary gland tumor. The tumor is composed of combination of four types of cells: (1) mucin-producing, (2) squamous, (3) intermediate, and (4) clear cells. Well-differentiated tumors have predominance of mucinous cells, while poorly differentiated have more solid and infiltrative pattern; and
  c. Apudomas are tumors arising from polypeptide-secreting cells of the diffuse neuroendocrine system.

SUMMARY

Classification based on	Subtypes	Description	Examples
Unicellular	Goblet cells	Single cell with upper portion appears empty (as mucus gets washed out while staining) and basal scanty cytoplasm with nucleus	Epithelium lining the intestines
Multicellular			
Type of ducts	Simple	Only one duct	Gastrointestinal (GIT)
	Compound	Branching of ducts	Salivary glands
Shape of secretory unit	Acinar	Glands with secretory unit round or oval in shape	Salivary glands
	Tubular	Secretory unit tubular in shape. The tube may be straight, coiled, or branched	Gastric glands
	Alveolar	Glands with secretory unit flask shaped. However, it may be noted that the terms acini and alveoli are often used as if they were synonymous	
Mode of secretion	Merocrine	The secretion is released by exocytosis	Salivary glands, some sweat glands, and pancreas
	Apocrine	Apical part of the cell is lost	Sweat glands in the axillae, areola and nipples of the breast, ear canal, eyelids, wings of the nostril, perianal region, and some parts of the external genitalia
	Holocrine	Whole cell is discharged as secretion	Sebaceous gland, tarsal gland
Nature of secretion	Serous	Secretion is protein in nature and watery	Pancreas
	Mucous	Cells secrete mucus rich in mucopolysaccharides, which is thick, viscous, and jelly-like protective lubricant known as mucin	Goblet cells, minor salivary glands of tongue and palate
	Mixed	Both mucus and serous acini present	Submandibular and sublingual glands

Exocrine gland may be: Unicellular, simple tubular, simple alveolar (or acinar), compound tubular, compound alveolar, and compound tubuloalveolar (or racemose)

CHAPTER 3: Epithelia and Glands

MULTIPLE CHOICE QUESTIONS

1. Stratified squamous epithelium tissues are present in:
    a. Thyroid gland and trachea
    b. Lungs and kidneys
    c. Urinary bladder and kidneys
    d. Mouth and esophagus
2. Transitional epithelium is present in:
    a. Stomach
    b. Urinary bladder
    c. Uterus
    d. Lungs
3. What do you call the simple squamous epithelium that lines the blood vessels?
    a. Epithelioid tissue
    b. Mesothelium
    c. Endothelium
    d. Transitional
4. What cell type makes up the mucosa of the gallbladder?
    a. Simple cuboidal
    b. Simple columnar
    c. Stratified squamous
    d. Transitional
5. What forms the brush border?
    a. Microvilli
    b. Cilia
    c. Stereocilia
    d. Flagella
6. Reproductive cells (germinal epithelium) are made up of which of the following epithelial tissue?
    a. Cuboidal
    b. Columnar
    c. Squamous
    c. Sensory
7. Urethra, vagina, and esophagus have a common inner lining of:
    a Squamous epithelium
    b. Ciliated epithelium
    c. Columnar epithelium
    d. Stratified squamous epithelium
8. Pavement epithelium is another name for:
    a. Simple cuboidal epithelium
    b. Simple ciliated epithelium
    c. Simple squamous epithelium
    d. Stratified epithelium
9. All of the following are the characteristic of epithelial tissues; *except*:
    a. They are highly vascular
    b. They rest on basement membrane
    c. They have very little intercellular spaces
    d. Cells have surface modifications
10. Outer layer of skin is made up of keratinized epithelium, this is because:
    a. It is exposed thus, subjected to wear and tear
    b. It covers the whole body
    c. It is thick
    d. It prevents the entry of pathogens
11. Epithelial tissues arise from:
    a. Ectoderm
    b. Endoderm
    c. Mesoderm
    d. All of the above
12. Goblet cell is a ____type of gland
    a. Mucus
    b. Serous
    c. Holocrine
    d. Apocrine
13. The cells which is contractile and present in acini or ducts are:
    a. Serous
    b. Mucus
    c. Goblet
    d. Myoepithelial
14. Salivary gland is unique in that, its secretion are controlled by:
    a. Hormones
    b. Nerves
    c. Chemicals
    d. All of the above
15. Sublingual gland is ____ type of gland.
    a. Serous
    b. Mucous
    c. Mixed
    d. None of the above
16. Which of the following is correct about serous glands?
    a. They are specialized for the synthesis, storage, and secretion of proteins
    b. They contain secretory granules in the apical cytoplasm and the secretion of granule content occurs by exocytosis
    c. Serous cells are pyramidal in shape
    d. All of the above
17. Serous demilunes are seen in which of the gland?
    a. Pancreas
    b. Submandibular
    c. Liver
    d. Gastric
18. Identify this
    a. Serous acini
    b. Mucous acini
    c. Serous demilunes
    d. Intercalated duct
19. When the whole cell disintegrates to release the secretion, it is called as ____ type of glands.
    a. Merocrine
    b. Apocrine
    c. Holocrine
    d. Cytocrine
20. Sebaceous gland is a type of:
    a. Merocrine
    b. Apocrine
    c. Holocrine
    d. Cytocrine
21. Interlobular ducts are lined by which of the epithelium?
    a. Squamous
    b. Cuboidal
    c. Columnar
    d. Pseudostratified

Answers

1. d	2. b	3. c	4. b	5. a	6. a	7. d	8. c	9. a
10. a	11. d	12. a	13. d	14. d	15. c	16. d	17. b	18. b
19. c	20. c	21. c						

CHAPTER 4

General Connective Tissue

Learning objectives

To study the:
- General features
- Classification of connective tissue (CT)
- Components of CT
- Different forms of connective tissue
- Functions of CT
- Connective tissue with special properties
- Applied histology

IDENTIFICATION POINTS

Loose areolar tissue
- Connective tissue (CT) components seen—fibers, cells, and ground substance
- Areolar pockets are seen due to loose arrangement of components
- Collagen fibers seen—arranged in bundles and are unbranched
- Elastic fibers—branched, single, and wavy
- Fibrocytes or blasts are seen dispersed among fibers
- Adipocytes are seen in groups.

Adipose tissue
- Signet ring-shaped cells seen—fat deposit pushes the cytoplasm to periphery with only bulge seen due to nucleus
- Cells arranged together in groups pressing against each other with thin rim of cytoplasm are seen
- Blood vessels are seen.

GENERAL FEATURES

- The term **connective tissue (CT)** is applied to a tissue that fills the interstices between more specialized elements.
- They are predominantly composed of intercellular substance (matrix) secreted by its cells.
- Present in almost every part of the body, it is conspicuous in some regions and scanty in others.
- This kind of CT is referred to as **general CT.**
- They are mesodermal in origin.
- They also have trophic and morphogenetic roles in growth and differentiation of surrounding tissues, mediate exchange of nutrients, metabolites, and waste products.

CLASSIFICATION OF CONNECTIVE TISSUE

Connective tissue can assume various forms depending upon the nature of the ground substance, and of the type of fibers and cells present. There are various kinds of classification of CTs. Based on the structure and function, it can be classified into:

- *Embryonic/fetal CT*:
  - Mucoid CT
  - Mesenchyme
- *Connective tissue proper*:
  - Loose CT
  - Dense CT—regular and irregular
- *Specialized CT*:
  - Cartilage
  - Bone
  - Adipose tissue
  - Blood
  - Hemolymphatic tissue.

COMPONENTS OF CONNECTIVE TISSUE

Connective tissue = Cells + Intercellular matrix (Fibers + Ground substance) (Fig. 4.1 and Flowchart 4.1).

Cells *are intrinsic components of CT. They can be broadly classified into two groups:*

1. *Resident cells/intrinsic component cells*: They are responsible for production and maintenance of extracellular matrix.

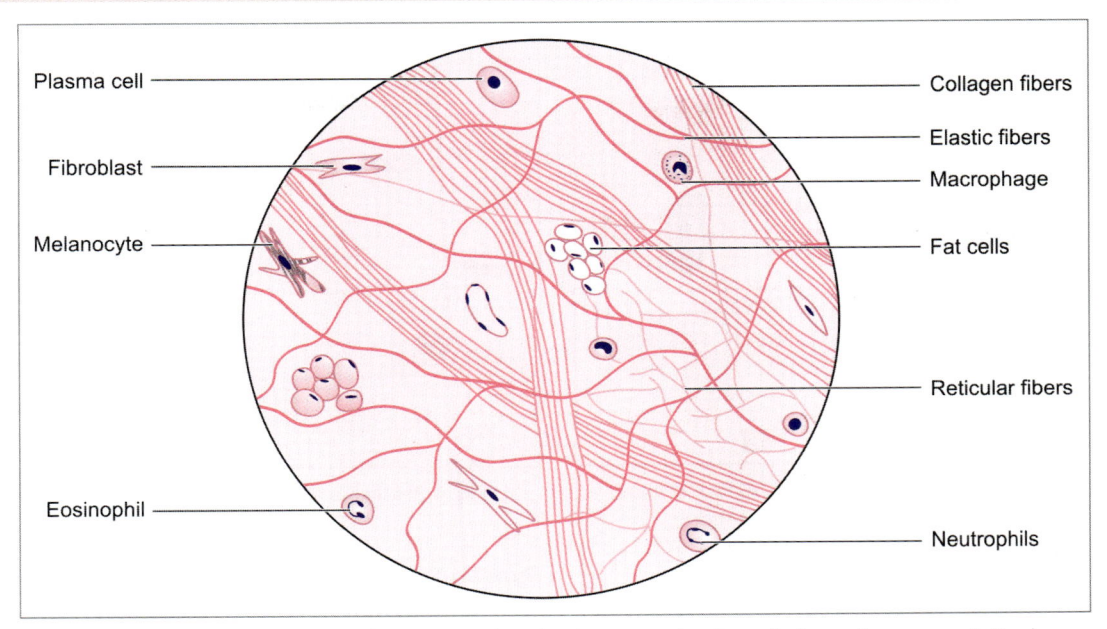

Fig. 4.1: Stretch preparation of omentum showing loose areolar tissue (schematic representation).

Flowchart 4.1: Basic components of connective tissue.

```
                Components of
                connective tissue
         ┌───────────┼───────────┐
         ▼           ▼           ▼
       Fibers       Cells    Intercellular
    • Collagen fibers         ground
    • Reticular fibers        substance
    • Elastic fibers
              ┌──────────┴──────────┐
              ▼                     ▼
    Intrinsic component cells   Migrant (extrinsic) cells
    • Fibroblasts               • Macrophage cells
    • Undifferentiated          • Mast cells
      mesenchymal cells         • Lymphocytes
    • Pigment cells             • Plasma cells
    • Adipocytes                • Monocytes
                                • Eosinophils
```

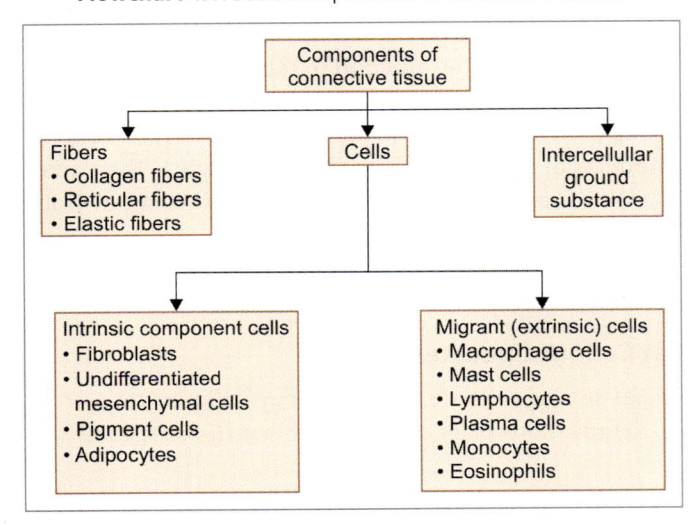

- Fibroblast
- Adult stem cells
- Fat cells
- Fixed macrophages
- Mast cells
- Pigment cells.

2. *Wandering/fluctuating/migrating cells extrinsic:* They bring out tissue reaction to injuries.
    - Free macrophages
    - Leukocytes
    - Plasma cells
    - Monocytes.

Fibroblasts

❖ These are the most numerous cells of CT.
❖ They are called fibroblasts because they are concerned with the production of fibers. Fibroblasts are present in close relationship to collagen fibers.
❖ Where associated with reticular fibers, they are usually called ***reticular cells***.
❖ In tissue sections the cells appear spindle-shaped, and the nucleus appears to be flattened. When seen from the surface, the cells show branching processes (Figs. 4.2A and B).
❖ The nucleus is large, euchromatic, and has prominent nucleoli.
❖ They are called fibrocytes when the cytoplasm is scanty, organelles are few, and the nucleus is heterochromatic.
❖ In contrast to fibrocytes, active fibroblasts have abundant cytoplasm (characteristic of cells actively engaged in protein synthesis). The endoplasmic reticulum, the Golgi complex, and mitochondria become much more conspicuous.
❖ Myofibroblasts share the features of fibroblasts and smooth muscle. They are elongated spindle-shaped cells with the bundles of actin filaments.

Functions

❖ Fibroblasts become very active when there is a need to lay down collagen fibers; for example, during wound repair, where they form granulation tissue with budding capillaries.

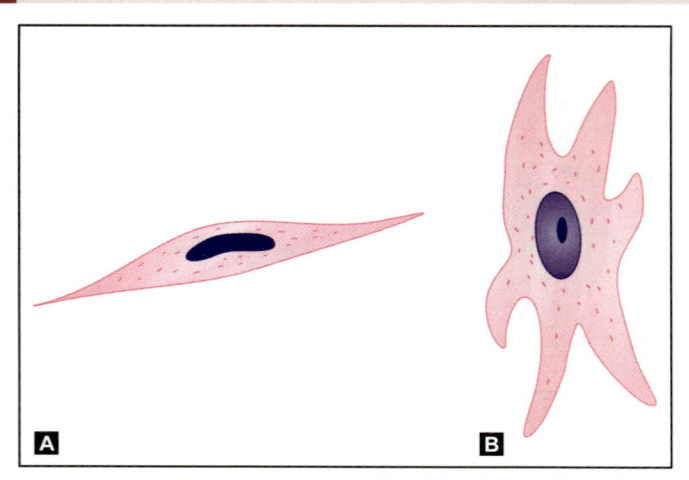

Figs. 4.2A and B: Structure of a fibroblast. (A) Profile view; (B) Structure view (schematic representation).

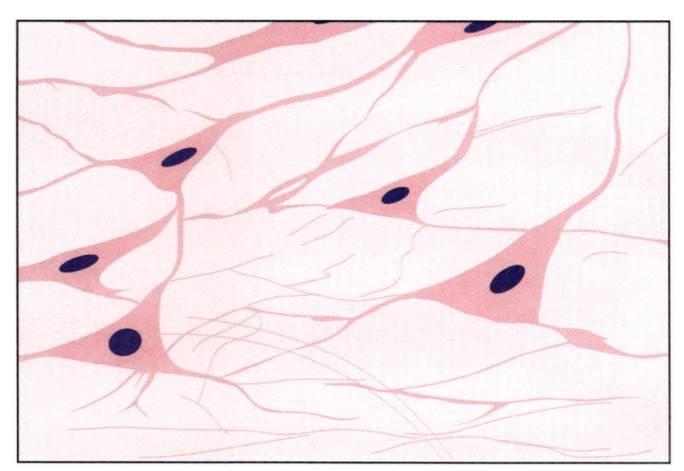

Fig. 4.3: Mesenchymal cells (schematic representation).

- They also produce ground substance.
- Fibroblasts are targets of various growth factors which influence cell growth and differentiation.
- In glands and lymphoid tissue, fibroblasts with reticular fibers form fibrocellular network called reticular tissue.
- Myofibroblasts help in wound contraction (Fig. 4.3).

Undifferentiated Mesenchymal Cells/Stem Cells

- Embryonic CT is called *mesenchyme*.
- It is made up of stellate small cells with slender branching processes that join to form a fine network.

Pigment Cells

- They are most abundant in CT of the skin, and in the choroid and iris of the eyeball.
- Pigment cells are easily distinguished as they contain brown pigment (melanin) in their cytoplasm and are called melanocytes.
- Melanocytes have rounded cell bodies and long processes. They contain melanin granules in a membrane-bound form called—melanosomes.
- The cells which cannot synthesize melanin but engulf them are called chromatophore (when they engulf melanin—melanophore).
- In contrast to melanocytes, *chromatophores* or *melanophores* are star-shaped (stellate) with long branching processes. They are probably modified fibroblasts.
- When melanin pigment is brownish-black, it is called—eumelanin and pheomelanin when it is reddish-yellow.

Functions

- Variations in the number of pigment cells, and in the amount of pigment in them account for the differences in the skin color of different races, and in different individuals (Fig. 4.4).
- Pigment cells prevent light from reaching other cells. The importance of this function in relation to the eyeball is obvious.
- Pigment cells in the skin protect deeper tissues from the effects of light (especially ultraviolet light). The darker skin of races living in tropical climates is an obvious adaptation for this purpose.
- Albinism is a condition where there is a complete absence of melanin pigment.

Fat Cells (Adipocytes)

- Fat-storing cells are called adipocytes/lipocytes.
- Aggregations of fat cells constitute *adipose tissue*.

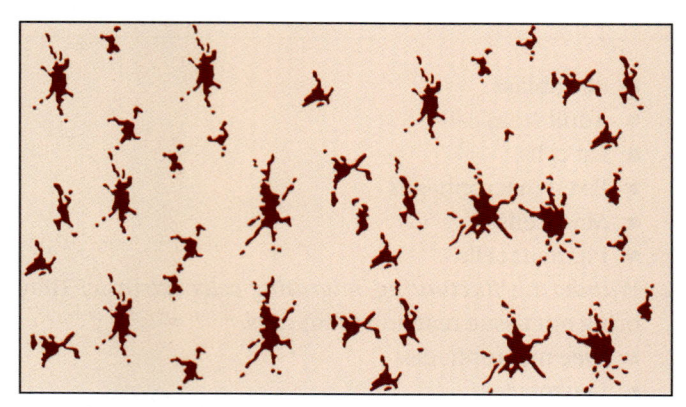

Fig. 4.4: Pigment cells (schematic representation).

CHAPTER 4: General Connective Tissue

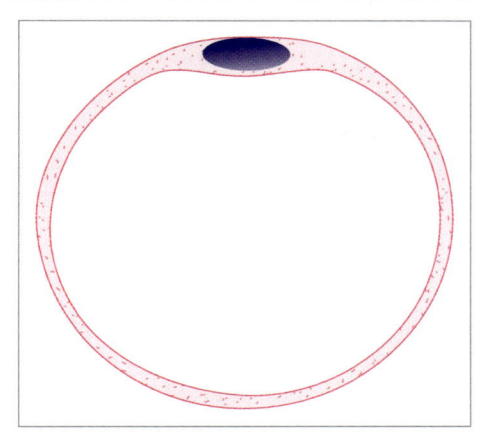

Fig. 4.5: Fat cell (schematic representation).

- Each fat cell contains a large droplet of fat, which almost fills it (Fig. 4.5). As a result, the cell becomes rounded (when several fat cells are closely packed they become polygonal because of mutual pressure).
- The cytoplasm of the cell forms a thin layer just deep to the plasma membrane.
- The nucleus is pushed against the plasma membrane and is flattened.
- In routine slide preparation, fat is dissolved by organic solvent, thus giving adipocytes signet ring appearance.
- Adipocytes are incapable of division.
- For more details, see the "Adipose Tissue" section.

Macrophage Cells

- Macrophage cells of CT are also called **histiocytes** or **clasmatocytes** (Fig. 4.6).
- Macrophage cells of CT belong to **mononuclear phagocyte system (MPS)**.
- They are derived from monocytes which migrate from blood.
- They have the ability to phagocytose (eat up) unwanted material (both organic and inorganic). Macrophages can be demonstrated by injecting the tissue with India ink (or trypan blue, or lithium carmine) particles of it are taken up into the cytoplasm of macrophages, thus making them easy to recognize.
- Macrophages are usually described as "fixed" when they are attached to fibers. Fixed macrophages resemble fibroblasts in appearance.
- They are called motile/nomadic macrophages when they are free, not attached to fibers. Free macrophages are rounded and have regular form.
- However, all macrophages are capable of becoming mobile when suitably stimulated.

- The nuclei of macrophages are smaller, heterochromatic and stain more intensely than those of fibroblasts. They are often kidney-shaped (Fig. 4.6).
- Cytoplasm is mildly basophilic. With the electron microscope (EM), the cytoplasm is seen to contain numerous lysosomes that help in "digesting" material phagocytosed by the macrophage.
- Sometimes, macrophages may fuse together to form multinucleated **giant cells**.
- Apart from direct phagocytic activity, macrophages play an important role in immunological mechanisms.

Mast Cells

- These are large round or oval cells (**mastocytes** or **histaminocytes**) (Fig. 4.7).
- The nucleus is small and centrally placed.
- Irregular microvilli (filopodia) are present on the cell surface.
- The distinguishing feature of these cells is the presence of numerous granules in the cytoplasm.

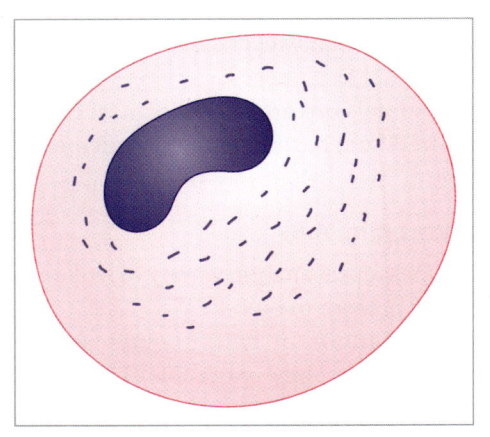

Fig. 4.6: Macrophage cell (histiocyte) (schematic representation).

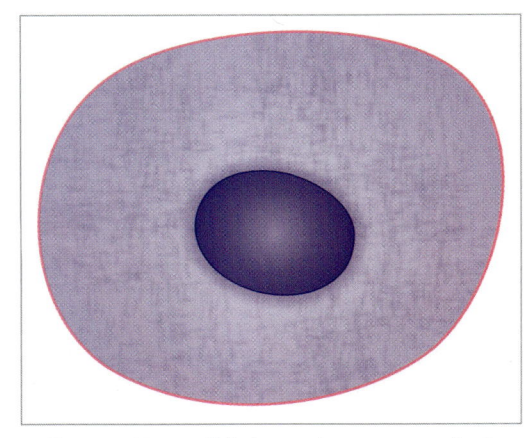

Fig. 4.7: Mast cell (schematic representation).

- The granules can be demonstrated with the periodic acid-Schiff (PAS) stain.
- In hematoxylin and eosin (H&E) stain, mast cells are seen with pale blue cytoplasm and round to oval nuclei. They also stain with dyes, such as toluidine blue or Alcian blue; with them the nuclei stain blue, but the granules stain purple to red (when components of a cell or tissue stain in a color different from that of the dye used, the staining is said to be *metachromatic*).
- On the basis of the staining reactions, the granules are known to contain acid mucopolysaccharides.
- With the EM, cytoplasm shows membrane-bound vesicles containing "granules."
- The granules are osmophillic substances containing heparin, histamine tryptase, and superoxide dismutase. The most important of these is histamine.
- Release of histamine is associated with the production of allergic reactions when a tissue is exposed to an antigen to which it is sensitive (because of previous exposure).
- They are most frequently seen around blood vessels and nerves.
- Mast cells are probably related in their origin to basophils of blood.
- Brain and spinal cord are devoid of mast cells, thus they are protected from harmful effects of edema and allergic reactions.

Lymphocytes (Fig. 4.8)

- Lymphocytes represent one variety of leukocytes (white blood cells) present in blood.
- Large aggregations of lymphocytes are present in lymphoid tissues. They reach CT from these sources, and are especially numerous when the tissue undergoes inflammation.
- Lymphocytes are small with rounded highly heterochromatic nuclei and thin rim of cytoplasm.
- They play an important role in defense of the body against invasion by bacteria and other organisms.
- They have the ability to recognize substances that are foreign to the host body and to destroy these invaders by producing antibodies against them.

- The lymphocytes are derived from stem cells present in bone marrow.
- Based on the presence of specific cluster of differentiation (CD) proteins, three major groups of cells are described. They are: (1) *T-lymphocytes*, (2) *B-lymphocytes* and (3) *Natural killer cells* (for more details, refer Lymphatic Tissue chapter).

Other Leukocytes

- Apart from lymphocytes, two other types of leukocytes may be seen in CT.
- *Monocytes* are closely related in function to the macrophages.
- *Eosinophils* (so called because of the presence of eosinophilic granules in the cytoplasm) are found in the CT of many organs (Fig. 4.9). They increase in number in allergic disorders.

Plasma Cells or Plasmatocytes

- They are round, relatively large cell with basophilic cytoplasm (Fig. 4.10).

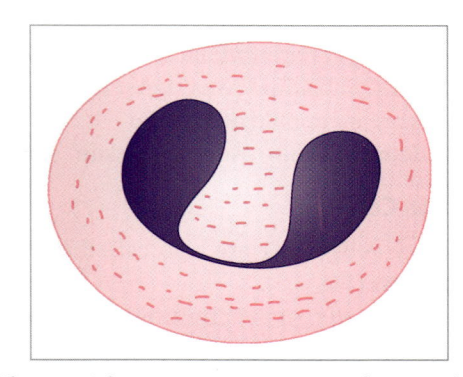

Fig. 4.9: Schematic representation of eosinophil.

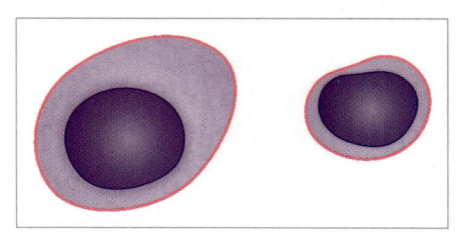

Fig. 4.8: Schematic representation of lymphocyte.

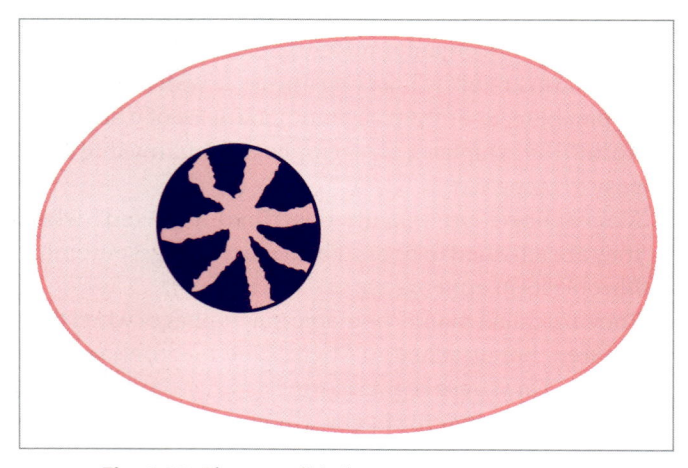

Fig. 4.10: Plasma cell (schematic representation).

CHAPTER 4: General Connective Tissue

- Basophilic cytoplasm is due to the fact that it has many rough endoplasmic reticulum in it, except for a small region near the nucleus where a well-developed Golgi complex is located.
- Nucleus is spherical and eccentric.
- The chromatin in its nucleus forms four or five clumps near the periphery (of the nucleus), thus giving the nucleus a resemblance to a **cartwheel appearance**.
- Both these features are indicative of the fact that plasma cells are engaged in considerable synthetic activity.
- They produce antibodies that may be discharged locally, may enter the circulation, or may be stored within the cell itself in the form of inclusions called **Russell's bodies**.
- Very few plasma cells can be seen in normal CT. Their number increases in the presence of certain types of inflammation.
- It is believed that plasma cells represent B-lymphocytes that have matured and have lost their power of further division.

> **Added Information**
>
> - When macrophages encounter foreign bodies, they may fuse to form large cell with many nuclei to engulf the foreign body. Such cells are called **Langerhans/epitheloid/foreign body giant cells.** Under MPS, macrophages are given different names in different tissue as follows:
>   - Macrophage/histiocyte—CT
>   - Kupffer cell—liver
>   - Osteoclast—bone
>   - Langerhans cell—skin
>   - Hofbauer cell—placenta
>   - Microglia—central nervous system
>   - Alveolar macrophage—lungs.
> - Mast cells and basophils arise from hemopoietic stem cell in bone marrow. At first, mast cells circulate in blood as agranular cells of monocyte appearance, after migrating into tissue, immature mast cells differentiate and produce their characteristic granules.
>   Two types of mast cells are described in human beings:
>   1. MC_{TC} type: They have granule-associated tryptase and chymase. These cells have cytoplasmic granules with lattice-like structure. For example, mast cells of skin, intestinal mucosa, breast, and axillary lymphnodes.
>   2. MC_T type: They have granule-associated tryptase. These cells have cytoplasmic granules with scroll-like structure. For example, mast cells of lung, intestinal mucosa.
> - T-lymphocytes: These cells arise from bone marrow, then migrates to thymus for maturation, and later moves to their destination (peripheral lymphoid tissue).

■ FIBERS OF CONNECTIVE TISSUE

The most conspicuous components of CT are the fibers within it. These are of three main types (Table 4.1): (1) Collagen, (2) Reticular and (3) Elastic fibers.

Table 4.1: Difference between collagen fibers and elastic fibers.

Collagen fibers	Elastic fibers
White in color	Yellow in color
Arranged in bundles	Arranged individually
Bundles branch	Individual fibers branch
Have straight ends	Have curled ends
Provides strength to the structure	Provides elasticity to the structure
Produced throughout the life	Produced only during fetal period

Collagen Fibers

- ***Collagen fibers*** are most numerous. They can be classified into various types. ***Reticular fibers*** were once described as a distinct variety of fibers, but they are now regarded as one variety of collagen fiber.
- With the light microscope, collagen fibers are seen in bundles (Figs. 4.11 and 4.12A). The bundles may be straight or wavy depending upon how much they are stretched. The bundles are made up of collections of individual collagen fibers which are 1–12 μm in diameter.
- The bundles often branch or anastomose with adjacent bundles, but the individual fibers do not branch.
- With the EM, each collagen fiber is seen to be made of fibrils that are 20–200 nm in diameter. Each fibril consists of a number of microfibrils (3.5 nm in diameter). At high magnifications of the EM, each fibril shows characteristics of cross-striations (or periods) after every 67 nm interval (in unfixed tissue).

Staining Characters

- Unstained collagen fibers in bundles appear white in color with the unaided eye.
- In sections stained with H&E, collagen fibers are stained light pink.
- With special methods, they assume different colors depending upon the dye used. Two commonly used methods are **Masson's trichrome** with which the fibers stain blue and the **Van Gieson** method with which they stain red. After silver impregnation, the fibers are stained brown.

Chemical Nature

- Collagen fibers are mainly made up of a protein called ***collagen***.
- Protein collagen in turn is made up of molecules of ***tropocollagen***.

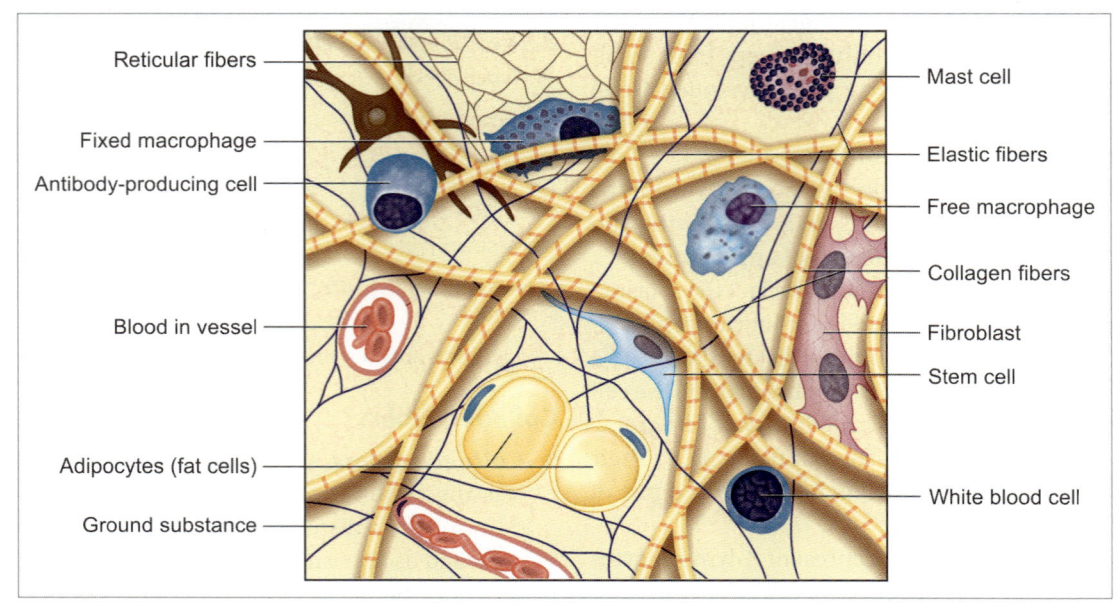

Fig. 4.11: Components of loose connective tissue (schematic representation).

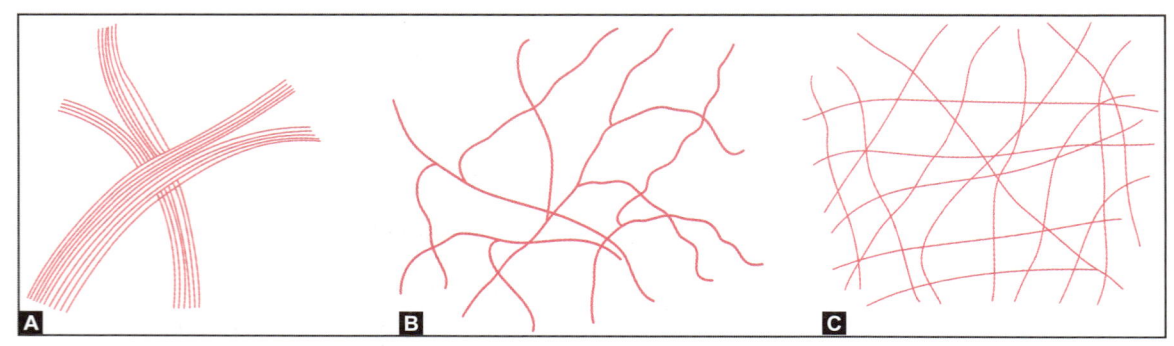

Figs. 4.12A to C: Fibers of connective tissue. (A) Collagen fibers; (B) Elastic fibers; (C) Reticular fibers (schematic representation).

- Microfibrils of collagen are the chains of tropocollagen molecules. Each molecule of tropocollagen is 300 nm in length. Within a fiber, the molecules of tropocollagen are arranged in a regular overlapping pattern which is responsible for producing the cross-striated appearance of the fibers.
- Each molecule of tropocollagen is made up of three polypeptide chains. The chains are arranged in the form of a triple helix. The polypeptide chains are referred to as procollagen.
- Each procollagen chain consists of a long chain of amino acids that are arranged in groups of three (triplets). Each triplet contains the amino acid glycine. The other two amino acids in each triplet are variable. Most commonly, these are hydroxyproline and hydroxylysine.

Physical Properties

Collagen fibers can resist considerable tensile forces (i.e. stretching) without significant increase in their length. At the same time, they are pliable and can bend easily.

Reticular Fibers

These fibers are a variety of collagen fibers and are composed of collagen type III. They show periodicity (striations) of 67 nm. They differ from typical (type I) collagen fibers as follows:

- They are much finer and have uneven thickness.
- They form a network (or reticulum) by branching, and by anastomosing with each other. They do not run in bundles (Fig. 4.12C).
- They can be stained specifically by silver impregnation, which renders them black. They can, thus, be easily

distinguished from type I collagen fibers which are stained brown. Because of their affinity for silver salts, reticular fibers are sometimes called ***argentophil fibers*** (Fig. 4.13).

* Reticular fibers contain more carbohydrates than type I fibers (which is probably the reason, why they are argentophil).

Functions

* Reticular fibers provide a supporting network in lymphoid organs, such as the spleen, lymph nodes, and bone marrow; most glands, including liver (Fig. 4.13) and kidneys.
* Reticular fibers form an essential component of all basement membranes.
* They are also found in relation to smooth muscle and nerve fibers. Reticular fibers are synthesized by fibroblasts and reticular cells (special variety of fibroblasts).

Elastic Fibers

* Elastic fibers are much fewer than those of collagen. They run singly (not in bundles), branch and anastomose with other fibers (Fig. 4.12B).
* Elastic fibers are thinner than those of collagen (0.1–0.2 µm) (*see* Fig. 4.1). In some situations, elastic fibers are thick (e.g. in the ligamenta flava). In other situations (as in walls of large arteries), they form fenestrated membranes.
* With the EM, each elastic fiber is seen to have a central amorphous core and an outer layer of fibrils (Fig. 4.14).

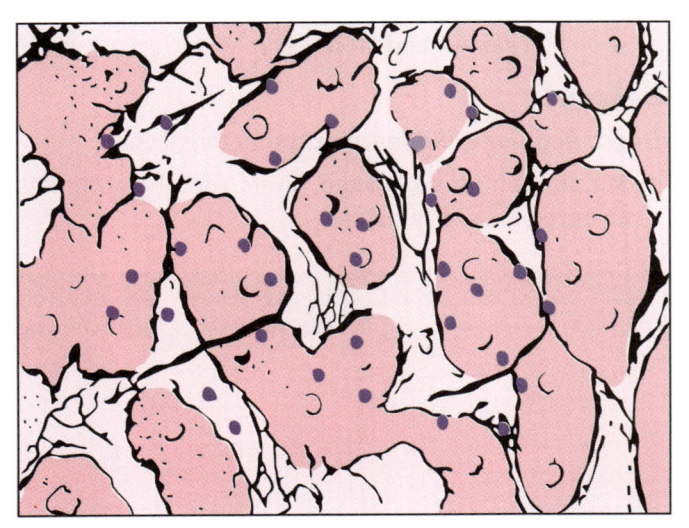

Fig. 4.13: Reticular fibers (black) forming a network in the liver. The white spaces represent sinusoids (schematic representation).

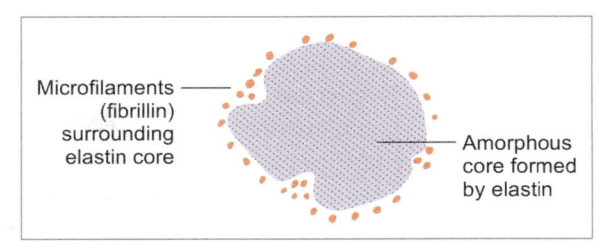

Fig. 4.14: Electron microscopy appearance of an elastic fiber as seen in transverse section (schematic representations).

* The outer fibrils are made up of a glycoprotein called ***fibrillin***. Periodic striations are not present in elastic fibers.

Staining Characters

Elastic fibers do not stain with the usual stains for collagen. They can be demonstrated by staining with **orcein**, with **aldehyde fuchsin**, and by **Verhoeff's method**.

Chemical Nature

* Elastic fibers are composed mainly of a protein called ***elastin*** that forms their central amorphous core.
* Elastin is made up of smaller units called ***tropoelastin***.
* Elastin contains a high quantity of the amino acids valine and alanine. Another amino acid called desmosine is found exclusively in elastic tissue. The outer fibrils of elastic fibers are composed of the glycoprotein fibrillin.

Production of Elastic Fibers

Elastic fibers of CT are produced by fibroblasts. In some situations, elastic tissue can be formed by smooth muscle cells.

Physical Properties

* Elastic fibers can be stretched (like a rubber band) and return to their original length when tension is released.
* They are highly refractile and are, therefore, seen as shining lines in unstained preparations. Relaxed elastic fibers do not show birefringence, but when stretched the fibers become highly birefringent.
* Unlike collagen, elastic fibers are not affected by weak acids or alkalies, or by boiling. However, they are digested by the enzyme **elastase**.

INTERCELLULAR GROUND SUBSTANCE OF CONNECTIVE TISSUE

* It is transparent homogenous viscous solution called ***ground substance or matrix***.

- It fills the space between cells and fibers.
- Ground substance is rich in protein–carbohydrate complexes or **proteoglycans**.
- Proteoglycans are complexes formed by protein and long-chained polysaccharides called **glycosaminoglycans (GAGs)**.
- Glycosaminoglycans are highly negatively charged and tend to take basic stain because of sulfate and carboxyl groups in them. The negative-charged molecules attract water and forms hydrated gel.
- In addition to proteoglycans, the ground substance also contains **structural glycoproteins**. Its main function is to facilitate adhesion between various elements of CT.
- Intercellular ground substance is synthesized by fibroblasts. Osteoblasts, chondroblasts, and even smooth muscle cells can also produce ground substance.
- Because of different sugar moieties and bondages, various GAGs are recognized. Different GAGs and the tissues in which each type is present are given in Table 4.2.

> **Added Information**
>
> With the exception of hyaluronic acid, all other GAGs listed in the Table 4.2 have the following features.
> - They are linked with protein (to form proteoglycans).
> - They carry sulfate groups (SO⁻) and carboxyl groups (COO⁻) which give them a strong negative charge.
> - The proteoglycans formed by them are in the form of long chains that do not fold. Because of this, they occupy a large space (or **domain**) and hold a large amount of water.
> - They also hold Na⁺ ions. Retained water and proteoglycans form a gel that gives a certain degree of stiffness to CT and helps it to resist compressive forces.
> - Because of the arrangement of molecules within it, ground substance acts like a sieve. The size of the pores of the sieve can be altered (by change in the orientation of molecules, and by change in the charges on them).
> - In this way, ground substance forms a selective barrier. This barrier function is very important in basement membranes. In the kidney, this barrier prevents large protein molecules from passing (from blood) into urine. However, exchange of gases is permitted in the lungs.

Hyaluronic Acid
- They are huge molecules with thousands of sugar moieties.
- Unlike other GAGs, they are not directly linked to proteins, by indirect linkages, it forms proteoglycan aggregates. They are devoid of sulfate groups.

Multiadhesive Glycoproteins
- These protein molecules are responsible for anchoring the extracellular matrix to cell surface and thus stabilizes it.
- They also regulate the functions of extracellular matrix.
- *Examples*—fibronectin, osteopontin, laminin, and tenascin.

DIFFERENT FORMS OF CONNECTIVE TISSUE

Loose Connective/Areolar Tissue
- It is so called because of the loosely arranged collagen fibers in it enclose small spaces (areolae—*L.* "little open space") which are filled with interstitial fluid.
- It has abundant ground substance, which makes it soft.
- It has numerous fibroblasts and macrophages along with other types of CT cells scattered between loosely arranged collagen and elastic fibers.
- Its main function is to bind different tissues together.
- *Areolar tissue* gets distorted easily; hence, it allows the tissue to move freely.
- *Examples*—endomysium, subperiosteal tissue, lamina propria of gastrointestinal tract (GIT), hypodermis, stroma of glands, and mesentery.

Dense CT

Dense Regular Collagenous Connective Tissue
- Mainly contains collagen fibers (or fiber bundles) arranged in orderly fashion.

Table 4.2: Different types of glycosaminoglycans in various tissues.

Tissues	Chondroitin sulfate	Dermatan sulfate	Heparan sulfate	Heparin	Keratan sulfate	Hyaluronic acid
Typical connective tissue	+	–	–	–	–	+
Cartilage	+	–	–	–	+	+
Bone	+	–	–	–	–	–
Skin	+	+	–	+	–	+
Basement membrane	–	–	+	–	–	–
Others	–	Blood vessels and heart	Lung arteries	Mast cells, lungs, and liver	Cornea, intervertebral discs	Synovial fluid

- Nuclei of some cells (mainly fibroblasts) are seen between the bundles of collagen. Nuclei are elongated in shape (elliptical).
- Ground substance is less in amount.
- *Examples*—*Tendon* of muscle, *ligaments* of joint, deep fascia, intermuscular septa, aponeuroses, the central tendon of the diaphragm, the fibrous pericardium, and dura mater (Plate 4.1).

Dense Irregular Connective Tissue (Dermis of Skin)

- In this CT, collagen bundles do not show such a regular arrangement, but interlace in various directions forming **dense irregular tissue.**
- Few cells (fibroblast) and less ground substance.
- *Examples*—Dermis, CT sheaths of muscles and nerves, capsules of glands, the sclera, the periosteum, and the adventitia of blood vessels (Plate 4.2 and Figure 4.15).

Adipose Tissue

Adipose tissue is an aggregation of fat cells also called adipocytes (Fig. 4.16).

Distribution

- It is found subcutaneously (superficial fascia) throughout the body except over the eyelid, auricle, penis, and scrotum. This subcutaneous layer of fat is called the **panniculus adiposus**. In women, it forms a thicker and more even layer: this is responsible for the soft contours of the female body.
- Subcutaneous fat is not present in animals that have a thick coat of fur.
- Adipose tissue fills several hollow spaces in the body. These include the orbits, the axillae, and the ischiorectal fossae.
- In the adult, much of the space in marrow cavities of long bones is filled by fat in the form of yellow bone marrow.
- Much fat is also present in synovial folds of many joints filling spaces that would otherwise have been empty during certain phases of movement.
- Fat is present around many abdominal organs, specially the kidneys (**perinephric fat**).
- Considerable amounts of fat may be stored in the greater omentum, and in other peritoneal folds.

Structure

- Adipocytes have single large fat globule, which occupies whole of the cytoplasm.
- In routine sections, the cells appear empty as the fat in them gets dissolved during preparation (treatment with fat solvents, such as xylene or benzene) of the section giving it a honeycomb appearance.
- The cytoplasm of the cell appears as a thin rim around the fat globule.
- The nucleus is flat and lies to one side (eccentric) giving it **signet ring** appearance.
- Fat cells may be scattered singly in some situations, but they are usually aggregated into groups that form lobules of adipose tissue.
- The cells are supported by reticular fibers, and the lobules are held together by areolar tissue.
- Adipose tissue is richly supplied with blood and is rich in enzyme systems.
- Fat cells are derived from specific cells (**lipoblasts**) arising from undifferentiated mesenchymal cells.
- Special stains, such as Sudan III, Sudan IV, stain them (fat droplets) dark (Plate 4.3).

Functions

- It acts as a storehouse of nutrition, fat being deposited when available in excess, and being removed when deficient in the diet.
- In many situations, fat performs a mechanical function. The fat around the kidneys keeps them in position. If

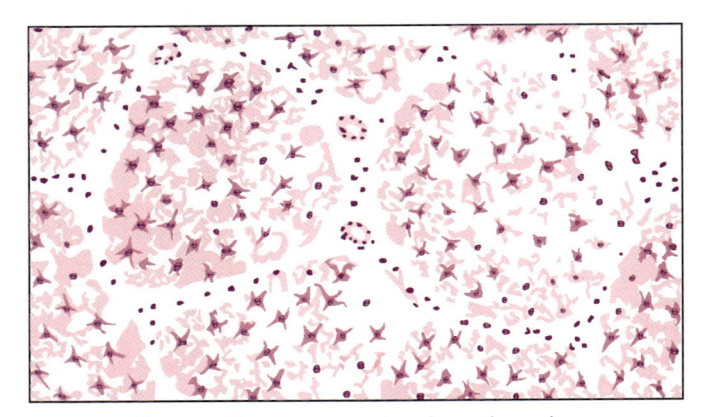

Fig. 4.15: Transverse section through tendon (schematic representation).

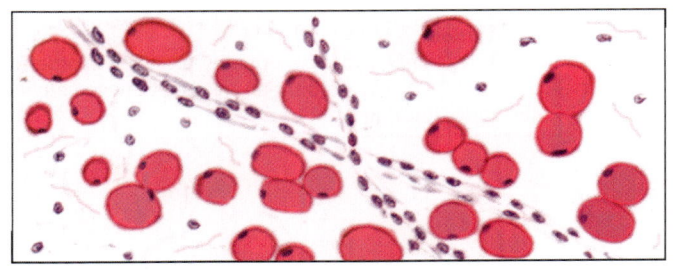

Fig. 4.16: Fat cells in a stretch preparation of omentum stained with a specific stain for fat (Sudan IV) (schematic representation).

Plate 4.1: Dense regular connective tissue

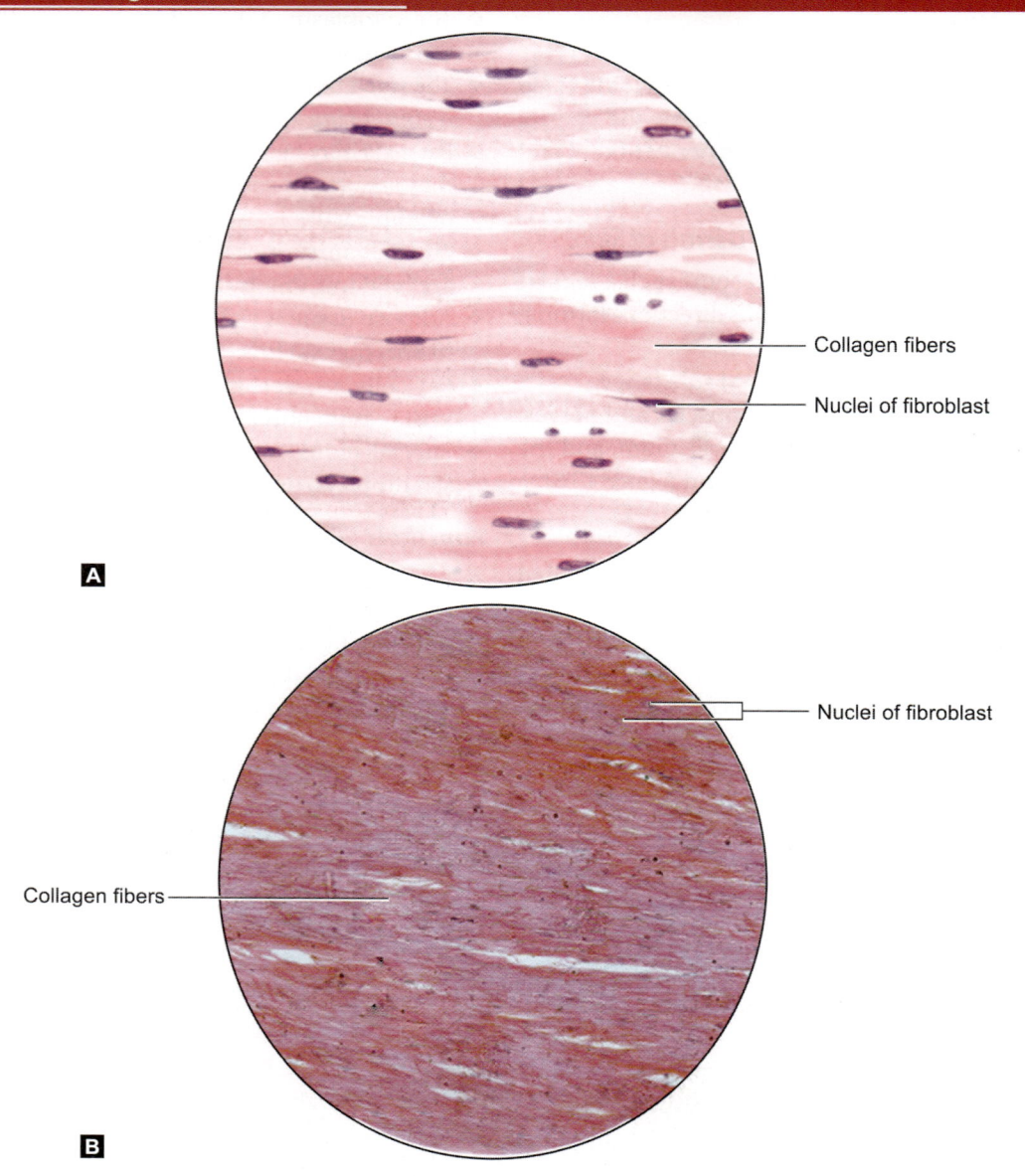

Dense regular connective tissue (Longitudinal section through a tendon): (A) As seen in drawing; (B) Photomicrograph.

Points of identification
- Presence of collagen fibers (or fiber bundles) arranged in orderly fashion parallel to each other
- Nuclei of some cells (mainly fibroblasts) are seen between the bundles of collagen. They are elongated (elliptical)
- Ground substance is less in amount.

CHAPTER 4: General Connective Tissue

Plate 4.2: Dense irregular connective tissue (Dermis of skin)

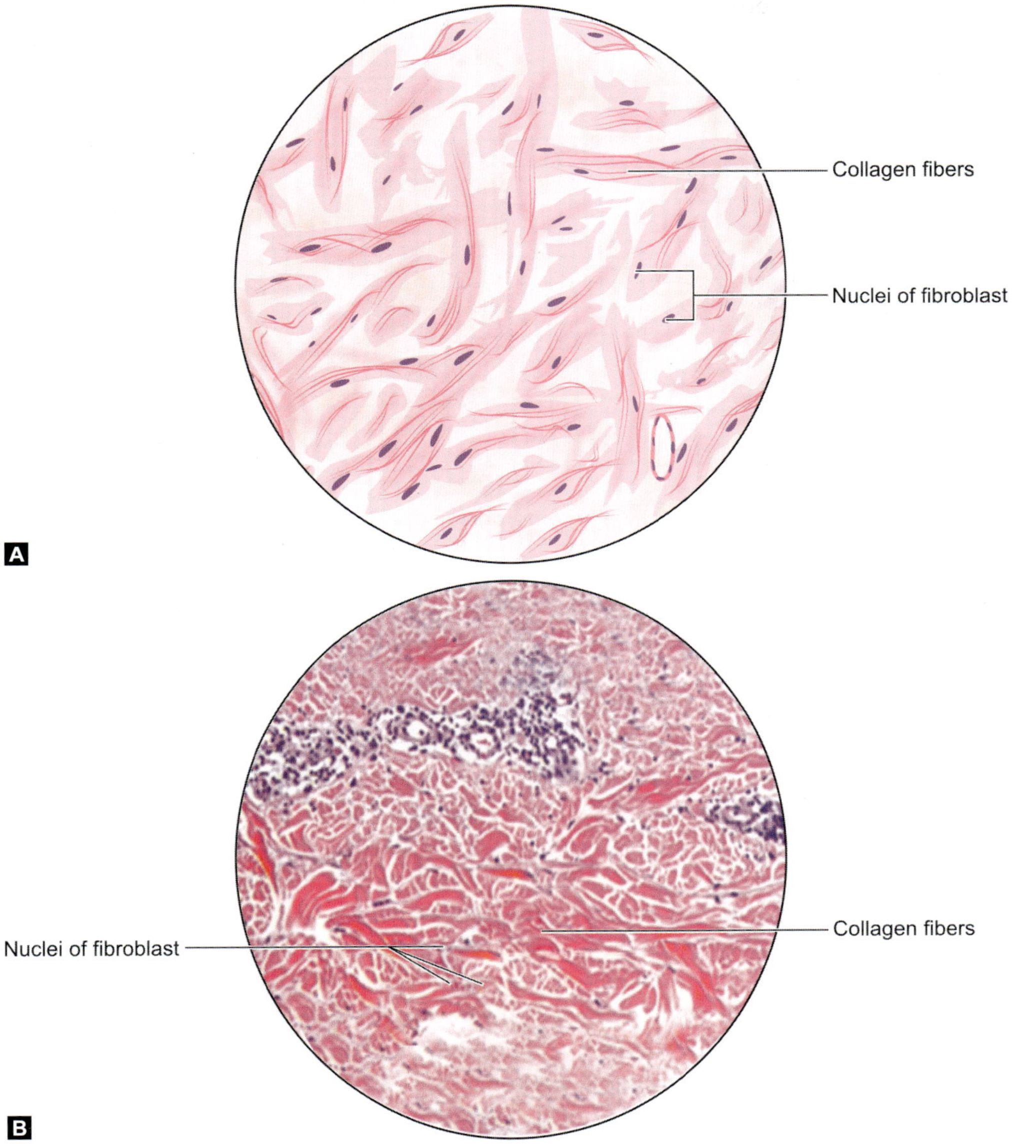

A — Collagen fibers; Nuclei of fibroblast

B — Nuclei of fibroblast; Collagen fibers

Dense irregular connective tissue (dermis of skin): (A) Drawing; (B) Photomicrograph.

Points of identification
- Irregularly arranged bundles of collagen fibers that stain pink. In stretch preparation they are seen in wavy bundles. Other fibers present (elastic, reticular) can be seen only with special stains
- Few cells (fibroblast) and less ground substance.

Plate 4.3: Adipose tissue

Adipose tissue: (A) As seen in drawing; (B) Photomicrograph (the arrows point to nuclei).

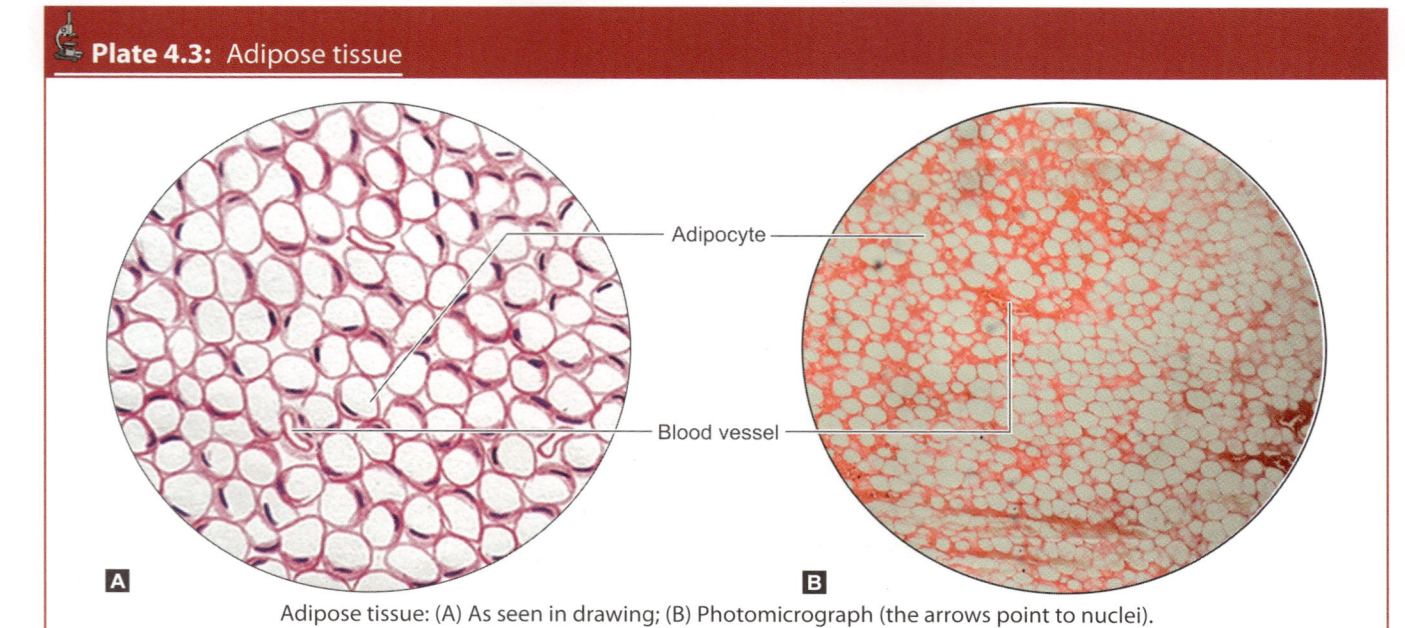

Points of identification
- Presence of fat cells. In routine sections the cells appear empty as the fat in them gets dissolved during preparation of the section giving it a honeycomb appearance
- The cytoplasm of each cell is seen as a pink rim
- The nucleus is flat and lies to one side (eccentric).

---

there is a sudden depletion of this fat, the kidneys may become mobile (***floating kidney***). The fat around the eyeball performs an important supporting function and allows the eyeball to move smoothly. In the palms and soles and over the buttocks, fat has a cushioning effect protecting underlying tissues from pressure. This fat is the last to be depleted in prolonged starvation.

❖ The subcutaneous fat has been regarded as insulation against heat loss and would certainly perform this function if the layer of adipose tissue is thick. The whale (a warm blooded mammal) can survive in very cold water because it has a very thick layer of subcutaneous fat.

❖ They also help in heat generation.

Types

Adipose tissue is of following two types:
1. Yellow (white) or unilocular adipose tissue (adult type)
2. Brown or multilocular adipose tissue (embryonic type).

The yellow adipose tissue is the adult type which has been described in detail above.

Brown adipose tissue

❖ It is brown in color.
❖ Cells are smaller than in typical adipose tissue.
❖ The fat in the cytoplasm occurs in the form of several small droplets. Hence, brown fat is also called ***multilocular adipose tissue*** (while the typical variety is described in Figs. 4.17A and B).
❖ The cytoplasm and nucleus of the cell are not pushed to the periphery.
❖ The cytoplasm contains numerous mitochondria (which are few in typical fat cells).
❖ Brown adipose tissue is abundant in the newborn, but most of it is lost during childhood.
❖ Brown fat is also abundant in hibernating animals in which it serves mainly as a heat generator when the animal comes out of hibernation.

FUNCTIONS OF CONNECTIVE TISSUE

❖ It holds together structures, such as skin, muscles, blood vessels, etc. It binds together various layers of hollow viscera. In the form of areolar tissue and reticular tissue, it forms a framework that supports the cellular elements of various organs, such as the spleen, lymph nodes, and glands, and provides capsules for them.
❖ The looseness of areolar tissue facilitates movement between structures connected by it. The looseness of

CHAPTER 4: General Connective Tissue

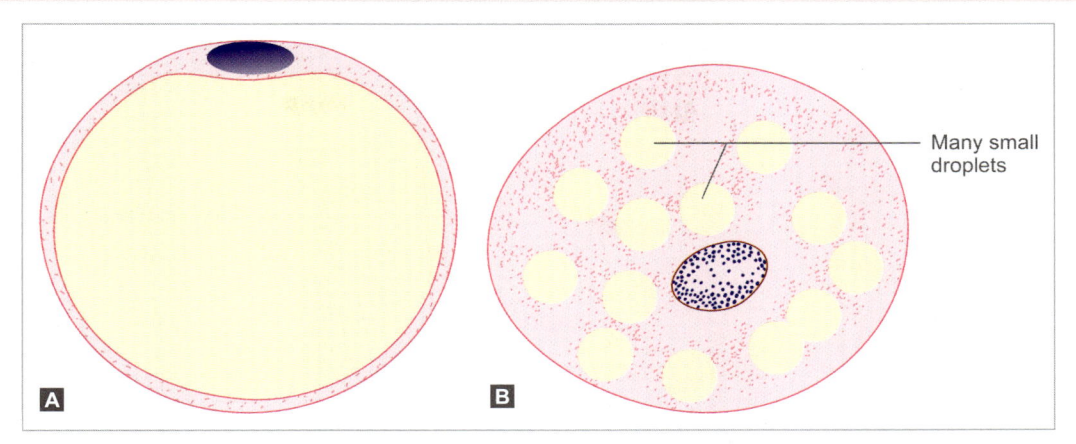

Figs. 4.17A and B: (A) Unilocular adipose tissue (white adipose tissue cell); (B) Multilocular adipose tissue (brown adipose tissue cell) (schematic representation).

superficial fascia enables the movement of skin over deep fascia. In hollow organs, this allows for mobility and stretching.
- In the form of deep fascia, CT provides a tight covering for deeper structures (especially in the limbs and neck) and helps to maintain the shape of these regions and also venous return of lower limb.
- In the form of ligaments, it holds bone ends together at joints.
- In the form of deep fascia, intermuscular septa, and aponeuroses, CT provides attachment for the origins and insertions of many muscles.
- In the form of tendons, it transmits the pull of muscles to their insertion.
- Thickened areas of deep fascia form retinacula that hold tendons in place at the wrist and ankle.
- Both areolar tissue and fascial membranes provide planes along which blood vessels, lymphatics, and nerves travel. The superficial fascia provides passage to vessels and nerves going to the skin and supports them.
- In the form of dura mater, it provides support to the brain and spinal cord.
- In the form of adipose tissue, it provides a store of nutrition. In cold weather, the fat provides insulation and helps to generate heat.
- Because of the presence of cells of the immune system (macrophages and plasma cells), CT helps the body to fight against invading foreign substances (including bacteria) by destroying them, or by producing antibodies against them.
- Because of the presence of fibroblasts, CT helps in laying down collagen fibers necessary for wound repair.
- By virtue of the presence of undifferentiated mesenchymal cells, CT can help in regeneration of tissues (e.g. cartilage and bone) by providing cells from which specialized cells can be formed.

CONNECTIVE TISSUE WITH SPECIAL PROPERTIES

Elastic Tissue
- It is specialized dense CT formed by elastic fibers.
- In contrast to fibrous tissue, which appears white, elastic tissue is yellow in color.
- Some ligaments like ligamentum nuchae, ligamentum flava and vocal ligament are examples.

Reticular Tissue
- It is loose CT made up of reticular fibers.
- In certain structures, such as lymph nodes, glands, etc., these fibers form supporting networks for the cells (see Fig. 4.13).
- In other tissues (e.g. bone marrow, spleen, and lymph nodes), the reticular network is closely associated with *reticular cells*. Most of these cells are fibroblasts, but some may be macrophages.

Mucoid Tissue
- The most conspicuous component of mucoid tissue is a jelly-like ground substance rich in hyaluronic acid.
- Scattered through this ground substance, there are star-shaped fibroblasts, some delicate collagen fibers, and some rounded cells (Fig. 4.18).
- This kind of tissue is found in the umbilical cord, vitreous humor of the eyeball.

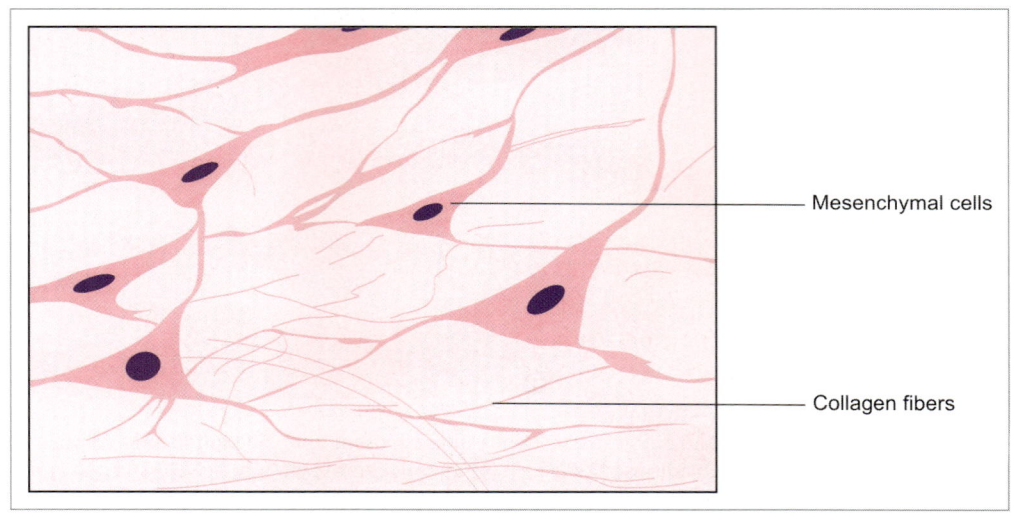

Fig. 4.18: Mucoid tissue (schematic representation).

> ### Added Information
>
> The mechanism of the production of collagen fibers by fibroblasts has been extensively studied. Collagen is also synthesized by chondroblasts of cartilage, osteoblasts of bone and smooth muscles of blood vessels. Amino acids necessary for the synthesis of fibers are taken into the cell. Under the influence of ribosomes, located on rough endoplasmic reticulum, the amino acids are bonded together to form polypeptide chains (α-chains) (Flowchart 4.2). A procollagen molecule is formed by joining together of three such chains. Molecules of procollagen are transported to the exterior of the cell where they are acted upon by enzymes (released by the fibroblast) to form tropocollagen. Collagen fibers are formed by the aggregation of tropocollagen molecules. Vitamin C and oxygen are necessary for collagen formation, and wound repair may be interfered with if either of these is deficient. In this connection, it may be noted that fibroblasts are themselves highly resistant to damaging influences and are not easily destroyed.
>
> There are observations that indicate that the orientation of collagen fibers depends on the stresses imposed on the tissue. If fibroblasts growing in tissue culture are subjected to tension in a particular direction, the cells exposed to the tension multiply faster than others; they orientate themselves along the line of stress and lay down fibers in that direction. It follows that in the embryo collagen fibers would tend to be laid down wherever they are required to resist a tensile force. In this way, tendons, ligaments, etc., will tend to develop wherever they are required. (This cannot, of course, be a complete explanation. Genetic factors must play a prominent role in development of these structures).

Flowchart 4.2: Scheme to show how collagen fibers are synthesized.

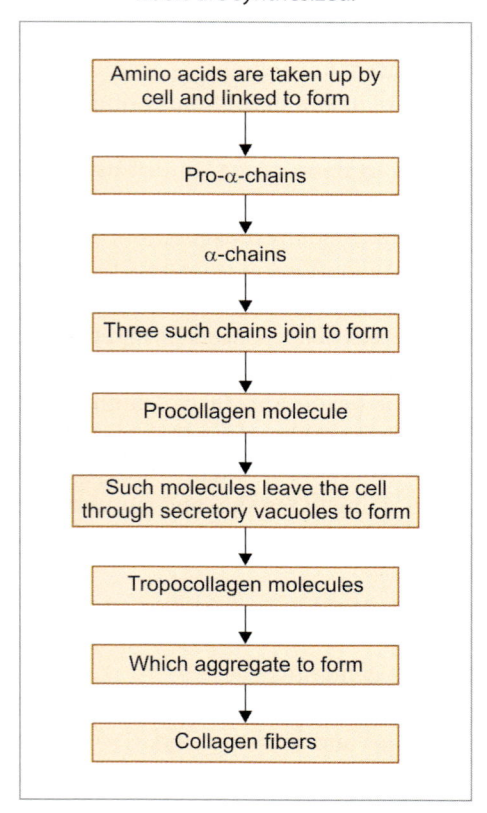

Amino acids are taken up by cell and linked to form
↓
Pro-α-chains
↓
α-chains
↓
Three such chains join to form
↓
Procollagen molecule
↓
Such molecules leave the cell through secretory vacuoles to form
↓
Tropocollagen molecules
↓
Which aggregate to form
↓
Collagen fibers

Types of Collagen

A single collagen molecule is made up of three polypeptide chains (triple helical structure) called as α chains. In each chain glycine is a compulsory amino acid along with any other two amino acids. The other two amino acids will be proline and hydroxyproline/hydroxylysine usually. Different arrangement of amino acids results in formation of more than 40 types of α chain, which vary in size. Based on various combinations of α chains 25 or more types of collagen have been identified. The types and their location is briefed in Flowchart 4.2 and Table 4.3.

APPLIED HISTOLOGY

Some Diseases of Connective Tissue

- **Osteogenesis imperfecta**: Disease of bone, due to the mutation of genes coding for collagen fibers. When collagen is not properly formed, bones are weak and break easily, one of the characteristic feature of the disease.
- **Ehlers-Danlos syndrome**: Here skin becomes abnormally extensible, and joints may be lax (because of improperly formed ligaments).
- **Marfan's syndrome**: This is due to defect in the genes coding for *fibrillin*, which is needed in the formation of extracellular matrix and elastic fibers. It affects almost all structures of the body.

Table 4.3: Types of collagen and their location.

Type	Location
I	Skin, tendon, sclera, bone, fascia
II	Vitreous humor of eye, intervertebral disc, cartilage
III	Skin, blood vessels, lung
IV	Basement membrane of epithelium
V	Mostly found with type I collagen, forms stroma
VI	Muscle, cartilage (matrix)
VII	Skin-mainly at the dermo-epidermal junction, uterus
VIII	Endothelium of blood vessels
IX	Vitreous humor, cartilage
X	Growing cartilages
XI	Vitreous humor, cartilage
XII	Skin, placenta, tendon and bone
XIII	Skin, neuromuscular junction
XIV	Skin, tendon and bone
XV	Surrounding the basement membrane, skeletal and cardiac muscles
XVI	Wide distribution
XVII	Epithelial tissue—mainly at junctions
XVIII	In structures surrounding the basement membrane
XIX	Basement membrane
XX	Cornea
XXI	Various structures containing type I collagen
XXII	At the junction of two tissues
XXIII	Heart, retina and metastatic cancer cells
XXIV	Bone, cornea
XXV	Brain
XXVI	Gonads
XXVII	Schwann cell, basement membrane

MULTIPLE CHOICE QUESTIONS

1. Wharton's jelly is an example for:
   a. Loose areolar tissue
   b. Dense connective tissue
   c. Mucoid connective tissue
   d. Adipose tissue
2. Cell responsible for wound contraction/scar retraction is:
   a. Clasmatocytes
   b. Plasma cells
   c. Myofibroblast
   d. Histiocytes
3. Type of collagen fibers present in the basement membrane is:
   a. IV
   b. II
   c. I
   d. V
4. Reticular fibers are seen in:
   a. Liver
   b. Lung
   c. Heart
   d. Spleen

Answers
1. c   2. c   3. a   4. d

CHAPTER 5

Cartilage

Learning objectives

To study the:
- Features of cartilage
- Perichondrium
- Components of cartilage
- Different types of cartilage with examples
- Applied histology

IDENTIFICATION POINTS

Hyaline cartilage	White fibrous cartilage	Elastic cartilage
❑ Ground glass appearance of matrix ❑ Chondrocytes arranged in group (cell nest) of 2 or more ❑ Perichondrium surrounding the cartilage.	❑ Bundles of collagen fibers with little ground substance ❑ Chondrocytes arranged in rows (of single cell thickness) between the fibers ❑ Absence of perichondrium.	❑ Branching and anastomosing elastic fibers in all direction ❑ Closely packed chondrocytes surrounded by amorphous ground substance ❑ Presence of perichondrium.

GENERAL FEATURES OF CARTILAGE

- Cartilage is an avascular connective tissue that forms the "skeletal" basis of some parts of the body, e.g. the auricle of the ear, or the lower part of the nose.
- Cartilage develops from mesenchyme.
- They are not rigid but firm enough to maintain the form of the structure.
- Cartilage contains cells and fibers embedded in homogeneous ground substance.
- Cells are relatively less and are called as **chondrocytes**.
- Three main types of cartilage can be recognized depending on the amount and variety of fibers in the matrix. These are: (1) **hyaline cartilage**, (2) **fibrocartilage**, and (3) **elastic cartilage**.
- *Growth of cartilage*: When cartilage grows by multiplication of cells throughout its substance, such a growth is called **interstitial growth**. Further, if a cartilage grows by addition of new cartilage over the surface of existing cartilage that is called **oppositional growth**.
- Cartilage has very limited ability for regeneration (after destruction by injury or disease). Defects in cartilage are usually filled in by fibrous tissue.

PERICHONDRIUM

- Perichondrium develops from mesenchymal cells that surround the developing cartilage.
- It has two layers: (1) **inner chondrogenic layer** and (2) **outer fibrous layer**.
- The undifferentiated mesenchymal cells in the **chondrogenic layer**, can proliferate and differentiate to form cartilage cells on the existing cartilage (oppositional growth).
- The cells in the outer layer differentiate to form fibroblast/fibrocytes which in turn produces fibers (collagen) thus, converting it to **fibrous layer**.

COMPONENTS OF CARTILAGE

Cartilage = Chondrocytes + Extracellular matrix (ground substance + fibers)

Like ordinary connective tissue, cartilage is made up of:
- Cells—chondrocytes
- Intercellular/extracellular matrix
- Fibers—collagen/elastic/reticular fibers.

Cartilage Cells

- Mature cells of cartilage are called as **chondrocytes**.
- They vary in size and shape with degree of maturation. Mature cells are large and rounded.
- They lie in spaces (or **lacunae**) present in the matrix.
- The nucleus is heterochromatic and organelles are less prominent. The cytoplasm of chondrocytes may also contain glycogen and lipids.
- Young metabolically active flat cells are called as **chondroblasts.** The nucleus is euchromatic. Mitochondria, endoplasmic reticulum (ER), and Golgi complex are prominent.

Ground Substance

- Ground substance forms major component and makes up to 95% of volume of the cartilage.
- The ground substance is made up of complex molecules containing proteins and carbohydrates (proteoglycans). Along with the water content, these molecules form a firm gel that gives cartilage its characteristic consistency.
- The carbohydrates are chemically **glycosaminoglycans** (GAGs).
- **Multiadhesive glycoproteins** bind chondrocytes and the matrix molecules.

Fibers of Cartilage

- The collagen fibers present in cartilage are (as a rule) chemically distinct from those in most other tissues.
- They are described as type II collagen.
- However, type I collagen is present in fibrocartilage and perichondrium. Elastic cartilage contains elastic fibers.

TYPES OF CARTILAGE

Hyaline Cartilage

- Hyaline cartilage is so called because it is translucent (*hyalos* = glass).
- Its matrix appears to be homogeneous, but using special techniques, many collagen fibers can be demonstrated.
- Hyaline cartilage has been compared to a tyre. The ground substance (corresponding to the rubber of the tyre) resists compressive forces, while the collagen fibers mainly type-II (corresponding to the treads of the tyre) resist tensional forces.
- Hyaline cartilage is surrounded by perichondrium but although articular cartilage is a hyaline cartilage, it is devoid of perichondrium.
- In hematoxylin and eosin-stained preparations, the matrix is stained blue, i.e. it is basophilic.
- The GAGs of ground substance includes chondroitin sulfate, keratin sulfate, and hyaluronic acid. In hyaline cartilage, the most important proteoglycan monomer is aggrecan (Plate 5.1).
- Toward the center of mass of hyaline cartilage, the chondrocytes are large and are usually present in groups (of two or more)—**cell nest (isogenous cell groups)**. The groups are formed by division of a single parent cell.
- Matrix around the cells is darkly stained called as **capsular matrix** and around the isogenous cell group as **territorial/lacunar matrix**.
- Toward the periphery of the cartilage, the cells are small and elongated in a direction parallel to the surface. Just under the perichondrium, the cells become indistinguishable from fibroblasts. The pale staining matrix separating cell nests is the **interstitial matrix**.
- In old people, hyaline cartilage can undergo calcification and degeneration. The costal cartilages or the large cartilages of the larynx are commonly affected.
- Examples: Costal cartilage, articular cartilage, thyroid cartilage, cricoid cartilage, arytenoid cartilage, tracheal rings, and large and smaller bronchi.

Functions

- By forming structural framework that provides support to various structures
- Forms cartilage model for developing fetal skeleton
- Forms articular cartilage.

Elastic Cartilage

- Elastic cartilage (or yellow fibrocartilage) is similar in many ways to hyaline cartilage.
- The main difference between hyaline cartilage and elastic cartilage is that instead of collagen fibers, the matrix contains numerous branching and anastomosing elastic fibers that form a network (Plate 5.2).
- The fibers are difficult to see in hematoxylin and eosin-stained sections, but they can be clearly visualized if special methods for staining elastic fibers are used.
- The surface of elastic cartilage is covered by perichondrium.
- Contrast to hyaline cartilage, elastic cartilage does not undergo calcification.

Plate 5.1: Hyaline cartilage

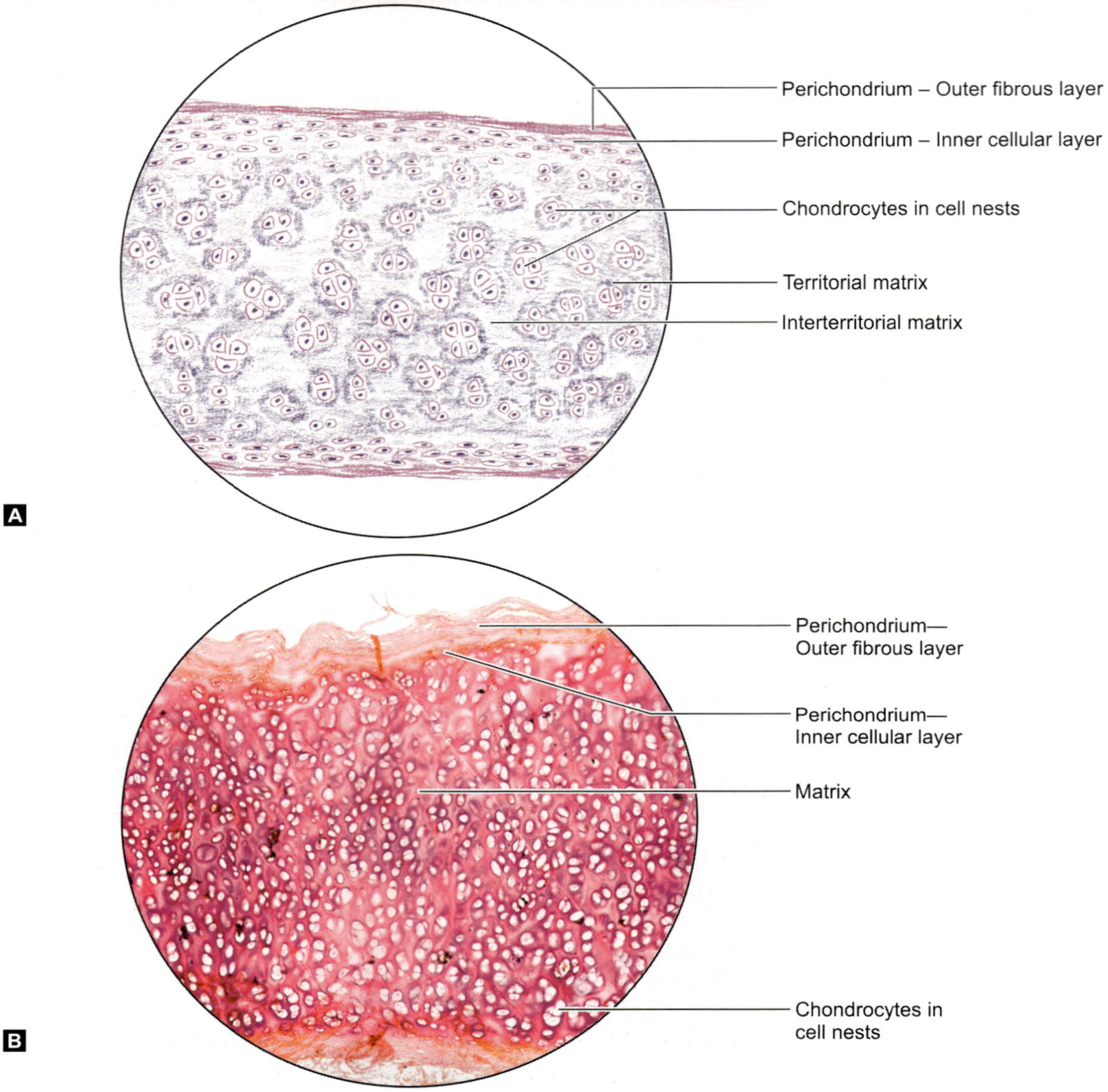
Perichondrium – Outer fibrous layer
Perichondrium – Inner cellular layer
Chondrocytes in cell nests
Territorial matrix
Interterritorial matrix
A
Perichondrium—Outer fibrous layer
Perichondrium—Inner cellular layer
Matrix
Chondrocytes in cell nests
B

Hyaline cartilage: (A) As seen in drawing; (B) Photomicrograph.
Courtesy: Balakrishna Shetty, Sweekritha H Poonja. HISTOLOGY Practical Manual, 4th edition. New Delhi: Jaypee Brothers Medical Publishers (P) Ltd; 2019. p. 17-18.

Points of identification

- Hyaline cartilage is characterized by isogenous groups of chondrocytes called as cell nest
- Chondrocytes are surrounded by a homogeneous basophilic matrix which separates the cells widely
- Chondrocytes increase in size from periphery to center
- Near the surface of the cartilage the cells are flattened and merge with the cells of the overlying connective tissue. This connective tissue forms the perichondrium
- Perichondrium displays an outer fibrous and inner cellular layer.

Examples

Auricle (or pinna) and of the lateral part of the external acoustic meatus, medial part of the auditory tube, epiglottis, and two small laryngeal cartilages (corniculate and cuneiform). The apical part of the arytenoid cartilage contains elastic fibers but the major portion of it is hyaline.

CHAPTER 5: Cartilage

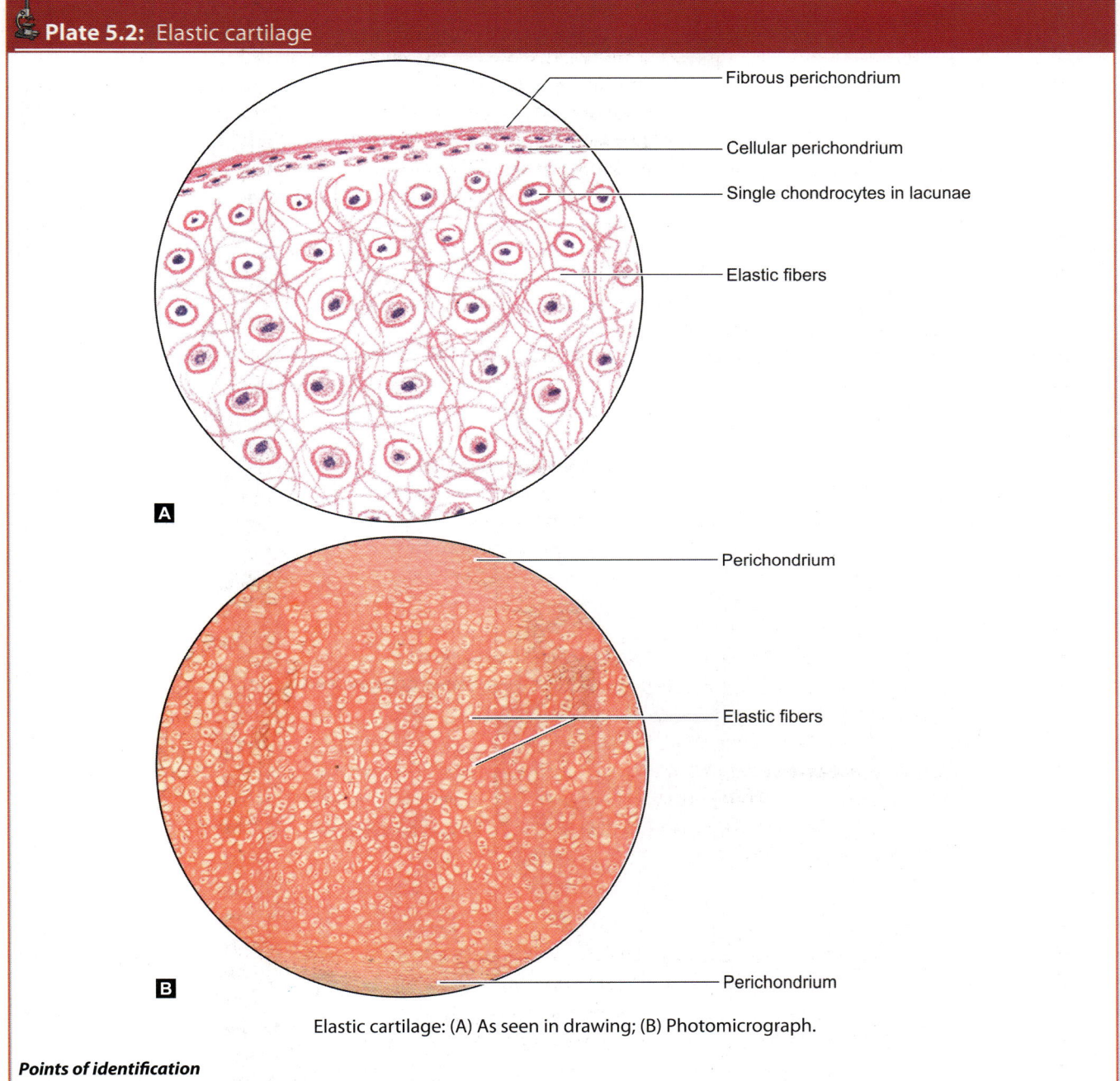

Plate 5.2: Elastic cartilage

Elastic cartilage: (A) As seen in drawing; (B) Photomicrograph.

Labels (A): Fibrous perichondrium; Cellular perichondrium; Single chondrocytes in lacunae; Elastic fibers

Labels (B): Perichondrium; Elastic fibers; Perichondrium

Points of identification
- Elastic cartilage is characterized by presence of chondrocytes within lacuna surrounded by bundles of elastic fibers
- Perichondrium is present showing an outer fibrous and inner cellular layer.

Function

Provides elasticity (flexibility) to the structures.

Fibrocartilage

- Fibrous cartilage (also called *white fibrocartilage*) looks very much like dense fibrous tissue (Plate 5.3).
- Since fibrocartilage is a transitional tissue between dense connective tissue and hyaline cartilage, lack of perichondrium helps in its proper blending with surrounding structure.
- The chondrocytes are similar to that of hyaline cartilage but arranged in single rows or in isogenous groups.

Plate 5.3: Fibrocartilage

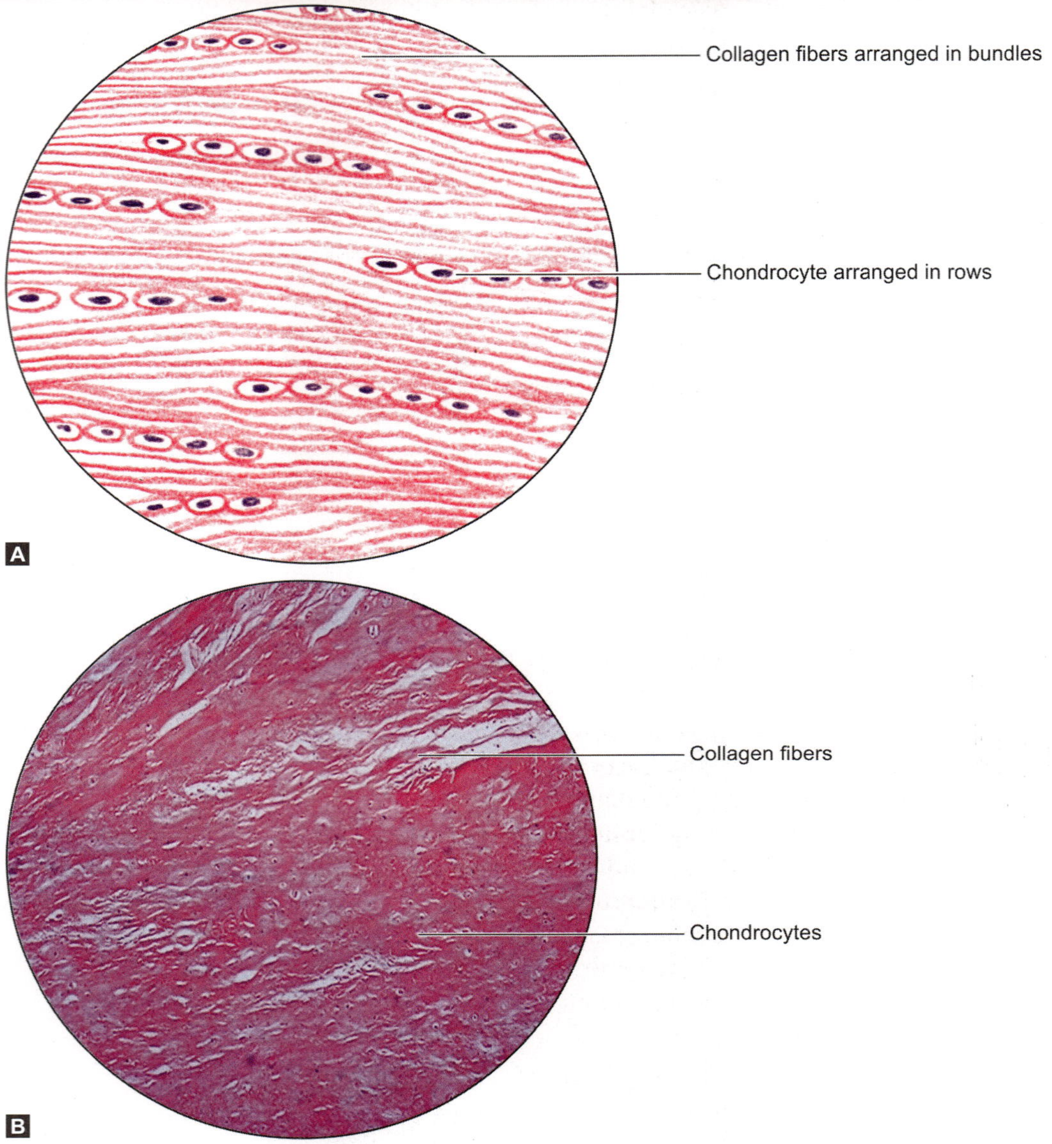

Fibrocartilage: (A) As seen in drawing; (B) Photomicrograph.

Points of identification
- Presence of prominent collagen fibers arranged in bundles with rows of chondrocytes intervening between the bundles
- Perichondrium is absent
- This kind of cartilage can be confused with the appearance of a tendon. However the chondrocytes in fibrocartilage are rounded but in a tendon, fibrocytes are flattended and elongated.

CHAPTER 5: Cartilage

- The matrix is pervaded by numerous collagen bundles both type I and type II, in between, there are some fibroblasts. The fibers merge with those of surrounding connective tissue. Their proportion varies with age.
- There is no perichondrium over the cartilage.
- The fibrocartilage undergoes calcification during repair process.

Examples
Intervertebral discs, symphysis pubis, menisci of the knee joint, and articular disc of sternoclavicular and temporomandibular joint.

Functions
- Offers resistance to both compression and shearing forces
- Acts as shock absorbers.

APPLIED HISTOLOGY

- **Osteoarthritis**: Osteoarthritis is an inflammatory disorder of joint due to degeneration of articular cartilage.
- **Achondroplasia**: One of the causes of dwarfism in early life is due to reduced proliferation of chondrocytes in the epiphyseal plates of long bones.
- **Cartilage-forming (chondroblastic) tumors**: The tumors which are composed of frank cartilage or derived from cartilage-forming cells are included in this group. This group comprises benign lesions like osteocartilaginous exostoses (osteochondromas), enchondroma, chondroblastoma and chondromyxoid fibroma, and a malignant counterpart, chondrosarcoma.
  - **Osteocartilaginous exostoses or osteochondromas**: These are the most common of benign cartilage-forming lesions. Exostoses arise from growth plate of long bones as exophytic lesions, most commonly lower femur and upper tibia and upper humerus.
  - **Enchondroma**: Enchondroma is the term used for the benign cartilage-forming tumor that develops centrally within the interior of the affected bone, while chondroma refers to the peripheral development of lesion.
  - **Chondroblastoma**: Chondroblastoma is a relatively rare benign tumor arising from the epiphysis of long bones adjacent to the epiphyseal cartilage plate. Most commonly affected bones are upper tibia and lower femur and upper humerus.
  - **Chondrosarcoma**: Chondrosarcoma is a malignant tumor of chondroblasts.

Added Information

- Being avascular tissue, cartilage receives nutrition through blood vessels found in cartilage canals. Each canal contains a small artery surrounded by numerous venules and capillaries. Cartilage cells receive their nutrition by diffusion from vessels in the perichondrium or in cartilage canals. Cartilage canals may also play a role in the ossification of cartilage by carrying bone forming cells into it.
- The greater part of the skeleton is cartilaginous in early fetal life. The ends of most long bones are cartilaginous at the time of birth, and are gradually replaced by bone. The replacement is completed only after full growth of the individual (i.e. by about 18 years of age). Replacement of cartilage by bone is called **ossification**. Ossification of cartilage has to be carefully distinguished from **calcification**, in which the matrix hardens because of the deposition of calcium saltsin it but true bone is not formed.
- Capsular matrix contains the highest concentration of sulfated proteoglycans, hyaluronan, and many multiadhesive glycoproteins (e.g. fibronectin, laminin, and decorin). Main type of fiber istype VI collagen fibrils whereas territorial matrix—type II collagen fibers.
- The first formed chondrocyte lives within the primary lacuna, when the same cell divides it forms daughter cells. The lacunae around each daughter cell are termed as secondary lacunae. Therefore, the secondary lacunae of cell nest lie within the primary lacunae.
- Growth of cartilage: The process of formation of cartilage is known as chondrogenesis. Main gene regulating is *SOX9*.The process starts with aggregation of chondrogenic mesenchymal cells. The place where hyaline cartilage is going to form there appears chondrogenic nodule, cells in them gets differentiated to form chondroblasts. Chondroblasts secrets the matrix and also lay down the essential fibers. Once they are completely surrounded by the matrix and locked in the lacunae, chondroblasts are referred as chondrocytes. The peripheral cells of the nodule form the perichondrium. Two types of growth are observed:
  1. *Interstitial growth*: Here the chondroblasts within the matrix divides and contribute for increase in size of the cartilage.
  2. *Oppositional growth*: Here the cells in the chondrogenic layer of the perichondrium differentiate into chondroblasts and lay down matrix and fibers on the existing cartilage.

SUMMARY

Features	*Hyaline cartilage*	*Elastic cartilage*	*Fibrocartilage*
Appearance	Ground glass	–	White
Main cells	Chondroblasts, chondrocytes	Chondroblasts, chondrocytes	Chondrocytes, fibroblasts
Fibers	Type II collagen	Type II collagen and elastic fibers	Type I and type II collagen
Perichondrium	Present	Present	Absent
Calcification	Occurs	No	Only during repair
Function	Protects against compression, provides cushion effect	Provides flexibility	Protects against deformation
Examples	Tracheal rings, costal cartilages, thyroid, cricoid, and base of arytenoid cartilage	Auditory tube, epiglottis, cuneiform and corniculate cartilage, and ear pinna	Intervertebral disks, symphysis pubis, menisci of the knee joint, and articular disc of sternoclavicular and temporomandibular joint

MULTIPLE CHOICE QUESTIONS

1. All the following are true, *except:*
   a. Elastic cartilage contains type II collagen
   b. Perichondrium is absent in fibrocartilage
   c. Hyaline cartilage does not undergo calcification
   d. Elastic cartilage provides flexibility
2. Territorial matrix is:
   a. Matrix around the chondrocytes
   b. Matrix surrounding the cell nests
   c. Matrix near the perichondrium
   d. Matrix between the cell nests
3. Hyaline cartilage is present in:
   a. Epiglottis
   b. Auricle
   c. Tracheal rings
   d. Intervertebral disc
4. Gene regulating chondrogenesis:
   a. *SOX9*
   b. *HLA-DRB1*
   c. *CAPN10*
   d. *BRCA1*
5. Core protein in hyaline cartilage is:
   a. Aggrecan
   b. Laminin
   c. Lumican
   d. Fibromodulin
6. Cartilage seen in intervertebral disc is:
   a. Hyaline cartilage
   b. Elastic cartilage
   c. White fibrocartilage
   d. None of the above
7. Fibers seen in hyaline cartilage are:
   a. Elastic fibers
   b. Reticular fibers
   c. Type II collagen fibers
   d. Type I collagen fibers

Answers
1. c   2. b   3. c   4. a   5. a   6. c   7. c

CHAPTER 6

Bone

Learning objectives

To study the:
- General features of bone and its function
- Components of bone
- Classification and structure of bone
- Formation of bone—ossification
- Growth of bone
- Applied histology

IDENTIFICATION POINTS

Bone (Transverse section)
- Haversian system made up of concentric lamellae, lacunae with osteocytes, Haversian (central) canal containing blood vessels and nerves are seen
- Three types of lamellae are seen—(1) circumferential, (2) concentric, and (3) interstitial
- Canaliculi radiate from lacunae
- Lacunae with osteocytes.

Bone (Longitudinal section)
- Volkmann's canal interconnecting Haversian systems is seen
- Lacunae with osteocytes.

INTRODUCTION

Bone is a hard and rigid form of connective tissue in which the extracellular matrix is impregnated with inorganic salts, mainly calcium phosphate and carbonate, which provide hardness.

GENERAL FEATURES

- Sclerous connective tissue specialized to provide support because of infiltration with inorganic salts.
- It is characterized by its rigidity, hardness, and power of regeneration and repair.
- Bone is a dynamic, living tissue, which constantly undergoes remodeling during an individual's life to help it adapt to changing physical, biochemical, and hormonal influences.
- **Functions:** (a) Bears weight; (b) Provides attachment for muscles and tendons thus, helps in movement; (c) Reservoir of minerals—calcium, phosphorus, and other ions; (c) Protects vital organs; and (d) Bone marrow within is hematopoietic tissue.

COMPOSITION OF BONE TISSUE

Like cartilage, bone is a modified connective tissue. It consists of bone cells (Figs. 6.1A to C) that are widely separated from one another by a considerable amount of intercellular substance. The latter consists of a homogeneous ground substance or matrix in which collagen fibers and mineral salts (mainly calcium and phosphorus) are deposited.

There are three types of cells in the bone: (1) *osteocytes* (mature bone cells), (2) *osteoblast* (bone forming cells),

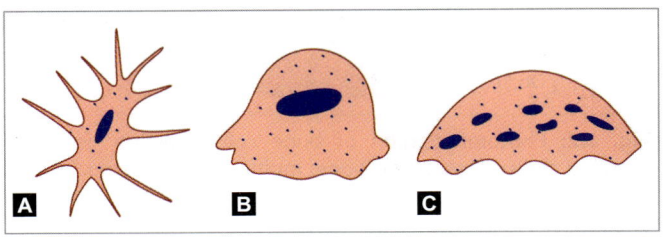

Figs. 6.1A to C: Bone cells. (A) Osteocyte; (B) Osteoblast; (C) Osteoclast (schematic representation).

and (3) *osteoclasts* or bone removing cells (Figs. 6.1 and 6.2). Other cells present include **osteoprogenitor cells** from which osteoblasts and osteocytes are derived; cells lining the surfaces of bone; cells belonging to periosteum; and cells of blood vessels and nerves which invade bone from outside.

Cells of Bone

- ❖ **Osteoprogenitor cells:**
  - Stem cells of mesenchymal origin
  - Can proliferate and convert themselves into osteoblasts whenever there is need for bone formation
  - Resemble fibroblasts in appearance
  - In the fetus, such cells are numerous at sites where bone formation is to take place. In the adult, osteoprogenitor cells are present over bone surfaces (on both the periosteal and endosteal aspects).
- ❖ **Osteoblasts:**
  - Bone forming cells derived from osteoprogenitor cells.
  - Found lining growing surfaces of bone, sometimes giving an epithelium-like appearance. However, on closer examination, it is seen that the cells are of varied shapes (oval, triangular, cuboidal, etc.) and that there are numerous gaps between adjacent cells.
  - The nucleus of an osteoblast is ovoid and euchromatic. The cytoplasm is basophilic because of the presence of abundant rough endoplasmic reticulum. This, and the presence of a well-developed Golgi complex, signifies that the cell is engaged in considerable synthetic activity. Numerous slender cytoplasmic processes radiate from each cell and come into contact with similar processes of neighboring cells.
  - Osteoblasts are responsible for laying down the organic matrix of bone including the collagen fibers. They are also responsible for the calcification of the matrix. Alkaline phosphatase present in the cell membranes of osteoblasts plays an important role in this function. Osteoblasts are believed to shed off *matrix vesicles* that possibly serve as points around which formation of hydroxyapatite crystals takes place. Osteoblasts may indirectly influence the resorption of bone by inhibiting or stimulating the activity of osteoclasts.
- ❖ **Osteocytes:**
  - The cells of mature bone.
  - Lie in the lacunae of bone and represent osteoblasts that have become "imprisoned" in the matrix during bone formation. Delicate cytoplasmic processes arising from osteocytes establish contacts with other osteocytes and with bone lining cells present on the surface of bone.
  - In contrast to osteoblasts, osteocytes have eosinophilic or lightly basophilic cytoplasm. This is to be correlated with the fact that these cells have negligible secretory activity and presence of only a small amount of endoplasmic reticulum in the cytoplasm.
  - Osteocytes are present in greatest numbers in young bone, the number gradually decreasing with age.
  - *Functions:* (1) It maintains the integrity of the lacunae and canaliculi, and thus, keeps open the channels for the diffusion of nutrition through bone, (2) They play a role in the removal or deposition of matrix and of calcium when required.
- ❖ **Osteoclasts:**
  - These are bone removing cells.
  - Found in relation to surfaces where bone removal is taking place (bone removal is essential for maintaining the proper shape of growing bone). At such locations, the cells occupy pits called **resorption bays** or *lacunae of Howship*.
  - Very large cells (20–100 μm or even more in diameter). They have numerous nuclei: up to 20 or more. The cytoplasm shows numerous mitochondria and

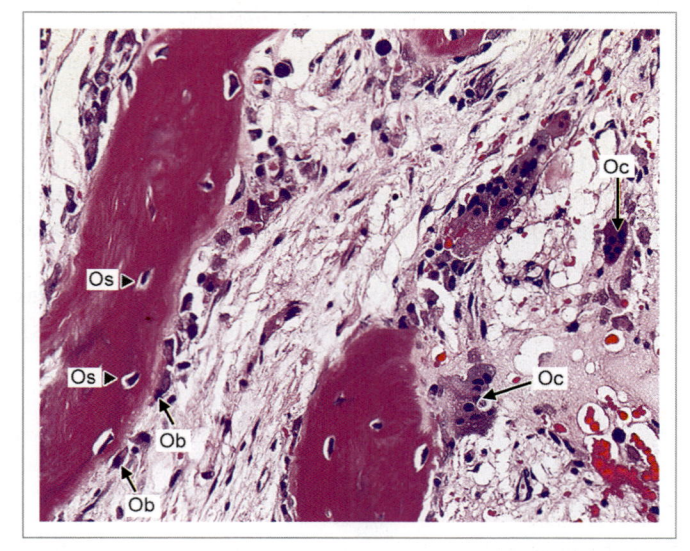

Fig. 6.2: Photomicrograph of bone cells showing osteoblast rimming the surface of the bone; multinucleated osteoclast and osteocyte. [Ob: osteoblast (short arrow); Oc: osteoclast (long arrow); Os: osteocyte (arrowhead)]

lysosomes containing acid phosphatase. At the sites of bone resorption, the surface of an osteoclast shows many folds that are described as a ***ruffled membrane.***

- Removal of bone by osteoclasts involves demineralization and removal of matrix. Bone removal can be stimulated by factors secreted by osteoblasts, by macrophages, or by lymphocytes. It is also stimulated by the parathyroid hormone.
- Recent studies have shown that osteoclasts are derived from monocytes of blood. It is not certain whether osteoclasts are formed by the fusion of several monocytes, or by repeated division of the nucleus, without division of cytoplasm.

Bone Lining Cells

These cells form a continuous epithelium-like layer on bony surfaces where active bone deposition or removal is not taking place. The cells are flattened. They are present on the periosteal surface as well as the endosteal surface. They also line spaces and canals within bone. It is possible that these cells can change to osteoblasts when bone formation is called for (in other words, many of them are osteoprogenitor cells).

Intercellular Substance

It is made up of fibers and ground substance (matrix). Matrix in turn is made up of organic and inorganic components.

Fibers

It forms 80–90% of organic component of bone. The ***collagen fibers*** are similar to those in connective tissue (type I collagen) (they are sometimes referred to as ***osteoid collagen***). The fibers are usually arranged in layers, the fibers within a layer running parallel to one another. Collagen fibers of bone are synthesized by osteoblasts.

Bone Matrix (Ground Substance)

The ground substance (or matrix) of bone consists of an organic matrix in which mineral salts are deposited.

Organic matrix

- This consists of a ground substance in which collagen fibers are embedded.
- The ***ground substance*** consists of glycosaminoglycans, proteoglycans, and water.
- Two special glycoproteins ***osteonectin*** and ***osteocalcin*** are present in large quantity. They bind readily to calcium ions and, therefore, play a role in the mineralization of bone. Vitamin D stimulates the synthesis of these proteins.
- Various other substances including chondroitin sulfates, phospholipids, and phosphoproteins are also present.
- The matrix of bone shows greater density than elsewhere immediately around the lacunae, forming capsules around them, similar to those around chondrocytes in cartilage. **The term *osteoid* is applied to the mixture of organic ground substance and collagen fibers (before it is mineralized).**

Inorganic ions

- The ions present are predominantly calcium and phosphorus (or phosphate). Magnesium, carbonate, hydroxyl, chloride, fluoride, citrate, sodium, and potassium are also present in significant amounts.
- Most of the calcium, phosphate, and hydroxyl ions are in the form of **needle-shaped crystals** that are given the name *hydroxyapatite* $[Ca_{10}(PO_4)_6(OH_2)]$. Hydroxyapatite crystals lie parallel to collagen fibers and contribute to the lamellar appearance of bone. Some amorphous calcium phosphate is also present.
- About 65% of the dry weight of bone is accounted for by inorganic salts, and 35% by organic ground substance and collagen fibers (note that these percentages are for dry weight of bone. In living bone, about 20% of its weight is made up by water). About 85% of the total salts present in bone are in the form of calcium phosphate, and about 10% in the form of calcium carbonate. 97% of total calcium in the body is located in bone.
- The calcium salts present in bone are not "fixed". There is considerable interchange between calcium stored in bone and that in circulation. When calcium level in blood rises, calcium is deposited in bone; and when the level of calcium in blood falls, calcium is withdrawn from bone to bring blood levels back to normal. These exchanges take place under the influence of hormones (parathormone produced by the parathyroid glands, and calcitonin produced by the thyroid gland).

BONE MEMBRANES

The external and internal surface of the bone is covered by the layers of connective tissue known as periosteum and endosteum, respectively.

Periosteum

- The external surface of any bone is, as a rule, covered by a membrane called periosteum (Fig. 6.3).
- The only parts of the bone surface devoid of periosteum are those that are covered with articular cartilage.

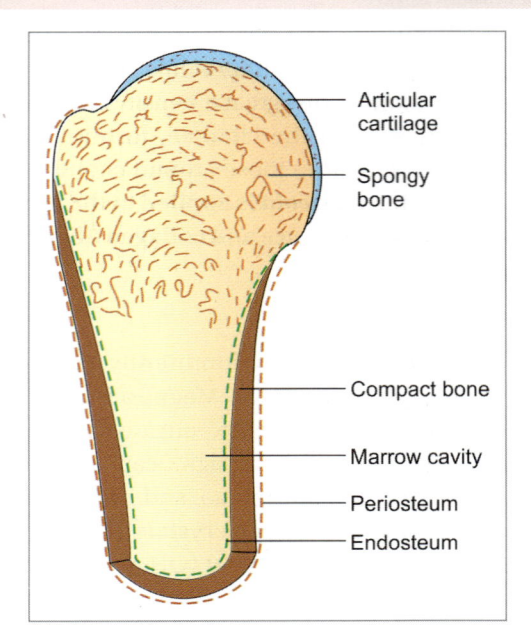

Fig. 6.3: Some features of bone structure as seen in a longitudinal section through one end of a long bone (schematic representation).

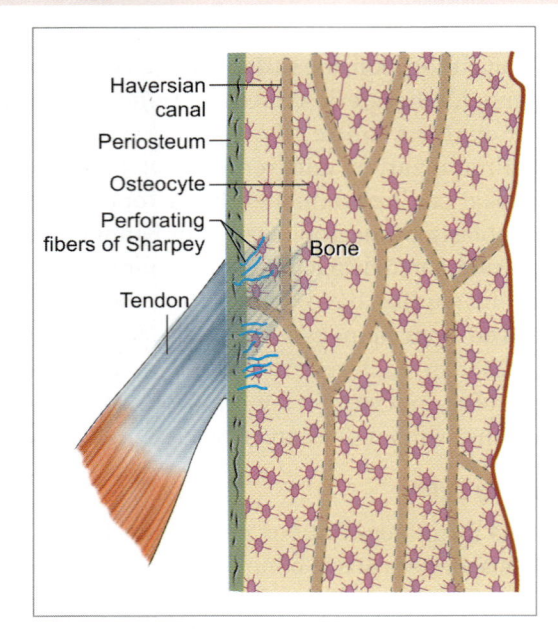

Fig. 6.4: Longitudinal section of compact bone.

- The periosteum consists of two layers, outer and inner. The outer layer is a fibrous membrane. The inner layer is cellular. In young bones, the inner layer contains numerous osteoblasts and is called the **osteogenetic layer** (this layer is sometimes described as being distinct from periosteum). In the periosteum covering, the bones of an adult osteoblasts are not conspicuous, but osteoprogenitor cells present here can form osteoblasts when need arises, e.g. in the event of a fracture.
- Periosteum is richly supplied with blood. Many vessels from the periosteum enter the bone and help to supply it.

Endosteum
- Thin layer of vascular connective tissue lining the medullary spaces of tubular bone and marrow spaces of cancellous bone.
- Also extend as lining into canaliculi of compact bone.
- Have osteogenic potential.

Functions of Periosteum and Endosteum
- It provides a medium through which muscles, tendons, and ligaments are attached to bone. In situations where very firm attachment of a tendon to bone is necessary, the fibers of the tendon continue into the outer layers of bone as the **perforating fibers of Sharpey** (Fig. 6.4). The parts of the fibers that lie within the bone are ossified; they have been compared to "nails" that keep the lamellae in place.
- Because of the blood vessels passing from periosteum into bone, the periosteum performs a nutritive function. This also forms reason for preserving them during bone surgeries.
- The osteoprogenitor cells in its deeper layer can form bone when required. This role is very important during development. It is also important in later life for the repair of bone after fracture.
- The fibrous layer of periosteum is sometimes described as a **limiting membrane** that prevents bone tissue from "spilling out" into neighboring tissues. This is based on the observation that if periosteum is torn, osteogenic cells may extend into surrounding tissue forming bony projections (**exostoses**). Such projections are frequently seen on the bones of old persons. The concept of the periosteum as a limiting membrane helps to explain how ridges and tubercles are formed on the surface of a bone. At sites where a tendon pulls upon periosteum, the latter tends to be lifted off from bone. The "gap" is filled by proliferation of bone leading to the formation of a tubercle (Such views are, however, hypothetical).
- It has rich nerve supply hence sensitive to pain.

Decalcification: Mineral salts can be removed from bone by treating it with weak acids. Chelating agents (e.g. ethylenediaminetetraacetic acid or EDTA) are also used. The process, called decalcification, is necessary for preparing sections of bone. When mineral salts are removed by decalcification, the tissue becomes soft and pliable. This shows that the rigidity of bone is mainly due to the presence of mineral salts in it.

CHAPTER 6: Bone

Calcination: Conversely, the organic substances present in bone can be destroyed by heat (as in burning). The process is called **calcination.** The form of the bone remains intact, but the bone becomes very brittle and breaks easily. It follows that the organic matter contributes substantially to the strength of bone. Resistance to tensile forces is mainly due to the presence of collagen fibers.

CLASSIFICATION AND STRUCTURE OF BONE

- *Based on the gross appearance of bone*: Compact bone and spongy bone.
- *Based on maturity*: Mature/lamellar bone and immature/woven bone.
- *Based on ossification*: Cartilaginous, membranous, and membranocartilaginous.

Compact Bone

The wall of the tube is made up of a hard dense material that appears, on naked eye examination, and shows a uniform smooth texture with no obvious spaces in it. This kind of bone is called *compact bone* (Plates 6.1 and 6.2).

The section of compact bone consists of the following:

- **Lamellae (lamella—singular):** Thin plate of bone consisting of collagen fibers and mineral salts that are deposited in a gelatinous ground substance. Even the smallest piece of bone is made up of several lamellae placed over one another (Fig. 6.5). They are of three types:
  1. **Circumferential lamellae**: Arranged parallel to the surface. Outer beneath the periosteum and inner around marrow cavity.
  2. **Concentric lamellae**: Arranged in the form of concentric rings that surround a narrow Haversian canal.
  3. **Interstitial lamellae**: Located between osteons at the angular intervals. They are the remnants of earlier formed osteons.
- **Lacunae:** Between adjoining lamellae, we see small flattened spaces or *lacunae*. Each lacuna contains one osteocyte. Spreading out from each lacuna, there are fine canals or *canaliculi* that communicate with those from other lacunae (Fig. 6.6). The canaliculi are occupied by delicate cytoplasmic processes of osteocytes. They network with each other and thus facilitate the diffusion of metabolic products between osteocytes.
- The unit of compact bone is **Haversian system or osteon**. Most of the lamellae are arranged in the form of concentric rings that surround a narrow **Haversian canal** present at the center of each ring. The Haversian canal is occupied by blood vessels, nerve fibers, and some cells. One Haversian canal and the lamellae around it constitute a **Haversian system** or *osteon* (Figs. 6.7 and 6.8). Compact bone consists of several such osteons.
- The longitudinal sections of compact bone (Fig. 6.8) has Haversian canals (and, therefore, the osteons) that

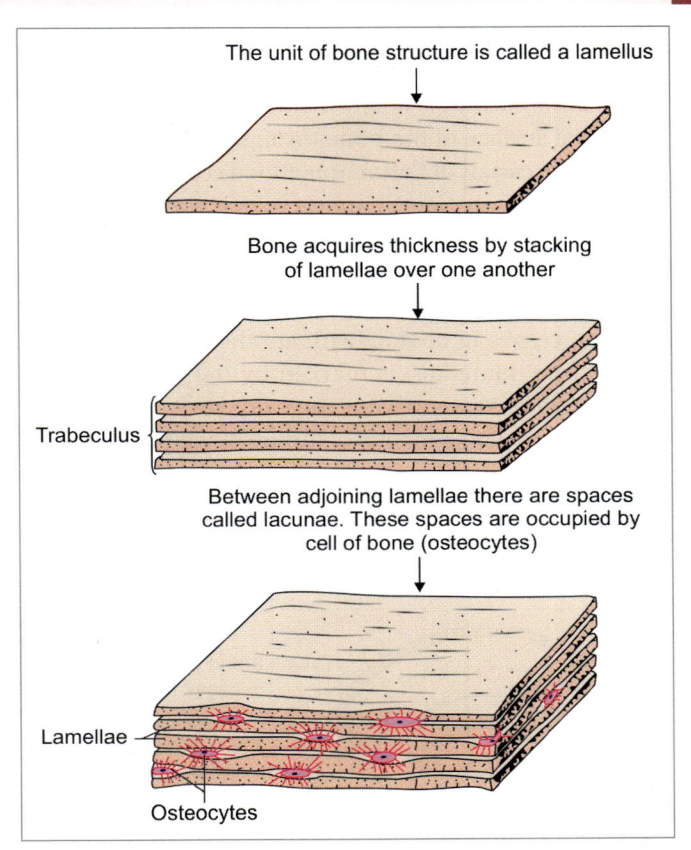

Fig. 6.5: How lamellae constitute bone (schematic representation).

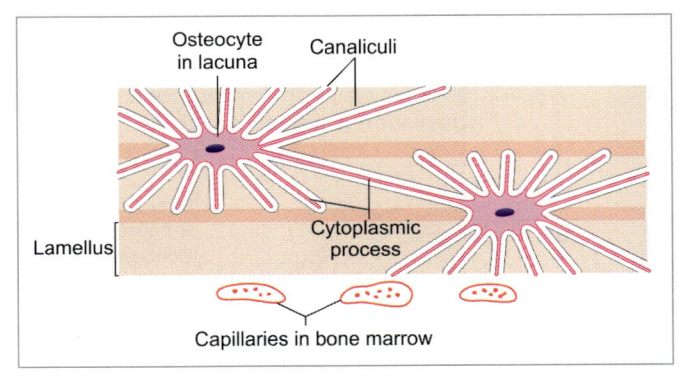

Fig. 6.6: Relationship of osteocytes to bone lamellae (schematic representation).

run predominantly along the length of the bone. The canals branch and anastomose with each other. They also communicate with the marrow cavity, and with the external surface of the bone through channels that are called **the canals of Volkmann.** Blood vessels and nerves pass through all these channels so that compact bone is permeated by a network of blood vessels that provide nutrition to it.

❖ **Cement line:** The place where the periphery of one osteon comes in contact with another osteon (or with interstitial lamellae) is marked by the presence of a cement line. Along this line there are no collagen fibers, the line consisting mainly of inorganic matrix.

Spongy/Cancellous Bone

❖ The shaft is tubular and encloses a large *marrow cavity*. The end of long bone and diploë of flat bones the marrow cavity does not extend. Instead made up of trabeculated network of tiny rods or plates of bone and containing numerous spaces, the whole appearance resembles to that of a sponge. This kind of bone is called *spongy or cancellous bone (cancel = cavity)*. **They do not have Haversian system.**

❖ The spongy bone at the bone ends is covered by a thin layer of compact bone, thus providing the bone ends with smooth surfaces (*see* Fig. 6.3). Small bits of spongy bone are also present over the wall of the marrow cavity.

❖ Cancellous bone is made up of a meshwork of bony plates or rods called trabeculae. Each trabeculus is made up of a number of lamellae (described above) between which there are lacunae containing osteocytes. Canaliculi, containing the processes of osteocytes, radiate from the lacunae (Fig. 6.9). The trabeculae enclose wide spaces that are filled in by bone marrow (Fig. 6.9 and Plate 6.1). They receive nutrition from blood vessels in the bone marrow.

❖ The trabeculae are covered externally by vascular endosteum containing osteoblasts, osteoclasts, and osteoprogenitor cells.

The marrow cavity and the spaces of spongy bone (present at the bone ends) are filled by a highly vascular tissue called *bone marrow*.

❖ *Red marrow*: At the bone ends, the marrow is red in color. Apart from blood vessels, this contains numerous masses of blood forming cells (*hematopoietic tissue*).

❖ *Yellow marrow*: In the shaft of the bone of an adult, the marrow is yellow. This is made up predominantly of fat cells. Some islands of hematopoietic tissue may be seen here also.

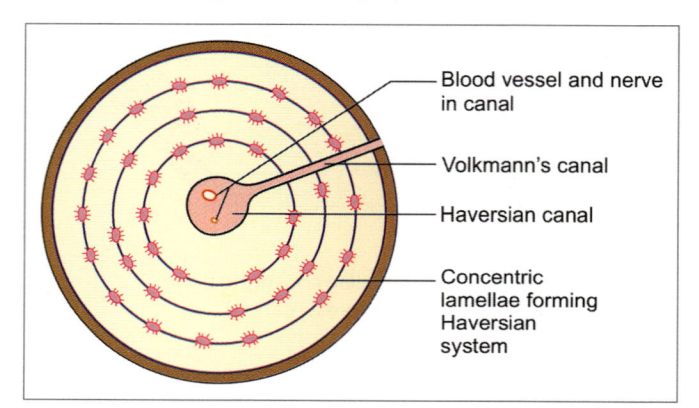

Fig. 6.7: Haversian system in compact bone (schematic representation).

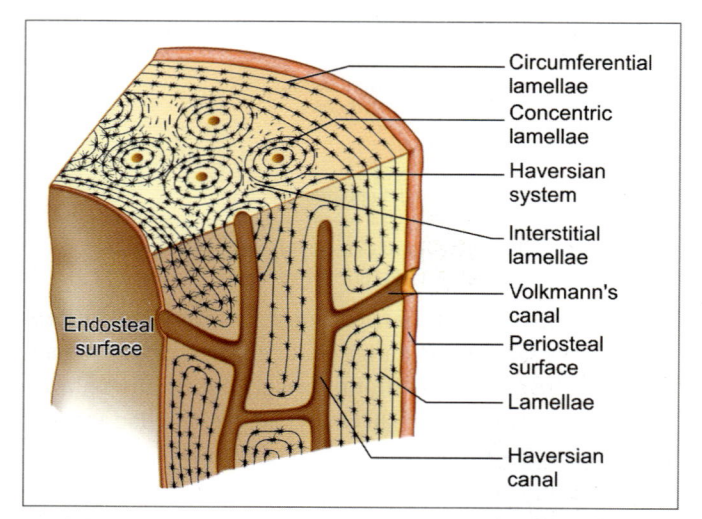

Fig. 6.8: Transverse section and longitudinal section through compact bone to show Haversian canals and the Volkmann's canal (schematic representation).

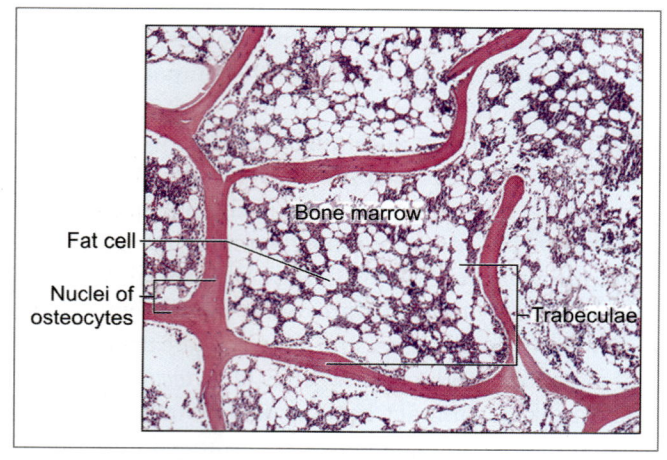

Fig. 6.9: Structure of cancellous bone (schematic representation).

CHAPTER 6: Bone

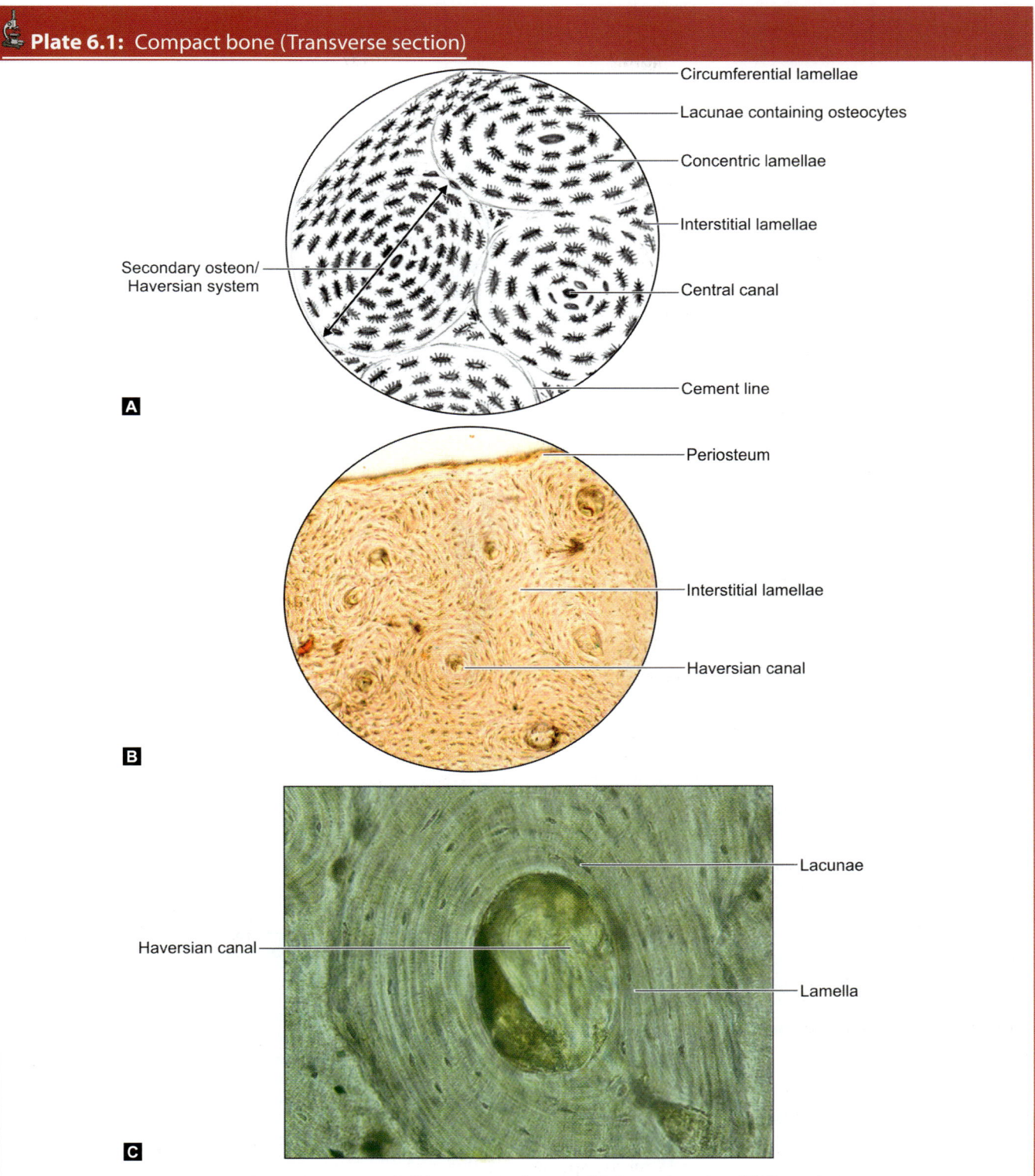

Plate 6.1: Compact bone (Transverse section)

A — labels: Circumferential lamellae; Lacunae containing osteocytes; Concentric lamellae; Interstitial lamellae; Central canal; Cement line; Secondary osteon/Haversian system

B — labels: Periosteum; Interstitial lamellae; Haversian canal

C — labels: Lacunae; Lamella; Haversian canal

Compact Bone (Transverse section): (A) As seen in drawing; (B) Ground section; (C) Haversian system.

Points of identification
- Haversian system made up of concentric lamellae, lacunae with osteocytes, Haversian (central) canal containing blood vessels and nerves are seen
- Three types of lamellae are seen—(1) circumferential, (2) concentric, and (3) interstitial
- Canaliculi radiate from lacunae.

Plate 6.2: Compact bone (Longitudinal section)

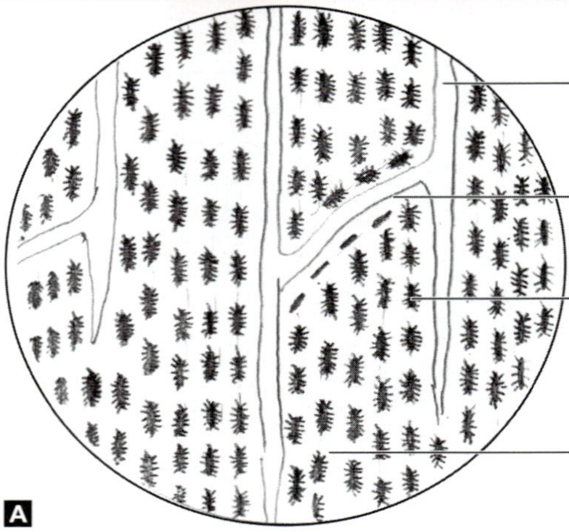

Compact bone (Longitudinal section): (A) Hand drawing; (B) Photomicrograph.

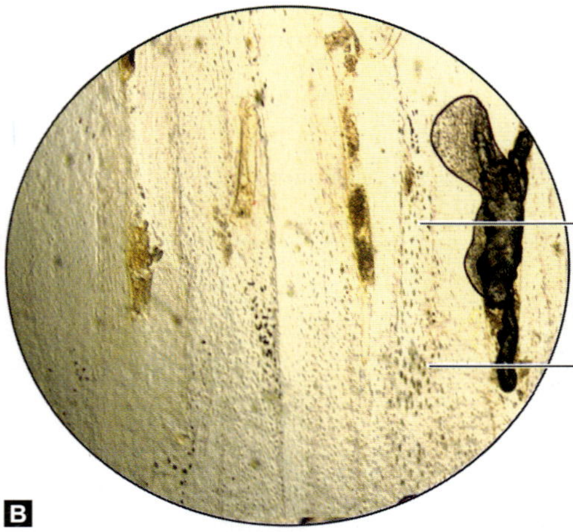

Labels: Haversian canal; Volkmann's canal; Osteocytes in lacunae; Lamellae; Lamella; Lacunae with osteocytes.

Points of identification
- Volkmann's canal interconnecting Haversian systems is seen
- Lacunae with osteocytes.

In bones of a fetus or of a young child, the entire bone marrow is red. The marrow in the shaft is gradually replaced by yellow marrow with increasing age.

Comparison between Cancellous and Compact Bone

There is an essential similarity in the structure of cancellous and compact bone. Both are made up of lamellae. The difference lies in the relative volume occupied by bony lamellae and by the spaces. In compact bone the spaces are small, and the solid bone is abundant with Haversian system, whereas in cancellous bone the spaces are large, and actual bone tissue is sparse (lamella do not form Haversian system) (Plate 6.2).

Added Information

Osteons
- During bone formation, the first formed osteons do not have a clear lamellar structure, but consist of woven bone. Such osteons are described as **primary osteons (or atypical Haversian systems)**. Subsequently, the primary osteons are replaced by **secondary osteons (or typical Haversian systems)** having the structure already described.
- The osteons run in a predominantly longitudinal direction (i.e. along the long axis of the shaft). However, this does not imply that osteons lie parallel to each other. They may follow a spiral course, may branch, or may join other osteons. In transverse sections, osteons may appear circular, oval, or ellipsoid.
- The number of lamellae in each osteon is highly variable. The average number is six.

Contd...

CHAPTER 6: Bone

Contd...

> - In an osteon collagen fibers in one lamellus usually run either longitudinally or circumferentially (relative to the long axis of the osteon). Typically, the direction of fibers in adjoining lamellae is alternately longitudinal and circumferential. It is because of this difference in the direction of fibers that the lamellar arrangement is obvious in sections. It has been claimed that in fact fibers in all lamellae follow a spiral course, the "longitudinal" fibers belonging to a spiral of a long "pitch"; and the "circumferential" fibers to the spirals of a short "pitch".
> - The various lacunae within an osteon are connected with one another through canaliculi that also communicate with the Haversian canal. The peripheral canaliculi of the osteon do not (as a rule) communicate with those of neighboring osteons: They form loops and turn back into their own osteon. A few canaliculi that pass through the cement line provide communications leading to interstitial lamellae.
> - The lacunae and canaliculi are only partially filled in by osteocytes and their processes. The remaining space is filled by a fluid that surrounds the osteocytes. This space is in communication with the Haversian canal and provides a pathway along which substances can pass from blood vessels in the Haversian canal to osteocytes.
> - When a transverse section of compact bone is examined with polarized light, each osteon shows two bright bands that cross each other. This phenomenon is called birefringence. It is an indication of the very regular arrangement of collagen fibers (and the crystals related to them) within the lamellus.
> - The lamellar appearance (*see* Fig. 6.5) of bone depends mainly on the arrangement of collagen fibers. The fibers of one lamellus run parallel to each other, but those of adjoining lamellae run at varying angles to each other. The ground substance of a lamellus is continuous with that of adjoining lamellae.

Classification Based on Histology

- **Lamellar bone:** Bone matrix contains thin sheets called as lamellae arranged parallel. It is also called secondary bone.
- **Woven bone:** The newly formed bone does not have a lamellar structure. The collagen fibers are present in bundles that appear to run randomly in different directions, interlacing with each other. Because of the interlacing of fiber bundles, this kind of bone is called ***woven bone***. It is also known as primary bone. All newly formed bone is woven bone. It is later replaced by lamellar bone.

FORMATION OF BONE—OSSIFICATION

- All bones are of mesodermal origin. The process of bone formation is called ***ossification***.
- Types: (a) ***Endochondral ossification***: The formation of most of the bones is preceded by the formation of a cartilaginous model, which is subsequently replaced by bone. This kind of ossification is called ***endochondral ossification***; and bones formed in this way are called ***cartilage bones***, (b) In some situations (e.g. the vault of the skull), formation of bone is not preceded by the formation of a cartilaginous model. Instead bone is laid down directly in a fibrous membrane. This process is called ***intramembranous ossification***; and bones formed in this way are called ***membrane bones***. The bones of the vault of the skull, the mandible, and the clavicle are membrane bones.

Intramembranous Ossification

The various stages in intramembranous ossification are as follows:

- At the site where a membrane bone is to be formed the mesenchymal cells become densely packed (i.e. a ***mesenchymal condensation*** is formed). The region becomes highly vascular. Some of the mesenchymal cells lay down the bundles of collagen fibers in the mesenchymal condensation. In this way a ***membrane is formed.***
- Some mesenchymal cells (possibly those that had earlier laid down the collagen fibers) enlarge and acquire a basophilic cytoplasm and may now be called ***osteoblasts*** (Fig. 6.10A). They come to lie along the bundles of collagen fibers. These cells secrete a gelatinous matrix in which the fibers get embedded. The fibers also swell up. Hence the fibers can no longer be seen distinctly. This mass of swollen fibers and matrix is called ***osteoid*** (Fig. 6.10B).
- Under the influence of osteoblasts, calcium salts are deposited in osteoid. As soon as this happens, the layer of osteoid can be said to have become one lamellus of bone (Fig. 6.10C).
- Over this lamellus, another layer of osteoid is laid down by osteoblasts. The osteoblasts move away from the lamellus to line the new layer of osteoid. However, some of them get caught between the lamellus and the osteoid (Fig. 6.10D). The osteoid is now ossified to form another lamellus. The cells trapped between the two lamellae become osteocytes (Fig. 6.10D).
- In this way a number of lamellae are laid down one over another, and these lamellae together form a trabeculus of bone (Fig. 6.10E).
- The first formed bone may not be in the form of regularly arranged lamellae. The elements are irregularly arranged and form woven bone.

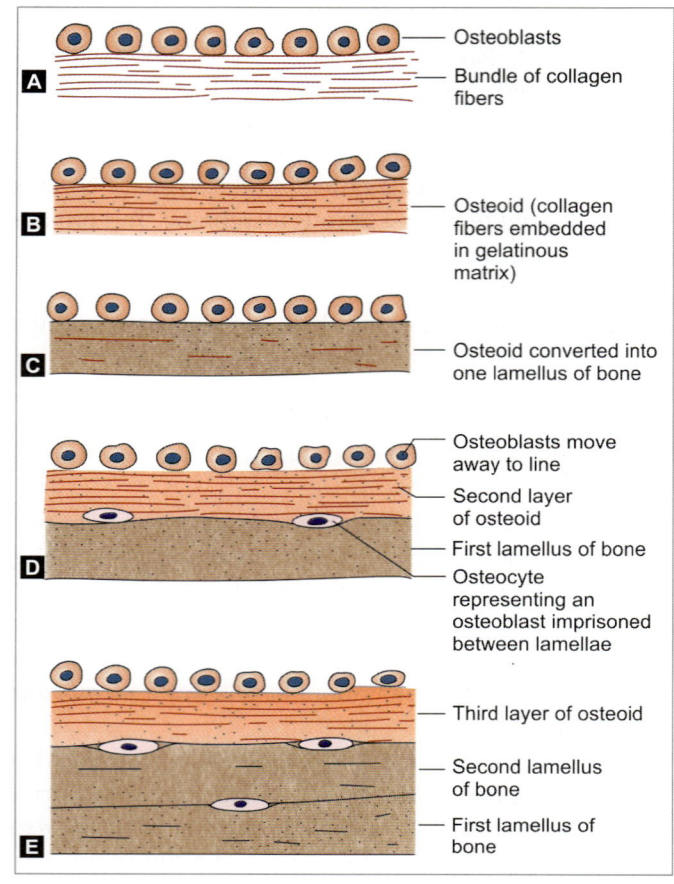

Figs. 6.10A to E: Scheme to show how bony lamellae are laid down over one another intramembranous ossification.

Endochondral Ossification

The essential steps in the formation of bone by endochondral ossification are as follows:

- At the site where the bone is to be formed, the mesenchymal cells become closely packed to form a mesenchymal condensation (Fig. 6.11A).
- Some mesenchymal cells become **chondroblasts** and lay down hyaline cartilage (Fig. 6.11B). Mesenchymal cells on the surface of the cartilage form a membrane called the perichondrium. This membrane is vascular and contains osteoprogenitor cells.
- The cells of the cartilage are at first small and irregularly arranged. However, in the area where bone formation is to begin, the cells enlarge considerably (Fig. 6.11C).
- The intercellular substance between the enlarged cartilage cells becomes calcified, under the influence of alkaline phosphatase, which is secreted by the cartilage cells. The nutrition to the cells is thus cut off, and they die, leaving behind empty spaces called *primary areolae* (Fig. 6.11C).
- Some blood vessels of the perichondrium (which may be called periosteum as soon as bone is formed) now invade the cartilaginous matrix. They are accompanied by osteoprogenitor cells. This mass of vessels and cells is called the **periosteal bud**. It eats away much of the calcified matrix forming the walls of the primary areolae, and thus creates large cavities called *secondary areolae* (Fig. 6.11D).
- The walls of secondary areolae are formed by thin layers of calcified matrix that have not dissolved. The osteoprogenitor cells become osteoblasts and arrange themselves along the surfaces of these bars, or plates, of calcified matrix (Fig. 6.11E).

  These osteoblasts now lay down a layer of ossein fibrils embedded in a gelatinous ground substance (i.e. osteoid), exactly as in intramembranous ossification (Fig. 6.11F). This osteoid is calcified, and a lamellus of bone is formed (Fig. 6.11G).
- Osteoblasts now lay down another layer of osteoid over the first lamellus. This is also calcified. Thus two lamellae of bone are formed. Some osteoblasts that get caught between the two lamellae become osteocytes. As more lamellae are laid down, bony trabeculae are formed (Figs. 6.11H and I).
- It may be noted that the process of bone formation in endochondral ossification is exactly the same as in intramembranous ossification. The calcified matrix of cartilage only acts as a support for the developing trabeculae and is not itself converted into bone.
- At this stage the ossifying cartilage shows a central region where bone has been formed. As we move away from this area, we see:
  - A region where cartilaginous matrix has been calcified and surrounds dead and dying cartilage cells.
  - A zone of hypertrophied cartilage cells in an uncalcified matrix.
  - Normal cartilage in which there is considerable mitotic activity.

In this way the formation of new cartilage keeps pace with the loss due to replacement by bone. The total effect is that the ossifying cartilage progressively increases in size.

Conversion of Cancellous Bone to Compact Bone

All newly formed bone is cancellous. It is converted into compact bone as follows.

CHAPTER 6: Bone

- Each space between the trabeculae of cancellous bone comes to be lined by a layer of osteoblasts. The osteoblasts lay down lamellae of bone as already described. The first lamellus is formed over the inner wall of the original space and is, therefore, shaped like a ring. Subsequently, concentric lamellae are laid down inside this ring thus forming an osteon. The original space becomes smaller and smaller and persists as a Haversian canal.
- The first formed Haversian systems are called *atypical Haversian systems* or *primary osteons*. These osteons do not have a typical lamellar structure, and their chemical composition may also be atypical.
- Primary osteons are soon invaded by blood vessels and by osteoclasts that bore a new series of spaces through them. These new spaces are again filled in by bony lamellae, under the influence of osteoblasts, to form *secondary osteons* (or *typical Haversian systems*). The process of formation and destruction of osteons takes place repeatedly as the bone enlarges in size and continues even after birth. In this way the internal structure of the

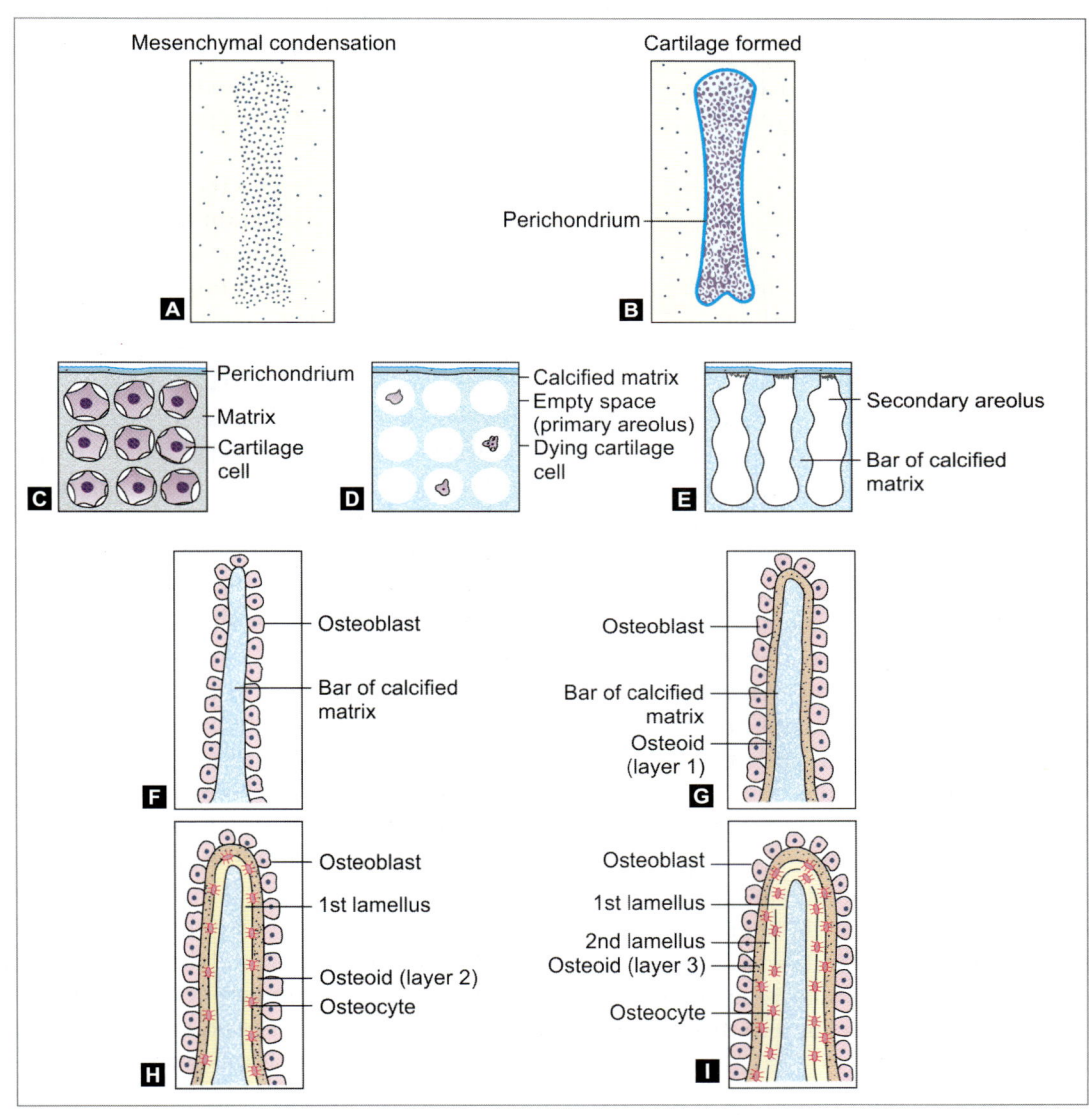

Figs. 6.11A to I: Endochondral ossification. Formation of cartilaginous model (schematic representation). (A and B) Formation of cartilaginous model; (C) Early stage, the cartilage cells are separated by matrix; (D) The matrix has calcified. Cartilage cells are dead leaving empty spaces called primary areolae; (E) Some primary areolae have fused to form larger spaces called secondary areolae; (F to I) Four stages in formation of bony lamellae.

bone can be repeatedly remodeled to suit the stresses imposed on the bone.
- Interposed in between osteons of the newest series, there will be remnants of previous generations of osteons. The interstitial lamellae of compact bone represent such remnants.
- When a newly created cavity begins to be filled in by lamellae of a new osteon, the first formed layer is atypical in that it has a very high density of mineral deposit. This layer can subsequently be identified as a ***cement line*** that separates the osteon from previously formed elements. As the cement line represents the line at which the process of bone erosion stops and at which the process of bone formation begins, it is also called a ***reversal line***. The cement lines are never present around primary osteons but are always present around subsequent generations of osteons.

HOW BONES GROW?

A hard tissue like bone can grow only by the deposition of new bone over existing bone, i.e. by apposition.

Growth of Bones of Vault of Skull

- In the bones of the vault of the skull (e.g. the parietal bone), ossification begins in one or more small areas called **centers of ossification** and forms following the usual process.
- At first, it is in the form of narrow trabeculae or spicules. These spicules increase in length by the deposition of bone at their ends. As the spicules lengthen, they radiate from the center of ossification to the periphery. Gradually the entire mesenchymal condensation is invaded by this spreading process of ossification, and the bone assumes its normal shape. However, even at birth, the radiating arrangement of trabeculae is obvious.
- The mesenchymal cells lying over the developing bone differentiate to form the periosteum.
- The embryonic parietal bone, formed as described above, has to undergo considerable growth. After ossification has extended into the entire membrane representing the embryonic parietal bone, this bone is separated from neighboring bones by intervening fibrous tissue (in the region of the sutures).
- Growth in size of the bone can occur by the deposition of bone on the edges adjoining sutures (Figs. 6.12 and 6.13). Growth in thickness and size of the bone also occurs when the overlying periosteum forms bone (by the process of intramembranous ossification described above) over the outer surface of the bone.
- Simultaneously, there is the removal of bone from the inner surface. In this way, as the bone grows in size, there is simultaneous increase in the size of the cranial cavity.

Development of a Typical Long Bone

- In the region where a long bone is to be formed the mesenchyme first lays down a cartilaginous model of the bone (Figs. 6.14A to C). This cartilage is covered by perichondrium. Endochondral ossification starts in the central part of the cartilaginous model (i.e. at the center of the future shaft). This area is called the ***primary center of ossification*** (Fig. 6.14D). Gradually, bone formation extends from the primary center toward the ends of shaft. This is accompanied by progressive enlargement of the cartilaginous model.
- Soon after the appearance of the primary center, and the onset of endochondral ossification in it, the perichondrium (which may now be called periosteum) becomes active. The osteoprogenitor cells in its deeper layer lay down bone on the surface of the cartilaginous model by ***intramembranous ossification***. This periosteal bone completely surrounds the cartilaginous shaft and is, therefore, called the ***periosteal collar*** (Figs. 6.14D and E). The periosteal collar is first formed only around the region of the primary center, but rapidly extends toward the ends of the cartilaginous model (Figs. 6.14F and G). It acts as a splint and gives strength to the cartilaginous model at the site where it is weakened by the formation of secondary areolae. We shall see that most of the shaft of the bone is derived from this periosteal collar and is, therefore, membranous in origin.
- At about the time of birth the developing bone consists of a part called the ***diaphysis*** (or shaft), that is bony, and has been formed by extension of the primary center of ossification, and ends that are cartilaginous (Fig. 6.14F). At varying times after birth, ***secondary centers*** of endochondral ossification appear in the cartilages forming the ends of the bone (Fig. 6.14G). These centers enlarge until the ends become bony (Fig. 6.14H). More than one secondary center of ossification may appear at either end. The portion of bone formed from one secondary center is called an ***epiphysis***.
- For a considerable time after birth the bone of the diaphysis and the bone of any epiphysis are separated by a plate of cartilage called the ***epiphyseal cartilage***, or ***epiphyseal plate***. This is formed by cartilage into which

CHAPTER 6: Bone

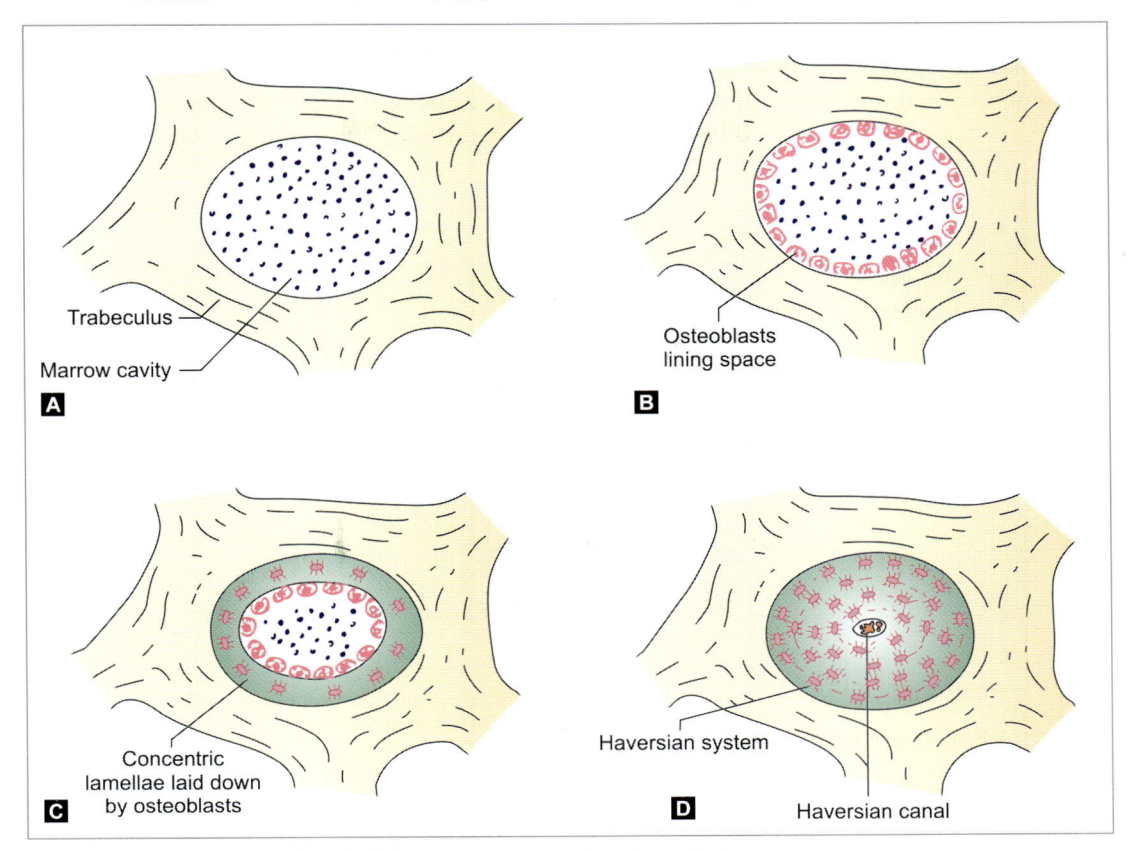

Figs. 6.12A to D: Scheme to show how skull bones grow.

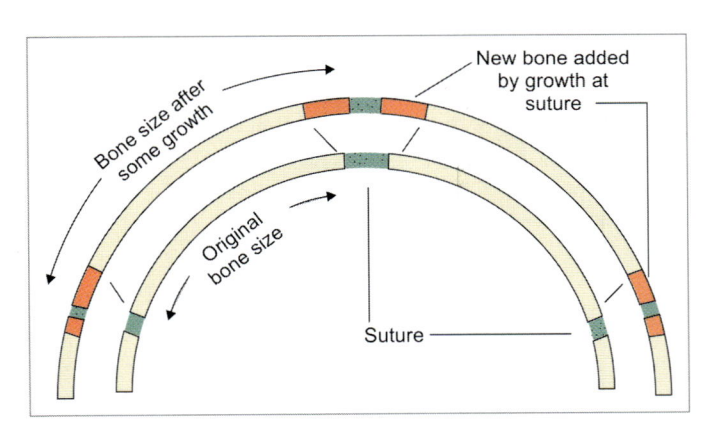

Fig. 6.13: Growth of skull bones at sutures.

ossification has not extended either from the diaphysis or from the epiphysis. We shall see that this plate plays a vital role in growth of the bone.

Growth of a Long Bone

❖ A growing bone increases both in length and in girth. The periosteum lays down a layer of bone around the shaft of the cartilaginous model. This periosteal collar gradually extends to the whole length of the diaphysis. As more layers of bone are laid down over it, the periosteal bone becomes thicker and thicker. However, it is neither necessary nor desirable for it to become too thick. Hence, osteoclasts come to line the internal surface of the shaft and remove bone from this aspect.

❖ As bone is laid down outside the shaft, it is removed from the inside. The shaft thus grows in diameter, and at the same time, its wall does not become too thick. The osteoclasts also remove trabeculae lying in the center of the bone that were formed by endochondral ossification. In this way a *marrow cavity* is formed.

❖ As the shaft increases in diameter, there is a corresponding increase in the size of the marrow cavity. This cavity also extends toward the ends of the diaphysis but does not reach the epiphyseal plate. Gradually, most of the bone formed from the primary center (i.e. of endochondral origin) is removed, except near the bone ends, so that the wall of the shaft is ultimately made up entirely of periosteal bone formed by the process of intramembranous ossification.

- To understand how a bone grows in length, we will now take a closer look at the **epiphyseal plate**. Depending on the arrangement of cells, three zones can be recognized (Fig. 6.15).

- *Zone of resting cartilage*: Here the cells are small and irregularly arranged.
- *Zone of proliferating cartilage*: This is also called the *zone of cartilage growth*. In this zone the cells

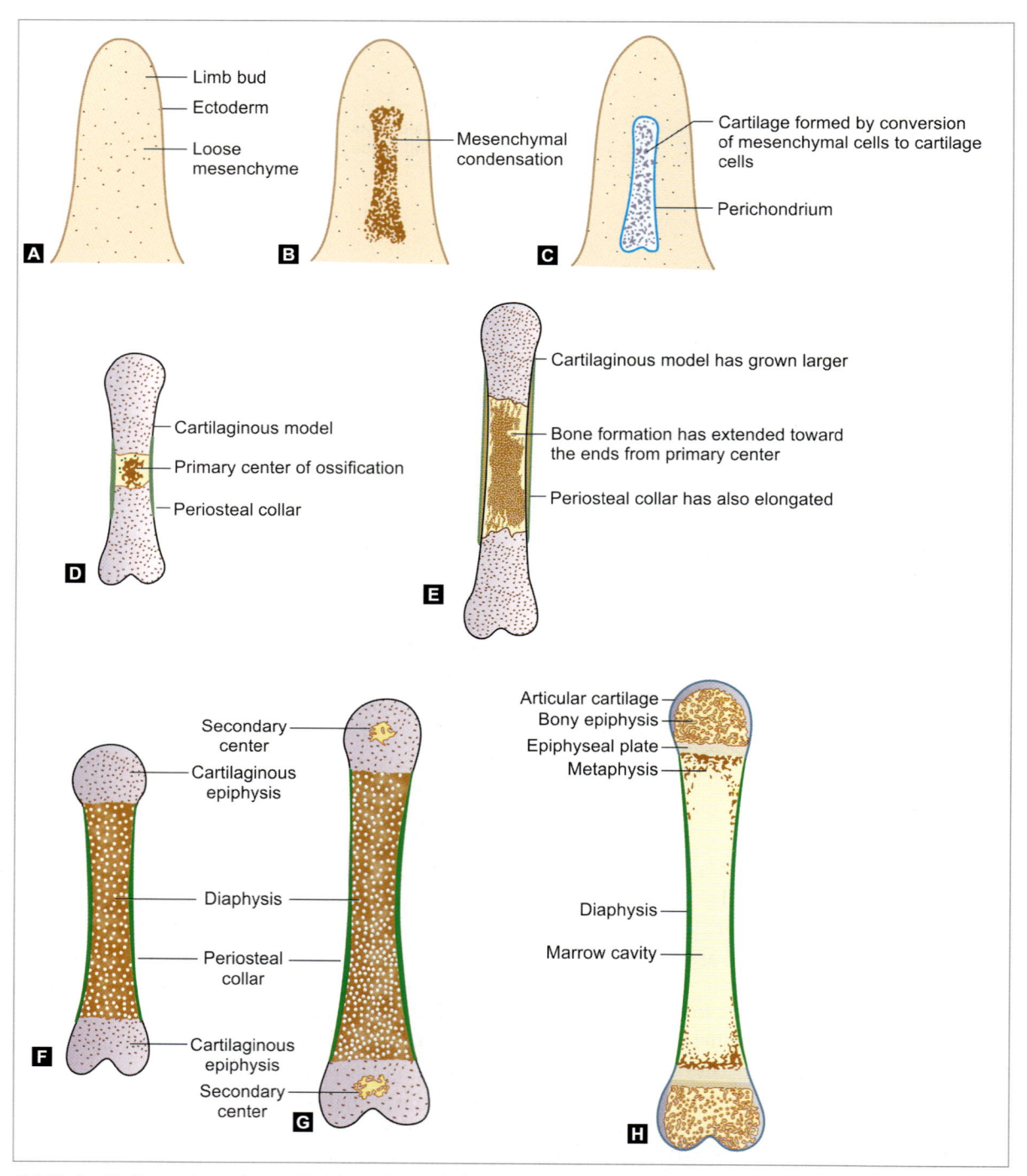

Figs. 6.14A to H: Formation of a typical long bone (schematic representation). (A to C) Establishment of cartilaginous model; (D and E) Formation of primary center of ossification and periosteal collar; (F and G) Formation of secondary centers of ossification; (H) Formation of bony epiphyses and epiphyseal plates.

CHAPTER 6: Bone

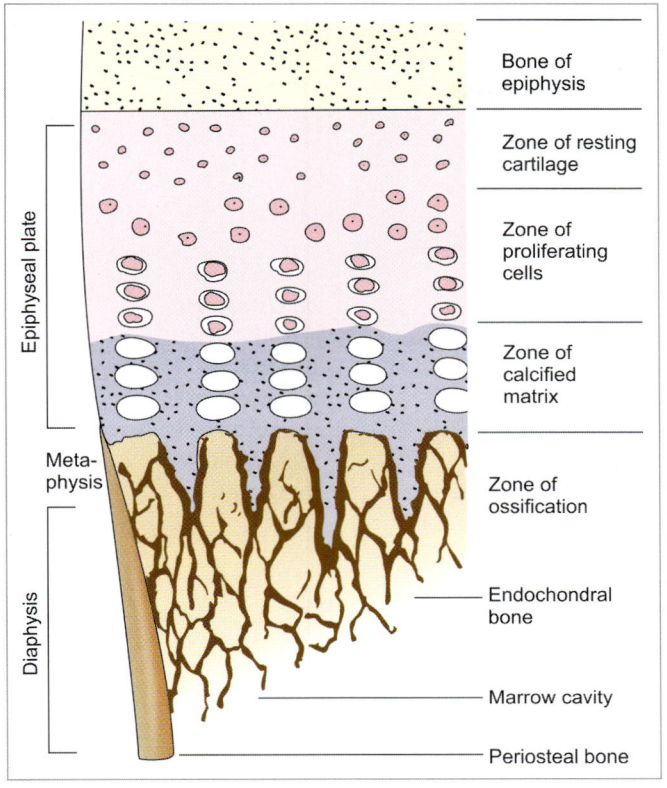

Fig. 6.15: Structure of an epiphyseal plate (schematic representation).

Metaphysis

The portion of the diaphysis adjoining the epiphyseal plate is called the metaphysis. It is a region of active bone formation and, for this reason, it is highly vascular. The metaphysis does not have a marrow cavity. Numerous muscles and ligaments are usually attached to the bone in this region. Even after bone growth has ceased, the calcium turnover function of bone is most active in the metaphysis, which acts as a storehouse of calcium. The metaphysis is frequently the site of infection (osteomyelitis) because blood vessels show hairpin bends, and blood flow is sluggish.

> ### Added Information
> **Wolff's law:** The structure of each part of a bone is adapted to these stresses bone being thickest along the lines of maximum stress, and absent in areas where there is no stress. This applies not only to the gross structure of a bone but also to its microscopic structure. The fact that the trabeculae of cancellous bone are arranged along the lines of stress has been recognized since long: this fact is known as Wolff's law. In some situations (e.g. at the upper end of the femur) the trabeculae appear to be arranged predominantly in two planes at right angles to each other. It has been suggested that trabeculae in one plane resist compressive forces, and those in the other direction resist tensile forces. In this context, it is interesting to note that a clear pattern of trabeculae is seen in the femur of a child only after it begins to walk.

are larger and undergo repeated mitosis. As they multiply, they come to be arranged in parallel columns, separated by bars of intercellular matrix.

- **Zone of calcification**: This is also called the *zone of cartilage transformation*. In this zone the cells become still larger, and the matrix becomes calcified. Next to the zone of calcification, there is a zone where cartilage cells are dead, and the calcified matrix is being replaced by bone. Growth in length of the bone takes place by continuous transformation of the epiphyseal cartilage to bone in this zone (i.e. on the diaphyseal surface of the epiphyseal cartilage). At the same time the thickness of the epiphyseal cartilage is maintained by the active multiplication of cells in the zone of proliferation.

❖ When the bone has attained its full length, cells in the cartilage stop proliferating. The process of calcification, however, continues to extend into it until the whole of the epiphyseal plate is converted into bone. The bone substance of the diaphysis and that of the epiphysis then become continuous. This is called ***fusion of the epiphysis***.

APPLIED HISTOLOGY

❖ **Osteopetrosis:** It is a disorder affecting osteoclasts in which they cannot resorb bone, which creates an imbalance between bone formation and bone resorption. These persons with display increased bone density.
❖ **Osteoporosis**
❖ **Rickets/Acromegaly**
❖ A benign tumor arising from osteoblasts is called an **osteoma**. A malignant tumor arising from the same cells is called an **osteosarcoma**. Osteosarcomas are most commonly seen in bones adjoining the knee joint. They can spread to distant sites in the body through the blood stream.
❖ **Paget's disease of bone or osteitis deformans**: Abnormal persistence of woven bone is a feature of Paget's disease. It was first described by Sir James Paget in 1877. Paget's disease of bone is an osteolytic and osteosclerotic bone disease of uncertain etiology involving one (monostotic) or more bones (polyostotic). The condition affects predominantly males over the age of 50 years. The bones are weak, and there may be deformities.

MULTIPLE CHOICE QUESTIONS

1. Which of the following provide a pathway for the diffusion of nutrients within compact bone?
   a. Canaliculi
   b. Lamellae
   c. Periosteum
   d. Lacunae
2. Which of the following cells is the precursor to bone forming cells?
   a. Osteogenic
   b. Osteoblast
   c. Chondroblast
   d. Osteoclast
3. When there is too little calcium in blood, which cells begin resorption of bone to release calcium to the blood?
   a. Osteocytes
   b. Osteoblast
   c. Osteoclast
   d. Osteogenic
4. Which of these features indicates that a bone is not mature?
   a. Articular cartilage
   b. Epiphyseal plate
   c. Medullary cavity
   d. Spongy bone
5. What is compact bone?
   a. Dense
   b. Spongy
   c. Cancellous
   d. Woven
6. What sits in a lacuna?
   a. Osteoclast
   b. Osteogenic
   c. Osteocyte
   d. Osteoblast
7. What cell is an immature bone cell?
   a. Osteoclast
   b. Osteon
   c. Osteocyte
   d. Osteoblast
8. What is the hollow area underneath an osteoclast called?
   a. Vacuole
   b. Lacuna
   c. Howship's lacuna
   d. Osteon

Answers
1. a   2. b   3. c   4. b   5. a   6. c   7. d   8. c

CHAPTER 7

Muscular Tissue

Learning objectives

To study the:
- Types of muscular tissue
- Skeletal muscle
- Cardiac muscle
- Smooth muscle
- Myoepithelial cells
- Applied histology

IDENTIFICATION POINTS

Skeletal muscle
- Long cylindrical fibers
- Alternate dark and light band causing striations
- Peripherally located multiple nuclei.

Smooth muscle
- Spindle-shaped cells with central flat nucleus
- Absence of striations.

Cardiac muscle
- Branched muscle fibers
- Central round single nucleus
- Presence of striations.

INTRODUCTION

Muscle tissue is one of the basic tissues that are specialized to shorten in length by contraction causing movement. It is in this way that virtually all movements within the body, or of the body in relation to the environment, are ultimately produced.

- Muscle tissue is made up basically of cells that are called *myocytes*. Myocytes are elongated in one direction and are, therefore, often referred to as *muscle fibers*.
- Myocytes are mesodermal in origin; exception: arrector pilorum, muscles of iris and myoepithelial cells which are ectodermal in origin.
- Each muscle fiber contains contractile proteins actin and myosin.
- The various cell organelles of muscle fibers have been given special terms, plasma membrane-sarcolemma, cytoplasm-sarcoplasm, smooth endoplasmic reticulum (ER)-sarcoplasmic reticulum, and mitochondria-sarcosome.
- Each muscle fiber is closely invested by connective tissue that is continuous with that around other muscle fibers. Because of this fact, the force generated by different muscle fibers gets added together. In some cases, a movement may be the result of simultaneous contraction of thousands of muscle fibers. The connective tissue framework of muscle also provides pathways along which blood vessels and nerves reach muscle fibers.

TYPES OF MUSCULAR TISSUE

Histologically, muscle is classified into three types:
1. *Skeletal muscle*:
    - Present mainly in the limbs and in relation to the body wall.
    - Because of its close relationship to the bony skeleton, it is called **skeletal muscle**.
    - When examined under a microscope, fibers of skeletal muscle show prominent transverse striations. Skeletal muscleis, therefore, also called **striated muscle**.
    - Skeletal muscle can normally be made to contract under our will (to perform movements we desire). It is, therefore, also called **voluntary muscle**. Skeletal muscle is supplied by somatic motor nerves.
2. *Smooth muscle*:
    - Present mainly in relation to viscera.
    - It is seen most typically in the walls of hollow viscera.
    - As fibers of this variety do not show transverse striations, it is called **smooth muscle**, or **nonstriated muscle**.

- As a rule, contraction of smooth muscle is not under our control; and smooth muscle is, therefore, also called **involuntary muscle**. It is supplied by autonomic nerves.
3. ***Cardiac muscle***:
    - Present exclusively in the heart.
    - It resembles smooth muscle in being involuntary; but it resembles striated muscle in that the fibers of cardiac muscle also show transverse striations.
    - Cardiac muscle has an inherent rhythmic contractility the rate of which can be modified by autonomic nerves that supply it.

Note: Some "skeletal" muscle has no relationship to the skeleton being present in situations such as the wall of the esophagus, or of the anal canal. The term striated muscle is usually treated as being synonymous with skeletal muscle, but we have seen that cardiac muscle also has striations. In many instances, the contraction of skeletal muscle may not be strictly voluntary (e.g. in sneezing or coughing; respiratory movements; maintenance of posture). Conversely, contraction of smooth muscle may be produced by voluntary effort as in passing urine.

SKELETAL MUSCLE

Microscopic Features

- ❖ Skeletal muscle is made up essentially of long, cylindrical "fibers". The length of the fibers is highly variable, the longest being as much as 30 cm in length. The diameter of the fibers also varies considerably (10–60 μm; usually 50–60 μm). Each "fiber" is really a syncytium (Fig. 7.1A) with hundreds of nuclei along its length (The "fiber" is formed, during development, by fusion of numerous myoblasts).
- ❖ The nuclei are elongated and lie along the periphery of the fiber, just under the cell membrane (which is called the **sarcolemma**). The cytoplasm (or **sarcoplasm**) is filled with numerous longitudinal fibrils that are called **myofibrils** (Fig. 7.1B). This pushes the nuclei to periphery underneath sarcolemma.
- ❖ The most striking feature of skeletal muscle fibers is the presence of transverse striations in them (Plate 7.1). After staining with hematoxylin, the striations are seen as alternate dark and light bands that stretch across the muscle fiber. The dark bands are called ***A-bands*** (anisotropic), while the light bands are called ***I-bands*** (isotropic) (Fig. 7.3). (As an aid to memory, note that "A" and "I" correspond to the second letters in the words dark and light).
- ❖ In addition to myofibrils, the sarcoplasm of a muscle fiber contains the usual cell organelles that tend to aggregate near the nuclei. Mitochondria are numerous. Substantial amounts of glycogen are also present. Glycogen provides energy for contraction of muscle.
- ❖ Skeletal muscle fibers are multinucleated because they are syncytium. In the embryo they are uninucleated entities in myoblasts. Later during development myoblasts fuse together and gives rise to multinucleated muscle fiber. Larger the length of fiber more will be the number of nuclei. This in turn helps to sufficient translation of mRNA to proteins and enzymes.
- ❖ **Organization:** Each muscle fiber is closely invested by connective tissue. This connective tissue supports muscle fibers and unites them to each other. Each muscle fiber is surrounded by delicate connective tissue that is called the **endomysium**. Individual fasciculi are surrounded by a stronger sheath of connective tissue called the **perimysium**. The entire muscle is surrounded by

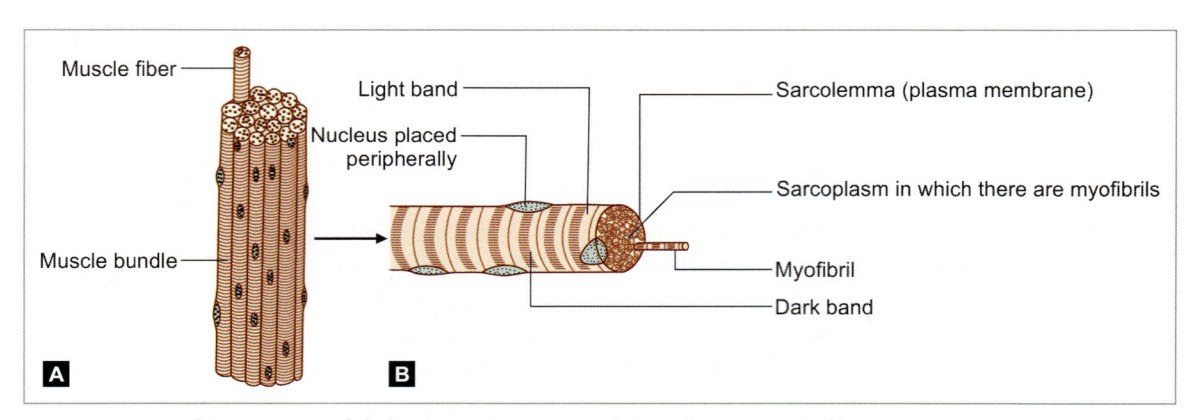

Figs. 7.1A and B: Structure of skeletal muscles: (A) Muscle bundle; (B) Muscle fiber (schematic representation).

CHAPTER 7: Muscular Tissue

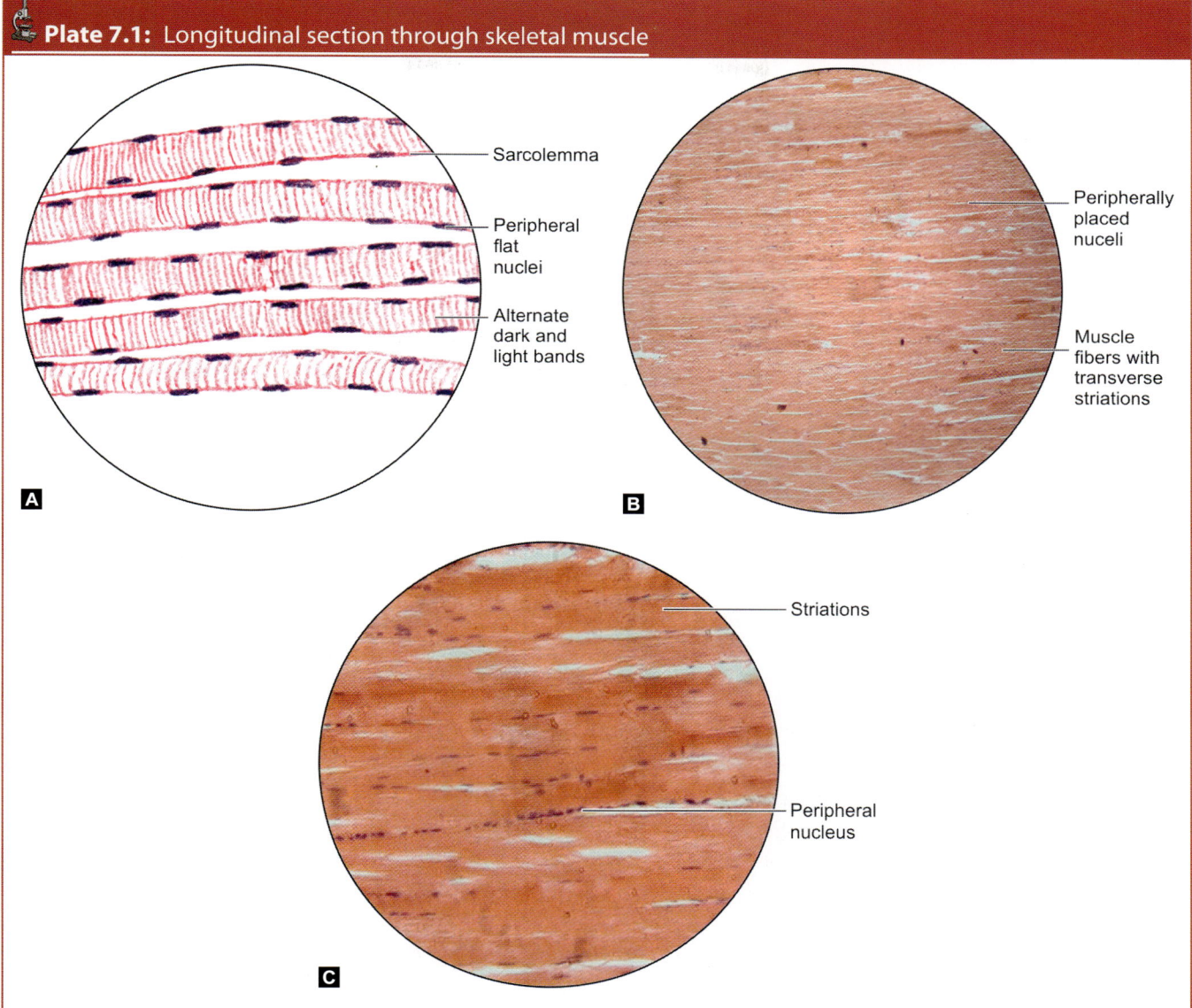

Plate 7.1: Longitudinal section through skeletal muscle

A — Sarcolemma; Peripheral flat nuclei; Alternate dark and light bands

B — Peripherally placed nuclei; Muscle fibers with transverse striations

C — Striations; Peripheral nucleus

Longitudinal section through skeletal muscle: (A) As seen in drawing; (B) Photomicrograph low power; (C) Photomicrograph high power.

Points of identification
- In a longitudinal section through skeletal muscle, the fibers are easily distinguished as they show characteristic transverse striations
- The fibers are long and parallel without branching
- Many flat nuclei are placed at the periphery
- The muscle fibers are separated by some connective tissue.

---

connective tissue called the ***epimysium*** (Fig. 7.2 and Plate 7.2). At the junction of a muscle with a tendon, the fibers of the endomysium, the perimysium, and the epimysium become continuous with the fibers of the tendon.

❖ Within a muscle, the muscle fibers are arranged in the form of bundles or fasciculi. The numbers of fasciculi in a muscle, and the number of fibers in each fasciculus, are both highly variable. In small muscles concerned with fine movements (like those of the eyeball, or those of the vocal folds), the fasciculi are delicate and few in number. In large muscles (in which strength of contraction is the main consideration), fasciculi are coarse and numerous.

❖ **Ultrastructure of striated muscle [under electron microscope (EM)]**: Each muscle fiber is covered by a

Plate 7.2: Transverse section through skeletal muscle

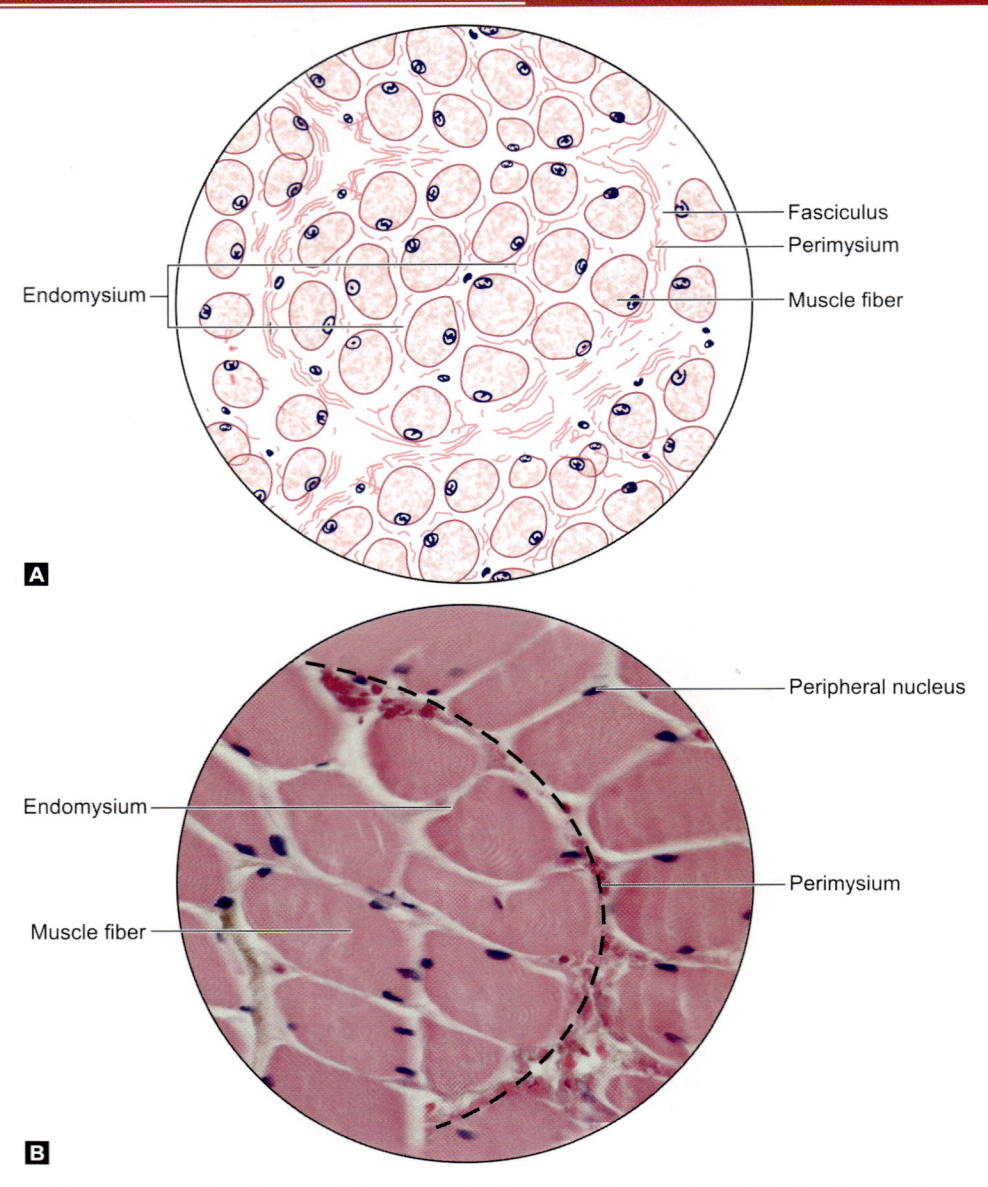

Transverse section through skeletal muscle: (A) As seen in drawing; (B) Photomicrograph.

Points of identification
The transverse section of a skeletal muscle fiber is characterized by:
- Fibers seen as irregularly round structures with peripheral nuclei
- Muscle fibers grouped into numerous fasciculi
- Dots within the fibers are myofibrils which are seen at higher magnification.

The connective tissue of the muscle consists of:
- **Epimysium**: Connective tissue sheath of muscle (not seen in photomicrograph)
- **Perimysium**: Connective tissue covering of each fascicle
- **Endomysium**: Loose connective tissue surrounding each muscle fiber.

CHAPTER 7: Muscular Tissue

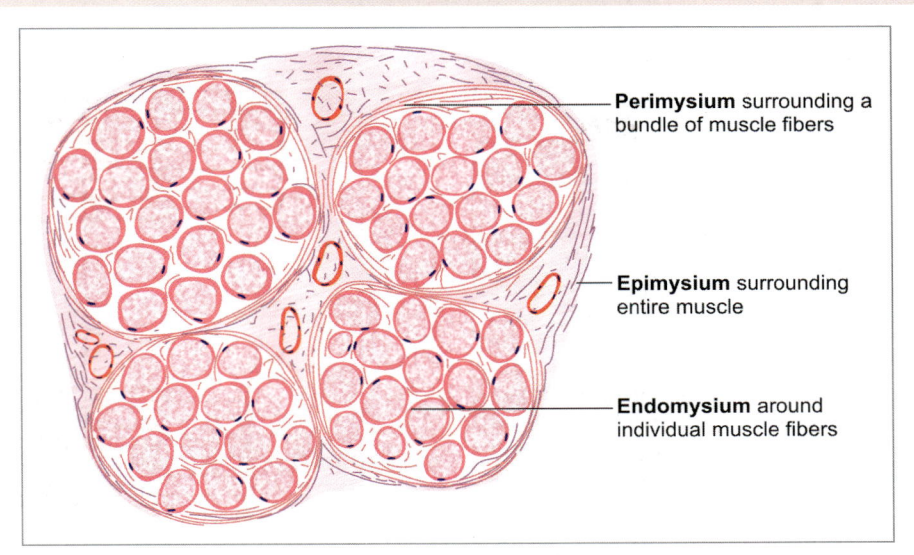

Fig. 7.2: Connective tissue present in relation to transverse section of skeletal muscle (schematic representation).

plasma membrane that is called the **sarcolemma**. The sarcolemma is covered on the outside by a basement membrane (also called the external lamina) that establishes an intimate connection between the muscle fiber and the fibers (collagen, reticular) of the endomysium. The cytoplasm (sarcoplasm) is permeated with myofibrils that push the elongated nuclei to a peripheral position. Between the myofibrils, there is an elaborate system of membrane-lined tubes called the sarcoplasmic reticulum. Elongated mitochondria (sarcosomes) and clusters of glycogen are also scattered among the myofibrils. Perinuclear Golgi bodies, ribosomes, lysosomes, and lipid vacuoles are also present.

- **Structure of myofibrils (Fig. 7.3):** When examined by EM, each myofibril is seen to be made of fine myofilaments. Each myofibril has alternating I and A bands seen under light microscopy. In good preparations (especially if the fibers are stretched), some further details can be made out. Running across the middle of each I-band there is a thin dark line called the **Z-band**. The middle of the A-band is traversed by a lighter band, called the **H-band** (or H-zone). Running through the center of the H-band, a thin dark line can be made out. This is the **M-band**. These bands appear to run transversely across the whole muscle fiber because corresponding bands in adjoining myofibrils lie exactly in alignment with one another. The part of a myofibril situated between two consecutive Z-bands is called a *sarcomere*. The cross striations seen in a myofibril under electron microscopy is due to the presence of orderly arrangement of *myofilaments* (contractile protein filaments) within it.

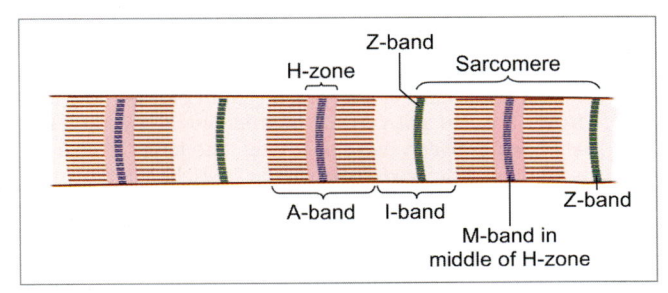

Fig. 7.3: Terminology of transverse bands in a myofibril. Note that the A-band is confined to one sarcomere, but the I-band is made up of parts of two sarcomeres that meet at the Z-band (schematic representation).

- **Structure of myofilaments:** There are two types of myofilaments in skeletal muscle, *myosin* and *actin*, made up of molecules of corresponding proteins (each myosin filament is about 12 nm in diameter, while an actin filament is about 8 nm in diameter. They are, therefore, referred to as thick and thin filaments, respectively). The arrangement of *myosin* and *actin* filaments within a sarcomere is shown in Figure 7.4. It will be seen that myosin filaments are confined to the A-band, the width of the band being equal to the length of the myosin filaments. The actin filaments are attached at one end to the Z-band. From here, they pass through the I-band and extend into the "outer" parts of the A-band, where they interdigitate with the myosin filaments. Note that the I-band is made up of actin filaments alone. The H-band represents the part of the A-band into which actin filaments do not extend. The Z-band is really a complicated network at which the actin filaments of adjoining sarcomeres meet. The M-band is produced by fine interconnections between adjacent myosin filaments.

> **Added Information**
>
> **Origin of terms I-band and A-band**
> We have seen that the light and dark bands of myofibrils (or of muscle fibers) are designated I-bands and A-bands, respectively. The letters "I" and "A" stand for the terms *isotropic* and *anisotropic*, respectively. These terms refer to the way in which any material (e.g. a crystal) behaves with regard to the transmission of light through it. Some materials refract light equally in all directions: they are said to be *isotropic*. Other materials that do not refract light equally in different planes are **anisotropic**. These qualities depend on the arrangement of the elements making up the material. In the case of muscle fibers, the precise reason for alternate bands being isotropic and anisotropic is not understood. The phenomenon is most probably due to peculiarities in arrangement of molecules within them. Although striations can be made out in unstained material using ordinary light, they are much better seen through a microscope using polarized light.
>
> **Significance of letters Z, H, and M**
> We have seen that the part of a myofibril between the two Z-bands is called a sarcomere. In other words, a Z band is a plate lying between two sarcomeres. The letter "Z" is from the German word *zwischenschiebe* (zwischen = between; schiebe = disc). The M-band is a plate lying in the middle of the sarcomere. The letter "M" is from the German word *mittleschiebe* (mittle = middle). The H-band (or zone) is named after Hensen who first described it.

Each *myosin filament* is made up of a large number of myosin molecules. Each molecule is made up of two units, each unit having a head and a tail (Fig. 7.5). The tails are coiled over each other. A myosin filament is a "bundle" of the tails of such molecules (Fig. 7.6). The heads project outward from the bundle as projections of the myosin filament. The projecting heads are arranged in a regular helical manner.

Because of the manner in which it is formed, each myosin fibril can be said to have a head end and a tail end. The tail end is attached to the M-line.

Each *actin* filament is really composed of two subfilaments that are twisted round each other (Fig. 7.7). Each subfilament is a chain of globular (rounded) molecules. These globular molecules are G-actin, and the chain formed by them is designated as **F-actin**. Each actin filament has a head end (that extends into the A-band) and a tail end that is anchored to the Z-line (through a protein called α-actinin). The filament also contains two other proteins called **tropomyosin** and **troponin**. Tropomyosin is in the form of a long fiber that winds around actin and stabilizes it.

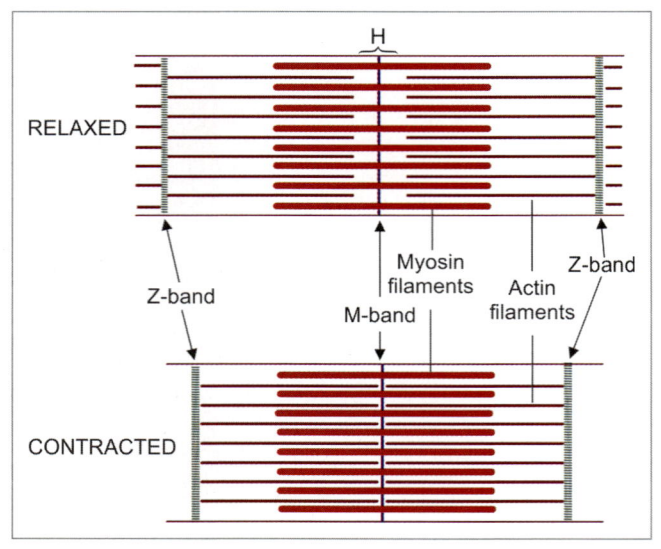

Fig. 7.4: Arrangement of myofilaments in sarcomere. Note that the width of the I-band becomes less, and that the H-zone disappears when the myofibril contracts (schematic representation).

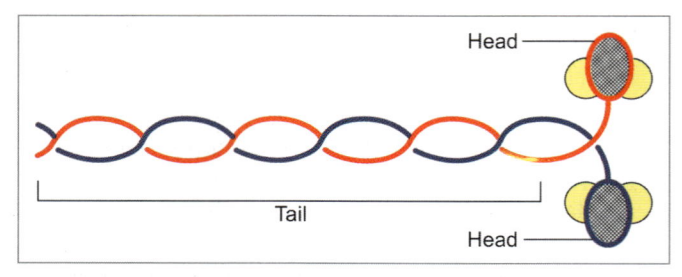

Fig. 7.5: Structure of a myosin molecule. Each molecule has two components (shown in red and blue) each consisting of a head and a tail. The tails are coiled over each other. The parts shown in red or blue are heavy myosin. Light myosin is shaded yellow (schematic representation).

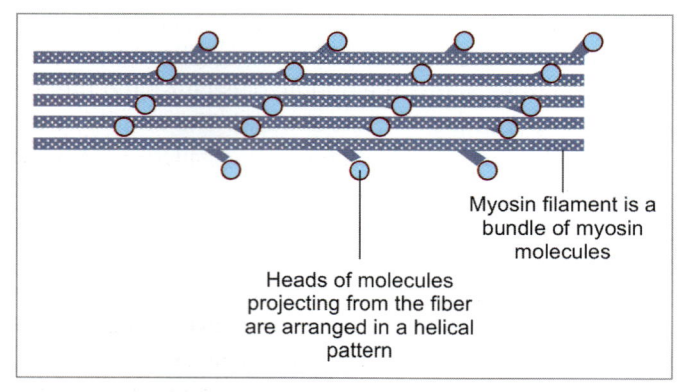

Fig. 7.6: Myosin filament made up of several molecules of myosin (schematic representation).

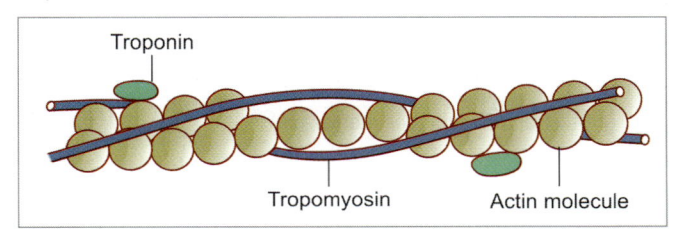

Fig. 7.7: Actin filament (F-actin) made up of globular molecules of G-actin (schematic representation).

Troponin is a complex made up of several fractions. These complexes are arranged regularly over the actin fiber and represent sites at which myosin binds to actin.

Contraction of Skeletal Muscle

During contraction, there is no shortening of individual thick and thin myofilaments; but there is an increase in the degree of overlap between the filaments. In an uncontracted myofibril, overlap between actin and myosin filaments is minimal. During contraction under the influence of energy released by adenosine triphosphate (ATP) and calcium released from sarcoplasmic reticulum, the fibril shortens by sliding in of actin filaments more and more into the intervals between the myosin filaments. As a result, the width of the I-band decreases, but that of the A-band is unchanged. The H-bands are obliterated in a contracted fibril.

Other Proteins Present in Skeletal Muscle

Several proteins other than actin and myosin are present in muscle. Some of them are as follows.
- ❖ *Actinin* is present in the region of Z discs. It binds the tail ends of actin filaments to this disc.
- ❖ *Myomesin* is present in the region of the M disc. It binds the tail ends of myosin filaments to this disc.
- ❖ *Titin* links the head ends of myosin filaments to the Z disc. This is a long and elastic protein that can lengthen and shorten as required. It keeps the myosin filament in proper alignment.
- ❖ *Desmin* is present in intermediate filaments of the cytoskeleton. It links myofibrils to each other, and also to the cell membrane.

Sarcoplasmic Reticulum

In the intervals between myofibrils, the sarcoplasm contains an elaborate system of tubules called the *sarcoplasmic reticulum* (Fig. 7.8). The larger elements of this reticulum run in planes at right angles to the long axes of the myofibrils, and form rings around each myofibril. At the level of every junction between an A and I band, the myofibril is encircled by a set of three closely connected tubules that constitute a *muscle triad*.

Muscle Triad

For purposes of description, each such triad can be said to be composed of an upper, a middle, and a lower tubule (Fig. 7.8). The upper and lower tubules of the triad are connected to the tubules of adjoining triads through a network of smaller tubules. There is one such network opposite each A-band, and another opposite each I-band. These networks, along with the upper and lower tubules of the triad, constitute the sarcoplasmic reticulum. This reticulum is a closed system of tubes.

The middle tube of the triad is an entity independent of the sarcoplasmic reticulum. It is called a *centrotubule* and belongs to what is called the *T-system* of membranes. The centrotubules are really formed by invagination of the sarcolemma into the sarcoplasm. Their lumina are, therefore, in communication with the exterior of the muscle fiber.

Contraction of muscle is dependent on release of calcium ions into myofibrils. In a relaxed muscle, these ions are strongly bound to the membranes of the sarcoplasmic reticulum. When a nerve stimulus reaches a motor endplate, the sarcolemma is depolarized. The wave of depolarization is transmitted to the interior of the muscle fiber through the centrotubules. As a result of this wave, calcium ions are released from the sarcoplasmic reticulum into the myofibrils causing their contraction.

Types of Skeletal Muscle Fibers

- ❖ From morphological, histochemical, and functional point of view, skeletal muscle fibers are of two types (Table 7.1):
  1. Red muscle fiber (because they are red in color).
  2. White muscle fiber.
- ❖ The color of red fibers is due to the presence (in the sarcoplasm) of a pigment called *myoglobin*. This pigment is similar (but not identical with) hemoglobin. It is present also in white fibers, but in much lesser quantity.
- ❖ As compared to white fibers, the contraction of red fibers is relatively slow. Hence, red fibers are also called *slow twitch fibers*, or *type I fibers*; while white fibers are also called *fast twitch fibers* or *type II fibers*.
- ❖ Red fibers are narrower than white fibers. Relative to the volume of the myofibrils, the sarcoplasm is more abundant. Probably because of this fact, the myofibrils,

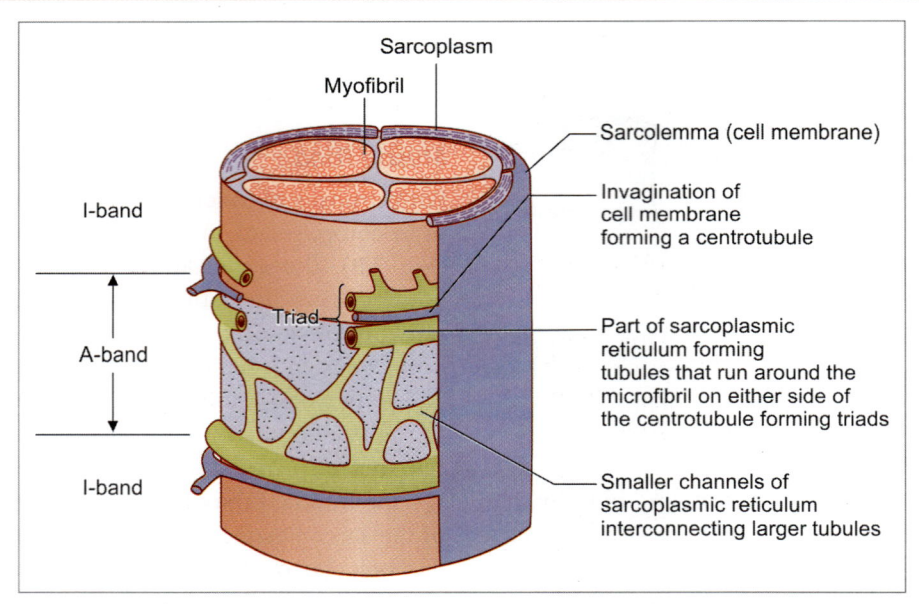

Fig. 7.8: Relationship of the sarcoplasmic reticulum and the T-tubes to a myofibril (schematic representation).

Table 7.1: Characteristics of red and white muscle fibers.

Red muscle fiber	White muscle fiber
Rich in myoglobin and cytochrome hence red in color	Less myoglobin and cytochrome hence white in color
Narrow in diameter with less defined striations and nuclei not always placed at the periphery	Broader in diameter, with well-defined striations and nuclei placed at the periphery
Volume of sarcoplasm is more than myofibrils. Sarcoplasm contains more glycogen	Volume of myofibrils is more. Sarcoplasm contains less glycogen
Numerous mitochondria but sarcoplasmic reticulum is less extensive	Few mitochondria with extensive sarcoplasmic reticulum
Slow and continuous contraction (not easily fatigued)	Rapid contraction (easily fatigued)
Rich blood supply	Poor blood supply
For example, predominate in postural muscles which have to remain contracted over long periods, e.g. erector spinae	For example, predominate in muscles responsible for sharp active movements, e.g. extraocular muscles and flight muscles in birds

and striations, are less well-defined; and the nuclei are not always at the periphery, but may extend deeper into the fiber. Mitochondria are more numerous in red fibers, but the sarcoplasmic reticulum is less extensive. The sarcoplasm contains more glycogen. The capillary bed around red fibers is richer than around white fibers. Differences have also been described in enzyme systems and the respiratory mechanisms in the two types of fibers. Fibers intermediate between red and white fibers have also been described.

❖ In some animals, complete muscles may consist exclusively of red or white fibers, but in most mammals, including man, muscles contain an admixture of both types. Although red fibers contract slowly, their contraction is more sustained, and they fatigue less easily. They predominate in the so-called postural muscles (which have to remain contracted over long periods), while white fibers predominate in muscles responsible for sharp active movements.

❖ Type II (white) fibers may be divided into type IIA and type IIB, the two types differing in their enzyme content, and in the chemical nature of their myosin molecules.

❖ In addition to color and speed of contraction, there are several other differences between red and white fibers. In comparison to white fibers, red fibers differ as follows.

Blood Vessels and Lymphatics of Skeletal Muscle

- Skeletal muscle is richly supplied with blood vessels. The main artery to the muscle enters it at the neurovascular hilus. Several other arteries may enter the muscle at its ends or at other places along its length.
- The arteries form a plexus in the epimysium and in the perimysium, and end in a network of capillaries that surrounds each muscle fiber. This network is richer in red muscle than in white muscle.
- Veins leaving the muscle accompany the arteries. A lymphatic plexus extends into the epimysium and the perimysium, but not into the endomysium.

Innervation of Skeletal Muscle

- The nerve supplying a muscle enters it (along with the main blood vessels) at an area called the **neurovascular hilus**. This hilus is usually situated nearer the origin of the muscle than the insertion.
- After entering the muscle, the nerve breaks up into many branches that run through the connective tissue of the perimysium and endomysium to reach each muscle fiber.
- The nerve fibers supplying skeletal muscle are axons arising from large neurons in the anterior (or ventral) gray columns of the spinal cord (or of corresponding nuclei in the brainstem). These **alpha-efferents** have a large diameter and are myelinated. Because of repeated branching of its axon, one anterior gray column neuron may supply many muscle fibers all of which contract when this neuron "fires".
- One anterior gray column neuron and the muscle fibers supplied by it constitute one **motor unit** (Fig. 7.9). The number of muscle fibers in one motor unit is variable. The units are smaller where precise control of muscular action is required (as in ocular muscles), and much larger in limb muscles where force of contraction is more important. The strength with which a muscle contracts at a particular moment depends on the number of motor units that are activated.
- The junction between a muscle fiber and the nerve terminal that supplies it is highly specialized and is called a **motor endplate** (discussed in detail later).
- Apart from the alpha efferents described earlier, every muscle receives smaller myelinated **gamma-efferents** that arise from gamma neurons in the ventral gray column of the spinal cord.
- These fibers supply special muscle fibers that are present within sensory receptors called **muscle spindles**. These

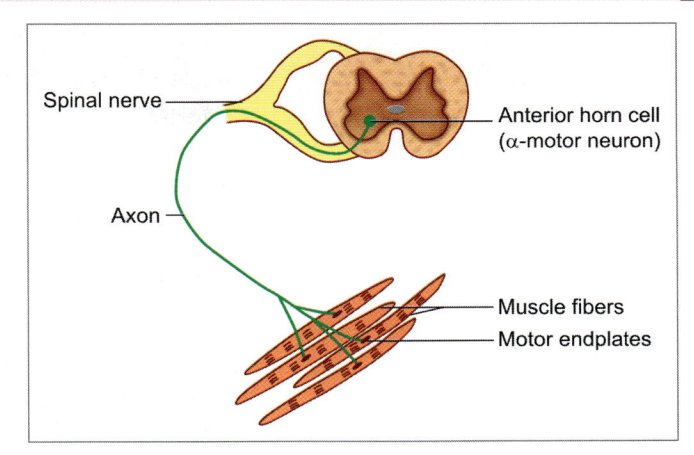

Fig. 7.9: Motor unit consisting of a number of muscle fibers innervated by a single motor neuron (schematic representation).

special muscle fibers are called **intrafusal fibers**. Nerves to muscles also carry autonomic fibers that supply smooth muscle present in the walls of blood vessels.

CARDIAC MUSCLE

The structure of cardiac muscle has many similarities to that of skeletal muscle; but there are important differences as well.

Similarities between Cardiac and Skeletal Muscles

- Like skeletal muscle, cardiac muscle is made up of elongated "fibers" within which there are numerous myofibrils (Plate 7.3). The myofibrils (and, therefore, the fibers) show transverse striations similar to those of skeletal muscle. A, I, Z, and H bands can be made out in the striations.
- The connective tissue framework, and the capillary network around cardiac muscle fibers are similar to those in skeletal muscle.
- With the EM, it is seen that myofibrils of cardiac muscle have the same structure as those of skeletal muscle and are made up of actin and myosin filaments. A sarcoplasmic reticulum, T-system of centrotubules, numerous mitochondria, and other organelles are present.

Differences between Cardiac and Skeletal Muscles

- The fibers of cardiac muscle do not run in strict parallel formation, but branch and anastomose with other fibers to form a network.

Plate 7.3: Cardiac muscle

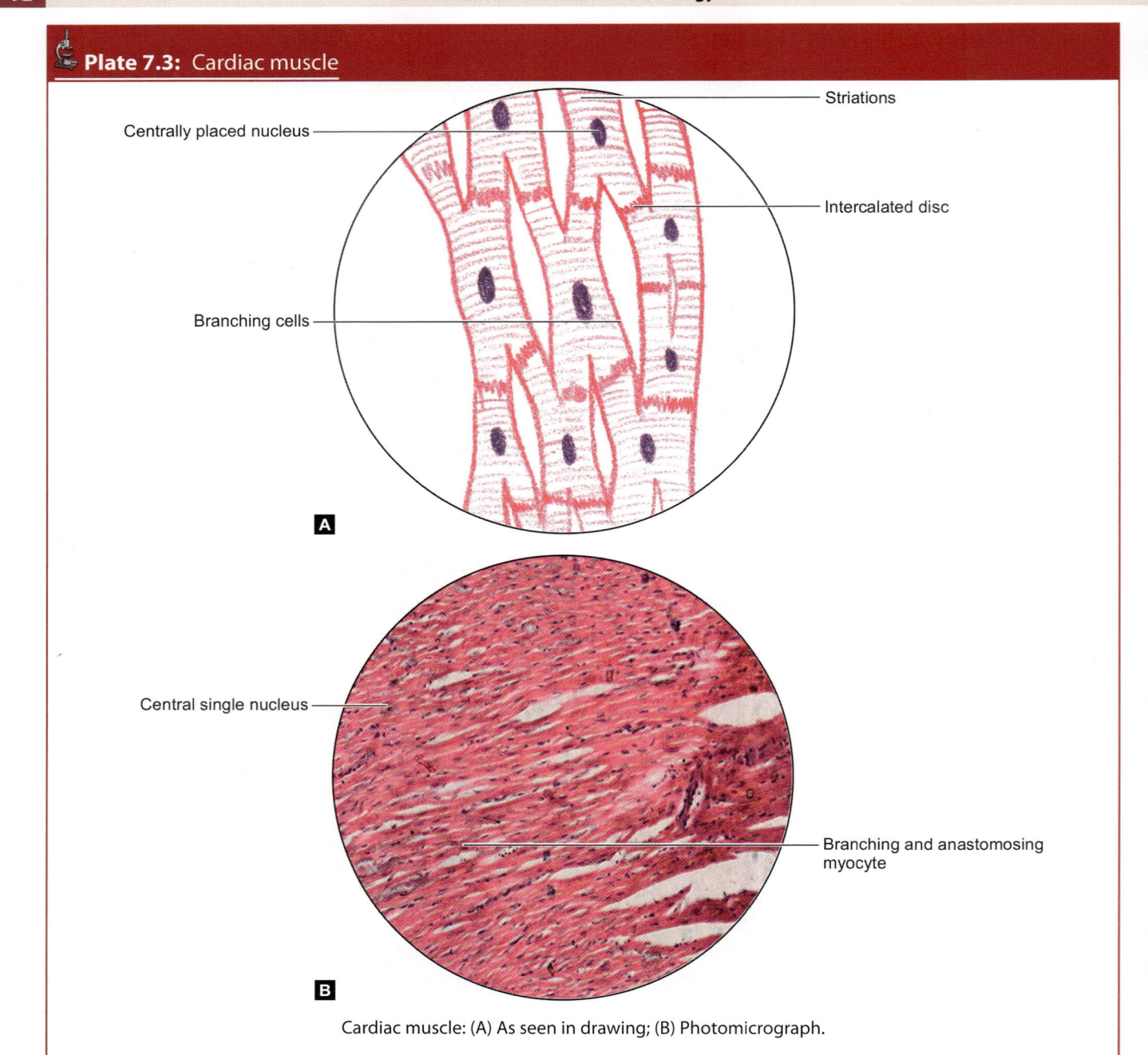

Cardiac muscle: (A) As seen in drawing; (B) Photomicrograph.

Points of identification
- The fibers are made up of "cells" each of which has a centrally placed nucleus and transverse striations
- A clear space called perinuclear halo is seen around the nucleus
- Adjacent cells are separated from one another by transverse lines called intercalated discs
- Fibers show branching
- Blood vessels are also seen.

CHAPTER 7: Muscular Tissue

- Each fiber of cardiac muscle is not a multinucleated syncytium as in skeletal muscle, but is a chain of cardiac muscle cells (or **cardiac myocytes**) each having its own nucleus. Each myocyte is about 80 μm long and about 15 μm broad.
- The nucleus of each myocyte is located centrally (and not peripherally as in skeletal muscle).
- The sarcoplasm of cardiac myocytes is abundant and contains numerous large mitochondria. The myofibrils are relatively few. At places, the myofibrils merge with each other. As a result of these factors, the myofibrils and striations of cardiac muscle are not as distinct as those of skeletal muscle. In this respect, cardiac muscle is closer to the red variety of skeletal muscle than to the white variety. Other similarities with red muscle are the presence of significant amounts of glycogen and of myoglobin, and the rich density of the capillary network around the fibers.
- With the EM, it is seen that the sarcoplasmic reticulum is much less prominent than in skeletal muscle. The centrotubules of the T-system lie opposite the Z-bands (and not at the junctions of A and I-bands as in skeletal muscle). The tubules are much wider than in skeletal muscle. Typical triads are not present. They are often replaced by **dyads** having one T-tube and one tube of the sarcoplasmic reticulum.
- With the light microscope, the junctions between adjoining cardiac myocytes are seen as dark staining transverse lines running across the muscle fiber. These lines are called **intercalated discs**. Sometimes, these discs do not run straight across the fibers, but are broken into a number of "steps" (Plate 7.3). The discs always lies opposite the I-bands. They are made of 3 types of cell junctions- Desmosomes/Macula densa (binds the filaments and joins the cells together there by prevents their seperation during contraction), Fascia adherens (anchoring sites for actin and connects neigbhouring sarcomeres) and gap junctions (helps in spread of action potential).
- Cardiac muscle is involuntary and is innervated by autonomic fibers (in contrast to skeletal muscle that is innervated by cerebrospinal nerves). Nerve endings terminate near the cardiac myocytes, but motor endplates are not seen.
- Isolated cardiac myocytes contract spontaneously in a rhythmic manner. In the intact heart, the rhythm of contraction is determined by a pacemaker located in the sinoatrial node. From here, the impulse spreads to the entire heart through a conducting system made up of a special kind of cardiac muscle.

> **Added Information**
>
> With the EM, it is seen that the intercalated discs are formed by cell membranes of adjacent myocytes, and by a layer of particularly dense cytoplasm present next to the cell membrane. The ends of actin filaments are embedded in this dense cytoplasm (Fig. 7.10). The cell membranes of adjoining myocytes are connected by numerous desmosomes, gap junctions, and tight junctions. Desmosomes link intermediate filaments present in the cytoskeleton of adjacent cells. Actin filaments of the cells end in relation to tight junctions. Gap junctions allow electrical continuity between adjacent myocytes, and thus, convert the cardiac muscle into a **physiological syncytium**.

SMOOTH MUSCLE

- Smooth muscle (also called **nonstriated, involuntary**, or **plain muscle**) is made up of long spindle-shaped cells (myocytes) having a broad central part and tapering ends.
- The nucleus, which is oval or elongated, lies in the central part of the cell. The length of smooth muscle cells (often called fibers) is highly variable (15–500 μm).
- With the light microscope, the sarcoplasm appears to have indistinct longitudinal striations, but there are no transverse striations.
- Smooth muscle is not striated because myofilaments are not arranged regularly along the length of spindle shaped cell.
- Smooth muscle cells are usually aggregated to form bundles, or fasciculi, that are further aggregated to form layers of variable thickness. In such a layer, the cells are so arranged that the thick central part of one cell is opposite the thin tapering ends of adjoining cells

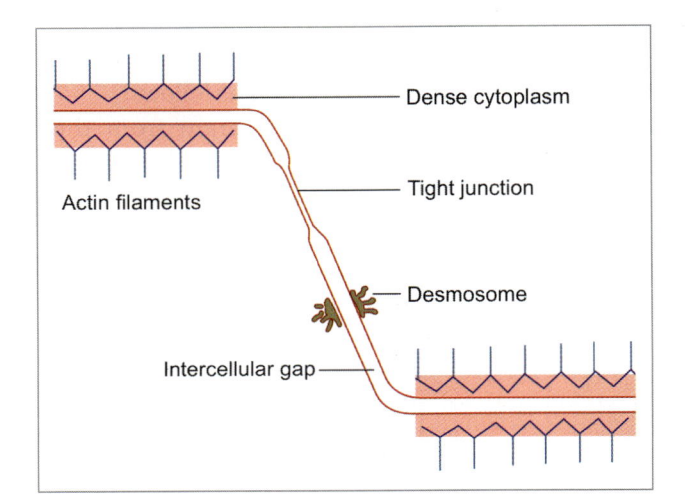

Fig. 7.10: Electron microscopic structure of part of an intercalated disc (schematic representation).

(Fig. 7.11). Aggregations of smooth muscle cells into fasciculi and layers are facilitated by the fact that each myocyte is surrounded by a network of delicate fibers (collagen, reticular, and elastic) that holds the myocytes together (Plate 7.4). The fibers between individual myocytes become continuous with the more abundant connective tissue that separates fasciculi or layers of smooth muscle.

Ultrastructure

- Each smooth muscle cell is bounded by a plasma membrane. Outside the plasma membrane, there is an external lamina to which the plasma membrane is adherent. Connective tissue fibers are attached to the lamina (through special proteins).
- Adjacent smooth muscle cells communicate through gap junctions.
- The longitudinal striations (seen with the light microscope) are due to the presence of delicate myofilaments. These myofilaments are composed mainly of the proteins actin and myosin, but these do not have the highly ordered arrangement seen in striated muscle. The actin filaments are also different from those in skeletal muscle. **Troponin is not present**.
- Apart from myofibrils, the sarcoplasm also contains mitochondria, a Golgi complex, some granular endoplasmic reticulum, free ribosomes, and intermediate filaments.
- A sarcoplasmic reticulum, similar to that in skeletal muscle, is present, but is not as developed.
- Numerous invaginations (caveolae) resembling endocytic vesicles are seen near the surface of each myocyte, but no endocytosis occurs here.

Contraction of Smooth Muscle

The mechanism of contraction of smooth muscle is different from that of skeletal muscle as follows:
- The myosin is chemically different from that in skeletal muscle. It binds to actin only if its light chain is phosphorylated. This phosphorylation of myosin is necessary for contraction of smooth muscle.

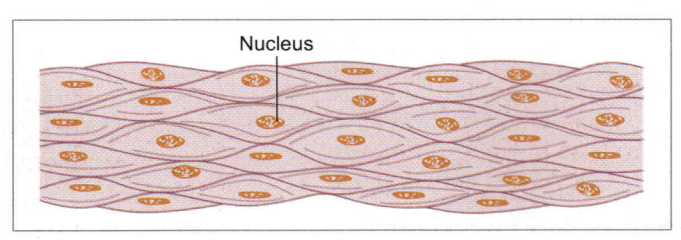

Fig. 7.11: Smooth muscle cells (schematic representation).

- As compared to skeletal muscle, smooth muscle needs very little ATP for contraction.
- The mechanisms regulating the flow of calcium ions into smooth muscle are different from those for skeletal muscle. Caveolae present on the surface of smooth muscle cells play a role in this process.
- Actin and myosin form bundles that are attached at both ends to the points on the cell membrane called anchoring points (or focal densities). When the muscle contracts, these points are drawn closer to each other. This converts an elongated smooth muscle cell in one that is oval.

Distribution

- Smooth muscle is seen most typically in the walls of hollow viscera including the stomach, the intestines, the urinary bladder, and the uterus.
- It is present in the walls of several structures that are in the form of narrow tubes, e.g. arteries, veins, bronchi, ureters, deferent ducts, uterine tubes, and the ducts of several glands.
- The muscles that constrict and dilate the pupil are made up of smooth muscle.
- Some smooth muscle is present in the orbit (orbitalis); in the upper eyelid (Muller's muscle); in the prostate; and in the skin of the scrotum (Dartos muscle). In the skin, delicate bundles of smooth muscle are present in relation to hair follicles. These bundles are called the *arrector pili* muscles.

Variations in Arrangement of Smooth Muscle

Smooth muscle fibers may be arranged in a variety of ways depending on functional requirements.
- In some organs (e.g. the gut), smooth muscle is arranged in the form of two distinct layers: (1) an inner circular and (2) an outer longitudinal. Within each layer, the fasciculi lie parallel to each other. Such an arrangement allows peristaltic movements to take place for propulsion of contents along the tube.
- In some organs (e.g. the ureter), the arrangement of layers may be reversed, the longitudinal layer being internal to the circular one. In yet other situations, there may be three layers: inner and outer longitudinal with a circular layer in between (e.g. the urinary bladder and vas deferens).
- In some regions (e.g. urinary bladder, uterus), the smooth muscle is arranged in layers, but the layers are not distinctly demarcated from each other. Even within

CHAPTER 7: Muscular Tissue

Plate 7.4: Smooth muscle

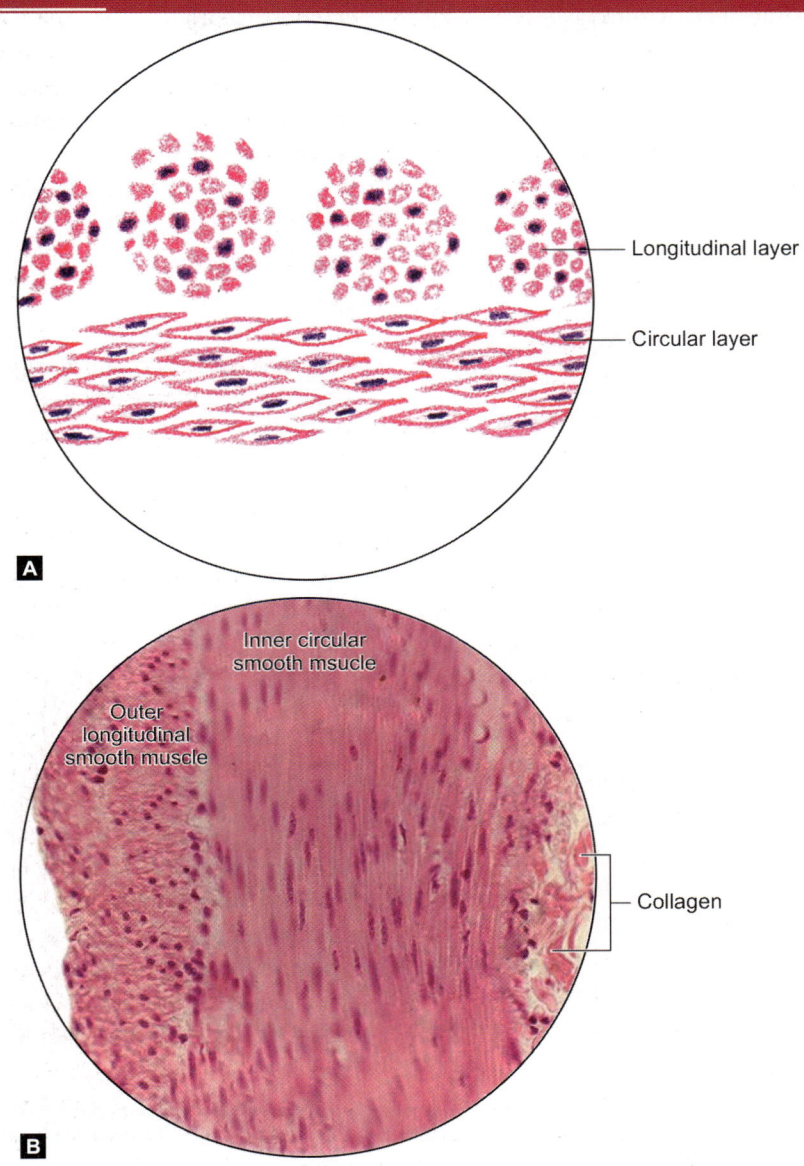

A — Longitudinal layer; Circular layer

B — Outer longitudinal smooth muscle; Inner circular smooth msucle; Collagen

Smooth muscle: (A) As seen in drawing; (B) Photomicrograph.

Points of identification
In the drawing, muscle is seen cut longitudinally as well as transversely.
- Loose connective tissue is seen above and below the layers of muscle.

In longitudinal section:
- The smooth muscle fibers are **spindle-shaped** cells with tapering ends
- The nucleus is elongated and centrally placed
- **No striations** are seen.

In transverse section:
- The spindle-shaped cells are cut at different places along the length resulting in various shapes and sizes of the cells
- The nucleus is seen in those cells which are cut through the center. Others do not show nuclei.

layers, the fasciculi tend to run in various directions and may form a network.
- In some tubes (e.g. the bile duct), a thick layer of circular muscle may surround a segment of the tube forming a **sphincter**. Contraction of the sphincter occludes the tube.
- In the skin, and in some other places, smooth muscle occurs in the form of narrow bands.

Innervation

Smooth muscle is innervated by autonomic nerves, both sympathetic and parasympathetic. The two have opposite effects. For example, in the iris, parasympathetic stimulation causes constriction of the pupil, and sympathetic stimulation causes dilatation. It may be noted that sympathetic or parasympathetic nerves may cause contraction of muscle at some sites, and relaxation at other sites.

Blood Vessels and Lymphatics

Blood vessels and lymphatics are present in smooth muscle, but the density of blood vessels is much less than in skeletal muscle (in keeping with much less activity) (Table 7.2).

MYOEPITHELIAL CELLS

- Apart from muscle, myoepithelial cells show the presence of contractile proteins (actin and myosin).
- **Myoepitheliocytes** (or **myoepithelial cells**) are present in close relation to secretory elements of some glands. They help to squeeze secretions out of secreting elements. Myoepithelial cells may be **stellate**, forming baskets around acini, or may be **fusiform**.
- Myoepitheliocytes are seen in salivary glands, the mammary glands, and sweat glands. These cells are of ectodermal origin.
- With the EM, they are seen to contain actin and myosin filaments. They can be localized histochemically, because they contain the protein **desmin** that is specific to muscle.
- Myoepithelial cells are innervated by autonomic nerves.

APPLIED HISTOLOGY

- **Muscle dystrophy:** Each muscle fiber contains a cytoskeleton. The fibers of the cytoskeleton are linked to actin fibers. The cytoskeleton is also linked to the external lamina through glycoproteins present in the cell membrane. Forces generated within the fiber are, thus, transmitted to the external lamina. The external lamina is in turn attached to connective tissue fibers around the muscle fiber. A number of proteins are responsible for these linkages. Genetic defects in these proteins can result in abnormalities in muscle (muscle dystrophy). One such protein is dystrophin, and its absence is associated with a disease called **Duchenne muscular dystrophy**.
- **Myasthenia gravis (MG)** is a neuromuscular disorder of autoimmune origin in which the acetylcholine receptors in the motor endplates of the muscles are damaged (Figs. 7.12A and B). The term **myasthenia** means "muscular weakness" and **gravis** implies "serious"; thus, both together denote the clinical characteristics of the disease. MG may be found at any age but adult women are affected more often than adult men in the ratio of 3:2. The condition presents clinically with muscular weakness and fatigability, initially in the ocular musculature but later spreads to involve the trunk and limbs.

Table 7.2: Differences between skeletal, cardiac, and smooth muscles.

Characteristics	Skeletal muscle	Cardiac muscle	Smooth muscle
Muscle fiber	Long, cylindrical, and unbranched	Short, narrow, and branched	Fusiform/spindle-shaped and unbranched
Control	Voluntary	Involuntary	Involuntary
Location	Muscle of skeleton, tongue, esophagus, and diaphragm	Heart, pulmonary veins, and superior and inferior vena cava	Vessels, organs, and viscera
Striations	Present (well-defined)	Present (poorly defined)	Absent
Nuclei	Multiple, flat, and located at periphery	Single, oval, and present in center	Single, oval, and present in center
Sarcoplasmic reticulum	Present (form triads)	Present (form dyad)	Absent
Intercalated disc	Absent	Present	Absent
Regeneration after injury	Seen (limited)	Not seen	Seen

CHAPTER 7: Muscular Tissue

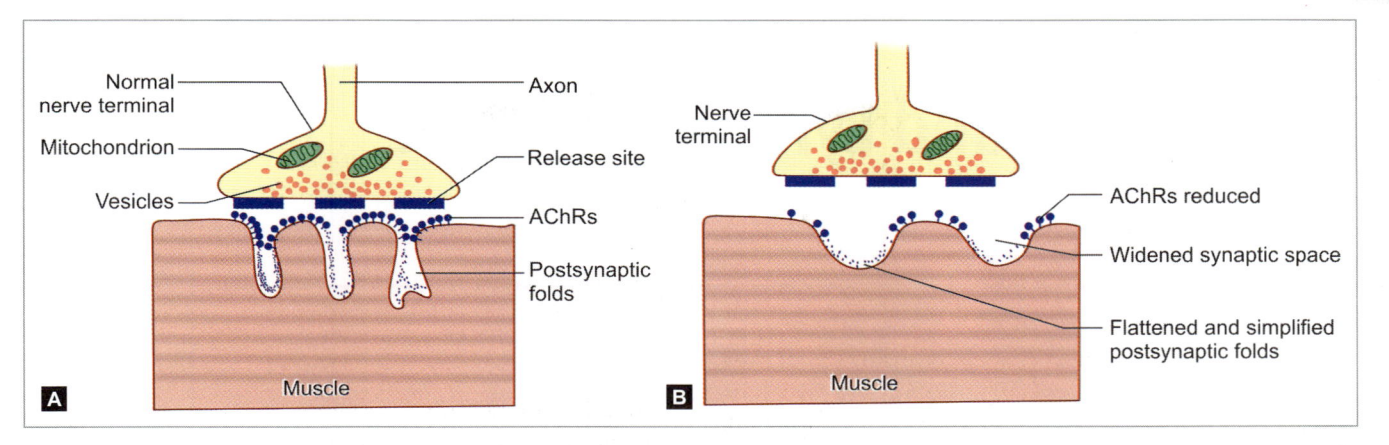

Figs. 7.12A and B: Neuromuscular junction in normal transmission. (A) In myasthenia gravis (MG); and (B) The junction in MG shows reduced number of acetylcholine receptors (AChRs), flattened and simplified postsynaptic folds, and a widened synaptic space but a normal nerve terminal (schematic representation).

- ❖ **Skeletal muscle tumors:** Rhabdomyoma and rhabdomyosarcoma are the benign and malignant tumors, respectively of striated muscle.
- ❖ **Muscle hypertrophy:** All varieties of muscle can hypertrophy when exposed to greater stress. Hypertrophy takes place by enlargement of existing fibers, and not by formation of new fibers. Skeletal muscle hypertrophies with exercise. Cardiac muscle hypertrophies, if the load on a chamber of the heart, is increased for any reason. An example is the hypertrophy of muscle in the wall of the left ventricle in hypertension. Hypertrophy of smooth muscle is seen most typically in the uterus where myocytes may increase from a length of about 15–20 μm at the beginning of pregnancy to as much as 500 μm toward the end of pregnancy.
- ❖ Smooth muscle and cardiac muscle have very little capacity for regeneration. Any defects produced by injury or disease are usually repaired by formation of fibrous tissue.
- ❖ Skeletal muscle fibers can undergo some degree of regeneration. They cannot divide to form new fibers. However, satellite cells present in relation to them (just deep to the external lamina) can give rise to new muscle fibers. Satellite cells are regarded as persisting myoblasts. When large segments of a muscle are destroyed, the gap is filled in by fibrous tissue.
- ❖ Excessive activity of smooth muscle is responsible for many symptoms. Constriction of bronchi leads to asthma. Spasm of smooth muscle can give rise to severe pain (colic) that may originate in the intestines (intestinal colic), ureter (renal colic), or bile duct (biliary colic). These symptoms can be relieved by drugs that cause relaxation of smooth muscle.

MULTIPLE CHOICE QUESTIONS

1. All the following are skeletal muscle type, *except*:
   a. Biceps brachii
   b. Diaphragm
   c. Esophagus
   d. Arrector pili
2. The part of a myofibril situated between two consecutive Z-bands is called:
   a. Sarcosome
   b. Sarcomere
   c. Sarcolemma
   d. Sarcoplasm
3. Origin of myocytes:
   a. Ectoderm
   b. Endoderm
   c. Mesoderm
   d. Neural crest
4. Contraction of muscle is dependent on release of:
   a. Ca^+
   a. K^+
   c. Mg^+
   d. Cl^-

Answers
1. c   2. b   3. c   4. a

CHAPTER 8

Lymphatics and Lymphoid Tissue

Learning objectives

To study the:
- Overview of lymphatic system
- Classification
- Lymph, lymph vessels and lymphocytes
- Lymphoid organs—structure of lymph node, spleen, thymus and palatine tonsil
- Applied histology

IDENTIFICATION POINTS

Lymph node	Spleen	Palatine tonsil	Thymus
☐ Capsule with subcapsular sinus ☐ Well demarcated cortex and medulla ☐ Cortex with aggregation of lymphatic follicles ☐ Medulla containing cords of lymphocytes with medullary sinuses.	☐ Presence of white pulp and red pulp ☐ White pulp with eccentric arteriole ☐ Cords of Billroth ☐ Numerous trabeculae with arteriole.	☐ Presence of tonsillar crypts ☐ Lined by stratified squamous nonkeratinized epithelium ☐ Subepithelial aggregation of lymphatic follicles ☐ Mucous glands (if present).	☐ Capsule with trabeculae ☐ Presence of incomplete lobules ☐ Lobules with cortex and medulla ☐ Hassall's corpuscles.

INTRODUCTION

- The lymphoid system includes lymphatic vessels and lymphoid tissue.
- When circulating blood reaches the capillaries, part of its fluid content passes into the surrounding tissues as tissue fluid. Most of this fluid reenters the capillaries at their venous ends. Some of it is, however, returned to the circulation through a separate system of **lymphatic vessels** (usually called **lymphatics**).
- The fluid passing through the lymphatic vessels is called **lymph**.
- The smallest lymphatic (or lymph) vessels are lymphatic capillaries that join together to form larger lymphatic vessels.
- The largest lymphatic vessel in the body is the **thoracic duct**. It drains lymph from the greater part of the body. The thoracic duct ends by joining the left subclavian vein at its junction with the internal jugular vein. On the right side, there is the **right lymphatic duct** that has a similar termination.
- The lymphatic system plays an important role in providing immunity.

CLASSIFICATION

Lymphoid tissue constitutes group of cells and organ like lymphocytes, thymus, bone marrow, spleen, etc. which are involved in protection of body surface and internal environment by combating noxious substances.

- *Primary lymphoid organs*: Here production and maturation of T- and B-lymphocytes takes place. They are **thymus** and **bone marrow**.
- *Secondary lymphoid organs:* Here the lymphocytes come in contact with the antigens, and then particular group of lymphocytes proliferate. They are lymphnode, spleen, mucosa-associated lymphoid tissue (MALT) such as Peyer's patch, vermiform appendix, and tonsil.

OTHER CLASSIFICATION

Lymphoid tissue may be broadly classified as:
- Diffuse lymphoid tissue
- Dense lymphoid tissue.

CHAPTER 8: Lymphatics and Lymphoid Tissue

Diffuse Lymphoid Tissue

Diffuse lymphoid tissue consists of diffusely arranged lymphocytes and plasma cells in the mucosa of large intestine, trachea, bronchi, and urinary tract.

Dense Lymphoid Tissue

It consists of an aggregation of lymphocytes arranged in the form of nodules. These nodules are found either as discrete encapsulated organs or in close association to the lining epithelium of the gut. Dense lymphoid tissue can therefore be divided as:

- ❖ **Discrete lymphoid organs**: These include thymus, lymph nodes, spleen, and tonsils.
- ❖ **Mucosa-associated lymphoid tissue**: Small numbers of lymphocytes may be present almost anywhere in the body, but significant aggregations are seen in relation to the mucosa of the respiratory, alimentary, and urogenital tracts. These aggregations are referred to as **MALT**. In the respiratory system the aggregations are relatively small and are present in the walls of the trachea and large bronchi called **bronchus-associated lymphoid tissue (BALT)**. **MALT** in the alimentary system also called **gut-associated lymphoid tissue (GALT)** and includes Peyer's patches of ileum, adenoids (located in the roof of pharynx), lingual tonsils in posterior one-third of tongue, palatine tonsils, and lymphoid nodules in vermiform appendix.

LYMPH

- ❖ Lymph is a transudate from blood and contains the same proteins as in plasma, but in smaller amounts and different proportions.
- ❖ Suspended in lymph, there are cells that are chiefly lymphocytes.
- ❖ Most of these lymphocytes are added to lymph as it passes through lymph nodes, but some are derived from tissues drained by the nodes.
- ❖ Large molecules of fat (chylomicrons) that are absorbed from the intestines enter lymph vessels. After a fatty meal, these fat globules may be so numerous that lymph becomes milky (and is then called *chyle*) (Fig. 8.1).

LYMPHATIC VESSELS

Lymph Capillaries

- ❖ Lymph capillaries (or lymphatic capillaries) begin blindly in tissues where they form a network.

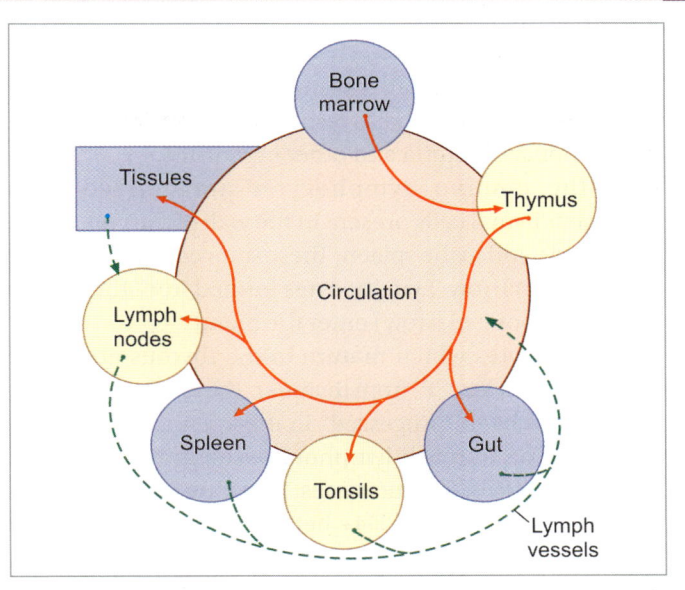

Fig. 8.1: Circulation of T-lymphocytes (schematic representation).

- ❖ The structure of lymph capillaries is basically similar to that of blood capillaries but has greater permeability.
- ❖ There is an inner lining of endothelium. The basal lamina is absent or poorly developed.
- ❖ Pericytes or connective tissue are not present around the capillary.
- ❖ Much larger molecules can pass through the walls of lymph capillaries. These include colloidal material, fat droplets, and particulate matter, such as bacteria.
- ❖ It is believed that these substances pass into lymph capillaries through gaps between endothelial cells lining the capillary, or by pinocytosis.
- ❖ Lymph capillaries are present in most tissues of the body. They are absent in avascular tissues (e.g. the cornea, hair, nails), in the splenic pulp, and in the bone marrow.

Larger Lymph Vessels

- ❖ The structure of the thoracic duct and of other larger lymph vessels is similar to that of veins.
- ❖ A tunica intima, media, and adventitia can be distinguished. Elastic fibers are prominent and can be seen in all the three layers.
- ❖ The media, and also the adventitia, contain some smooth muscle. In most vessels the smooth muscle is arranged circularly, but in the thoracic duct, the muscle is predominantly longitudinal.
- ❖ Numerous valves, similar to those in veins, are present in small as well as large lymphatic vessels. They are more numerous than in veins. The valves often give lymph vessels a beaded appearance.

LYMPHOCYTES

- Lymphocytes are an essential part of the *immune system* of the body that is responsible for defense against invasion by bacteria and other organisms.
- In the embryo, lymphocytes are derived from mesenchymal cells present in the wall of the yolk sac, in the liver, and in the spleen. These stem cells later migrate to bone marrow. Lymphocytes formed from these stem cells (in bone marrow) enter the blood.
- Lymphocytes which mature in the thymus are called *T-lymphocytes* ("T" from thymus). These T-lymphocytes, that have been "processed" in the thymus, re-enter the circulation to reach lymphoid tissue in lymph nodes, spleen, tonsils, and intestines. There are four main types of T lymphocytes—CD4+ helper cells, CD8+ cytotoxic cells, memory T cells and natural killer T cells.
- Lymphocytes of a second group arising from stem cells in bone marrow enter the bloodstream and directly go to lymphoid tissues (other than the thymus). Such lymphocytes are called *B-lymphocytes* ("B" from *bursa of Fabricus*, a diverticulum of the cloaca in birds: in birds, B-lymphocytes are formed here). B-lymphocytes are seen in lymphatic nodules. The germinal centers are formed by actively dividing B-lymphocytes. While the dark rims of lymphatic nodules are formed by dense aggregations of resting B-lymphocytes. Like T-lymphocytes, B-lymphocytes also circulate between lymphoid tissues and the bloodstream (Fig. 8.2).

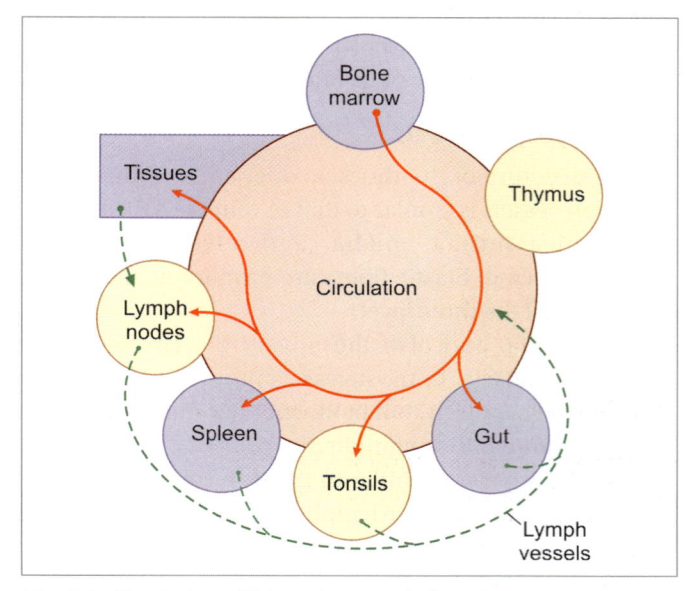

Fig. 8.2: Circulation of B-lymphocytes (schematic representation).

Functions of Lymphocytes

- Lymphocytes help to destroy microbes by producing substances called *antibodies*. These are protein molecules that have the ability to recognize a "foreign" protein (i.e. a protein not normally present in the individual). The foreign protein is usually referred to as an *antigen*.
- Antigen can be neutralized only by a specific antibody. This function of antibody production is done by *B-lymphocytes*. When stimulated by the presence of antigen, the cells enlarge and get converted to plasma cells. The plasma cells produce antibodies. Antibodies are also called *immunoglobulins (Igs)*. Igs are of five main types, viz. IgG, IgM, IgA, IgE, and IgD. B-lymphocytes defend the body through blood-borne antibodies thus provides *humoral immunity*.
- T-lymphocytes have surface receptors that recognize specific antigens (there being many varieties of T-lymphocytes; each type recognizing a specific antigen). When exposed to a suitable stimulus, the T-lymphocytes multiply and form large cells that can destroy abnormal cells by direct contact, or by producing cytotoxic substances called *cytokines* or *lymphokines*. T-lymphocytes are responsible for cell-mediated immune responses (*cellular immunity*).

LYMPH NODES

General Features

- Lymph nodes are small masses of lymphatic tissue along the course of lymphatic vessels.
- Lymph from any part of the body (with some exceptions) passes through one or more lymph nodes before entering the bloodstream. Lymphocytes are added to lymph in these nodes.
- Lymph nodes act as filters removing bacteria and other particulate matter from lymph. Each group of lymph nodes has a specific area of drainage.
- Each lymph node consists of a connective tissue framework, and of numerous lymphocytes and other cells, that fill the interstices of the network. The entire node is bean shaped, the concavity constituting a hilum through which blood vessels enter and leave the node. Several lymph vessels enter the node on its convex aspect. Usually, a single lymph vessel leaves the node through its hilum (Fig. 8.3).

Microscopic Features

- When a section through a lymph node is examined (at low magnification), it is seen that the node has an outer

CHAPTER 8: Lymphatics and Lymphoid Tissue

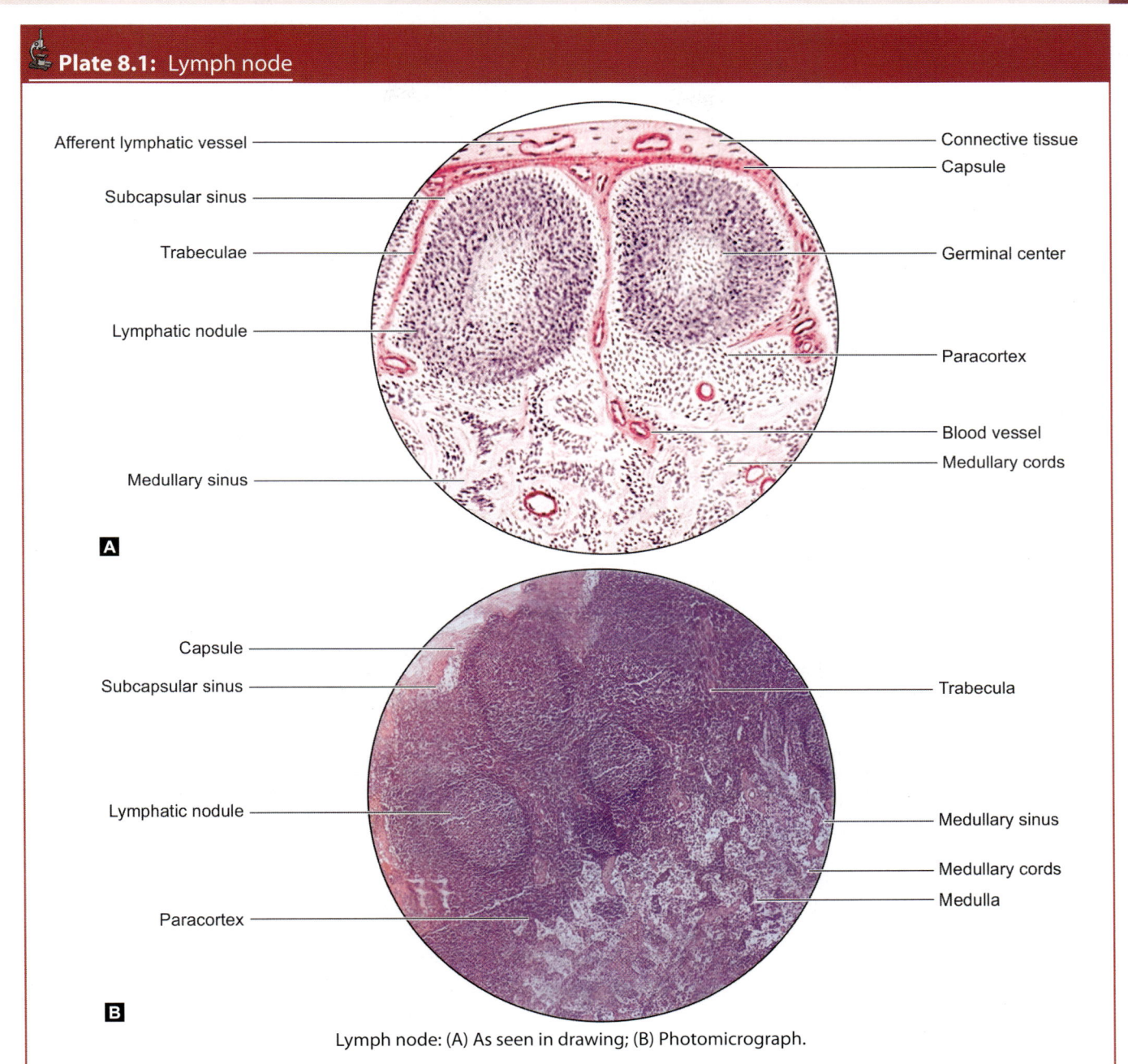

Plate 8.1: Lymph node

Labels (A):
- Afferent lymphatic vessel
- Subcapsular sinus
- Trabeculae
- Lymphatic nodule
- Medullary sinus
- Connective tissue
- Capsule
- Germinal center
- Paracortex
- Blood vessel
- Medullary cords

A

Labels (B):
- Capsule
- Subcapsular sinus
- Lymphatic nodule
- Paracortex
- Trabecula
- Medullary sinus
- Medullary cords
- Medulla

B

Lymph node: (A) As seen in drawing; (B) Photomicrograph.

Points of identification
- A thin capsule surrounds the lymph node and sends in trabeculae
- Just beneath the capsule a clear space is seen. This is the subcapsular sinus
- A lymph node has an outer cortex and an inner medulla
- The cortex is packed with lymphocytes. A number of rounded lymphatic follicles (or nodules) are present. Each nodule has a pale staining germinal center surrounded by a zone of densely packed lymphocytes
- Within the medulla the lymphocytes are arranged in the form of anastomosing cords. Several blood vessels can be seen in the medulla.

Note: All lymphoid tissue are easily recognized due to presence of aggregation of dark staining nuclei. The nuclei belong to lymphocytes.

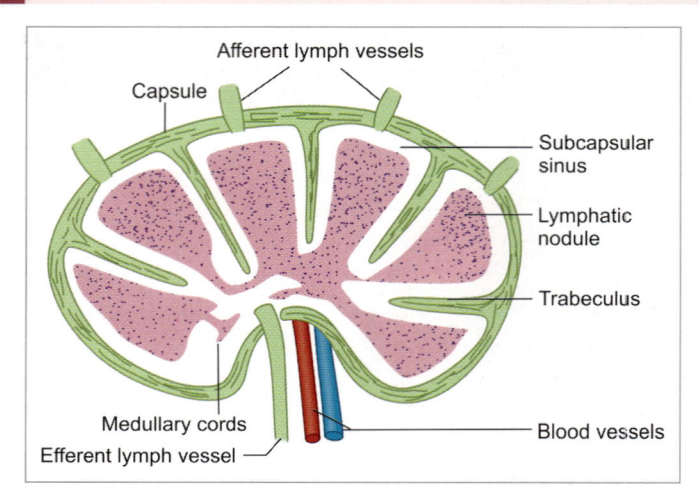

Fig. 8.3: Some features of the structure of a lymph node (schematic representation).

zone that contains densely packed lymphocytes, and therefore stains darkly: this part is the **cortex**. The cortex does not extend into the hilum.

* Surrounded by the cortex, there is a lighter staining zone in which lymphocytes are fewer, called *medulla* (Plate 8.1).
* A lymph node is surrounded by a *capsule*. The capsule consists mainly of collagen fibers. Some elastic fibers and some smooth muscle may be present.
* Just beneath the capsule is the **subcapsular sinus** (Fig. 8.3).
* A number of *septa* (or *trabeculae*) extend into the node from the capsule and divide the node into lobules.
* The hilum is occupied by a mass of dense fibrous tissue.
* A delicate network of reticular fibers occupies the remaining spaces forming a fibrous/reticular framework within the node. Associated with the network, there are reticular cells, macrophages, dendritic cells, and follicular dendritic cells.

Cortex

* Within the cortex, there are several rounded areas that are called **lymphatic follicles** or **lymphatic nodules** within the reticular framework.
* Lymphatic nodules which are aggregations of small lymphocytes are called **primary nodules**, and those with **germinal center** are called **secondary nodules**.
* Germinal center is the central lightly stained region of the lymphatic nodules. They mainly contain immature proliferating lymphocytes (lymphoblasts). Germinal center indicates the response of the nodules to the antigen.
* Small lymphocytes encircle this germinal center and form a ring called as **mantle zone/corona**.
* It is mainly in the superficial part of the cortex where the lymphatic nodules are seen so it is otherwise called as nodular cortex/superficial cortex.
* Region between the nodular cortex and the medulla is called **deep/paracortex**. It is mainly populated by the major portion of T-lymphocytes of lymph node; hence, it is also called as thymus-dependent cortex.

Medulla

* Within the medulla, the lymphocytes are arranged in the form of branching and anastomosing cords called medullary cords. The cords are separated by medullary sinuses.
* Contained within the reticular framework, the medullary cords contain mainly B-lymphocytes, macrophages, dendritic cells, and plasma cells.

Circulation of Lymph through Lymph Nodes

* The entire lymph node is pervaded by a network of reticular fibers. Most of the spaces of this network are packed with lymphocytes. At some places, however, these spaces contain relatively few cells and form channels through which lymph circulates.
* These channels known as sinuses are lined by endothelium, but their walls allow free movement of lymphocytes and macrophages into and out of the channels.
* Afferent lymphatics reaching the convex outer surface of the node enter an extensive **subcapsular sinus** (Fig. 8.3). From this sinus a number of radial cortical sinuses run through the cortex toward the medulla.
* Reaching the medulla the sinuses join to form larger medullary sinuses. In turn the medullary sinuses join to form (usually) one, or more than one, efferent lymph vessel through which lymph leaves the node.
* Lymph passing through the system of sinuses comes into intimate contact with macrophages present in the node. Bacteria and other particulate matter are removed from lymph by these cells. Lymphocytes freely enter or leave the node through these channels.

Blood Supply of Lymph Nodes

* Arteries enter the lymph node at the hilum. They pass through the medulla to reach the cortex where they end in arterioles and capillaries. These arterioles and capillaries are arranged as loops that drain into venules.

CHAPTER 8: Lymphatics and Lymphoid Tissue

- Postcapillary venules in lymph nodes are unusual in that they are lined by cuboidal endothelium (they are, therefore, called **high endothelial venules**).
- This "high" endothelium readily allows the passage of lymphocytes between the bloodstream and the surrounding tissue.
- These endothelial cells bear receptors that are recognized by circulating lymphocytes. Contact with these receptors facilitates passage of lymphocytes through the vessel wall.

Functions

- Lymph nodes are the centers of lymphocyte production. Both B-lymphocytes and T-lymphocytes are produced here by multiplication of pre-existing lymphocytes. These lymphocytes pass into lymph and thus reach the bloodstream.
- Bacteria and other particulate matter are removed from lymph through phagocytosis by macrophages. Antigens thus carried into these cells are "presented" to lymphocytes stimulating their proliferation. In this way, lymph nodes play an important role in the immune response to antigens.
- Plasma cells (representing fully mature B-lymphocytes) produce antibodies against invading antigens, while T-lymphocytes attack cells that are "foreign" to the host body.

SPLEEN

General Features

- The spleen is the largest lymphoid organ of the body.
- It is a blood-forming organ in fetal life and blood-destroying organ in postnatal life [graveyard of red blood cells (RBCs)].
- Since it is in the bloodstream, it filters the blood from bloodborne antigens and microorganisms.

Structure Connective Tissue Framework

- Except at the hilum, the surface of the spleen is covered by a layer of peritoneum (referred to as the **serous coat**). Deep to the serous layer, the organ is covered completely by a **capsule** (Plate 8.2).
- **Trabeculae** arising from the capsule extend into the substance of the spleen and form network.
- The capsule and trabeculae are made up of fibrous tissue in which elastic fibers are abundant.
- The spaces between the trabeculae are pervaded by a network of reticular fibers, embedded in an amorphous matrix.
- Fibroblasts (reticular cells) and macrophages are also present in relation to the reticulum. The interstices of the reticulum are pervaded by lymphocytes, blood vessels and blood cells, and by macrophages.

Circulation Through the Spleen

Knowledge of vasculature is essential to understand the histology of spleen.

- On reaching the hilum of the spleen, the splenic artery divides into about five branches that enter the organ independently.
- Each branch divides and subdivides as it travels through the trabecular network.
- Arterioles arising from this network leave the trabeculae to pass into the intertrabecular spaces. For some distance, each arteriole is surrounded by a dense sheath of lymphocytes. These lymphocytes constitute the **white pulp** of the spleen.
- The arteriole then divides into a number of straight vessels that are called **penicilli**.
- Penicillar arterioles either open into the red pulp (**open circulation**) or they open into the splenic sinusoids (**closed circulation**) (Fig. 8.4).
- Veins from these sinusoids and the red pulp end in the trabecular veins.
- The sinusoids of the spleen are lined by modified endothelium. The cells are elongated and are banana-shaped called as **stave cells**. With the electron microscopy a system of ultramicroscopic fibrils is seen to be present in their cytoplasm. The fibrils may help to alter the shape of the endothelial cells thus opening or closing gaps between adjoining cells.
- The spleen acts as a filter for worn-out RBCs. Normal erythrocytes can change shape and pass easily through narrow passages in penicilli and ellipsoids. However, cells that are aged are unable to change shape and are trapped in the spleen where they are destroyed by macrophages.

Parenchyma

The interior of the spleen shows round white areas (white pulp) surrounded by red matrix (red pulp).

White Pulp

- The white pulp is made up of aggregations of lymphocytes that surround a small artery or arterioles.
- In hematoxylin and eosin (H&E) staining, white pulp appears basophilic because of dense heterochromatin of the lymphocytes.

Plate 8.2: Spleen

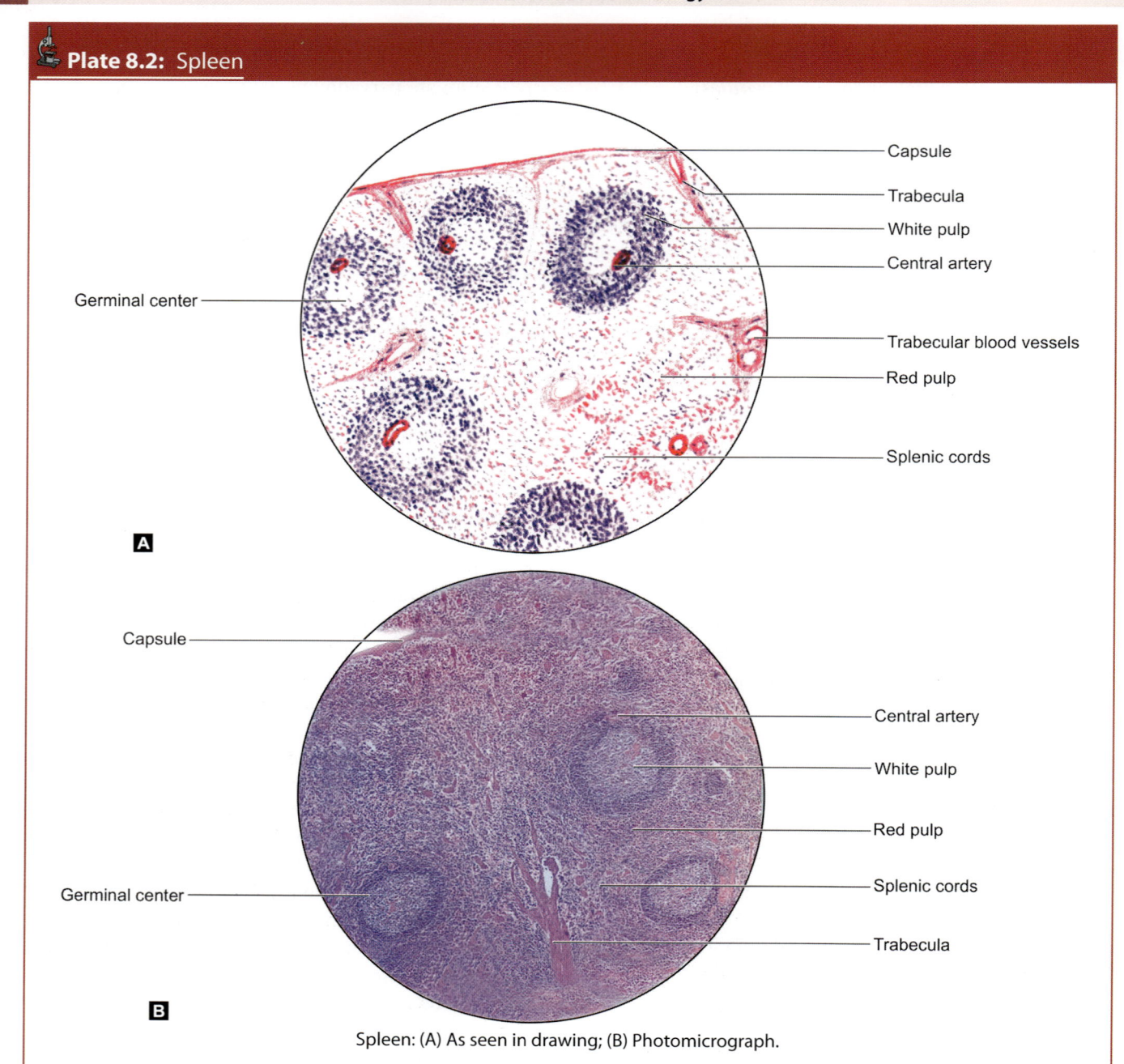

Spleen: (A) As seen in drawing; (B) Photomicrograph.

Labels (A): Capsule, Trabecula, White pulp, Central artery, Trabecular blood vessels, Red pulp, Splenic cords, Germinal center.

Labels (B): Capsule, Central artery, White pulp, Red pulp, Splenic cords, Trabecula, Germinal center.

Points of identification
- The spleen is characterized by a thick capsule with trabeculae extending from it into the organ (not shown in photomicrograph)
- The substance of the organ is divisible into the red pulp in which there are diffusely distributed lymphocytes and numerous sinusoids; and the white pulp in which dense aggregations of lymphocytes are present. The latter are in the form of cords surrounding arterioles
- When cut transversely the cords resemble the lymphatic nodules of lymph nodes, and like them they have germinal centers surrounded by rings of densely packed lymphocytes. However, the nodules of the spleen are easily distinguished from those of lymph nodes because of the presence of an arteriole in each nodule
- This arteriole occupies an eccentric position in the nodule

Note: Observe that this organ is full of lymphocytes. In the drawing also see the cords of densely packed lymphocytes around arteriole.

CHAPTER 8: Lymphatics and Lymphoid Tissue

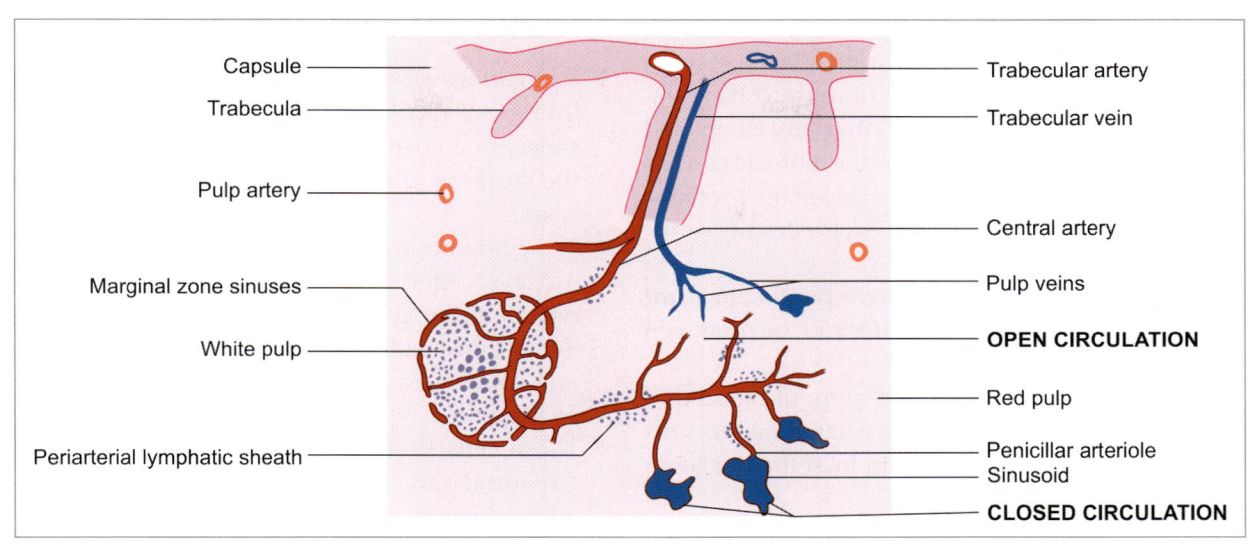

Fig. 8.4: The splenic circulation (schematic representation).

- Within the white pulp, the branch of splenic artery is called central artery (though eccentric in position). The lymphocyte aggregation around the central artery constitutes the periarterial lymphatic sheath (PALS).
- Localized expansions of PALS are called as nodules. The splenic nodules which have quite large germinal enters in reaction to antigen exposures are called as ***malpighian bodies***. More than one arteriole may be present in relation to one germinal center.
- The functional significance of the white pulp is similar to that of cortical tissue of lymph nodes. Lymphatic nodules of the white pulp are the aggregations of B-lymphocytes. The germinal centers are the areas where B-lymphocytes are dividing. Lymphocytes of the PALS are chiefly T-lymphocytes.

Red Pulp

- Red pulp is a modified lymphoid tissue infiltrated with all the cells of circulating blood.
- It is like a sponge permeated by spaces (splenic sinusoids) lined by reticular cells.
- The intervals between the spaces are filled by B-lymphocytes, T-lymphocytes, macrophages, and blood cells.
- Endothelium lining the sinusoids has processes, which makes contact with the adjacent cells.
- These cells appear to be arranged as cords (***splenic cords*** of Billroth). The cords form a network.
- The zone of red pulp immediately surrounding white pulp is the ***marginal zone***. This zone has a rich network of sinusoids. Numerous antigen-presenting cells (APCs) are found close to the sinusoids.

- This region seems to be specialized for bringing antigens confined to circulating blood (e.g. some bacteria) into contact with lymphocytes in the spleen so that an appropriate immune response can be started against the antigens (Such contact does not take place in lymph nodes. Antigens reach lymph nodes from tissues, through lymph). Surgical removal of the spleen (splenectomy) reduces the ability of the body to deal with bloodborne infections.
- The central artery like in white pulp divides and redivides to form straight arterioles then capillaries. Some capillaries are surrounded by macrophages and are called as sheathed capillaries.
- Blood from these capillaries directly drain into reticular meshwork of splenic cords and then into splenic sinuses. This type of circulation is called as ***open circulation***, which effectively exposes the blood to macrophages before they reach the splenic sinuses.
- In other species, blood from the sheathed capillaries directly opens into splenic sinuses, which is called as ***closed circulation***.
- Blood from the spaces of red pulp is collected by wide sinusoids that drain into trabecular veins.

Functions

- Like other lymphoid tissues, the spleen is a center where both B-lymphocytes and T-lymphocytes multiply and play an important role in immune responses. As stated above, the spleen is the only site where an immune response can be started against antigens present in circulating blood (but not present in tissues).

- The spleen contains the largest aggregations of macrophages of the mononuclear phagocyte system. In the spleen the main function of these cells is the destruction of red blood corpuscles that have completed their useful life. This is facilitated by the intimate contact of blood with the macrophages because of the presence of an open circulation. Macrophages also destroy worn-out leukocytes, and bacteria.
- In fetal life the spleen is a center for the production of *all* blood cells. In later life, only lymphocytes are produced here.
- The spleen is often regarded as a store of blood that can be thrown into the circulation when required. This function is much less important in man than in some other species.

THYMUS

- The thymus is a lymphoepithelial bilobed organ which is usually not seen in dissection hall cadavers (because of atrophy in old people, and because of rapid autolysis after death).
- The organ is also not accessible for clinical examination (as it lies deep to the manubrium sterni).
- At birth the thymus weighs 10–15 g. The weight increases to 30–40 g at puberty. Subsequently, much of the organ is replaced by fat. However, the thymus is believed to produce T-lymphocytes throughout life.
- The thymus has rich blood supply. It does not receive any lymph vessels but gives off efferent vessels.
- All other lymphoid organs originate exclusively from mesenchyme but thymus has dual embryonic origin.

Structure

- The thymus consists of right and left lobes that are joined together by fibrous tissue.
- Each lobe has a connective tissue capsule. Connective tissue septa passing inward from the capsule incompletely subdivide the lobe into a large number of lobules (Plate 8.3).
- The capsule and trabeculae contain blood vessels, efferent lymphatic vessels and nerves.
- Each lobule is about 2 mm in diameter. It has an outer cortex and an inner medulla. The medulla of adjoining lobules is continuous.
- Thymic cortex is darkly stained because of the densely packed developing T-lymphocytes called *thymocytes*.
- Both the cortex and medulla contain cells of two distinct lineages as described below.

Epithelioreticular Cells (Epitheliocytes)

- Embryologically these cells are derived from endoderm lining the third pharyngeal pouch. The cells form sheets that cover the internal surface of the capsule, the surfaces of the septa, and the surfaces of blood vessels.
- The epitheliocytes lying deeper in the lobule develop processes that join similar processes and form a reticulum. It may be noted that this reticulum is cellular, unlike the reticulum formed by reticular fibers in lymph nodes and spleen. Epithelial cells of the thymus are not phagocytic.
- These cells share features of reticular by providing structural reticulum and epithelial cells by having intercellular junctions and intermediate fibers.
- On the basis of structural differences, six types of epitheliocytes are recognized.
- Type 1 epitheliocytes line the inner aspect of the capsule, the septa, and blood vessels and form **blood–thymus barrier** that prevents antigens (present in blood and connective tissue) from reaching lymphocytes present in the thymus. Hence, blood–thymus barrier is formed by:
    - Tight junction between endothelial cells
    - Basal lamina of endothelial cells
    - Perivascular connective tissue
    - Basal lamina of epitheliocytes
    - Type 1 epitheliocytes.
- Type 2 epitheliocytes are star shaped with prominent nucleus. Type 2 and type 3 cells are present in the outer and inner parts of the cortex, respectively. They compartmentalize the cortex for developing lymphocytes. Cortical epitheliocytes are also described as ***thymic nurse cells***. They destroy lymphocytes that react against self-antigens.
- Type 4 cells lie in the deepest parts of the cortex, and also in the medulla. They form barrier between cortex and medulla.
- Type 5 cells have darkly stained nucleus and provide structural framework in the medulla.
- Type 6 cells form the characteristic feature of the thymic medulla—***Hassall's corpuscles***. These corpuscles are pink stained small rounded structures with concentrically arranged epitheliocytes intermingled with keratohyalin and lipid droplets. The central core is formed by degenerating epitheliocytes and macrophages. The functional significance of the corpuscles of Hassall is not understood. Recent studies have shown that they produce substances which help in lymphocyte differentiation and maturation.

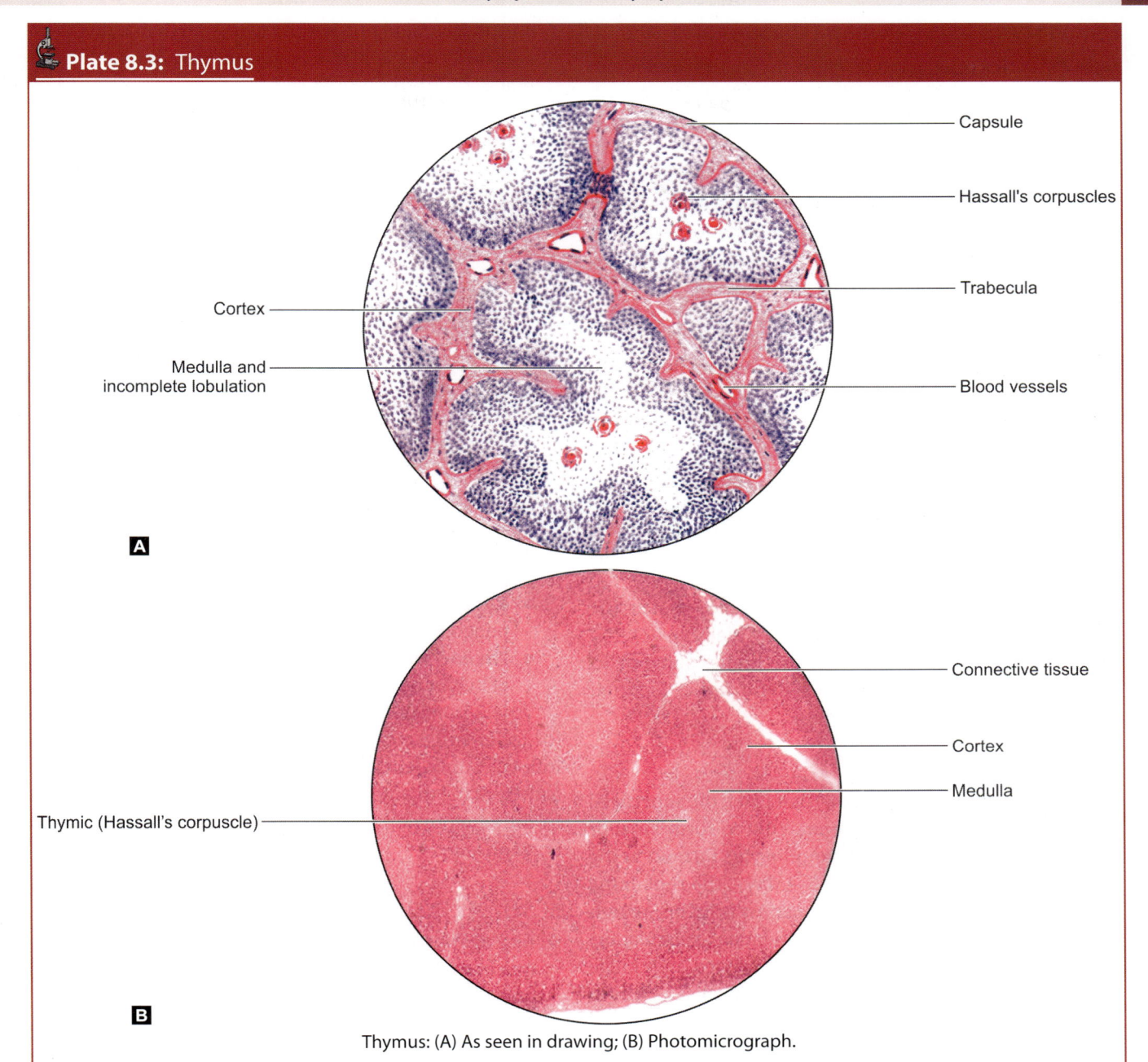

CHAPTER 8: Lymphatics and Lymphoid Tissue

Plate 8.3: Thymus

A — Labels: Capsule, Hassall's corpuscles, Trabecula, Blood vessels, Cortex, Medulla and incomplete lobulation

B — Labels: Connective tissue, Cortex, Medulla, Thymic (Hassall's corpuscle)

Thymus: (A) As seen in drawing; (B) Photomicrograph.

Points of identification
- The thymus is made up of lymphoid tissue arranged in the form of distinct lobules. The presence of this lobulation enables easy distinction of the thymus from all other lymphoid organs
- The lobules are partially separated from each other by connective tissue septae
- In each lobule an outer darkly stained cortex (in which lymphocytes are densely packed); and an inner lightly stained medulla (in which the cells are diffuse) are present
- Whereas the cortex is confined to one lobule, the medulla is continuous from one lobule to another
- The medulla contains pink staining rounded masses called the corpuscles of Hassall.

Lymphocytes of the Thymus (Thymocytes)

- In the cortex of each lobule of the thymus, the reticulum formed by epithelial cells is densely packed with lymphocytes. Stem cells formed in bone marrow travel to the thymus.
- In the thymus, they lie in the superficial part of the cortex and divide repeatedly to form small lymphocytes. Lymphatic nodules are not present in the normal thymus.
- The medulla of each lobule also contains lymphocytes, but these are less densely packed than in the cortex. As a result, the epithelial reticulum is more obvious in the medulla than in the cortex.
- As thymocytes divide, they pass deeper into the cortex, and into the medulla.
- Ultimately, they leave the thymus by passing into blood vessels and lymphatics.

Macrophages

- Apart from epithelial cells and lymphocytes, the thymus contains a fair number of macrophages (belonging to the mononuclear phagocyte system).
- They are placed subjacent to the capsule, at the corticomedullary junction, and in the medulla.
- The subcapsular macrophages are highly phagocytic. Deeper lying macrophages are dendritic cells. Their significance is considered below.

Functions of the Thymus

- Stem cells (from bone marrow) that reach the superficial part of the cortex divide repeatedly to form smaller lymphocytes. Total 90% of lymphocytes formed in the thymus are destroyed within 3–4 days. The remaining lymphocytes, which react only against proteins foreign to the body, are thrown into the circulation as circulating, immunologically competent T-lymphocytes. They lodge themselves in secondary lymph organs, such as lymph nodes, spleen, etc., where they multiply to form further T-lymphocytes of their own type when exposed to the appropriate antigen. Hence thymus is regarded as a *primary lymphoid organ* (along with bone marrow), where schooling of lymphocytes takes place to recognize self and foreign antigen.
- Within the thymus, lymphocytes are not allowed to come into contact with foreign antigens, because of the presence of the *blood–thymic barrier*. It has also been said that because of this, thymocytes do not develop into large lymphocytes or into plasma cells and do not form lymphatic nodules.
- The proliferation of T-lymphocytes and their conversion into cells capable of reacting to antigens probably takes place under the influence of hormones produced by epithelial cells of the thymus. Hormones produced by the thymus may also influence lymphopoiesis in peripheral lymphoid organs. This influence appears to be especially important in early life, as lymphoid tissues do not develop normally if the thymus is removed. Thymectomy has much less influence after puberty as the lymphoid tissues have fully developed by then.
- A number of hormones produced by the thymus have now been identified as follows. They are produced by epitheliocytes.
  - *Thymulin* enhances the function of various types of T-cells, especially that of suppressor cells.
  - *Thymopoietin* stimulates the production of cytotoxic T-cells. The combined action of thymulin and thymopoietin allows precise balance of the activity of cytotoxic and suppressor cells.
  - *Thymosin alpha-1* stimulates lymphocyte production, and also the production of antibodies.
  - *Thymosin beta-4* is produced by mononuclear phagocytes.
  - *Thymic humoral factor* controls the multiplication of helper and suppressor T-cells.

Apart from their actions on lymphocytes, hormones (or other substances) produced in the thymus probably influence the adenohypophysis and the ovaries. In turn the activity of the thymus is influenced by hormones produced by the adenohypophysis, by the adrenal cortex, and by sex hormones.

MUCOSA-ASSOCIATED LYMPHOID TISSUE

- Aggregations of lymphocytes seen in relation to the mucosa of the respiratory, alimentary, and urogenital tracts are referred to as *MALT*.
- The total volume of MALT is more or less equal to that of the lymphoid tissue present in lymph nodes and spleen.
- Mucosa-associated aggregations of lymphoid tissue have some features in common, which are as follows:
  - These aggregations are in the form of one or more lymphatic follicles (nodules) having a structure similar to nodules of lymph nodes. Germinal centers may be present.
  - Diffuse lymphoid tissue (termed the *parafollicular zone*) is present in the intervals between the nodules. The significance of the nodules and of the diffuse

aggregations of lymphocytes is the same as already described in the case of lymph nodes.
- The nodules consist predominantly of B-lymphocytes, while the diffuse areas contain T-lymphocytes.
- These masses of lymphoid tissue are present in very close relationship to the lining epithelium of the mucosa in the region concerned and lie in the substantia propria. Larger aggregations extend into the submucosa. Individual lymphocytes may infiltrate the epithelium and may pass through it into the lumen.
- The aggregations are not surrounded by a capsule, nor do they have connective tissue septa. A supporting network of reticular fibers is present.
- As a rule, these masses of lymphoid tissue do not receive afferent lymph vessels and have no lymph sinuses. They do not, therefore, serve as filters of lymph. However, they are the centers of lymphocyte production. Lymphocytes produced here pass into lymph nodes of the region through efferent lymphatic vessels. Some lymphocytes pass through the overlying epithelium into the lumen.

Mucosa-associated Lymphoid Tissue in the Respiratory System

In the respiratory system the aggregations are relatively small and are present in the walls of the trachea and large bronchi. The term **BALT** is applied to these aggregations.

Mucosa-associated Lymphoid Tissue in the Alimentary System

This is also called GALT. In the alimentary system, examples of aggregations of lymphoid tissue are tonsils, Peyer's patches, and lymphoid nodules in vermiform appendix.

TONSILS

- Near the junction of the oral cavity with the pharynx, there are a number of collections of lymphoid tissues that are referred to as **tonsils**.
- The largest of these are the right and left **palatine tonsils**, present on either side of the oropharyngeal isthmus. (In common usage the word—tonsils—refers to the palatine tonsils). Another midline collection of lymphoid tissue, the **pharyngeal tonsil**, is present on the posterior wall of the pharynx.
- Smaller collections are present on the dorsum of the posterior part of the tongue (**lingual tonsils**), and around the pharyngeal openings of the auditory tubes (**tubal tonsils**).
- They together form **Waldeyer's ring**.

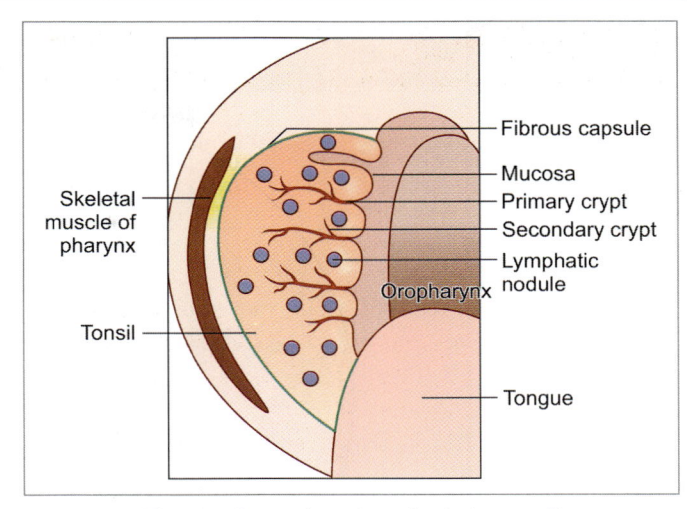

Fig. 8.5: Coronal section of palatine tonsil (schematic representation).

Palatine Tonsils

- Each palatine tonsil consists of diffuse lymphoid tissue in which lymphatic nodules are present.
- The lymphoid tissue is covered by stratified squamous nonkeratinized epithelium, continuous with that of the mouth and pharynx (Fig. 8.5 and Plate 8.4).
- This epithelium extends into the substance of the tonsil in the form of several **tonsillar crypts**.
- The lumen of a crypt usually contains some lymphocytes that have traveled into it through the epithelium.
- Desquamated epithelial cells and bacteria are also frequently present in the lumen of the crypt.

FURTHER READING

Mononuclear Phagocyte System

- Distributed widely through the body, there are a series of cells that share the property of being able to phagocytose unwanted matter, including bacteria and dead cells.
- These cells also play an important role in defense mechanisms, and in carrying out this function, they act in close collaboration with lymphocytes.
- With the discovery of a close relationship between these cells and mononuclear leukocytes of blood, the term **mononuclear phagocyte system** (or **monocyte phagocyte system**) has come into common usage.

Cells of Mononuclear Phagocyte System

The various cells that are usually included in the mononuclear phagocyte system are as follows.
- Monocytes of blood and their precursors in bone marrow (monoblasts, promonocytes).
- Macrophage cells (histiocytes) of connective tissue.

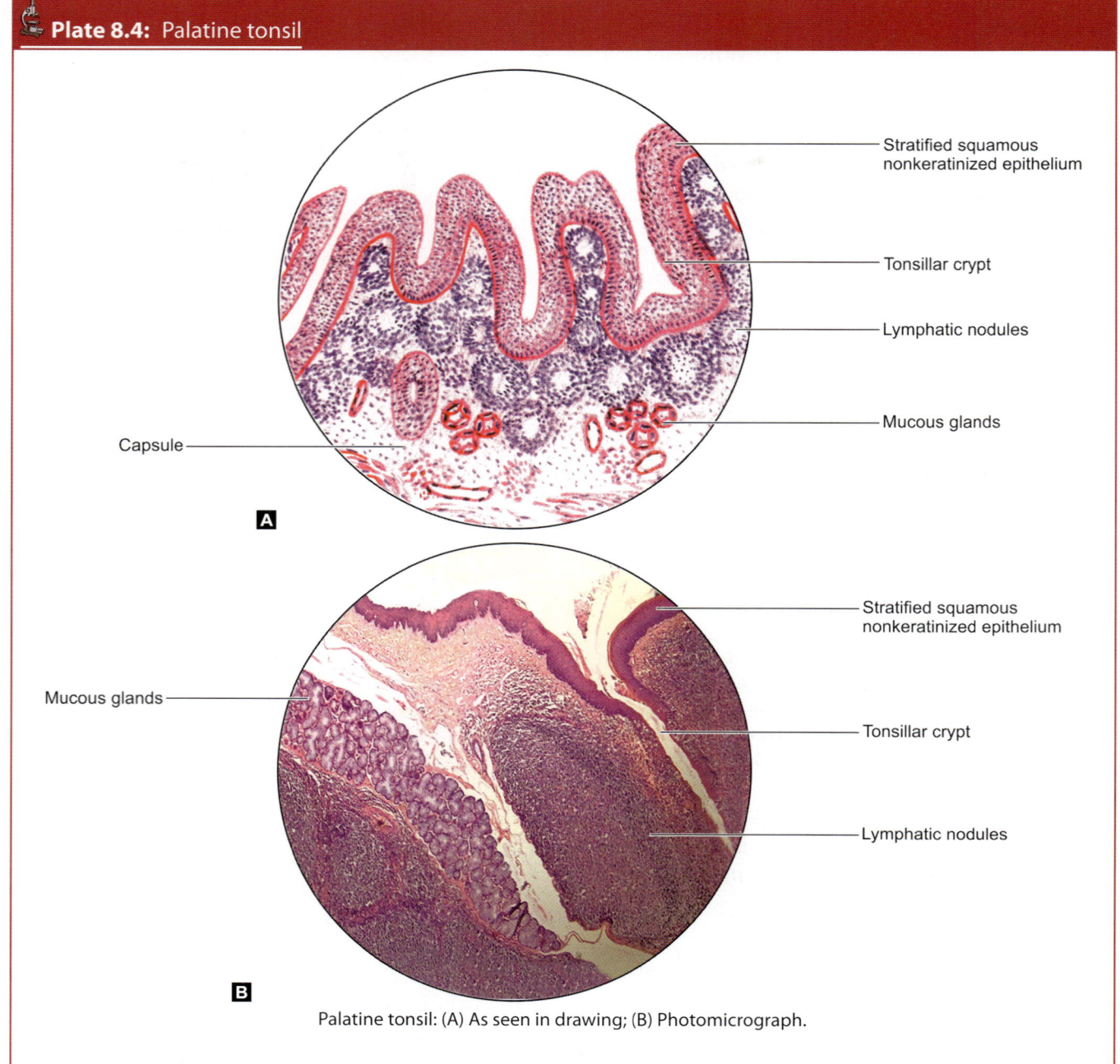

Plate 8.4: Palatine tonsil

Labels (A, drawing): Stratified squamous nonkeratinized epithelium; Tonsillar crypt; Lymphatic nodules; Mucous glands; Capsule

Labels (B, photomicrograph): Stratified squamous nonkeratinized epithelium; Tonsillar crypt; Lymphatic nodules; Mucous glands

Palatine tonsil: (A) As seen in drawing; (B) Photomicrograph.

Points of identification
- Palatine tonsil is an aggregation of lymphoid tissue that is readily recognized by the fact that it is covered by a stratified squamous epithelium
- At places the epithelium dips into the tonsil in the form of deep crypts
- Deep to the epithelium there is diffuse lymphoid tissue in which typical lymphatic nodules can be seen.

- Littoral cells (von Kupffer cells) interspersed among cells lining the sinusoids of the liver; and cells in the walls of sinusoids in the spleen and lymph nodes.
- Microglial cells of the central nervous system.
- Macrophages in pleura, peritoneum, alveoli of lungs, spleen, and in synovial joints.
- Free macrophages present in pleural, peritoneal, and synovial fluids.
- Dendritic cells of the epidermis and similar highly branched cells in lymph nodes, spleen, and thymus. These are now grouped as *APCs* (*see* below).

CHAPTER 8: Lymphatics and Lymphoid Tissue

Structure of cells

All cells of the mononuclear phagocyte system have some features in common.

- They are large (15–25 μm) in diameter. The nucleus is euchromatic. Granular and agranular endoplasmic reticulum, Golgi complex, and mitochondria are present, as are endocytic vesicles and lysosomes. The cells have irregular surfaces that bear filopodia (irregular microvilli). Most of the cells are more or less oval in shape, but the dendritic cells are highly branched.
- Macrophages often form aggregations. In relation to the peritoneum and pleura, such aggregations are seen as ***milky spots***; and in the spleen, they form ellipsoids around small arteries. When they come in contact with large particles, macrophages may fuse to form multinuclear giant cells (***foreign body giant cells***).
- In the presence of organisms, such as tubercle bacilli, the cells may transform to ***epithelioid cells***. (These are involved in T-cell-mediated immune responses).

From a functional point of view, mononuclear phagocytes are divided into two main types.

1. With the exception of dendritic cells, all the cell types are classified as ***highly phagocytic cells***.
2. The dendritic mononuclear phagocytes (now called dendritic APCs) are capable of phagocytosis, but their main role is to initiate immune reactions in lymphocytes present in lymph nodes, spleen, and thymus (in the manner discussed above). It has been postulated that ***all*** dendritic cells are primarily located in the skin. From here they pick up antigens and migrate to lymphoid tissues where they stimulate lymphocytes against these antigens. They are therefore referred to as APCs. Most APCs are derived from monocytes, but some are derived from other sources.

Functions of the Mononuclear Phagocyte System

Participation in defense mechanisms

As already stated, the cells have the ability to phagocytose particulate matter, dead cells, and organisms. In the lungs, alveolar macrophages engulf inhaled particles and are seen as ***dust cells***. In the spleen and liver, macrophages destroy aged and damaged erythrocytes.

Role in immune responses

- All mononuclear phagocytes bear antigens on their surface [class II major histocompatibility complex (MHC) antigens]. Antigens phagocytosed by macrophages are partially digested by lysosomes. Some remnants of these pass to the cell surface where they form complexes with the MHC antigens. This complex has the ability to stimulate T-lymphocytes.
- Certain T-lymphocytes produce macrophage-activating factors (including interleukin-2) that influence the activity of macrophages. Macrophages when thus stimulated synthesize and secrete cytokines that stimulate the proliferation and maturation of further lymphocytes.
- When foreign substances (including organisms) enter the body, antibodies are produced against them (by lymphocytes). These antibodies adhere to the organisms. Macrophages bear receptors (on their surface) that are able to recognize these antibodies. In this way, macrophages are able to selectively destroy such matter by phagocytosis, or by the release of lysosomal enzymes.

From the above, it will be seen that lymphocytes and macrophages constitute an integrated immune system for defense of the body.

- When suitably stimulated mononuclear phagocytes secrete a tumor-necrosing factor which is able to kill some neoplastic cells.
- Macrophages influence the growth and differentiation of tissues by producing several growth factors and differentiation factors.

APPLIED HISTOLOGY

Lymph Node

- **Lymphangitis** is inflammation of the lymphatics. Lymphangitis may be acute or chronic.
- **Acute lymphangitis** occurs in the course of many bacterial infections. The most common organisms are b-hemolytic streptococci and staphylococci. When this happens in vessels of the skin, the vessels are seen as red lines that are painful.
- **Chronic lymphangitis** occurs due to persistent and recurrent acute lymphangitis or from chronic infections, such as tuberculosis, syphilis, and actinomycosis.
- **Lymphedema** is the swelling of soft tissues due to localized increase in the quantity of lymph. It may be primary (idiopathic) or secondary (obstructive). Secondary lymphedema is more common and may be due to lymphatic invasion by malignant tumor, Postirradiation fibrosis, Parasitic infestations, e.g. in filariasis of lymphatics producing elephantiasis. Rupture of dilated large lymphatics may result in the escape of milky chyle into the peritoneum (**chyloperitoneum**), into the pleural cavity (**chylothorax**), into pericardial cavity (**chylopericardium**), and into the urinary tract (**chyluria**).

- Infection in any part of the body can lead to enlargement and inflammation of the lymph nodes draining the area. The inflammation of lymph nodes is called **lymphadenitis**.
- Carcinoma (cancer) usually spreads from its primary site either by growth of malignant cells along lymph vessels, or by "loose" cancer cells passing through lymph to nodes into which the area drains. This leads to enlargement of the lymph nodes of the region. Examination of lymph nodes gives valuable information about the stage of the cancer. In surgical excision of cancer, lymph nodes draining the region are usually removed.

Spleen

Splenomegaly: Enlargement of spleen is termed splenomegaly. It occurs in a wide variety of disorders which increase the cellularity and vascularity of the organ. Many of the causes are exaggerated forms of normal splenic function.

Causes of Splenomegaly

- Infections: Malaria, leishmaniasis.
- Disorders of immunoregulation: Rheumatoid arthritis, systemic lupus erythematosus.
- Altered splenic blood flow: Cirrhosis of liver, portal vein obstruction, splenic vein obstruction.
- Lymphohematogenous malignancies: Hodgkin's disease, non-Hodgkin's lymphomas.
- Diseases with abnormal erythrocytes: Thalassemias, spherocytosis, sickle cell disease.
- Storage diseases: Gaucher's disease, Niemann-Pick's disease.
- Miscellaneous: Amyloidosis, primary and metastatic splenic tumors.

Thymus

- Enlargement of the thymus is often associated with a disease called **myasthenia gravis**. In this condition, there is great weakness of skeletal muscle.
- Myasthenia gravis is due to disturbance of the immune system. There are some proteins to which acetyl choline released at motor end plates gets attached. In myasthenia gravis, antibodies are produced against these proteins rendering them ineffective. Myasthenia gravis is, thus, an example of a condition in which the immune system begins to react against one of the body's own proteins. Such conditions are referred to as **autoimmune diseases**.
- In many such cases the thymus is enlarged, and removal of the thymus may result in considerable improvement in some cases.

Tonsils

Tonsillitis is the infection of palatine tonsils. The palatine tonsils are often infected. It is a common cause of sore throat. Frequent infections can lead to considerable enlargement of the tonsils, especially in children. Such enlarged tonsils may become a focus of infection, and their surgical removal (**tonsillectomy**) may then become necessary.

MULTIPLE CHOICE QUESTIONS

1. Blood–thymus barrier is formed by:
   a. Type 3 epitheliocytes
   b. Type 2 epitheliocytes
   c. Type 1 epitheliocytes
   d. Type 4 epitheliocytes
2. Modified endothelial cells lining the splenic sinusoids are:
   a. Pericytes
   b. Stave cells
   c. Thymocytes
   d. Reticulocytes
3. PALS are characteristic features of:
   a. Thymus
   b. Spleen
   c. Tonsil
   d. Lymph node
4. Following are true about white pulp, *except*:
   a. Contains eccentric arteriole
   b. Also known as Malpighian corpuscles
   c. Formed by aggregation of lymphocytes
   d. They are found in thymus
5. Hassall's corpuscles are formed by:
   a. Type 3 epitheliocytes
   b. Type 6 epitheliocytes
   c. Type 1 epitheliocytes
   d. Type 4 epitheliocytes
6. Schooling of lymphocytes occurs at:
   a. Thymus
   b. Lymph node
   c. Spleen
   d. Tonsil
7. Cords of Billroth are present in:
   a. Thymus
   b. Lymph node
   c. Spleen
   d. Tonsil
8. Germinal center indicates all, *except*:
   a. Activation of lymphocytes
   b. Antibody production
   c. Differentiation of plasma cells
   d. Degeneration of lymphocytes

Answers
1. c   2. b   3. c   4. d   5. b   6. a   7. c   8. d

CHAPTER 9

Nervous Tissue

Learning objectives

To study the:
- Components of nervous system with classification
- Structure of a neuron and its types
- *Neuroglia*—types, structure, and function
- Myelination
- Structure of peripheral nerve/optic nerve
- *Ganglia*—autonomic and spinal
- Applied histology

IDENTIFICATION POINTS

Peripheral nerve	Optic nerve	Sensory/dorsal nerve root ganglia	Autonomic ganglia
☐ Each nerve fiber is covered by endoneurium ☐ Each bundle of nerve fibers is covered by perineurium ☐ Each nerve is covered by epineurium ☐ Cut section of axon with myelin sheath and Schwann cell nucleus.	☐ Covered by meninges—dura mater, arachnoid mater, and pia mater ☐ Central retinal artery and vein are seen ☐ Pial septa divides the nerve into bundles.	☐ Unipolar neurons with centrally placed nucleus ☐ Neurons are presented in a group between the bundles of nerve fibers ☐ Prominent satellite cells are seen.	☐ Multipolar neurons with eccentrically placed nucleus ☐ Neurons are scattered between the nerve fibers.

INTRODUCTION

The nervous system is a specialized type of tissue that has property of ability to conduct impulses rapidly from one part of the body to another. Nerve cells can convert information obtained from the environment into codes that can be transmitted along their axons. By such coding, the same neuron can transmit different kinds of information.

The total number of neurons in the human brain is estimated at more than 1 trillion. Nervous tissue is composed of neurons and neuroglia.

- ❖ **Neurons** are the specialized cells that constitute the structural and functional unit of nervous system.
- ❖ **Neuroglia:** Supporting connective tissue cells present in nervous system.

It has been taught that lymph vessels are not present, but the view has recently been challenged.

The nervous system may be divided into the *central nervous system (CNS)*, made up of the brain and spinal cord, the *peripheral nervous system (PNS)*, consisting of the peripheral nerves and the ganglia associated with them, and the ***autonomic nervous system***, consisting of the ***sympathetic*** and the ***parasympathetic nervous systems*** (Flowchart 9.1).

STRUCTURE OF A NEURON

Neurons are responsible for the receptive, integrative, and motor functions of the nervous system. Neurons vary considerably in size, shape, and other features. However, most of them have some major features in common, and these are described below.

Neuron is made up of the following parts:
- ❖ Cell body/soma/perikaryon
- ❖ *Processes/neurites*—single axon and multiple dendrites

Cell Body/Soma/Perikaryon

A neuron consists of a ***cell body*** that gives off a variable number of ***processes*** (Fig. 9.1).

Flowchart 9.1: Anatomical classification of nervous system.

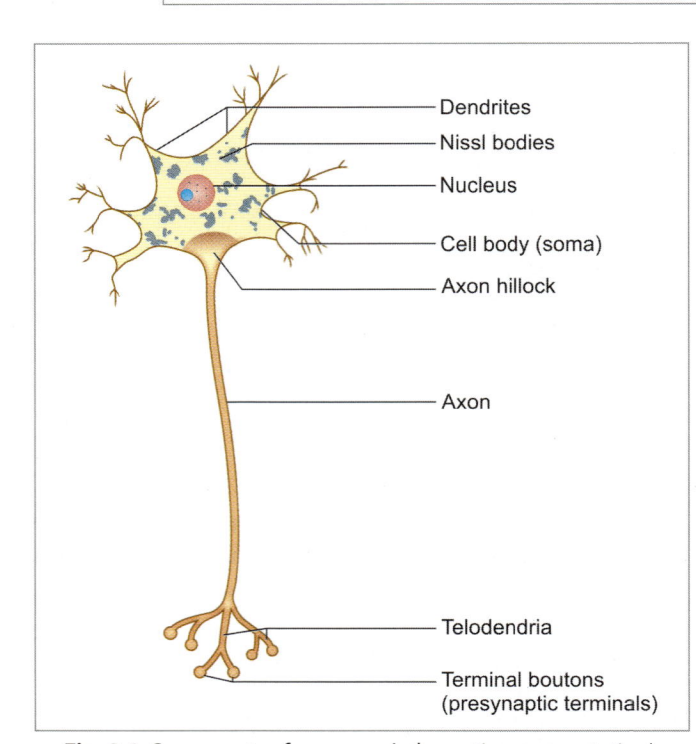

Fig. 9.1: Some parts of a neuron (schematic representation).

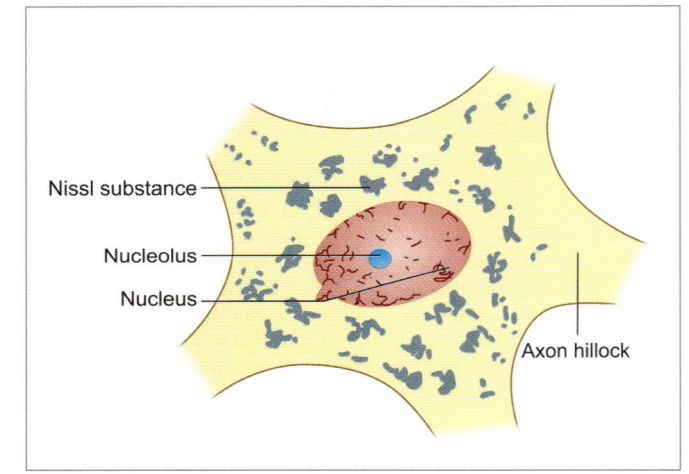

Fig. 9.2: Neuron stained to show Nissl substance. Note that the Nissl substance extends into the dendrites but not into the axon.

Cytoplasm: Like a typical cell, it consists of a mass of cytoplasm surrounded by a cell membrane. The cytoplasm contains a large central nucleus with a prominent nucleolus, highly developed rough endoplasmic reticulum, numerous mitochondria, lysosomes, and a Golgi complex (Fig. 9.2).

Nissl Substance

- The cytoplasm shows the presence of a granular material that stains intensely with basic dyes; this material is the ***Nissl substance*** (also called Nissl bodies or granules) (Fig. 9.2).
- When examined by electron microscope (EM), these bodies are seen to be composed of rough surfaced endoplasmic reticulum (Fig. 9.3). The presence of abundant granular endoplasmic reticulum is an indication of the high level of protein synthesis in neurons. The proteins are needed for maintenance and repair, and for the production of neurotransmitters and enzymes.

Neurofibrils

- Another distinctive feature of neurons is the presence of a network of fibrils permeating the cytoplasm (Fig. 9.4).
- These ***neurofibrils*** are seen when prepared by silver impregnation.

CHAPTER 9: Nervous Tissue

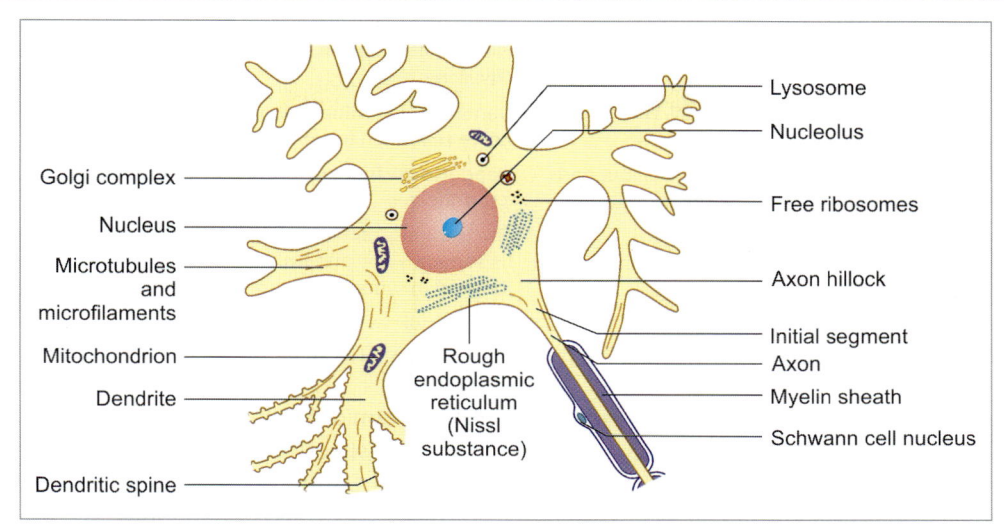

Fig. 9.3: Some features of the structure of a neuron as seen by electron microscope (schematic representation).

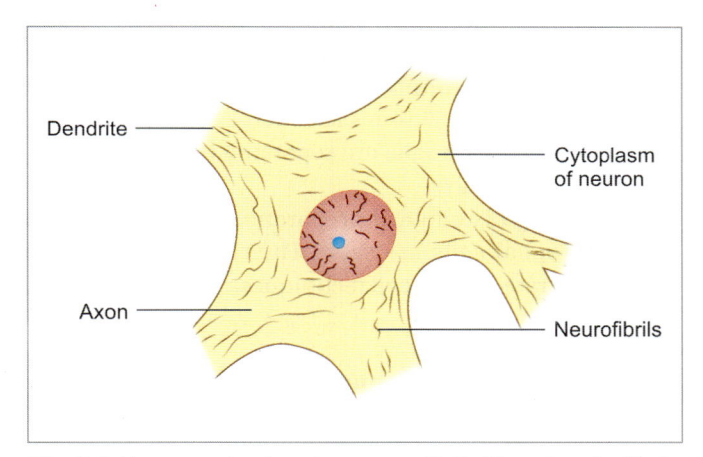

Fig. 9.4: Neuron stained to show neurofibrils. Note that the fibrils extend into both axons and dendrites.

- When seen under EM, it shows microfilaments, microtubules and neurofilaments (The centrioles present in neurons may be concerned with the production and maintenance of microtubules).

Axon Hillock and Initial Segment

- The axon hillock and the initial segment of the axon are of special functional significance. This is the region where action potentials are generated (spike generation), resulting in conduction along the axon. The initial segment is unmyelinated. It often receives axo-axonal synapses that are inhibitory. The plasma membrane here is rich in voltage-sensitive channels.

Some neurons contain pigment granules, e.g. neuromelanin in neurons of the substantia nigra. Aging neurons contain a pigment lipofuscin made up of residual bodies derived from lysosomes.

Neurites

The processes arising from the cell body of a neuron are called *neurites.* These are of two kinds, number of short branching processes called **dendrites** and one longer process called an *axon* (Table 9.1).

Axon

The axon may extend for a considerable distance away from the cell body.
- The longest axons may be as much as 1 meter long.
- Each axon has a uniform diameter and is devoid of Nissl substance. The Nissl-free zone extends for a short distance into the cell body: this part of the cell body is called the *axon hillock*. The part of the axon just beyond the axon hillock is called the *initial segment.*
- The cytoplasm within the axon is called axoplasm, and its cell membrane is called axolemma.
- The axoplasm contains all the cell organelles of neurons cell body except ribosomes. Hence, proteins synthesized in the cell body are continuously transported toward the axon terminals by a process called axoplasmic transport.
- In an axon the impulse travels *away from the cell body*.
- Axons constitute what are commonly called *nerve fibers*. The bundles of nerve fibers found in CNS are called as *nerve tracts,* while the bundles of nerve fibers found in PNS are called *peripheral nerves*.

An axon (or its branches) can terminate in two ways. Within the CNS, it always terminates by coming in intimate

Table 9.1: Differences between axons and dendrites.

Axon	Dendrites
Axon is a single, long, and thin process of a nerve cell, which terminates away from the nerve cell body	Dendrites are multiple, short, thick, and tapering processes of the nerve cell which terminate near the nerve cell body
Axon rarely branches at the right angle (axon collaterals) but ends by dividing into many fine processes called axon terminals	Dendrites are highly branched. Their branching pattern forms a dendritic tree
It has uniform diameter and smooth surface	The thickness of dendrite reduces as it divides repeatedly. Its surface is not smooth, but it bears many small spine-like projections for making synaptic contacts with the axons of other nerve cells
It is free of Nissl granules	Nissl granules are present in dendrites
The nerve impulses travel away from the cell body	The nerve impulses travel toward the cell body

relationship with another neuron, the junction between the two neurons being called a **synapse**. Outside the CNS, the axon may end in relation to an effector organ (e.g. muscle or gland), or may end by synapsing with neurons in a peripheral ganglion.

Dendrites (Dendron Means Tree)

- They are short processes of neuron and terminate near the cell body
- They are irregular in thickness, and Nissl granules extend into them
- They bear numerous small spines that are of variable shape
- In a dendrite, the nerve impulse travels **toward the cell body** (Table 9.1).

> **Added Information**
>
> **Axoplasmic flow**
>
> The cytoplasm of neurons is in constant motion. Movements of various materials occur through axons. This **axoplasmic flow** takes place both away from and toward the cell body. The flow away from the cell body is greater. Some materials travel slowly (0.1–2 mm a day) constituting a **slow transport**. In contrast, other materials (mainly in the form of vesicles) travel 100–400 mm a day constituting a **rapid transport**. The proteins present in dendrites and axons are not identical. This fact is used for the immunocytochemical identification of dendrites in tissue sections. A protein microtubule-associated protein-2 (MAP-2) is present exclusively in dendrites and helps in their identification.

NEUROGLIA

In addition to neurons, the nervous system contains several types of supporting cells called neuroglia (Flowchart 9.2).

Neuroglial Cells

- Astrocytes, oligodendrocytes, and microglia found in the parenchyma of the brain and spinal cord and ependymal cells lining the ventricular system.
- Schwann cells (lemmocytes) or peripheral glia forming myelin sheaths around axons of peripheral nerves. It is important to note that both neurilemma and myelin sheaths are the components of Schwann cells.
- Capsular cells or satellite cells or capsular gliocytes that surround neurons in peripheral ganglia.
- All neuroglial cells are much smaller in size than neurons. However, they are far more numerous. It is interesting to note that the number of glial cells in the brain and spinal cord is 10–50 times as much as that of neurons. Neurons and neuroglia are separated by a very narrow extracellular space.
- In ordinary histological preparations, only the nuclei of neuroglial cells are seen. Their processes can be demonstrated by special techniques.

Astrocytes

- These are small star-shaped cells that give off a number of processes (Fig. 9.5). The processes are often flattened into leaf-like laminae that may partly surround neurons and separate them from other neurons. The processes frequently end in expansions in relation to blood vessels or in relation to the surface of the brain. Small swellings called **gliosomes** are present on the processes of astrocytes. These swellings are rich in mitochondria.
- The processes of astrocytes are united to those of other astrocytes through gap junctions. Astrocytes communicate with one another through calcium channels. Such communication plays a role in the regulation of synaptic activity and in the metabolism of neurotransmitters and neuromodulators.
- Astrocytes are of two types: (1) Fibrous and (2) Protoplasmic.
  a. **Fibrous astrocytes** are seen mainly in white matter. Their processes are thin and are asymmetrical.

CHAPTER 9: Nervous Tissue

Flowchart 9.2: Types of neuroglia found in central and peripheral nervous systems.

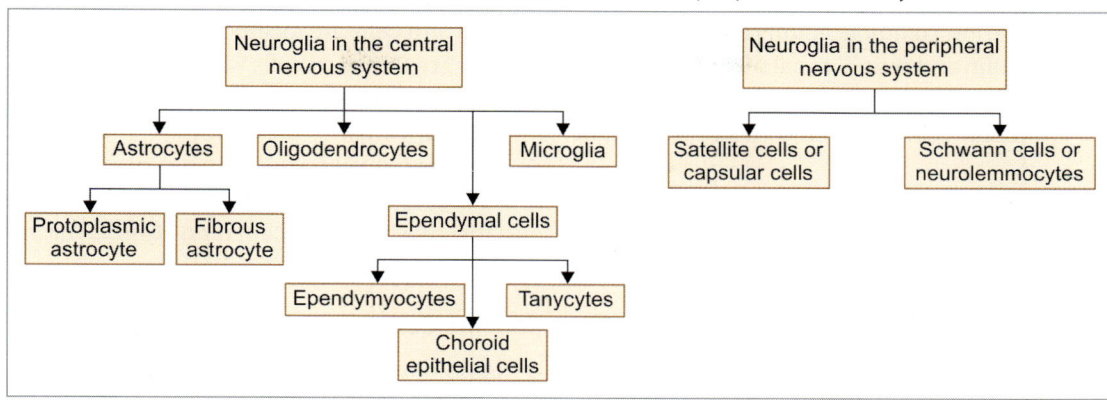

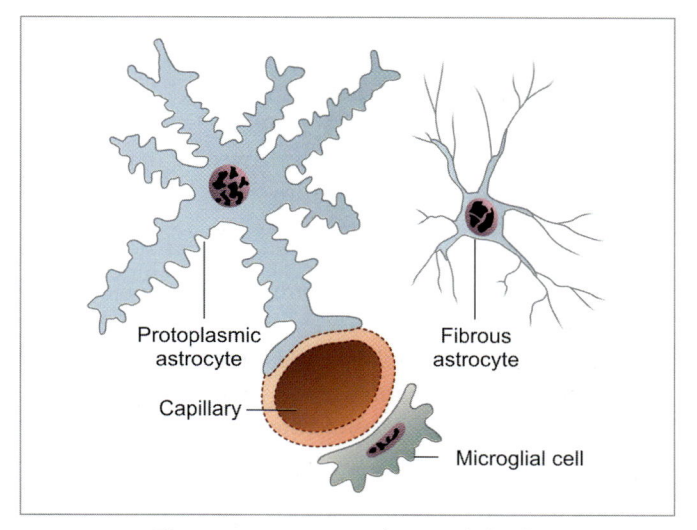

Fig. 9.5: Astrocytes and microglial cells (schematic representation).

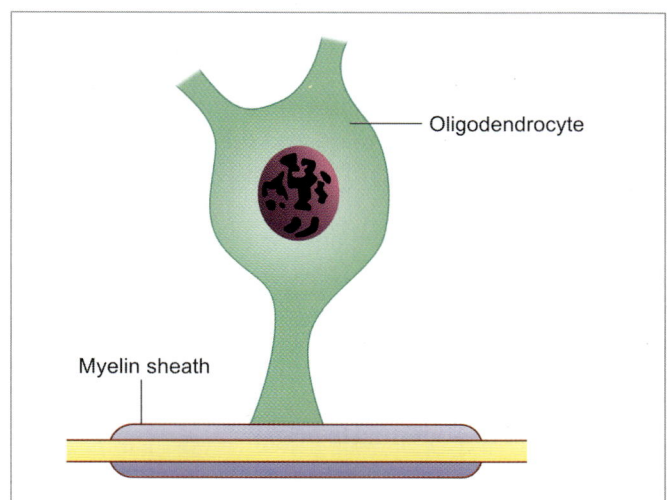

Fig. 9.6: Oligodendrocyte giving off a process that forms a segment of the myelin sheath of an axon (schematic representation).

b. **Protoplasmic astrocytes** are seen mainly in gray matter. Their processes are thicker than those of fibrous astrocytes and are symmetrical.
c. **Intermediate forms** between fibrous and protoplasmic astrocytes are also present. Protoplasmic extensions of astrocytes surround the nodes of Ranvier.

Functions
- Biochemical support of endothelial cells
- They help in the formation of blood–brain barrier
- Provision of nutrients to the nervous tissue
- Maintenance of extracellular ion balance
- Help in repair process by forming cellular scar tissue (**gliosis**)
- They serve as insulators and prevent neuronal impulses from spreading in unwanted directions

- They are believed to help in maintaining a suitable metabolic environment for the neurons. They can absorb neurotransmitters from synapses, thus, terminating their action.

Oligodendrocytes
- These cells are rounded or pear-shaped bodies with relatively few processes (oligo—scanty) (Fig. 9.6).
- These cells provide myelin sheaths to nerve fibers that lie within the brain and spinal cord. Their relationship to nerve fibers is basically similar to that of Schwann cells to peripheral nerve fibers.

Function
Oligodendrocytes provide myelin sheaths to nerve fibers within the CNS for fast conduction of nerve impulses.

Ependymal Cells

- Ependymal cells are low columnar epithelial cells lining the ventricles of the brain and central canal of the spinal cord.
- The specialized ependymal cells in choroid plexuses (choroidal epithelial cells) secrete cerebrospinal fluid (CSF).
- In some regions, these cells are ciliated that helps in the movement of CSF.
- Modifications of the ependymal cells in the ventricle help in the formation of choroid plexus and CSF.
- The ependymal cells lining the floor of the fourth ventricle have long basal processes and are termed "*tanycytes*".

Functions

- It secretes CSF and helps in maintaining the chemical composition of the CSF.
- Ependymal cells are concerned in the exchange of material between the brain and the CSF at the brain–CSF barrier. The blood in the capillaries of the choroid plexus is filtered through choroid epithelial cells at the blood–CSF barrier to secrete CSF.

Microglia

- These are the smallest neuroglial cells (Fig. 9.5). The cell body is flattened with short processes.
- They are the members of the mononuclear phagocyte system and mesodermal in origin.
- They are more numerous in gray matter than in white matter.

Functions

- They act as phagocytes in clearing debris and damaged structures and become active after damage to nervous tissue by trauma or disease.
- They also protect nervous system from viruses, microorganisms, and tumor formation.

Schwann Cells

- Schwann cells are located in PNS and envelop axons.
- They are flattened cells with flattened nucleus.
- They form either myelinated or unmyelinated coverings over the axons.
- They form myelin sheath in peripheral nervous system.
- Axon may be myelinated or unmyelinated. Axons having a myelin sheath are called ***myelinated axons***.
- They are derived from neural crest.

Satellite Cells

- Satellite glial cells are the principal glial cells found in the PNS, specifically in sensory, sympathetic, and parasympathetic ganglia.
- They help to regulate and stabilize the environment around ganglion cell bodies.
- They are derived from neural crest.
- They supply nutrients to the surrounding neurons and also act as protective, cushioning cells (Fig. 9.2).

Myelin Sheath

- It is an insulating sheath surrounding the axons outside the axolemma.
- In PNS, myelin sheath is formed by **Schwann cells** and in CNS by an ***oligodendrocyte***.
- Many Schwann cells surround the axons to form a myelin sheath in PNS, and single oligodendrocyte provides myelin sheath for many axons in CNS.

Formation of myelin sheath

- An axon lying near a Schwann cell invaginates into the cytoplasm of the Schwann cell. In this process, the axon comes to be suspended by a fold cell membrane of the Schwann cell: this fold is called the ***mesaxon*** (Figs. 9.7A and B). In some situations, the mesaxon becomes greatly

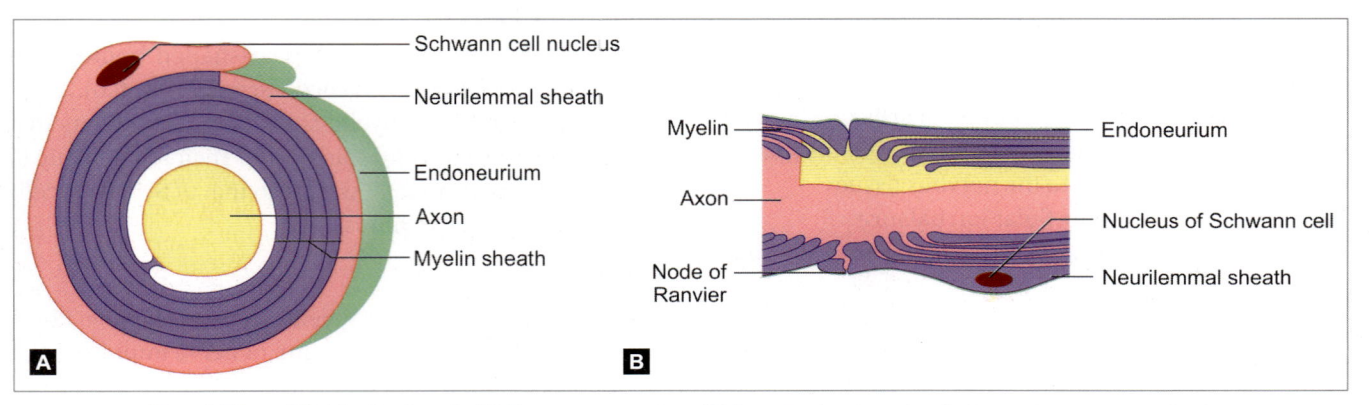

Figs. 9.7A and B: Myelin sheath: (A) Transverse section; (B) Longitudinal section (schematic representation).

elongated and comes to be spirally wound around the axon, which is thus surrounded by several layers of cell membrane.
❖ Lipids are deposited between the adjacent layers of the membrane. These layers of the mesaxon, along with the lipids, form the *myelin sheath*.
❖ Outside the myelin sheath, a thin layer of Schwann cell cytoplasm persists to form an additional sheath that is called the *neurilemma* (neurilemmal sheath or Schwann cell sheath).
❖ The presence of a myelin sheath increases the velocity of conduction. It also reduces the energy expended in the process of conduction.
❖ An axon is related to a large number of Schwann cells over its length (Fig. 9.8). Each Schwann cell provides the myelin sheath for a short segment of the axon. At the junction of any two such segments, there is a short gap in the myelin sheath. These gaps are called the *nodes of Ranvier* and it is the junction between the myelin sheath of two different Schwann cells.
❖ The nodes of Ranvier have great physiological importance. When an impulse travels down a nerve fiber, it jumps from one node to the next. This is called *saltatory conduction* (in unmyelinated neurons, the impulse travels along the axolemma. Such conduction is much slower than saltatory conduction and consumes more energy).
❖ The segment of myelin sheath between two nodes of Ranvier is called *internode*, and a single Schwann cell will myelinate an internode.
❖ Myelin contains protein, lipids, and water. The main lipids present include cholesterol, phospholipids, and glycosphingolipids. Other lipids are present in smaller amounts.

Functions of the myelin sheath

❖ The presence of a myelin sheath increases the velocity of conduction.
❖ It reduces the energy expended in the process of conduction.
❖ It is responsible for the color of the white matter of the brain and spinal cord and provides insulation to the neurons.

Unmyelinated Axons

There are the axons that are devoid of myelin sheaths. These *unmyelinated axons* invaginate into the cytoplasm of Schwann cells, but the mesaxon does not spiral around them (Figs. 9.9 and 9.10), and several such axons may invaginate into the cytoplasm of a single Schwann cell (Table 9.2).

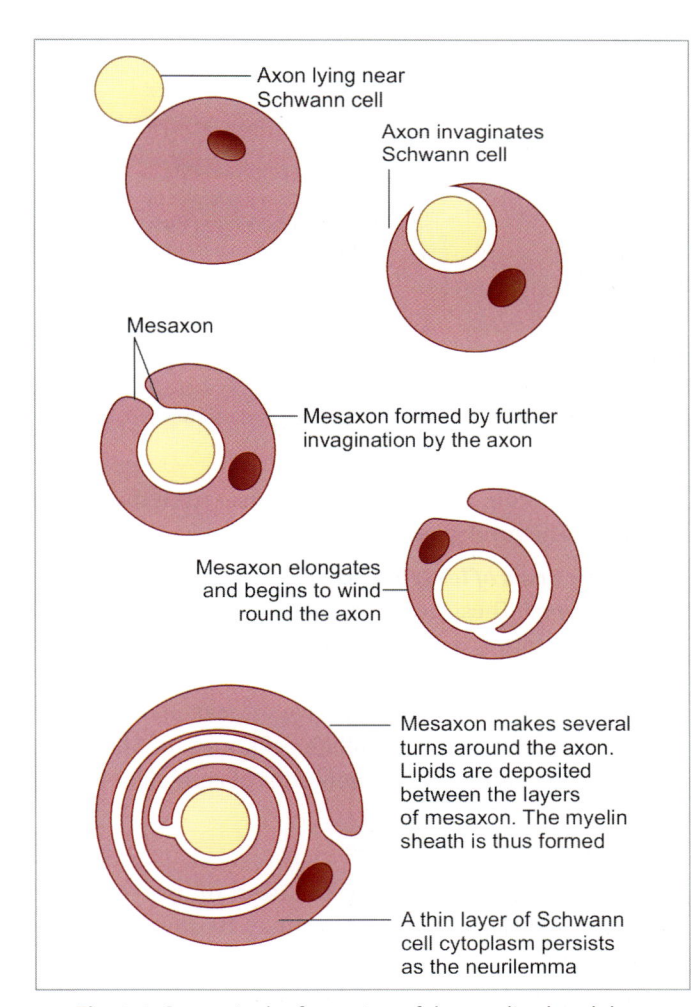

Fig. 9.8: Stages in the formation of the myelin sheath by a Schwann cell (schematic representation).

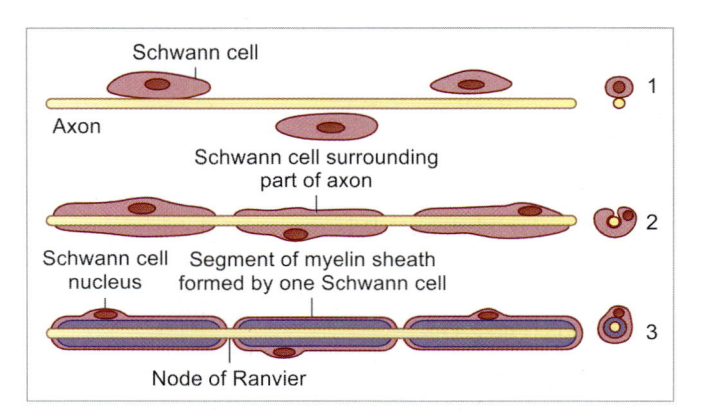

Fig. 9.9: One Schwann cell forms a short segment of the myelin sheath (schematic representation).

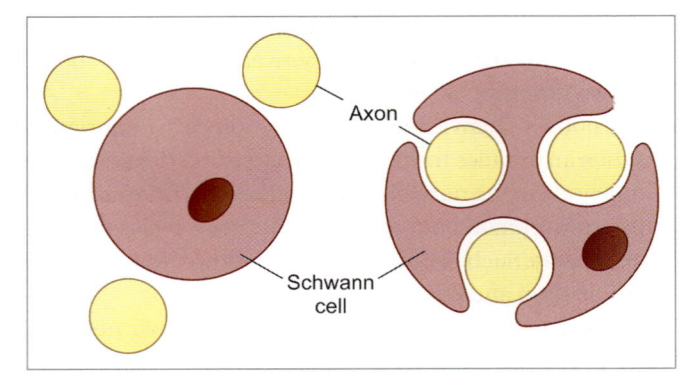

Fig. 9.10: Relationship of unmyelinated axons to Schwann cells (schematic representation).

Table 9.2: Differences between myelinated and unmyelinated nerve fibers.

Myelinated nerves	Unmyelinated nerves
Axons are of large diameter	Axons are of small diameter
Axons surrounded by concentric layers of Schwann cell plasma membrane	Axons surrounded by cytoplasm of Schwann cells
Single axon is surrounded by many Schwann cells	Single or group of axons are invaginated by single Schwann cell
Nerve impulse jumps from one node to other node called as saltatory conduction	Nerve impulse travels uniformly along the axolemma
Conduction is fast and consumes less energy	Conduction is slow and consumes more energy

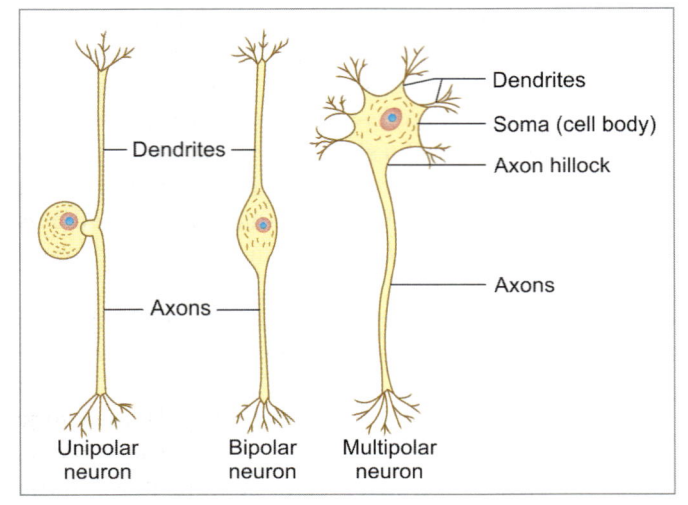

Fig. 9.11: Unipolar, bipolar, and multipolar neurons (schematic representation).

Table 9.3: Morphological classification of neurons.

Morphology	Location and example
According to polarity:	
❏ Unipolar/ pseudounipolar	❏ Sensory neurons of dorasl root ganglia and cranial nerve ganglia
❏ Bipolar	❏ Bipolar cells of retina, and sensory ganglia of vestibulocochlear nerve
❏ Multipolar	❏ Motor neuron and interneuron
According to size of nerve fiber:	
❏ Golgi type I	❏ Purkinje cells of cerebellum, anterior horn cells of spinal cord, and pyramidal cells of cerebral cortex
❏ Golgi type II	❏ Cerebral and cerebellar cortex

TYPES OF NEURONS (TABLE 9.3)

I. **On the basis of number of processes:**
- ❖ **Unipolar/Pseudounipolar:** These neurons have single process. After a very short course, this process divides into two. One of the divisions represents the axon; the other is functionally a dendrite, but its structure is indistinguishable from that of an axon, e.g. neurons in dorsal root ganglion (Fig. 9.11).
- ❖ **Bipolar neurons:** These neurons have only one axon and one dendrite, e.g. neurons in vestibular and spiral ganglia.
- ❖ **Multipolar neurons:** It is the most common type of neurons; the neuron gives off several processes, i.e. these neurons have one axon and many dendrites, e.g. motor neurons (Fig. 9.11).

II. **On the basis of function:**
- ❖ **Sensory neuron:** They carry impulses from receptor organ to the CNS.
- ❖ **Motor neuron:** They transmit impulses from the CNS to the muscles and glands.

III. **On the basis of length of axons:**
- ❖ **Golgi type I:** These neurons have long axons and connect remote regions, e.g. pyramidal cells of motor cortex in cerebrum.
- ❖ **Golgi type II:** These neurons have short axons which end near the cell body, e.g. stellate cells, cells of Martinotti of cerebral cortex and granule cells of cerebellar cortex.

PERIPHERAL NERVES

Peripheral nerves are the bundles of nerve fibers (axons) outside the CNS. These may be myelinated or unmyelinated.
- ❖ Nerve fibers carry impulses from the spinal cord or brain to peripheral structures, such as muscle or gland, are

called **efferent** or **motor** fibers. Efferent fibers are axons of neurons located in the gray matter of the spinal cord or of the brainstem.
- Nerve fibers carry impulses from peripheral organs to the brain or spinal cord are called **afferent** fibers. Afferent nerve fibers are processes of neurons that are located in ganglia.

Microscopic Structure of Peripheral Nerves

- Nerve fibers (myelinated or unmyelinated) are arranged in the form of bundles surrounded by connective tissue coverings.
- Each nerve fiber with its Schwann cell and basal lamina is surrounded by a layer of connective tissue called the **endoneurium** (Fig. 9.12 and Plate 9.1). The endoneurium contains type II collagen fibers, fibroblasts, Schwann cells, endothelial cells, and macrophages.
- Many nerve fibers together form bundles or **fasciculi**. Endoneurium holds adjoining nerve fibers together and facilitates their aggregation to form **fasciculi**. Each fasciculus is surrounded by a thicker layer of connective tissue called the **perineurium**. The perineurium is made up of layers of flattened cells separated by the layers of collagen fibers. Flattened cells are joined at their edges by tight junctions, this controls diffusion of substances in and out of axons (nerve-blood barrier).
- Many fasciculi are held together by a fairly dense layer of connective tissue that surrounds the entire nerve and is called the **epineurium**. It is made up of fibroblast, collagen fibers, and adipose tissue which give cushioning effect to the nerve.
- Nuclei seen in the section of axon is of Schwann cells and fibrocytes. The Schwann cells myelinate and surrounds individual axons, or encloses unmyelinated axons.

Optic Nerve (Plate 9.2)

- It belongs to CNS. It is second cranial nerve—a special sensory nerve.
- It is an outgrowth of brain—hence covered by meninges: dura mater, arachnoid mater, and pia mater which are separated from each other by subdural and subarachnoid spaces.
- It is made up of bundles of myelinated axons of ganglion cells of retina.
- In the center of the intraorbital part of the optic nerve lie the central retinal vessels enclosed in their envelope.
- The myelin sheath of optic nerve is formed by oligodendrocytes as it belongs to CNS.

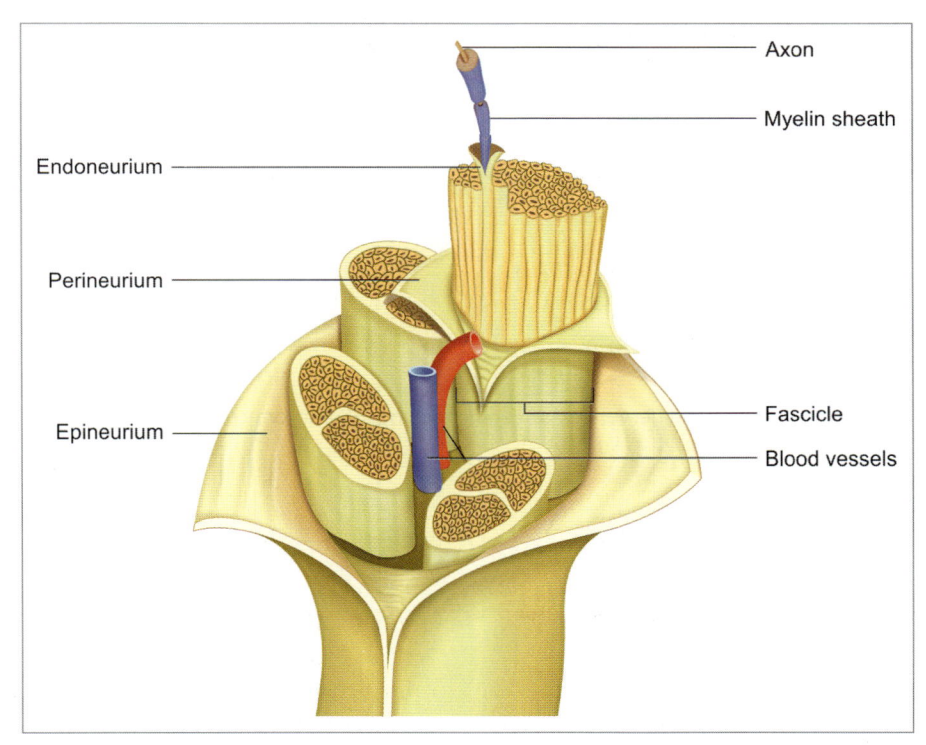

Fig. 9.12: Basic anatomy of peripheral nerves.

Plate 9.1: Peripheral nerve

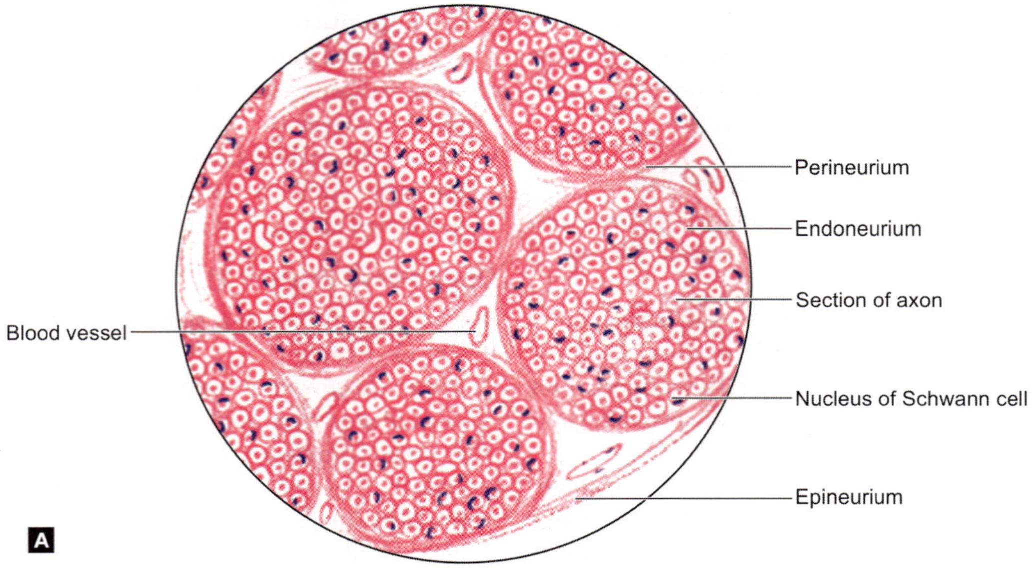

Peripheral nerve: (A) As seen in drawing; (B) Photomicrograph.

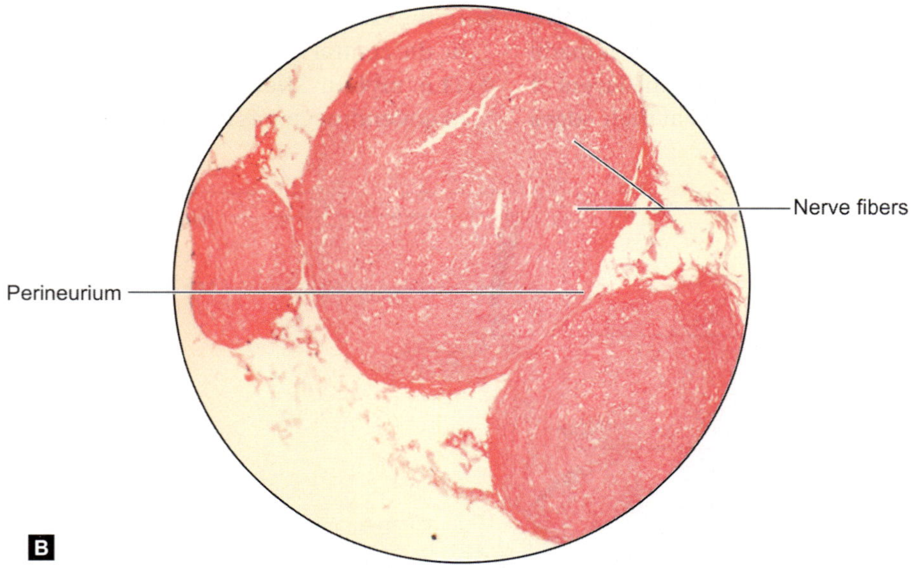

Points of identification
- Each nerve fiber is covered by endoneurium
- Each bundle of nerve fibers is covered by perineurium
- Each nerve is covered by epineurium
- Cut section of axon with myelin sheath and Schwann cell nucleus.

CHAPTER 9: Nervous Tissue 123

Plate 9.2: Optic nerve

Optic nerve: (A) As seen in drawing; (B) Photomicrograph.

Points of identification
- Covered by meninges—dura mater, arachnoid mater, and pia mater
- Central retinal artery and vein are seen
- Pial septa divides the nerve into bundles.

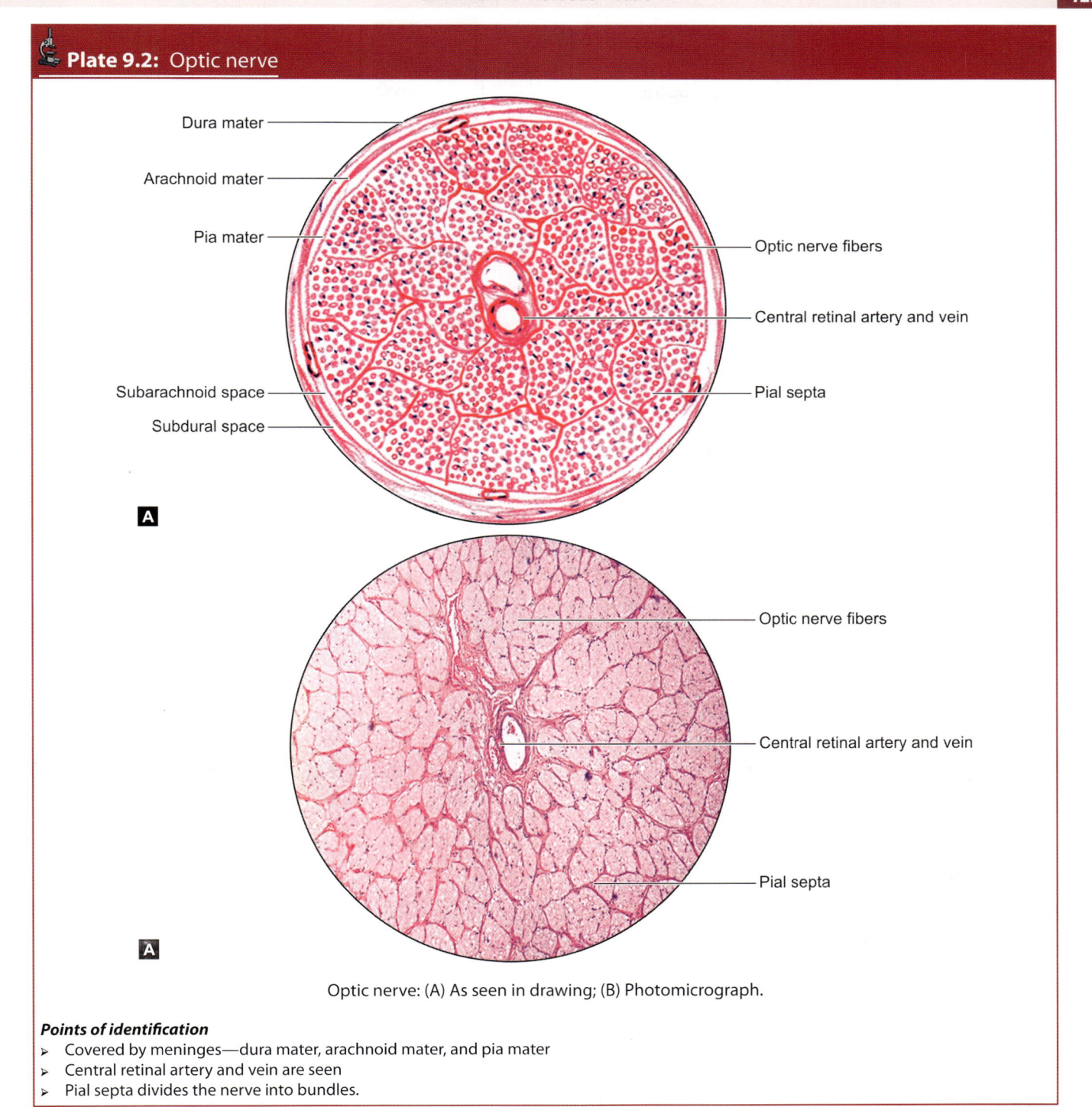

❖ The pia mater, attached directly to the optic nerve sends septa which divides the nerve into bundles/fascicles and guide the blood vessels to the nerve fibers.
❖ At the eyeball, the dura fuses with the sclera while the arachnoid and pia mater merge with the choroid. Connective tissue septa, which arise from the pia mater, separate the fiber bundles in the optic nerve.
❖ Since it is an extension of CNS, any changes in intracranial pressure is reflected in optic disc and nerve.

Added Information

Synapse

Synapses are the sites of junction between the neurons. Synapses can be broadly classified into:
- *Chemical synapses*: Synapses involving the release of neurotransmitters are referred to as **chemical synapses**.
- *Electrical synapses*: At some sites, one cell may excite another without the release of a transmitter. At such sites, adjacent cells have the direct channels of communication through which ions can pass from one cell to another altering their electrical status. Such synapses are called **electrical synapses**.

Classification of a chemical synapse based on neuronal elements taking part

Synapses may be of various types depending upon the parts of the neurons that come in contact.
- **Axodendritic synapse**: It is the most common type of synapse. In this type, an axon terminal establishes contact with the dendrite of a receiving neuron to form a synapse (Fig. 9.13A).
- **Axosomatic synapse**: The axon terminal synapses with the cell body (Fig. 9.13B).
- **Axoaxonal synapse**: The axon terminal synapses with the axon of the receiving neuron. An axoaxonal synapse may be located either on the initial segment (of the receiving axon) or just proximal to an axon terminal (Fig. 9.13C).

Contd...

Contd...

- **Dendroaxonic synapse**: In some parts of the brain (for example, the thalamus), we see some synapses in which the presynaptic element is a dendrite, instead of an axon, which synapses with the axon of the receiving neuron.
- **Dendrodendritic synapse**: Synapse between two dendrites.
- **Somatosomatic synapse**: The soma of a neuron may synapse with the soma of another neuron.
- **Somatodendritic synapse**: Synapse between a soma and a dendrite.

GANGLIA

Aggregations of cell bodies of neurons, placed outside the CNS, are known as ganglia. Ganglia are of two main types: *sensory* and *autonomic*.

Sensory Ganglia (Plate 9.3)

Gross Structure

- ❖ Sensory ganglia are the collection of cell bodies of sensory neurons.
- ❖ Sensory ganglia are associated with the dorsal nerve roots of spinal nerves called dorsal nerve root ganglia and with 5th, 7th, 8th, 9th, and 10th cranial nerves.

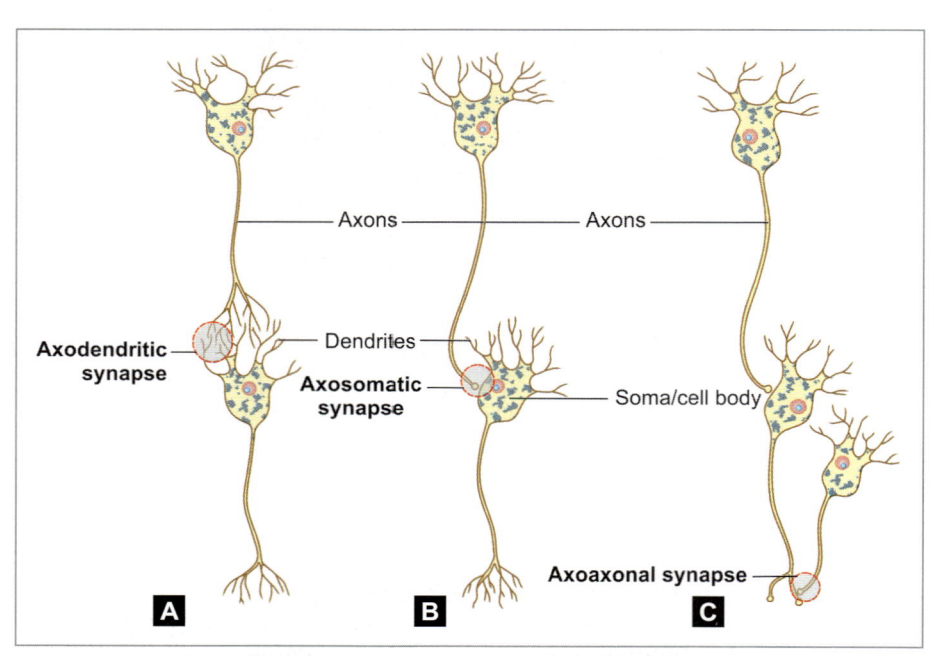

Figs. 9.13A to C: Various types of chemical synapses. (A) Axodendritic synapse; (B) Axosomatic synapse; and (C) Axo-axonal synapse (schematic representation).

CHAPTER 9: Nervous Tissue

Plate 9.3: Sensory ganglia

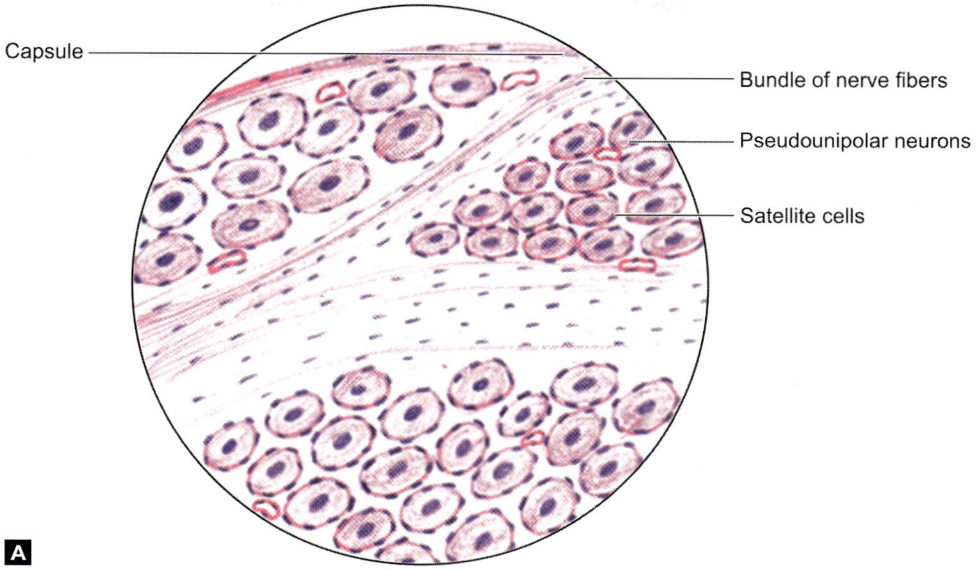

Labels (A, drawing): Capsule; Bundle of nerve fibers; Pseudounipolar neurons; Satellite cells

Labels (B, photomicrograph): Capsule; Pseudounipolar neurons in clusters; Blood vessel; Bundle of nerve fibers

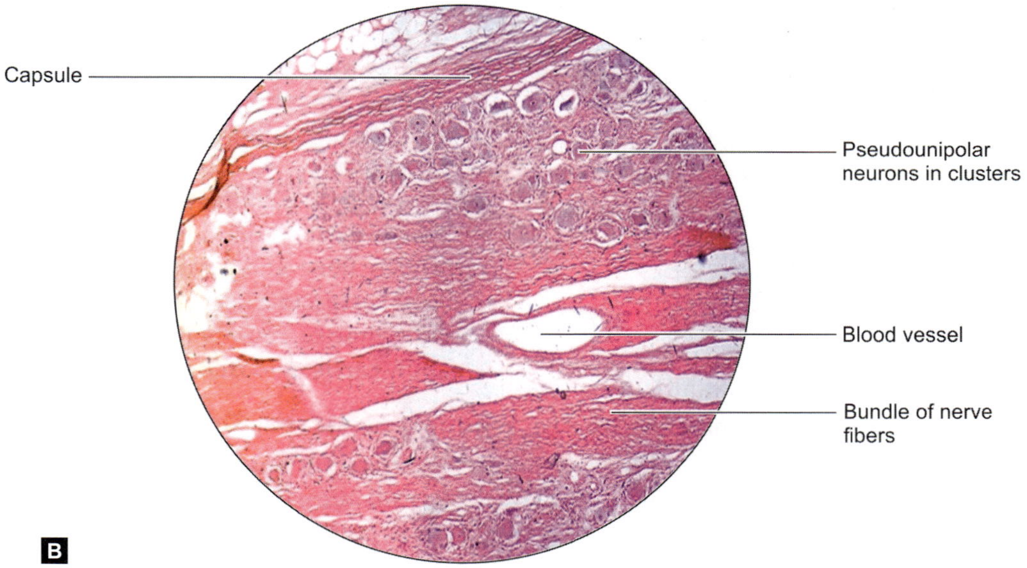

Sensory ganglia: (A) As seen in drawing; (B) Photomicrograph.

Points of identification
- Unipolar neurons with centrally placed nucleus
- Neurons are presented in a group between the group of nerve fibers
- Prominent satellite cells are seen.

❖ Neurons in these ganglia are of the unipolar type (except in the case of ganglia associated with the vestibulocochlear nerve in which they are bipolar).

❖ The peripheral process of each neuron forms an afferent (or sensory) fiber of a peripheral nerve. The central process enters the spinal cord or brainstem.

Histology
❖ The ganglion is covered the outside by a connective tissue capsule, and the entire ganglion is pervaded by fine connective tissue.

❖ The unipolar neurons with centrally placed nucleus are large and arranged in groups chiefly at the periphery of the ganglion (Plate 9.2). The groups of cells are separated by the groups of myelinated nerve fibers.

* The cell body of each neuron is surrounded by a layer of flattened capsular cells or satellite cells. Outside the satellite cells, there is a layer of delicate connective tissue (The satellite cells are continuous with the Schwann cells covering the processes arising from the neuron. The connective tissue covering each neuron is continuous with the endoneurium).

Autonomic Ganglia (Plate 9.4)

Gross Structure

* They are concerned with the nerve supply of smooth muscle or of glands.
* The pathway for this supply consists of two neurons: (1) preganglionic and (2) postganglionic.
* The cell bodies of preganglionic neurons are always located within the spinal cord or brainstem. Their axons leave the spinal cord or brainstem and terminate by synapsing with postganglionic neurons, the cell bodies of which are located in autonomic ganglia.
* Autonomic ganglia are, therefore, aggregations of the cell bodies of postganglionic neurons.
* Autonomic ganglia are subdivisible into two major types: (1) *sympathetic* and (2) *parasympathetic*.
* The neurons of autonomic ganglia are multipolar neurons, and they are smaller than those in sensory ganglia (Plate 9.3).

Histology

* The ganglion is covered outside by a thin capsule and permeated by connective tissue (intramural ganglia have no capsule).
* The multipolar neurons with eccentrically placed nucleus are not arranged in definite groups as in sensory ganglia but are scattered throughout the ganglion. The nerve fibers are nonmyelinated and thinner. They are, therefore, much less conspicuous than in sensory ganglia.
* Satellite cells are present around the neurons of autonomic ganglia, but they are not so well defined.
* The Nissl substance of the neurons is much better defined in autonomic ganglia than in sensory ganglia.

Table 9.4: Difference between sensory and autonomic ganglia.

Sensory ganglia	Autonomic ganglia
Cell bodies are large	Cell bodies are smaller
Unipolar type of neuron except in vestibulocochlear nerve (bipolar)	Multipolar type of neuron
Neurons with centrally placed nucleus	Neurons with eccentrically placed nucleus
Cell bodies of the neurons are arranged in groups	Cell bodies of the neuron does not form definite groups
Myelinated nerve fibers are arranged in bundles	Unmyelinated nerve fibers are scattered
Prominent satellite cells	Satellite cells are less prominent
Well-defined connective tissue capsule	Poorly defined or absent connective tissue capsule

* In sympathetic ganglia the neuronal cytoplasm synthesizes catecholamines; and in parasympathetic ganglia, it synthesizes acetylcholine (Table 9.4).

APPLIED HISTOLOGY

* The regeneration of neurons do not occur in CNS as myelination is by oligodendrocytes. Hence in multiple sclerosis, myelin formed from oligodendrocytes undergoes degeneration, while myelin from Schwann cells is spared.
* The epineurium contains fat that cushions nerve fibers. Loss of this fat in bedridden patients can lead to pressure on nerve fibers and paralysis.
* Blood vessels to a nerve travel through the connective tissue that surrounds it. Severe reduction in blood supply can lead to *ischemic neuritis* and pain.

Tumors of Nervous Tissue

* Precursors of neural cells can give rise to medulloblastomas. Once mature neurons are formed, they lose the power of mitosis and do not give origin to tumors.
* Certain tumors called germinomas appear near the midline, mostly near the third ventricle. They arise from germ cells that also give rise to teratomas.
* Most tumors of the brain arise from neuroglial cells. Astrocytomas are most common. Oligodendromas are also frequent.
* Tumors can also arise from ependyma and from Schwann cells (Figs. 9.14A and B).

CHAPTER 9: Nervous Tissue

Plate 9.4: Autonomic ganglia

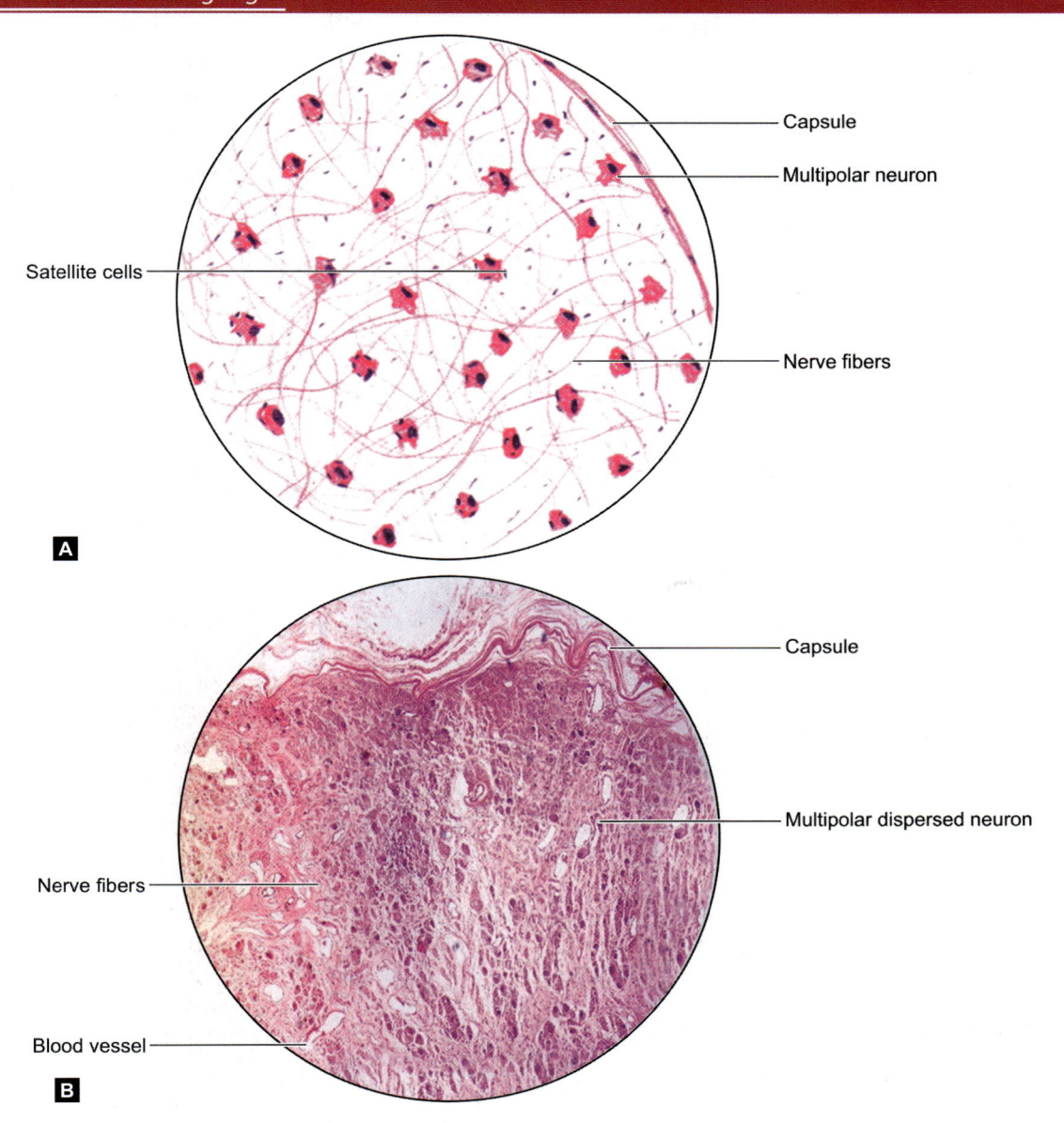

Autonomic ganglia: (A) As seen in drawing; (B) Photomicrograph.

Points of identification
- Multipolar neurons with eccentrically placed nucleus
- Neurons are scattered between the nerve fibers.

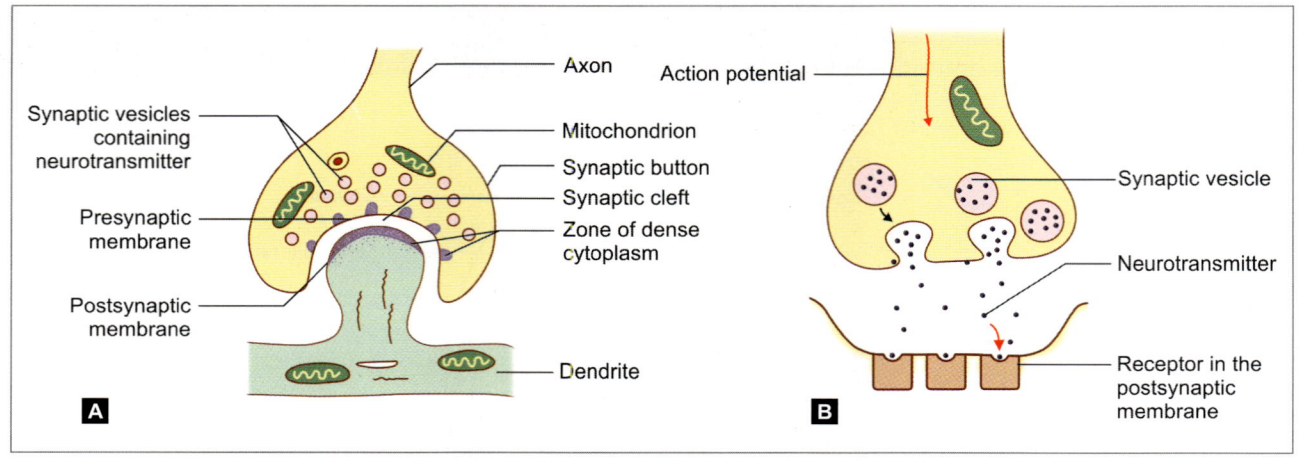

Figs. 9.14A and B: (A) Structure of a typical chemical synapse as seen under electron microscope; (B) Mechanism of synaptic transmission (schematic representation).

MULTIPLE CHOICE QUESTIONS

1. All the following statements are true, *except*:
   a. Spinal ganglia have unipolar neurons
   b. Autonomic ganglia have multipolar neurons
   c. Spinal ganglia have continuous sheath of satellite cells
   d. Autonomic ganglia has centrally placed nucleus
2. All of the following statements regarding myelination are true, *except*:
   a. Schwann cells are responsible for myelination in PNS
   b. Oligodendrocytes are responsible for myelination in CNS
   c. Initial segments are myelinated
   d. Myelination helps in saltatory conduction of impulses
3. The gap between two adjacent myelin segments along an axon is called the:
   a. Axolemma   b. Axonal cleft
   c. Choroid plexus   d. Node of Ranvier
4. Schwann cell membrane wrapped many times around an individual axon is called:
   a. Axolemma   b. Myelin sheath
   c. Perikaryon   d. Node of Ranvier
5. A group of nerve cell bodies located outside the CNS is called a:
   a. Ganglion   b. Nucleus
   c. Node   d. Myelin
6. White matter appears white because of the:
   a. Absence of blood vessels
   b. Absence of glial cells
   c. Presence of many collagen fibers
   d. Presence of many myelinated axons
7. A single Schwann cell forms myelin around one and only one axon, while a single oligodendroglial cell forms myelin around several separate axons.
   a. True   b. False
8. Endoneurium, perineurium, and epineurium are the connective tissues which ensheath axons, axon bundles, and peripheral nerves.
   a. True   b. False
9. Which of the following glial cell types is believed to be functionally related to macrophages?
   a. Astroglia   b. Oligodendroglia
   c. Microglia   d. Schwann cells
10. Which of the following cell types lines the central canal of the spinal cord and the ventricular system of the brain?
    a. Astroglia
    b. Microglia
    c. Schwann cells
    d. Ependymal cells

Answers
1. d   2. c   3. d   4. b   5. a   6. d   7. a   8. a   9. c
10. d

CHAPTER 10

Cardiovascular System

Learning objectives

To study the:
- Components of cardiovascular system
- Structure of blood vessels
- Applied histology

IDENTIFICATION POINTS

Large-sized artery	*Medium-sized artery*	*Large-sized vein*
❑ The tunica intima, media and adventitia can be made out, and are sharply demarcated ❑ Media made up mainly of elastic fibers in the form of fenestrated concentric membranes ❑ The internal elastic lamina is not distinct. ❑ Adventitia is relatively thin with greater proportion of elastic fibers.	❑ The tunica intima, media, and adventitia can be made out and can be sharply demarcated ❑ Intima is well developed and internal elastic lamina is prominent ❑ Media predominantly is made up of smooth muscle fibers arranged concentrically.	❑ The vein has a thinner wall and a larger lumen than the artery ❑ The tunica intima, media, and adventitia can be made out, but are not distinctly demarcated ❑ The media is thin and contains a much larger quantity of collagen fibers than arteries. The amount of elastic tissue is less ❑ The adventitia is relatively thick and contains bundles of longitudinal muscle fibers.

INTRODUCTION

- The cardiovascular system consists of the heart and blood vessels.
- The blood vessels that take blood from the heart to various tissues are called **arteries**. The smallest arteries are called **arterioles**. Arterioles open into a network of **capillaries** that pervade the tissues. Exchanges of various substances between the blood and the tissues take place through the walls of capillaries. At some places, capillaries are replaced by slightly different vessels called **sinusoids**.
- Blood from capillaries (or from sinusoids) is collected by small **venules** that join to form **veins**.
- The veins return blood to the heart.
- Blood vessels deliver nutrients, oxygen, and hormones to the cells of the body and remove metabolic base products and carbon dioxide from them.

BASIC STRUCTURE OF A BLOOD VESSEL

Wall of arteries/veins is made of three layers. From within outward, they are as follows:

1. **Tunica intima**: It is the innermost layer, made of three components:
   i. *Endothelium*—simple squamous epithelium lining the intima
   ii. *Basal lamina*—basement membrane of the lining cells
   iii. *Subendothelial connective tissue*—loose connective tissue beneath the endothelium.
   Tunica intima is limited by a fenestrated layer of elastic tissue called *internal elastic lamina*.
2. **Tunica media**: This layer consists of concentrically arranged smooth muscle cells, elastic fibers, and reticular fibers. Their concentration depends on the nature of the vessel, i.e. artery/vein. It is separated from tunica adventitia by fenestrated layer of elastic tissue *external elastic lamina*.
3. **Tunica adventitia**: It is the outer most layer of a vessel wall. It consists of longitudinally arranged collagen and reticular fibers, which gradually merges with the connective tissue of the surrounding structures. Thus it mainly anchors the blood vessel to the neighboring

structures. In large vessels, this layer contains network of blood vessels providing nutrition to them called *vasa vasorum* and network of autonomic nerves controlling their lumen diameter, *nervi vasorum*.

Endothelium

- They are monolayer of flattened polygonal cells, resting on basement membrane.
- It lines the inner surface of the heart and blood vessels.
- Many endothelial cells show invaginations of the cell membrane (on both internal and external surfaces). Sometimes the inner and outer invaginations meet to form channels passing right across the cell (seen typically in small arterioles). These features are seen in situations where vessels are highly permeable.
- Adjoining endothelial cells are linked by tight junctions, and also by gap junctions.
- Externally, they are supported by a basal lamina.

Functions of Endothelium

Apart from providing a smooth internal lining to heart and blood vessels, endothelial cells perform a number of other functions as follows:

- Maintenance of selective permeability barrier between the blood and intestinal fluid. Hence, they allow simple diffusion of O_2, CO_2; active transport of glucose, amino acids, electrolytes, and receptor-mediated endocytosis of low-density lipoprotein (LDL), cholesterol.
- Luminal surface is coated with glycocalyx; it also secretes anticoagulants, and antithrombogenic agents, such as heparin, tissue plasminogen activator (TPA), etc. form nonthrombogenic barrier.
- Modulates blood flow and vascular resistance by secreting vasoconstrictors [endothelin, angiotensin-converting enzyme (ACE)] and vasodilators [nitric oxide (NO), prostacyclins].
- Secretes and stores Von Willebrand factor (vWF) as rod-like inclusions like *Weibel–Palade bodies*. vWF plays an important role in platelet adhesion during vessel wall injury.
- Regulates immune response.
- Synthesizes growth factors.
- Maintains extracellular matrix (ECM).
- Antibodies to vWF serve as marker for tumors arising from endothelium.

Subendothelial Connective Tissue

- It is thin but variable.
- It is also termed as lamina propria. In smallest vessels, they are replaced by pericytes.
- It contains fibrocollagenous ECM, few fibroblasts, and occasionally smooth muscle cells.
- Von Willebrand factor concentrates in this layer and participates in clotting whenever endothelium is injured.

Smooth Muscle Cells

- They are spindle-shaped cells with elongated nuclei.
- Contraction of smooth muscle will cause reduction of vessel's lumen and hence raises the pressure on the proximal side.
- They synthesize and secrete elastin, collagen, and other components of ECM.
- Alters rigidity of vessel wall without causing constriction and thus affects distensibility of wall and propagates pulse.
- Mesenchymal cells are multifunctional in arteries, migrates and proliferates to replace damaged endothelium.
- They undergo fatty degeneration and form atheromatous plaques.

STRUCTURE OF ARTERIES

Elastic Artery/Large-sized Artery

- They are large conducting vessels.
- The innermost layer is called the **tunica intima** (tunica = coat). It consists of:
  - An endothelial lining.
  - A thin layer of glycoprotein which lines the external aspect of the endothelium and is called the **basal lamina**.
  - A delicate layer of subendothelial connective tissue—consisting contractile smooth muscle cells which is responsible for forming ECM, collagen and elastic fibers of this layer.
  - Tunica intima is limited by a layer of elastic tissue **internal elastic lamina**, which is less prominent due to underlying tunica media.
- Outside the tunica intima lies the thickest middle layer **tunica media**.
- The tunica media consists predominantly of elastic tissue and few smooth muscle fibers. The elastic fibers form fenestrated concentric lamellae alternating with smooth muscle cells. The number of lamellae of elastic fibers is directly proportional with the diameter of the artery and age of the individual.
- Some collagen fibers are also present in this layer, but fibroblasts are absent.
- In hypertension, the size and number of elastic lamellae increases due to increased blood pressure (BP).

CHAPTER 10: Cardiovascular System

- Tunica media is limited by a membrane formed by elastic fibers—***external elastic lamina***.
- The outermost layer is called the ***tunica adventitia***. This coat consists of connective tissue in which collagen fibers are prominent. This layer prevents undue stretching or distension of the artery (Plate 10.1).
- *Examples*—aorta, carotid artery, subclavian artery, axillary artery, and iliac artery.

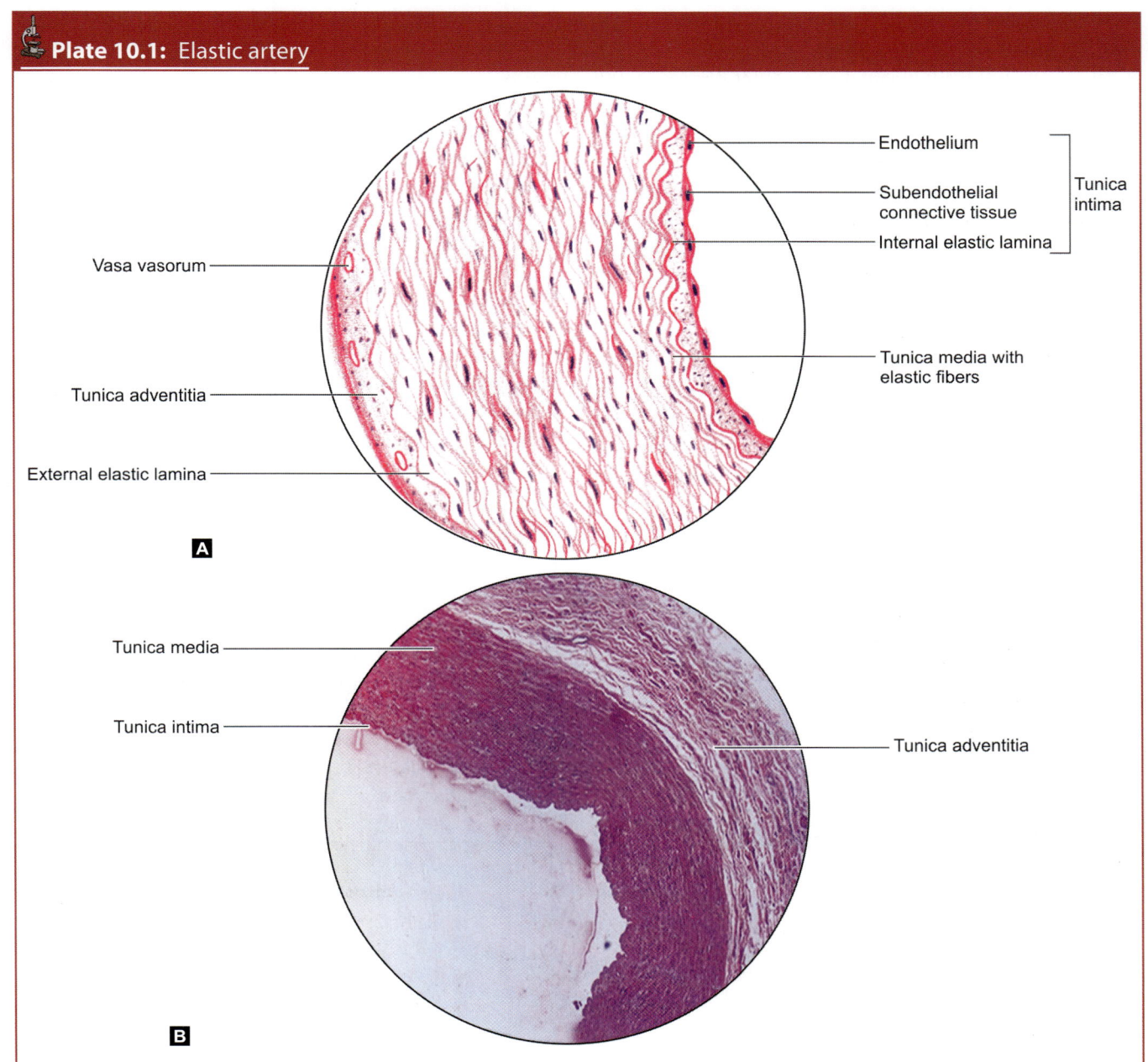

Plate 10.1: Elastic artery

Elastic artery: (A) As seen in drawing; (B) Photomicrograph.

Points of identification
Elastic artery is characterized by presence of:
- Tunica intima consisting of endothelium, subendothelial connective tissue, and internal elastic lamina
- The first layer of elastic fibers is called the internal elastic lamina. The internal elastic lamina is not distinct from the elastic fibers of media
- Well developed subendothelial layer in tunica intima
- Thick tunica media with many elastic fibers and some smooth muscle fibers
- Tunica adventitia containing collagen fibers with several elastic fibers
- Vasa vasorum in the tunica adventitia (Not seen in this slide).

Muscular Arteries/Medium-sized Arteries

- As the arterial tree divides and redivides, the size of the artery decreases. After the elastic artery, the next member in the hierarchy is muscular artery.
- The muscular arteries have more smooth muscle fibers in the media than elastic fibers.
- The transition from elastic to muscular arteries is not abrupt. There is a gradual reduction in elastic fibers and increase in smooth muscle content in the media from elastic artery to muscular artery.
- Muscular arteries can alter the size of the lumen because of the contraction or relaxation of smooth muscle in its wall; therefore, they regulate the amount of blood flowing into the regions supplied by them; hence, they are also called as *distributing arteries*.
- *Tunica intima:* The structure of tunica intima is like elastic artery with endothelium, lining the lumen (Table 10.1). Endothelial cells resting on basement membrane with underlying connective tissue. The internal elastic lamina in the muscular arteries is more prominent due to underlying smooth muscle fibers in the muscular media.
- *Tunica media:* It is made up mainly of smooth muscles and some elastic fibers in between. Longitudinally arranged muscle is present in the media of arteries that undergo repeated stretching or bending. Examples of such arteries are the coronary, carotid, axillary, and palmar arteries.
- *Tunica adventitia:* It mainly consists of collagen fibers, fibroblasts, and elastic fibers. In addition, they will have vasa vasorum and nervosa. The adventitia of muscular artery is relatively thicker than that of elastic artery (Plate 10.2).

ARTERIOLES

- When traced distally, muscular arteries progressively decrease in caliber till they have a diameter of about 100 µm.
- They become continuous with arterioles (Fig. 10.1). The larger or *muscular arterioles* are 100–50µm in diameter.
- Arterioles less than 50 µm in diameter are called *terminal arterioles*.
- All the three layers, i.e. (1) tunica adventitia, (2) tunica media, and (3) tunica intima are thin as compared to arteries.
- In arterioles, the adventitia is made up of a thin network of collagen fibers.
- Arterioles are the main regulators of peripheral vascular resistance.
- Contraction and relaxation of the smooth muscles present in the walls of the arterioles can alter the peripheral vascular resistance (or BP) and the blood flow.

Muscular arterioles can be distinguished from true arteries:
- By their small diameter.
- They do not have an internal elastic lamina. They have a few layers of smooth muscle in their media.

Terminal arterioles can be distinguished from muscular arterioles as follows:
- They have a diameter less than 50 µm, the smallest terminal arterioles having a diameter as small as 12 µm.
- They have only a thin layer of muscle in their walls.
- They give off lateral branches (called meta-arterioles) to the capillary bed.

Table 10.1: Differences between elastic artery and muscular artery.

Layers	Elastic artery	Muscular artery
Adventitia	It is relatively thin with greater proportion of elastic fibers	It consists of thin layer of fibroelastic tissue
Media	It is made up mainly of elastic tissue in the form of fenestrated concentric membranes. There may be as many as 50 layers of elastic membranes	It is made up mainly of smooth muscles arranged in circular manner
Intima	It is made up of endothelium, subendothelial connective tissue, and internal elastic lamina the subendothelial connective tissue contains more elastic fibers. The internal elastic lamina is not distinct.	Intima is well developed, especially internal elastic lamina which stands out prominently

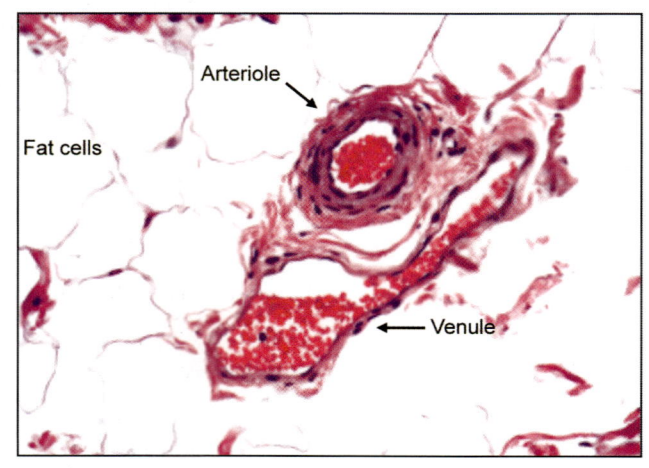

Fig. 10.1: Photomicrograph showing an arteriole and a venule.

CHAPTER 10: Cardiovascular System

Plate 10.2: Muscular (medium size) artery

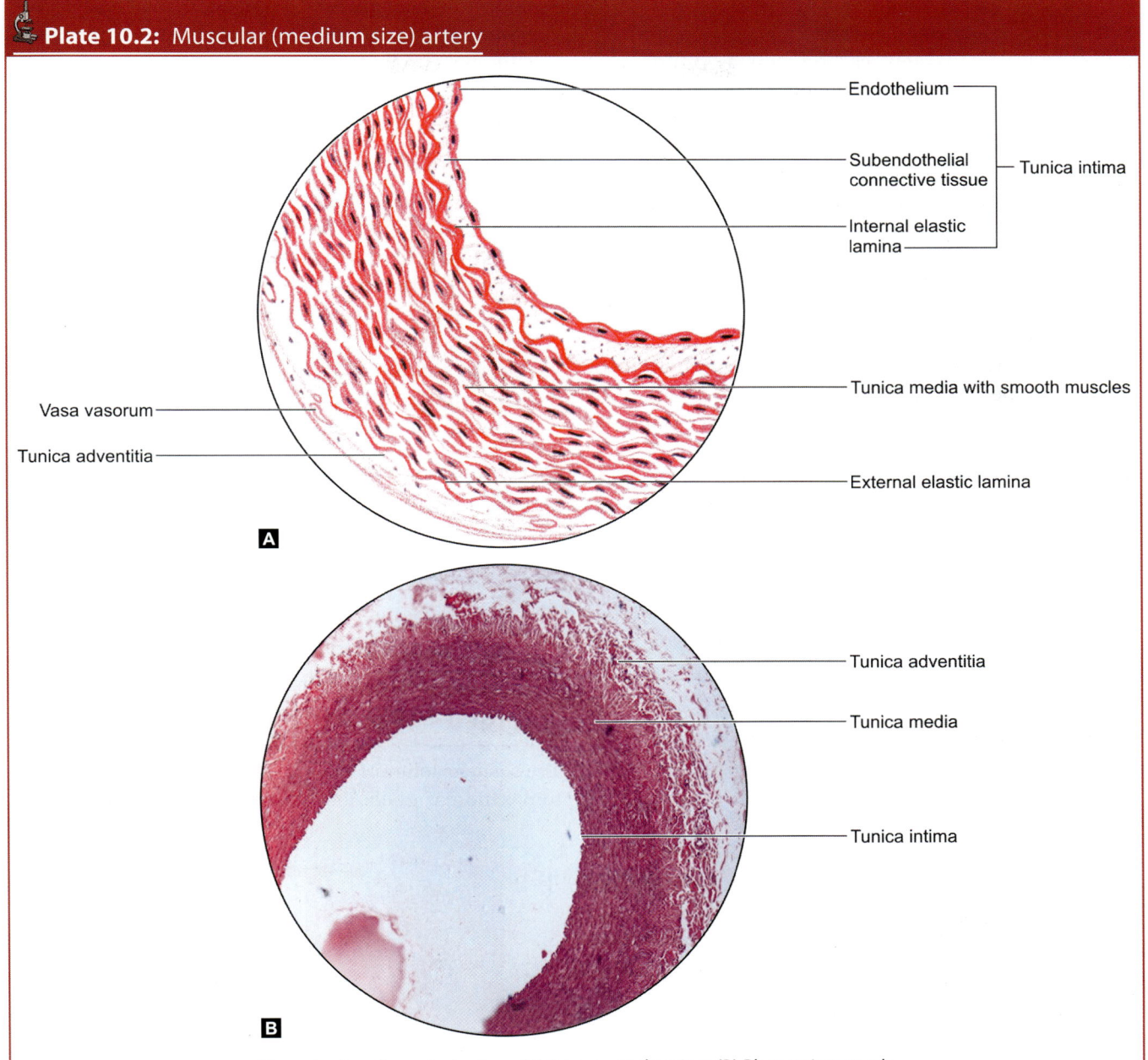

Muscular (medium size) artery: (A) As seen in drawing; (B) Photomicrograph.

Points of identification
- In muscular arteries, the tunica intima is made up of endothelium and internal elastic lamina, which is thrown into wavy folds due to contraction of smooth muscle in the media
- Tunica media is composed mainly of smooth muscle fibers arranged circularly
- Tunica adventitia contains collagen fibers and few elastic fibers.

The initial segment of each lateral branch is surrounded by a few smooth muscle cells. These muscle cells constitute the ***precapillary sphincter***. This sphincter regulates the flow of blood to the capillaries.

CAPILLARIES

- Terminal arterioles are continued into a capillary plexus that pervades the tissue supplied.

- Capillaries are the smallest blood vessels.
- The average diameter of a capillary is 8 μm.
- Exchanges (of oxygen, carbon dioxide, fluids, and various molecules) between blood and tissue take place through the walls of the capillary plexus (and through postcapillary venules).
- The arrangement of the capillary plexus and its density varies from tissue to tissue, the density being greatest in tissues having high metabolic activity.

Structure of Capillaries

- The wall of a capillary is lined by endothelial cells resting on the basal lamina.
- Overlying the basal lamina there is a delicate network of reticular fibers and cells.
- In some capillaries, specialized branching cells may be present called as *pericytes*.
- Pericyte or adventitial cells contain contractile filaments in the cytoplasm. They mainly provide support to the capillary wall and control the lumen size.

Types of Capillaries (Figs. 10.2 to 10.4)

There are three types of capillaries:
1. Continuous
2. Discontinuous
3. Fenestrated.

Continuous Capillaries

- In this type, the ends of endothelial cells fuse and form continuous capillary wall.
- In continuous capillaries, exchange of material between blood and tissue take place through the cytoplasm of endothelial cells
- Continuous capillaries are seen in the skin, connective tissue, muscle, lungs, and brain.

Fenestrated Capillaries (Figs. 10.3A and B)

- In this type, the capillary wall has fenestrations.
- The "fenestrations" are closed by a thin diaphragm (which may represent greatly thinned out cytoplasm of an endothelial cell, or only the basal lamina).
- Some fenestrations represent areas where endothelial cell cytoplasm has pores passing through the entire thickness of the cell.
- Fenestrated capillaries are seen in renal glomeruli, intestinal villi, endocrine glands, and pancreas.

Discontinuous Capillaries

- They are organ specific, also called as sinusoidal capillaries (Figs. 10.4A and B).
- They are found in spleen, liver, and bone marrow.
- They show gaps between the neighboring endothelial cells.
- They are more irregular and of larger diameter.
- They are associated with specialized cells of the tissue.

VEINS

The basic structure of veins is similar to that of arteries. The tunica intima, media, and adventitia can be distinguished,

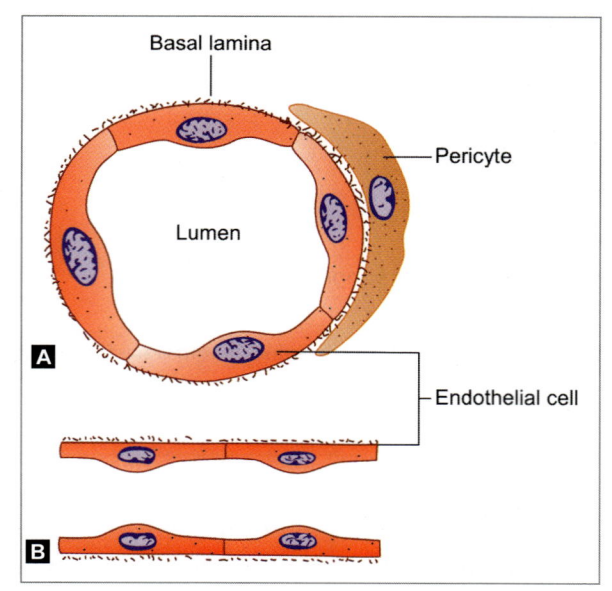

Figs. 10.2A and B: Structure of continuous capillary. (A) Circular section; (B) Longitudinal section (schematic representation).

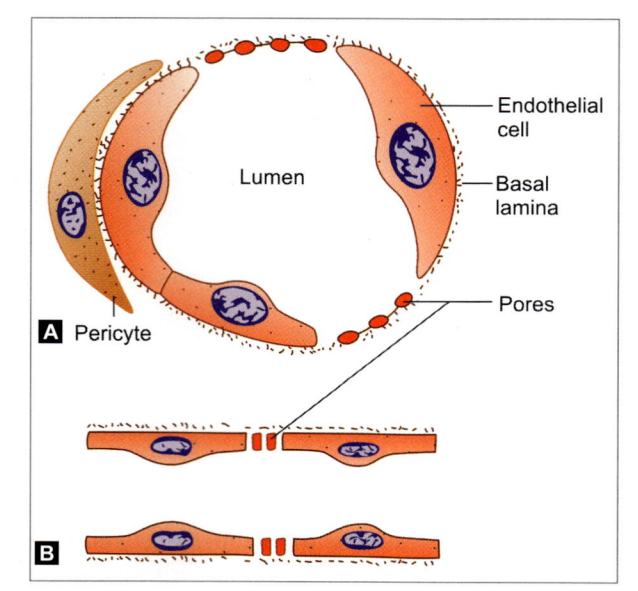

Figs. 10.3A and B: Structure of fenestrated capillary. (A) Circular section; (B) Longitudinal section (schematic representation).

CHAPTER 10: Cardiovascular System

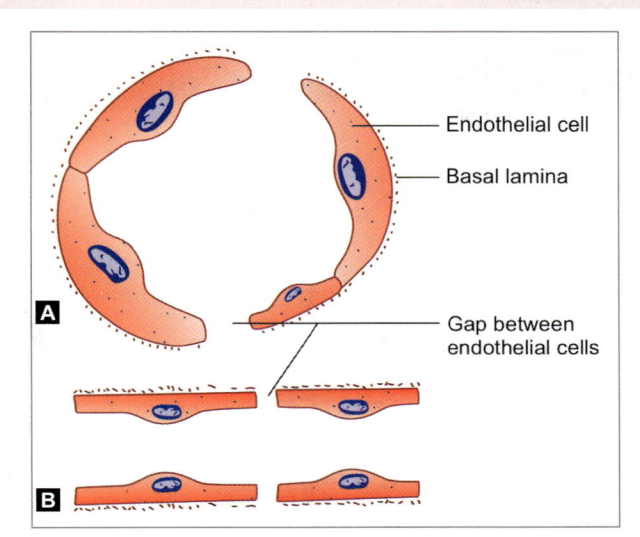

Figs. 10.4A and B: Structure of sinusoid. (A) Circular section; (B) Longitudinal section (schematic representation).

especially in large veins. The structure of veins differs from that of arteries in the following aspects:
- The wall of a vein is thinner than that of an artery having the same-sized lumen.
- The tunica media contains more collagen fibers than that of arteries. The amount of elastic fibers or of smooth muscle is much less.
- Because of the above mentioned differences, the wall of a vein is easily compressed. After death, veins are usually collapsed. In contrast, arteries retain their patency.
- In arteries the tunica media is usually thicker than the adventitia. In contrast the adventitia of veins is thicker than the media (especially in large veins). In some large veins (e.g. the inferior vena cava), the adventitia contains a considerable amount of elastic and muscle fibers that run in a predominantly longitudinal direction. These fibers facilitate elongation and shortening of the vena cava with respiration. This is also facilitated by collagen fibers in the adventitia which form a meshwork that spirals around the vessel.
- A clear distinction between the tunica intima, media, and adventitia cannot be made out in small veins as all these layers consist predominantly of fibrous tissue.
- Muscle is conspicuous by its complete absence in venous spaces of erectile tissue, in veins of cancellous bone, dural venous sinuses, retinal veins, and placental veins (Plate 10.3).

Valves of Veins
- Most veins contain valves that allow the flow of blood toward the heart, but prevent its regurgitation in the opposite direction.
- Typically, each valve is made up of two semilunar cusps. Each cusp is a fold of endothelium within which there is some connective tissue that is rich in elastic fibers.
- Valves are absent in very small veins, venae cavae, veins within the cranial cavity, and vertebral canal.
- Flow of blood through veins is assisted by the contractions of muscle in their walls. It is also assisted by the contraction of surrounding muscles, especially when the latter are enclosed in deep fascia.

VENULES

- The smallest veins, into which capillaries drain, are called *venules* (Fig. 10.1).
- They are 20–30 μm in diameter. Their walls consist of endothelium, basal lamina, and a thin adventitia consisting of longitudinally running collagen fibers.
- Flattened or branching cells called **pericytes** may be present outside the basal laminae of small venules (called **postcapillary venules**), while some muscle may be present in larger vessels (***muscular venules***).
- The walls of venules (especially those of postcapillary venules) have considerable permeability, and exchanges between blood and surrounding tissues can take place through them.
- In particular, venules are the sites at which lymphocytes and other cells may pass out of (or into) the bloodstream.

NUTRITION AND INNERVATION OF BLOOD VESSELS

- The walls of small blood vessels receive adequate nutrition by diffusion from blood in their lumina.
- The walls of large- and medium-sized vessels are supplied by small arteries called ***vasa vasorum*** (literally "vessels of vessels"; singular = ***vas vasis***).
- Vasa vasorum supply the adventitia and the outer part of the media (since diffusion becomes difficult from lumen if wall thickness > 1mm). These layers of the vessel wall also contain many lymphatic vessels.
- Blood vessels have a fairly rich supply by autonomic nerves (sympathetic).
- The nerves (Nervi vasorum) are unmyelinated. Most of the nerves are vasomotor and supply smooth muscle. Their stimulation causes vasoconstriction in some arteries, and vasodilatation in others. Some myelinated sensory nerves are also present in the adventitia.
- Coronary arteries are the largest vaso vasorum in the body.

Plate 10.3: Large-sized vein

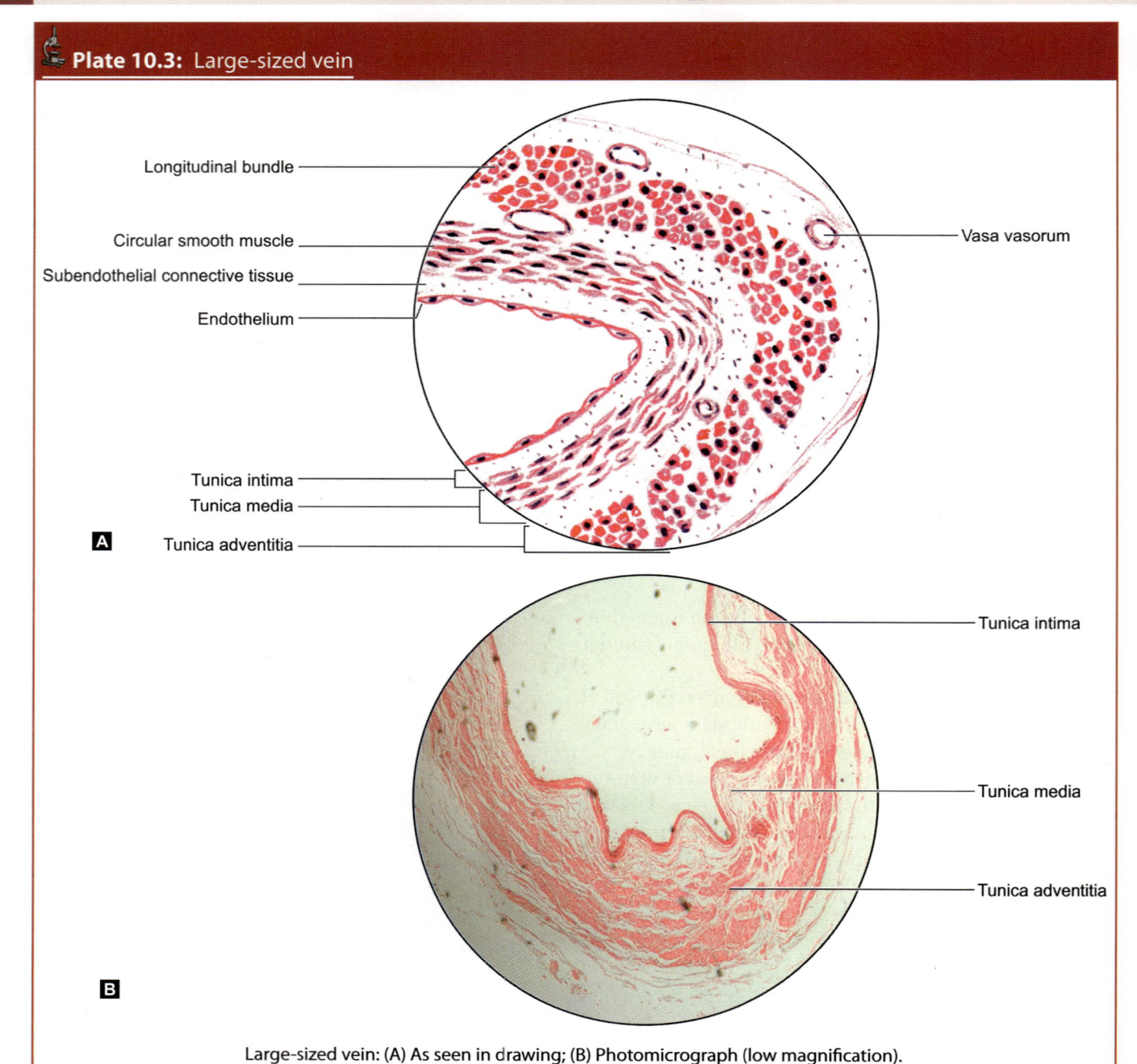

Large-sized vein: (A) As seen in drawing; (B) Photomicrograph (low magnification).

Points of identification
- The vein has a thinner wall and a larger lumen than the artery
- The tunica intima, media, and adventitia can be made out, but they are not sharply demarcated
- The media is thin and contains a much larger quantity of collagen fibers than arteries. The amount of elastic tissue or of muscle is much less
- The adventitia is relatively thick and contains considerable amount of elastic and muscle fibers.

Note: The luminal surface appears as a dark line, with an occasional nucleus along it.

Arteriovenous Anastomoses

- In many parts of the body, small arteries and veins are connected by direct channels that constitute arteriovenous anastomoses. These channels may be straight or coiled.
- Their walls have a thick muscular coat that is richly supplied with sympathetic nerves.
- When the anastomoses are patent, blood is short circuited from the artery to the vein so that very little blood passes through the capillary bed.
- However, when the muscle in the wall of the anastomosing channel contracts, its lumen is occluded so that all blood now passes through the capillaries.
- Arteriovenous anastomoses are found in the skin of the nose, lips, fingertips, and external ear, mucous membrane of the alimentary canal, nose, and the erectile tissue of penis and clitoris.
- They are also seen in the tongue, thyroid, and sympathetic ganglia.
- In some regions, we see arteriovenous anastomoses of a special kind. The vessels taking part in these anastomoses are in the form of a rounded bunch covered by connective tissue. This structure is called a *glomus* (Fig. 10.5). Each glomus consists of an afferent artery, one or more coiled (S-shaped) connecting vessels, and an efferent vein.

Function

Arteriovenous anastomoses in the skin help in regulating body temperature, by increasing blood flow through capillaries in warm weather and decreasing it in cold weather to prevent heat loss.

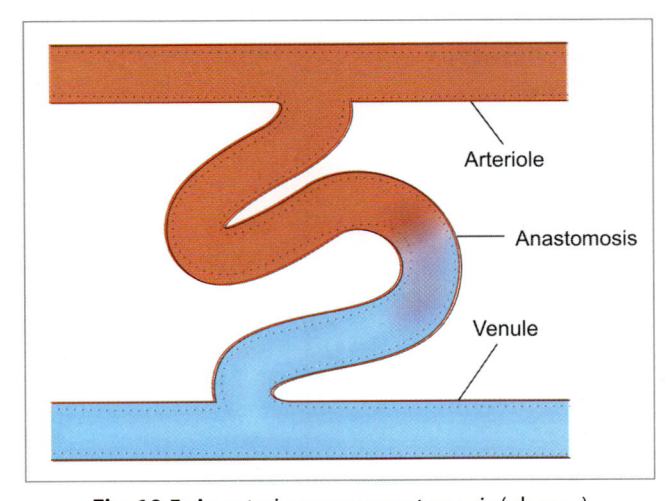

Fig. 10.5: An arteriovenous anastomosis (glomus) (schematic representation).

HEART

The heart is a muscular organ that pumps blood throughout the blood vessels to various parts of the body by repeated rhythmic contractions.

Structure

There are three layers in the wall of the heart:
1. The innermost layer is called the **endocardium**. It corresponds to the tunica intima of blood vessels. It consists of a layer of endothelium that rests on a thin layer of delicate connective tissue. Outside this, there is a thicker **subendocardial layer** of connective tissue.
2. The main thickness of the wall of the heart is formed by a thick layer of cardiac muscle called **myocardium**.
3. The external surface of the myocardium is covered by the **epicardium** (or **visceral layer of serous pericardium**). It consists of a layer of connective tissue that is covered, on the free surface, by a layer of flattened mesothelial cells.

FURTHER READING

Arteriovenous Anastomoses

They are few and inefficient in the newborn. In old age, again, arteriovenous anastomoses of the skin decrease considerably in number. It is because of this reason, temperature regulation is not efficient in the newborn as well as in old persons.

Precapillary Sphincters and Thoroughfare Channels

Arteriovenous anastomoses control blood flow through relatively large segments of the capillary bed. Much smaller segments can be individually controlled as follows:

- Capillaries arise as side branches of terminal arterioles. The initial segment of each such branch is surrounded by a few smooth muscle cells that constitute a *precapillary sphincter* (Fig. 10.6). Blood flow, through any part of the capillary bed, can be controlled by the precapillary sphincter.
- In many situations, arterioles and venules are connected (apart from capillaries) by some channels that resemble capillaries but have a larger caliber. These channels run a relatively direct course between the arteriole and venule. Isolated smooth muscle fibers may be present on their walls. These are called *thoroughfare channels* (Fig. 10.6).
- At times when most of the precapillary sphincters in the region are contracted (restricting flow through

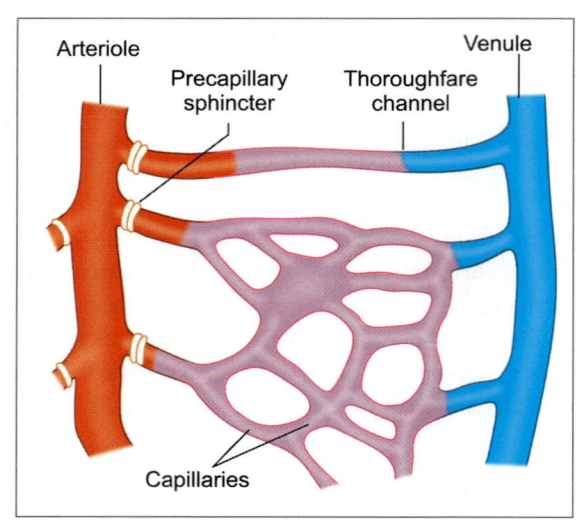

Fig. 10.6: Precapillary sphincters and thoroughfare channels (schematic representation).

capillaries), blood is short circuited from arteriole to venule through the thoroughfare channels. A thoroughfare channel and the capillaries associated with it are sometimes referred to as a *microcirculatory unit*.

APPLIED HISTOLOGY

1. **Atherosclerotic lesions** develop primarily in the tunica intima of large elastic arteries following endothelial injury, which leads to endothelial dysfunction and the formation of **atheromatous plaques**, which is the main risk factor for myocardial infarction, stroke, etc.
2. **Chronic hypertension** (BP >140/90 mm Hg) causes pressure overload on the cardiac muscle, leading to left ventricular hypertrophy. In small muscular arteries and arterioles, lumen size is reduced because of both contraction and hyperplasia of smooth muscles in the tunica media, thereby increasing the vascular resistance.
3. **Varicose veins** are permanently dilated and tortuous superficial veins of the lower extremities, especially the long saphenous vein and its tributaries. About 10–12% of the general population develops varicose veins of lower legs, with the peak incidence in fourth and fifth decades of life. Adult females are affected more commonly than the males, especially during pregnancy. This is attributed to venous stasis in the lower legs because of compression on the iliac veins by pregnant uterus.
4. **Angioma** benign tumors derived from the cells of vessel wall (blood/lymphatic vessel). *Hemangioma* benign tumor of small blood vessels. *Types*—capillary and cavernous hemangioma.
5. A **glomus tumor** is a rare neoplasm arising from the **glomus** body and mainly found under the nail, on the fingertip or in the foot.

MULTIPLE CHOICE QUESTIONS

1. Following are the layers of blood vessels, *except*:
   a. Tunica adventitia
   b. Tunica media
   c. Tunica albuginea
   d. Tunica intima
2. Pericytes are seen in:
   a. Elastic artery
   b. Muscular artery
   c. Large-sized vein
   d. Postcapillary venules
3. Vessels responsible for peripheral resistance are:
   a. Elastic artery
   b. Arterioles
   c. Large-sized vein
   d. Venules
4. Deep vein thrombosis mainly involves:
   a. Elastic artery
   b. Medium-sized vein
   c. Large-sized vein
   d. Postcapillary venules

Answers
   1. c   2. d   3. b   4. c

CHAPTER 11

Skin and its Appendages

Learning objectives

To study the:
- Functions of skin
- Types of skin with location
- Layers of skin
- Glands related to skin
- Appendages of skin
- Blood and nerve supply of skin
- Applied histology

IDENTIFICATION POINTS

Thin (hairy) skin
- Skin is made up of epidermis and dermis
- Epidermis has five layers: stratum basale, granulosum (single layer), spinosum (thin), lucidum (thin or absent) and corneum (thin)
- Epidermis is stratified squamous keratinized epithelium
- Hair follicles, arrector pili, sebaceous and sweat glands are present in the dermis.

Thick (non-hairy) skin
- Skin is made up of epidermis and dermis
- Epidermis has five layers: stratum basale, granulosum (4 to 5 layers), spinosum (prominent), lucidum (thick) and corneum (very thick)
- Dermis is thinner and does not contain hairs, sebaceous glands, or apocrine sweat glands.

INTRODUCTION

The skin forms the external covering of the body. It is the largest organ constituting 15–20% of total body mass.

FUNCTIONS

- It provides covering for the underlying soft tissues: Protection against injury, bacterial invasion, and desiccation.
- Absorption of ultraviolet rays from sun and the synthesis of vitamin D: Melanin—a dark-colored light-sensitive pigment that is found in the skin.
- Thermoregulation.
- Excretion through sweat glands.
- Largest sensory organ: Pressure/touch, heat/cold, and pain through somatic sensory receptors.
- Immunity, i.e. the role of the skin within the immune system by Langerhans cells of epidermis, phagocytic cells, and epidermal dendritic cells.
- Palm and sole have ridges and sulci and the pattern assumed by these ridges and sulci are known as dermatoglyphics. They are unique for each individual, and it is used for personal identification.

TYPES OF SKIN

There are two types of skin (Table 11.1):
1. **Thin or hairy skin:** In this type of skin, epidermis is very thin. It contains hair and is found in all other parts of body except palms and soles (Plate 11.1).
2. **Thick or glabrous skin:** In this type of skin, it has no hair and epidermis is very thick with a thick layer of stratum corneum. It is found in palms of hands and soles of feet (Plate 11.2).

Table 11.1: Difference between thick and thin skin.

Thin skin	Thick skin
Location: Entire body except palm and sole	*Location*: Where there is a lot of abrasion—fingertips, palm, and the sole
Epidermis is thin with only four layers (stratum lucidum layer is absent)	Epidermis is thick with all five layers
Dermis is thicker, which makes thin skin easier to suture, if it gets damaged. Contains hair follicle, sebaceous, and apocrine sweat glands	Dermis is thinner and does not contain hairs, sebaceous glands, or apocrine sweat glands
Sweat glands are more	Sweat glands are less
Arrector pili muscle is present	Arrector pili muscle is absent

Plate 11.1: Thin skin or hairy skin

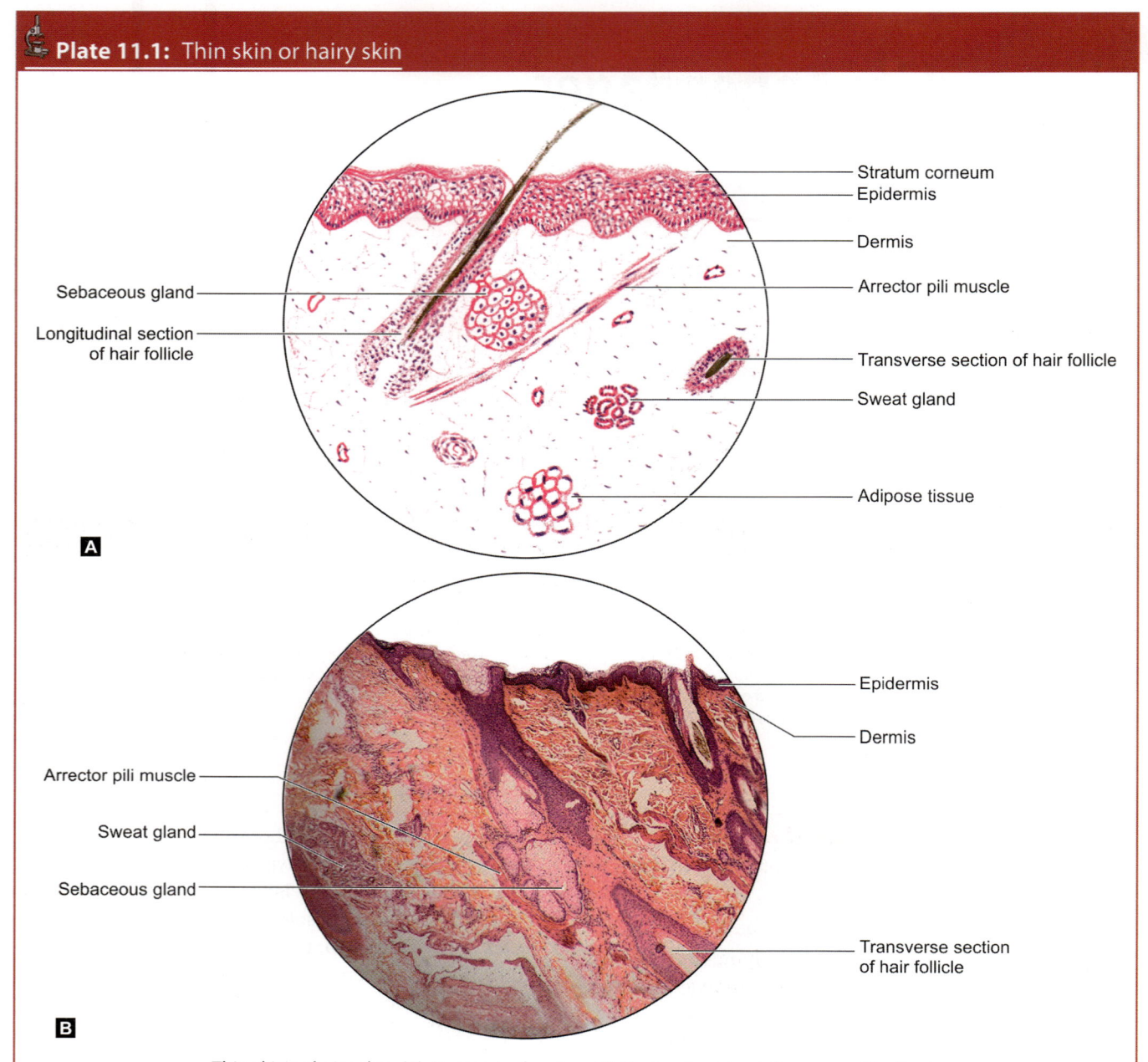

Thin skin or hairy skin: (A) As seen in drawing; (B) Photomicrograph (low magnification).

Points of identification
- Presence of thin epidermis made up of keratinized stratified squamous epithelium (stratum corneum is thin)
- Hair follicles, sebaceous glands and sweat glands are present in the dermis
- It is found in all others parts of body except palms and soles.

CHAPTER 11: Skin and its Appendages 141

Plate 11.2: Thick skin

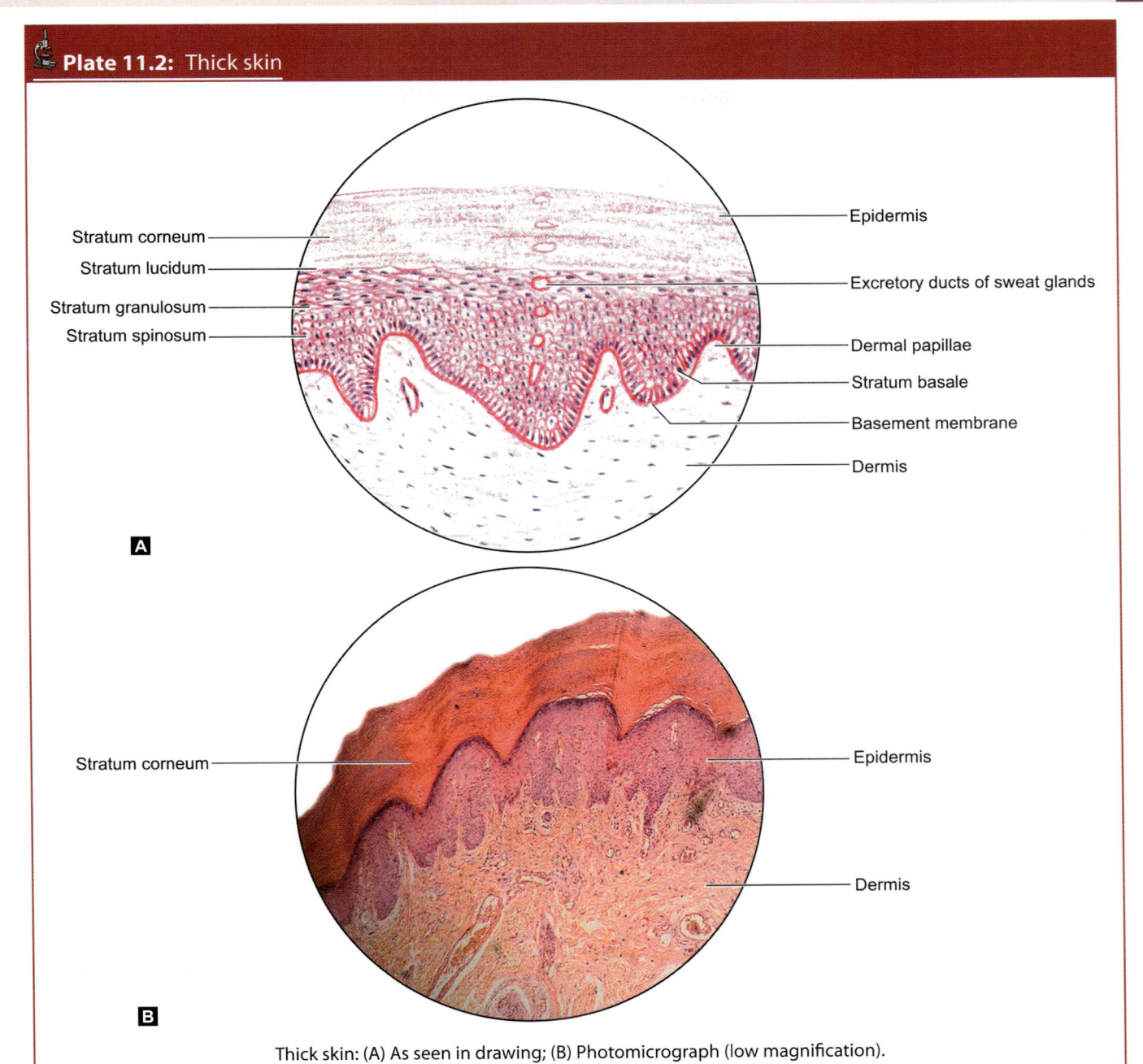

Labels (A, drawing):
- Stratum corneum
- Stratum lucidum
- Stratum granulosum
- Stratum spinosum
- Epidermis
- Excretory ducts of sweat glands
- Dermal papillae
- Stratum basale
- Basement membrane
- Dermis

Labels (B, photomicrograph):
- Stratum corneum
- Epidermis
- Dermis

Thick skin: (A) As seen in drawing; (B) Photomicrograph (low magnification).

Points of identification
- Presence of thick epidermis made up of keratinized stratified squamous epithelium (stratum corneum is very thick)
- Hair follicles and sebaceous glands are absent in dermis
- Sweat glands are present in the dermis
- It is found in palms of hands and soles of feet.

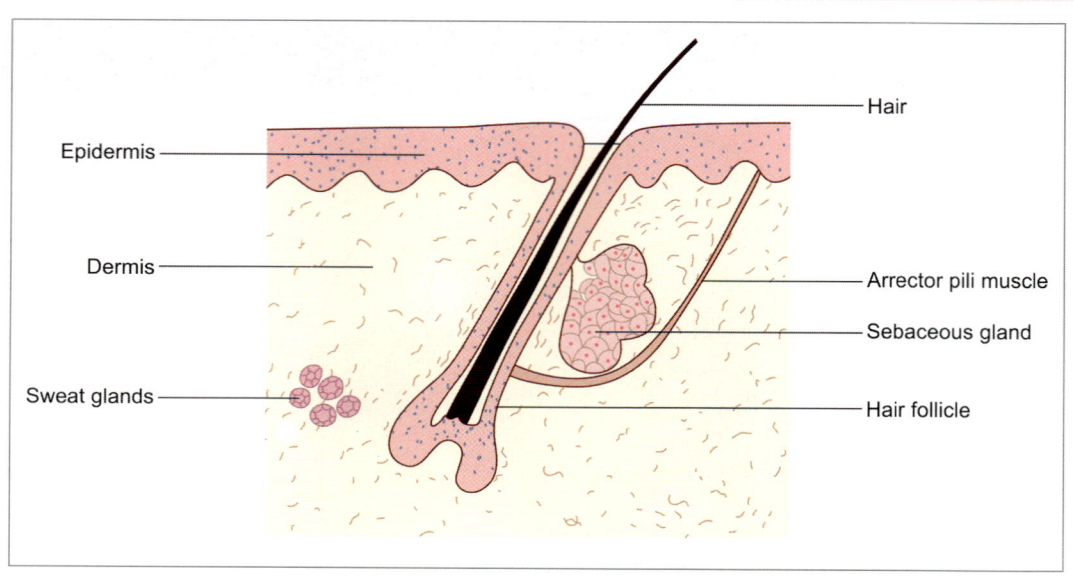

Fig. 11.1: Thin skin (schematic representation).

STRUCTURE OF SKIN

The skin consists of two layers.
- A superficial layer, the *epidermis*, is made up of stratified squamous epithelium.
- A deeper layer, the *dermis*, is made up of connective tissue (Fig. 11.1).
- The dermis rests on subcutaneous tissue (*subcutis*). This is sometimes described as a third layer of skin.
- In sections through the skin, the line of junction of the two layers is not straight but is markedly wavy because of the presence of numerous finger-like projections of dermis upward into the epidermis. These projections are called *dermal papillae*. The downward projections of the epidermis (in the intervals between the dermal papillae) are sometimes called *epidermal papillae* (Fig. 11.2).

Epidermis

The epidermis is derived from ectoderm and composed of stratified squamous keratinized epithelium (Figs. 11.3 and 11.4).

Layers of Epidermis

It is made up of five layers from within outward:
1. *Stratum basale*
2. *Stratum spinosum*

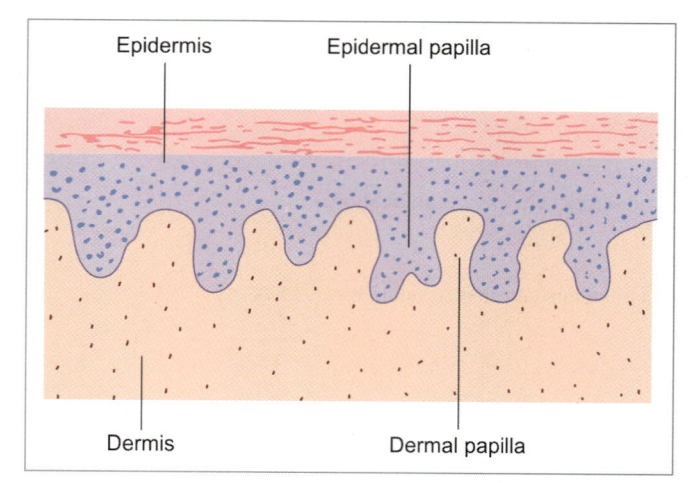

Fig. 11.2: Dermal and epidermal papillae (schematic representation).

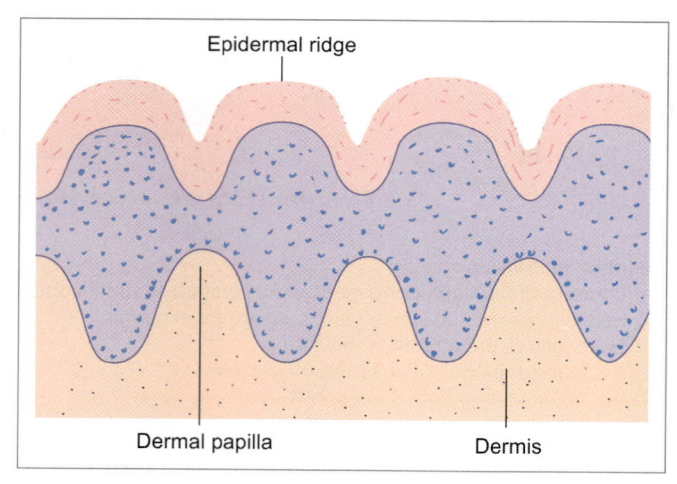

Fig. 11.3: Epidermal ridges (schematic representation).

CHAPTER 11: Skin and its Appendages

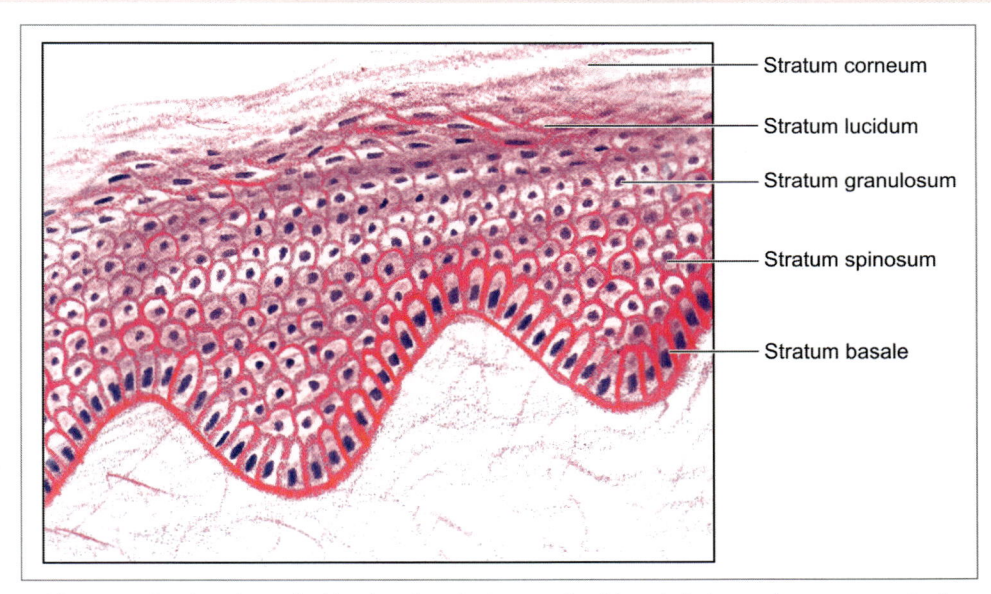

Fig. 11.4: Section through skin showing the layers of epidermis (schematic representation).

3. *Stratum granulosum*
4. *Stratum lucidum*
5. *Stratum corneum*.
   - **Stratum basale/stratum germinativum**
     - It is the deepest or **basal layer** of epidermis.
     - It is made up of a single layer of cuboidal to columnar cells with basophilic cytoplasm and large nucleus that rests on a basal lamina.
     - It contains stem cells that undergo mitosis and are responsible for the renewal of epidermal cells. Human epidermis is renewed about every 15–30 days depending on the region and age. The basal layer is therefore called the **germinal layer**.
   - **Stratum spinosum**
     - Above the basal layer, there are several layers of polygonal keratinocytes that constitute the **stratum spinosum** (or **malpighian layer**).
     - The cells of this layer are attached to one another by numerous desmosomes. During routine preparation of tissue for sectioning the cells retract from each other except at the desmosomes. As a result the cells appear to have a number of "spines." Hence, this layer is called the stratum spinosum, and the keratinocytes of this layer are also called **prickle cells** (Fig. 11.5).
     - Some mitoses may be seen in the deeper cells of the stratum spinosum, hence is included with the basal cell layer as the **germinative zone** of the epidermis.
   - **Stratum granulosum**
     - Above the stratum spinosum, there are one to five layers of flattened cells that are characterized by the presence of deeply staining granules in their cytoplasm called as keratohyalin granules.
     - The granules in them consist of a protein called **keratohyalin** (precursor of keratin).
     - The nuclei of cells in this layer are condensed and dark staining (pyknotic).
   - **Stratum lucidum**: Superficial to the stratum granulosum, there is the **stratum lucidum** (lucid = clear). This layer is so called because it appears

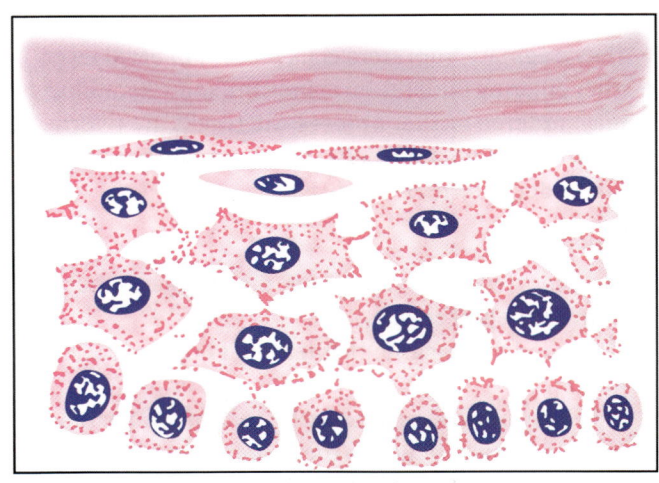

Fig. 11.5: Cells of the stratum spinosum showing typical spines (schematic representation).

homogeneous, the cell boundaries being extremely indistinct. Traces of flattened nuclei are seen in some cells.

- **Stratum corneum**
  - It is the most superficial layer of the epidermis.
  - It is acellular.
  - It is made up of flattened scale-like elements (squames)/dead cells containing keratin filaments embedded in protein. The squames are held together by a glue-like material which contains lipids and carbohydrates. The presence of lipid makes this layer highly resistant to permeation by water.
- The thickness of the stratum corneum is greatest where the skin is exposed to maximal friction, e.g. on the palm and sole.

Note: The stratum basale and stratum granulosum are called as germinative zone, andstratum corneum, the stratum lucidum, and the stratum granulosum are collectively referred to as the **zone of keratinization**, or as the **cornified zone.** The stratum granulosum and the stratum lucidum are well formed only in thick nonhairy skin (e.g. on the palms). They are usually absent in thin hairy skin.

Cells of Epidermis

The epidermis consists of two types of cells: (1) keratinocytes and (2) nonkeratinocytes (melanocytes, dendritic cell of Langerhans, and cells of Merkel).

Keratinocytes

- Keratinocytes are the predominant cell type of epidermis.
- They produce keratin.
- They originate from stem cells present in basal layer.
- After entering the stratum spinosum, some keratinocytes may undergo further mitoses. Such cells are referred to as **intermediate stem cells**. Thereafter, keratinocytes do not undergo further cell division.

Melanocytes

- Melanocytes are derived from melanoblasts that arise from the neural crest.
- They produce melanin pigment that imparts coloration to skin.
- They may be present among the cells of the germinative zone, or at the junction of the epidermis and the dermis. Each melanocyte gives off many processes; each of which is applied to a cell of the germinative zone.
- Melanin granules formed in the melanocyte are transferred to surrounding nonmelanin-producing cells through these processes. Because of the presence of processes, melanocytes are also called **dendritic cells** (Fig. 11.6).

Dendritic cells of Langerhans

- Langerhans cells are antigen-presenting cells located among the cells of the stratum spinosum.
- Represent 2–4% of cell population.
- Called dendritic cells because of the long processes. These cells are also found in oral mucosa, vagina, and thymus. These cells belong to the mononuclear phagocyte system.
- The dendritic cells of Langerhans originate in bone marrow and are a part of the mononuclear phagocytic system.
- They play an important role in protecting the skin against viral and other infections.
- It is believed that when the cells are stimulated, they take up antigens in the skin and transport them to lymphoid tissues.
- Under the electron microscopy (EM), dendritic cells are seen to contain characteristic elongated vacuoles that have been given the name **Langerhans bodies**, or **Birbeck bodies**.
- They play a role in controlling the rate of cell division in the epidermis. They increase in number in chronic skin disorders, particularly those resulting from allergy.

Cells of Merkel

- The basal layer of the epidermis contains specialized sensory cells called the cells of Merkel which may serve as mechanoreceptor.

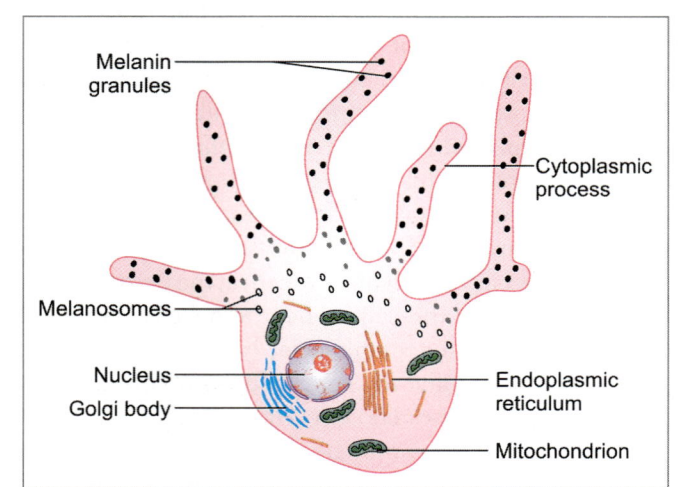

Fig. 11.6: Melanocyte showing dendritic processes (schematic representation).

- They are derived from neural crest cells.
- Sensory nerve endings are present in relation to these cells.

Dermis

The dermis is made up of irregular collagenous dense connective tissue. It is derived from mesoderm and divided into two layers.

1. ***Papillary layer:*** The papillary layer forms the superficial layers of dermis and includes the dense connective tissue of the dermal papillae. These papillae are best developed in the thick skin of the palms and soles. Each papilla contains a capillary loop. Some papillae contain tactile corpuscles.
2. ***Reticular layer:*** The reticular layer of the dermis is the deep layer of dermis and consists mainly of thick bundles of type I collagen fibers. It also contains considerable numbers of elastic fibers. Intervals between the fiber bundles are usually occupied by adipose tissue. The dermis rests on the superficial fascia through which it is attached to deeper structures. It contains epidermally derived structures, such as sweat glands, hair follicles, and sebaceous glands.

BLOOD SUPPLY OF THE SKIN

- Blood vessels to the skin are derived from a number of arterial plexuses. The deepest plexus is present over the deep fascia and one more plexus just below the dermis (***rete cutaneum*** or ***reticular plexus***), and a third plexus just below the level of the dermal papillae (***rete subpapillare***, or ***papillary plexus***). Capillary loops arising from this plexus pass into each dermal papilla.
- Blood vessels do not penetrate into the epidermis. The epidermis derives nutrition entirely by diffusion from capillaries in the dermal papillae. Veins from the dermal papillae drain into a venous plexus lying on deep fascia.
- A special feature of the blood supply of the skin is the presence of numerous arteriovenous anastomoses that regulate blood flow through the capillary bed and thus help in maintaining body temperature.

NERVE SUPPLY OF THE SKIN

- The skin is richly supplied with sensory nerves, and dense networks of nerve fibers are seen in the superficial parts of the dermis.
- Sensory nerves end in relation to various types of specialized terminals, such as free nerve endings, Meissner's corpuscles, Pacinian corpuscles, and Ruffini's corpuscles.
- In contrast to blood vessels, some nerve fibers do penetrate into the deeper parts of the epidermis.
- Skin also receives autonomic nerves that supply smooth muscle in the walls of blood vessels, the arrectores pilorum muscles, and myoepithelial cells present in relation to sweat glands. They also provide a secretomotor supply to sweat glands. In some regions (nipple, scrotum), nerve fibers innervate smooth muscle present in the dermis.

APPENDAGES OF THE SKIN

The appendages of the skin are the hair, nails, sebaceous glands, and sweat glands. The mammary glands may be regarded as highly specialized appendages of the skin.

Hair

- A hair may be regarded as a modified part of the stratum corneum of the skin.
- Hair is present on the skin covering almost the whole body. The sites where they are not present include the palms, the soles, the ventral surface and sides of the digits, and some parts of the male and female external genitalia.

Parts of Hair

- Each hair consists of a part (of variable length) that is seen on the surface of the body, and a part anchored in the thickness of the skin. The visible part is called the ***shaft***, and the embedded part is called the ***root***.
- The root has an expanded lower end called the ***bulb***. The bulb is invaginated from below by part of the dermis that constitutes the ***hair papilla***. The root of each hair is surrounded by a tubular sheath called the ***hair follicle*** (Fig. 11.7). The follicle is made up of several layers of cells that are derived from the layers of the skin.
- Hair roots are always attached to skin obliquely. As a result, the emerging hair is also oblique and easily lies flat on the skin surface.

Structure of Hair Shaft

It consists of three layers:

1. ***Cuticle***: The surface of the hair is covered by a thin membrane called the ***cuticle*** that is formed by flattened cornified cells.
2. ***Cortex***: It lies deep to the cuticle. The cortex is acellular and is made up of keratin.
3. ***Medulla***: An outer cortex and an inner medulla can be made out in large hair, but there is no medulla in thin hair. In thick hair the medulla consists of cornified cells of irregular shape.

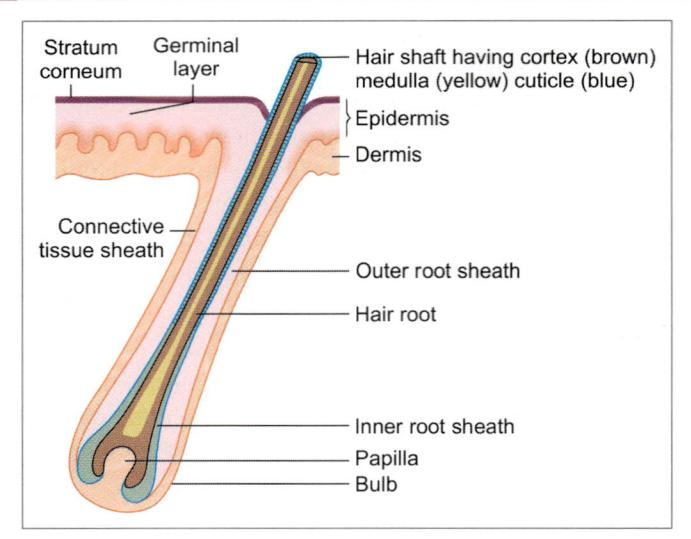

Fig. 11.7: Scheme to show some details of a hair follicle (schematic representation).

The cornified elements making up the hair contain melanin that is responsible for their color. Both in the medulla and in the cortex of a hair, minute air bubbles are present: they influence its color. The amount of air present in a hair increases with age and, along with the loss of pigment, is responsible for graying of hair.

Structure of Hair Follicle

The hair follicle may be regarded as a part of the epidermis that has been invaginated into the dermis around the hair root. Its innermost layer that immediately surrounds the hair root is, therefore, continuous with the surface of the skin; while the outermost layer of the follicle is continuous with the dermis.

The wall of the follicle consists of three main layers. From within outward, it is as follows (Fig. 11.8):
1. The ***inner root sheath*** present only in the lower part of the follicle
2. The ***outer root sheath*** that is continuous with the stratum spinosum
3. A connective tissue sheath derived from the dermis.

Note: The inner and outer root sheaths are derived from epidermis.

Inner root sheath

- The innermost layer is called the ***cuticle***. It lies against the cuticle of the hair and consists of flattened cornified cells.
- Next, there are one to three layers of flattened nucleated cells that constitute ***Huxley's layer***, or the ***stratum epithelial granulosum***. Cells of this layer contain large eosinophilic granules (***trichohyaline granules***).
- The outer layer (of the inner root sheath) is made up of a single layer of cubical cells with flattened nuclei. This is called ***Henle's layer***, or the ***stratum epithelial pallidum***.

Outer root sheath

- The outer root sheath is continuous with the stratum spinosum of the skin. At the lower end of the follicle, the cells of this layer become continuous with the hair bulb.
- The cells of the hair bulb also correspond to those of the stratum spinosum and constitute the ***germinative matrix***. They give rise to cells of the inner root sheath.

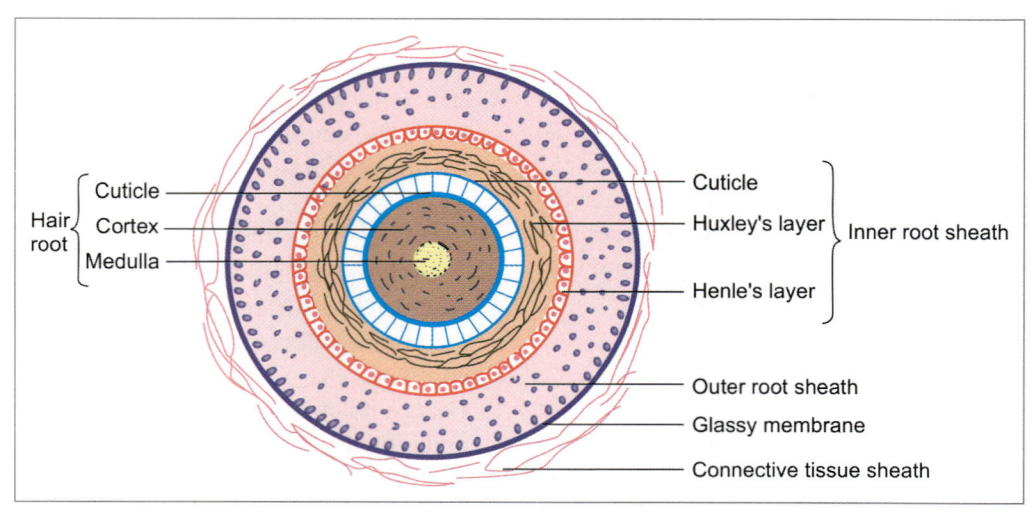

Fig. 11.8: Various layers to be seen in a hair follicle (schematic representation).

CHAPTER 11: Skin and its Appendages

- The outer root sheath is separated from the connective tissue sheath by a basal lamina that appears structureless and is, therefore, called the **glassy membrane**.

Connective tissue sheath

- The **connective tissue sheath** is made up of tissue continuous with that of the dermis.
- The tissue is highly vascular, and contains numerous nerve fibers that form a basket-like network round the lower end of the follicle.

Arrector Pili Muscles

- These are bands of smooth muscle attached at one end to the dermis, just below the dermal papillae, and at the other end, to the connective tissue sheath of a hair follicle.
- The arrector pili muscles pass obliquely from the lower part of the hair follicle toward the junction of the epidermis and dermis.
- It lies on that side of the hair follicle that forms an obtuse angle with the skin surface. A sebaceous gland lies in the angle between the hair follicle and the arrector pili.
- Contraction of the muscle pulls the hair follicle vertical (from its original oblique position) relative to the skin surface. Simultaneously the skin surface overlying the attachment of the muscle becomes depressed, while surrounding areas become raised and the skin takes on the appearance of "goose flesh". These reactions are seen during exposure to cold, or during emotional excitement, when the "hair stand on end".
- Upon the contraction of the arrector pili muscle the sebaceous gland is pressed upon, and its secretions are squeezed out into the hair follicle.
- The arrector pili muscles receive a sympathetic innervation.

Sebaceous Glands

- Sebaceous glands are holocrine type of glands and present in dermis in close association with hair follicles.
- Each gland consists of a number of alveoli that are connected to a broad duct that opens into a hair follicle (Plates 11.1 and 11.3). Each alveolus is pear shaped. It consists of a solid mass of polyhedral cells and has hardly any lumen (Fig. 11.9).
- The outermost cells are small and rest on a basement membrane. The inner cells are larger, more rounded, and filled with lipid.
- The secretion of sebaceous glands is called **sebum**. Its oily nature helps to keep the skin and hair soft. It helps to prevent the dryness of the skin and also makes it resistant to moisture.
- At some places, sebaceous glands occur independently of hair follicles. Such glands open directly on the skin surface. They are found around the lips, and in relation to some parts of the male and female external genitalia.
- The tarsal (Meibomian) glands of the eyelid are modified sebaceous glands.
- Montgomery's tubercles present in the skin around the nipple (areola) are also sebaceous glands.
- Secretion by sebaceous glands is not under nervous control.

Sweat Glands

Sweat glands produce sweat or perspiration. They are present in the skin over most of the body. They are of two types:
1. Typical or merocrine sweat glands
2. Atypical or apocrine sweat glands.

Typical Sweat Glands

- Typical sweat glands are of the merocrine variety. They are most numerous in the palm and sole, the forehead and scalp, and the axillae.
- The sweat glands are simple, coiled tubular glands whose duct opens at the skin surface.
- The lower end of the tube is highly coiled on itself and forms the **body** or **fundus** or secretory part of the gland. Secretory part is present in the reticular layer of the dermis (Fig. 11.10).

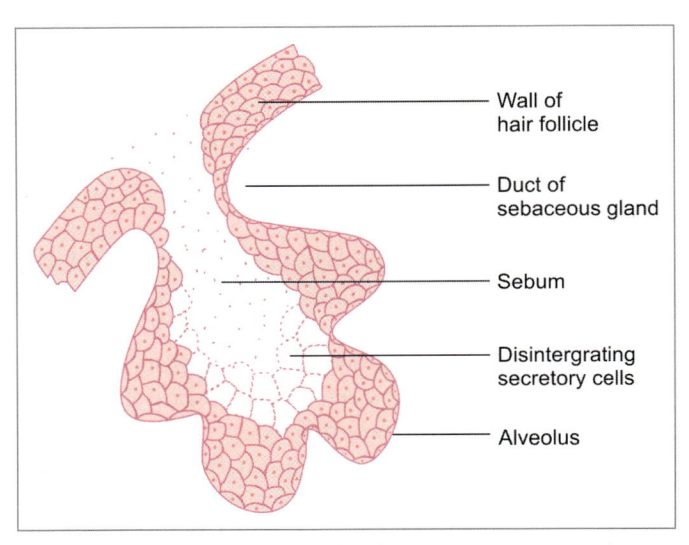

Fig. 11.9: Sebaceous gland (schematic representation).

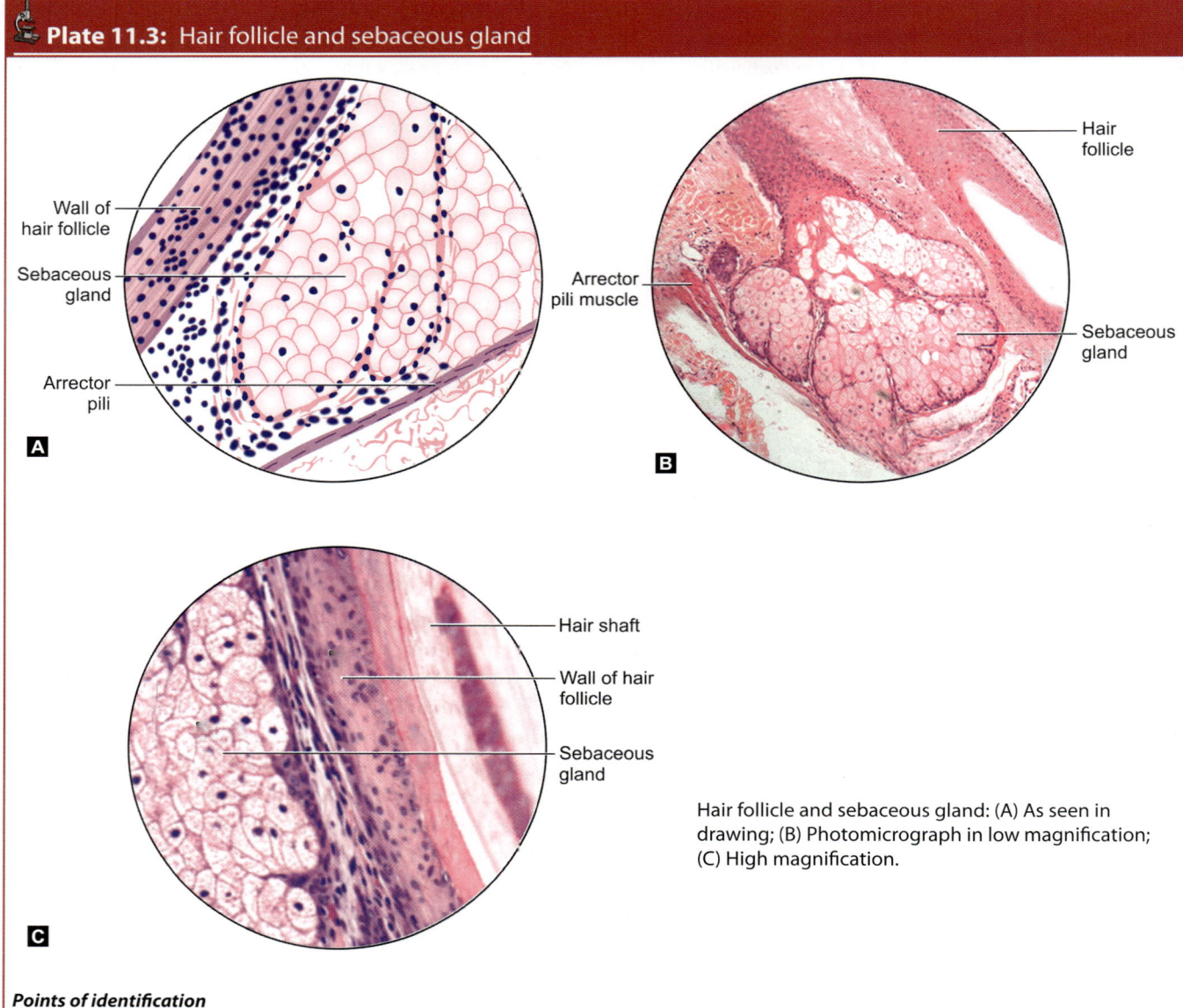

Plate 11.3: Hair follicle and sebaceous gland

A — Labels: Wall of hair follicle; Sebaceous gland; Arrector pili

B — Labels: Hair follicle; Arrector pili muscle; Sebaceous gland

C — Labels: Hair shaft; Wall of hair follicle; Sebaceous gland

Hair follicle and sebaceous gland: (A) As seen in drawing; (B) Photomicrograph in low magnification; (C) High magnification.

Points of identification
- In figures small areas of skin at higher magnification are shown
- The parts of a sebaceous gland and hair follicle containing a hair root can be seen
- Each sebaceous gland consists of a number of alveoli that open into a hair follicle
- Each alveolus is pear shaped. It consists mainly of a solid mass of polyhedral cells.

- In the secretory part is lined by cuboidal to low columnar cells. Sometimes, the epithelium may appear to be pseudostratified.
- The part of the tube connecting the secretory element to the skin surface is the **duct**. It runs upward through the dermis to reach the epidermis. Within the epidermis the duct follows a spiral course to reach the skin surface. The orifice is funnel shaped. On the palms, soles, and digits the openings of sweat glands lie in rows on epidermal ridges.
- In larger sweat glands flattened contractile, **myoepithelial cells** (Fig. 11.11) are present between the epithelial cells and their basal lamina.
- In the duct is lined by stratified cuboidal epithelium.
- Sweat glands (including the myoepithelial cells) are innervated by cholinergic nerves.
- Two types of cells are seen in the secretory part. **Dark cells** are pyramidal shape and contain secretory granules and **clear cells** without any granules. Dark cells secretion is mucoid, whereas clear cells secretion is watery.

CHAPTER 11: Skin and its Appendages

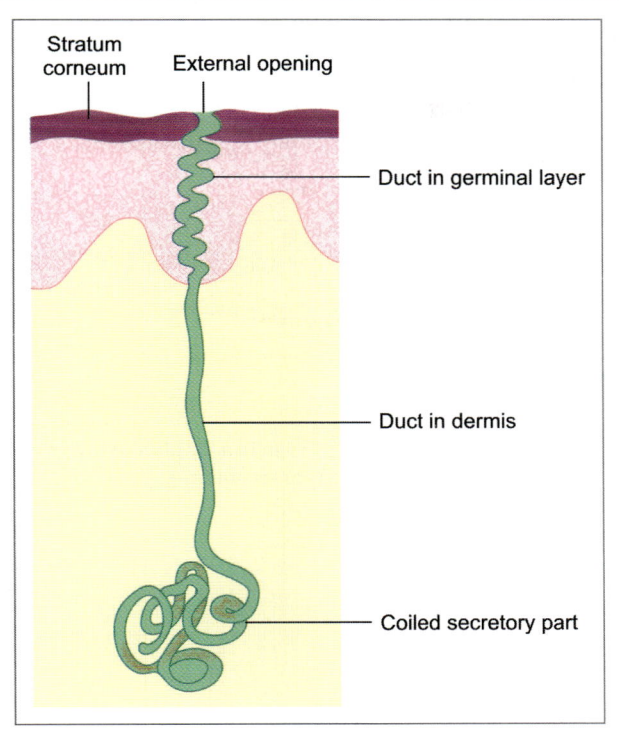

Fig. 11.10: Parts of a typical sweat gland (schematic representation).

- They are present in some parts of the body, such as the axilla, the areola and nipple, the perianal region, the glans penis, and some parts of the female external genitalia.
- Apocrine sweat glands are much larger compared to merocrine they are fully developed only after puberty.
- Unlike merocrine, the secretory part of these glands branch.
- Their ducts open not on the skin surface but into hair follicles.
- Secretory part is lined by epithelium of varying height: it may be squamous, cuboidal, or columnar.
- The secretions of apocrine sweat glands are viscous and contain proteins. They are odorless, but after bacterial decomposition, they give off body odors that vary from person to person.
- Innervated by an adrenergic nerve endings.
- Wax-producing *ceruminous glands* of the external acoustic meatus and *ciliary glands* of the eyelids are modified apocrine sweat glands.

Nails

- Nails are present on fingers and toes.
- They provide a rigid support for the finger tips. This support increases the sensitivity of the finger tips and increases their efficiency in carrying out delicate movements.
- The nail represents a modified part of the zone of keratinization of the epidermis. It is usually regarded as a much thickened continuation of the stratum lucidum,

Atypical Sweat Glands

- Atypical sweat glands are of the apocrine variety (apical parts of the secretory cells are shed off as part of their secretion).

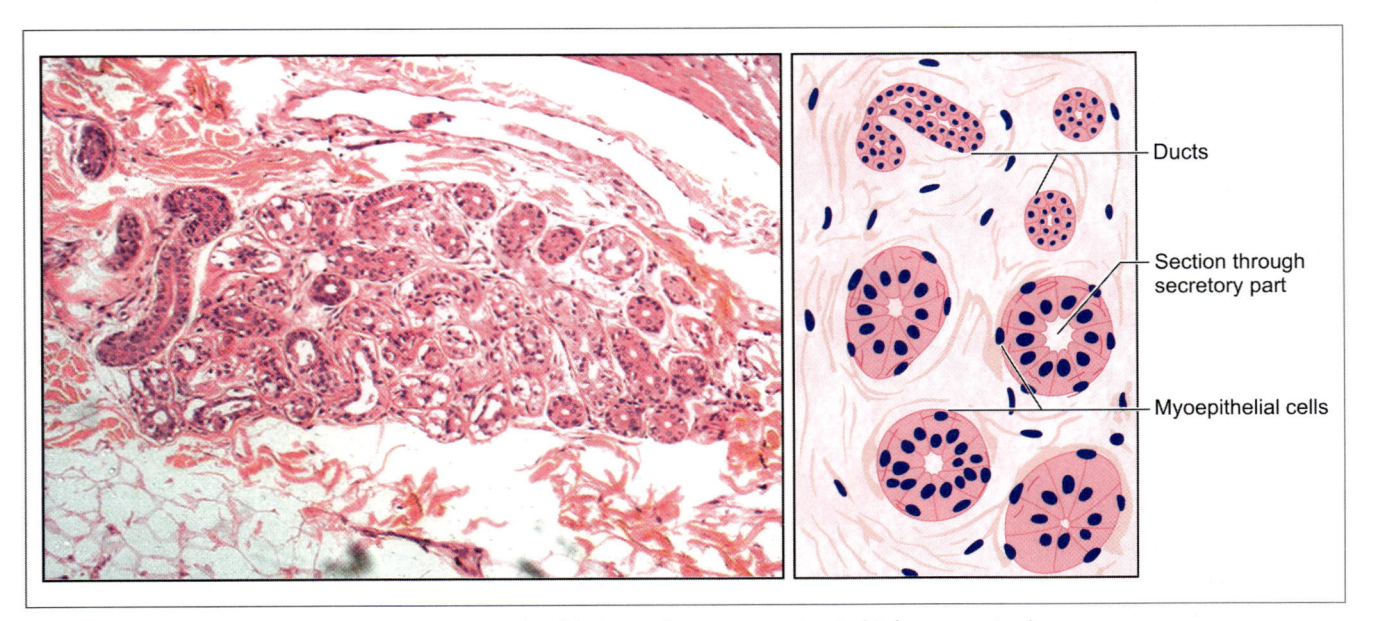

Fig. 11.11: Sweat gland (schematic representation in high power view).

but it is more like the stratum corneum in structure. The nail substance consists of several layers of dead, cornified, "cells" filled with keratin.
- Nail consists of body and root. The main part of a nail is called its **body**. The proximal part of the nail is implanted into a groove on the skin and is called the **root** (or **radix**).
- The tissue on which the nail rests is called the **nail bed**. The nail bed is highly vascular, and that is why, the nails look pink in color (Figs. 11.12 and 11.13).

Added Information
- Basal cells are mitotically active, and it shows mitotic figures. Mitosis occurs during night, and histological specimens are procured during day so they are not seen in the slides.
- The color of skin is influenced by the amount of melanin present. It is also influenced by some other pigments present in the epidermis, and by pigments hemoglobin and oxyhemoglobin present in blood circulating through the skin. The epidermis is sufficiently translucent for the color of blood to show through, especially in light-skinned individuals. That is why the skin becomes pale in anemia, blue when oxygenation of blood is insufficient, and pink while blushing.
- The time elapsing between the formation of a keratinocyte in the basal layer of the epidermis and its shedding off from the surface of the epidermis is highly variable. It is influenced by many factors including skin thickness, and the degree of friction on the surface. On the average, it is 40–50 days. In some situations, it is seen that flakes of keratin in the stratum corneum are arranged in regular columns (one stacked above the other). It is believed that localized areas in the basal layer of the epidermis contain groups of keratinocytes, all derived from a single stem cell. It is also believed that all the cells in the epidermis overlying this region are derived from the same stem cell. Such groups of cells, all derived from a single stem cell, and stacked in layers passing from the basal layer to the surface of the epidermis, constitute **epidermal proliferation units**. One dendritic cell (*see* below) is present in close association with each such unit.
- **Growth of nails:** Nails undergo constant growth by proliferation of cells in the germinal matrix. Growth is faster in hot weather than in cold. Finger nails grow faster than toe nails. Nail growth can be disturbed by serious illness or by injury over the nail root, resulting in transverse grooves or white patches in the nails. These grooves or patches slowly grow toward the free edge of the nail. If a nail is lost by injury, a new one grows out of the germinal matrix if the latter is intact.

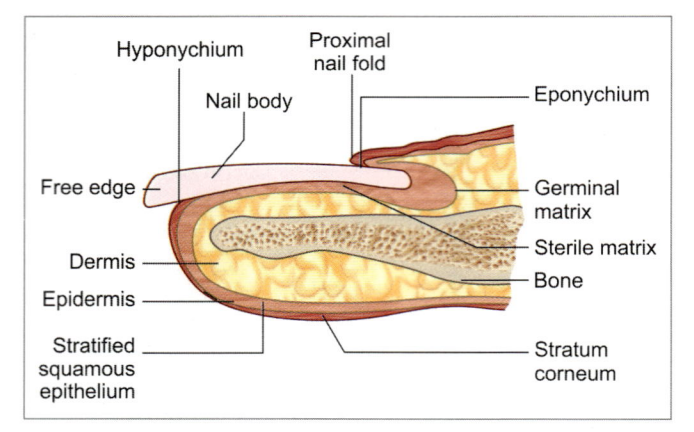

Fig. 11.12: Parts of a nail as seen in a longitudinal section (schematic representation).

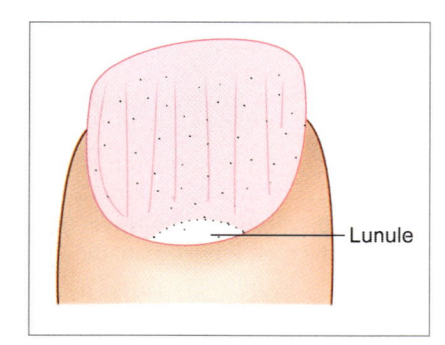

Fig. 11.13: Lunule of a nail (schematic representation).

increase in the epidermal thickness and rapid renewal of epidermis.
- **Acne vulgaris:**
  - It is a very common chronic inflammatory disease involving the sebaceous glands and hair follicles, found predominantly in adolescents in both sexes.
  - The flow of the sebum is continuous and a disturbance in the normal secretion and flow leading to obstruction and results in acne.
- **Albinism:** Hereditary inability of the melanocytes to synthesize melanin. Skin is not protected from solar radiation therefore increased incidence of skin cancers.
- **Vitiligo:** It is a disease that results from the immune system killing melanocytes. This results in the depigmentation of skin.
- **Onychia:** It is the inflammation of nail folds and shedding of nail resulting due to the introduction of microscopic pathogens through small wounds.
  - **Paronychia:** It is caused due to bacterial or fungal infection producing change in the shape of nail plate.

APPLIED HISTOLOGY

- **Psoriasis:** There is an increase in the number of proliferating cells and decrease in the cycle time of the cells in the stratum basale and spinosum leading to

CHAPTER 11: Skin and its Appendages

- **Koilonychia:** It is caused due to iron deficiency or vitamin B_{12} deficiency and is characterized by abnormal thinness and concavity (spoonshape) of the nails.
❖ The fiber bundles in the reticular layer of the dermis mostly lie parallel to one another. In the limbs the predominant direction of the bundles is along the long axis of the limb; while on the trunk and neck, the direction is transverse. The lines along which the bundles run are often called *cleavage lines*. The cleavage lines are of importance to the surgeon as incisions in the direction of these lines gape much less than those at right angles to them.
❖ The dermis contains considerable amounts of elastic fibers. Atrophy of elastic fibers occurs with age and is responsible for the loss of elasticity and wrinkling of the skin.
❖ **Linea gravidarum:** If skin is rapidly stretched, fiber bundles in the dermis may rupture scar tissue which can be seen in the form of prominent white lines (anterior abdominal wall in pregnancy).
❖ **Tumors:**
  - **Malignant melanoma:** Tumors arising from melanocytes.
  - **Basal cell carcinoma:** Tumors arising from the basal cells of stratum basale.
  - **Squamous cell carcinoma:** Tumors from the squamous cells of stratum spinosum. Squamous cell carcinoma may arise on any part of the skin and mucous membranes lined by squamous epithelium but are more likely to occur on sun-exposed parts in older people.

MULTIPLE CHOICE QUESTIONS

1. What is the prickle layer of the skin?
   a. Lucidum
   b. Corneum
   c. Spinosum
   d. Granulosum
2. Which of the following statements about the sebaceous glands is true?
   a. They control the body temperature
   b. They are always associated with hair follicles
   c. They are abundant on the face only
   d. They are a source of new hairs
3. The dermis is made up of two layers:
   a. Adipose tissue and basal layer
   b. Papillary layer and horny layer
   c. Papillary and reticular layers
   d. Inner layer and granular layer
4. Melanin protects the skin from:
   a. Pathogenic bacteria
   b. Electric heat
   c. Steam heat
   d. Ultraviolet rays
5. The main function of sebum is to prevent the skin from:
   a. Losing moisture
   b. Becoming dirty
   c. Losing color
   d. Becoming blemished
6. Name the sublayers of the epidermis from the inside outward:
   a. Basal, corneum, spinosum, lucidum, and granulosum
   b. Basal, spinosum, granulosum, lucidum, and corneum
   c. Basal, spinosum, granulosum, corneum, and lucidum
   d. Basal, granulosum, lucidum, corneum, and spinosum

Answers
   1. c   2. b   3. c   4. d   5. a   6. b

CHAPTER 12

Salivary Glands

Learning objectives

To study the:
- Classification of salivary glands with example
- Composition of salivary gland
- Structure of serous, mixed, and mucous salivary glands
- Applied histology

IDENTIFICATION POINTS

Parotid gland	Submandibular gland	Sublingual gland
❑ Only serous acini are present, which contain basophilic zymogen granules and are darkly stained	❑ Mixed salivary gland, predominantly serous with a few mucous acini	❑ Predominantly mucous acini are present with few serous acini
❑ Intercalated and striated (intralobular) ducts are seen	❑ Serous demilunes are present	❑ Intercalated and interlobular duct can be seen
❑ Interlobular duct can be seen	❑ Intercalated and striated (intralobular) ducts are seen	❑ It also contains adipocytes.
❑ It also contains adipocytes.	❑ Interlobular duct can be seen	
	❑ Striated ducts are more prominent than those in parotid gland.	

■ SALIVARY GLANDS

There are two main groups of salivary glands: (1) major and (2) minor.

1. **Major salivary glands**: Three paired glands: (1) parotid, (2) submandibular and (3) sublingual. They are **branched tubuloalveolar glands**.
2. **Minor salivary glands** are numerous and are widely distributed in the mucosa of oral cavity. Some of the minor salivary glands are the Von Ebner's gland in tongue, buccal glands in cheeks and labial glands in lips.

Structural Organization

Basically, a salivary gland consists of stroma, parenchyma, and a duct system which carries the secretions into the oral cavity.

Stroma

The connective tissue capsule provides septa and divides the glands into lobes and lobules. The blood vessels and nerves traverse through the connective tissue septa. Large ducts of the glands are also present in it.

Parenchyma

Parenchyma has two components: (1) the secretory part and (2) conducting part.

Secretory part

- Salivary glands are compound tubuloalveolar glands (racemose glands). Their secretory elements (also referred to as **end pieces** or as the **portio terminalis**) may be rounded (acini), pear-shaped (alveoli), tubular, or a mixture of these (tubuloacinar, tubuloalveolar).
- Salivon–Basic secretary unit which includes acini, intercalated duct, and excoretory duct.
- The acini are made up of either **serous** or **mucous** cells. A salivary gland may have only one type of acini, or there may be a mixture of both serous and mucous acini, these are called mixed acini.
- A secretory unit, or gland, with only one type of cell (serous or mucous) is said to be **homocrine**. If it contains more than one variety of cells, it is said to be **heterocrine**.

- **Serous acini**: Serous cells are usually arranged in the form of rounded acini. As a result, each cell is roughly pyramidal having a broadbase and a narrow apex with a single, **round**, and basally located nucleus. The nucleus is pushed to basal region due to accumulated secretory granules of apical region. The apical region is eosinophilic due to accumulation of zymogen granules; cytoplasm is basophilic due to cell organelles. Hence exhibit bipolar staining.
- **Mucous cells**: Mucous cells are usually arranged in the form of **tubular secretory**. The cells lining mucous cells tend to be columnar rather than pyramidal with a flattened nucleus at the basal part of the cell. The cytoplasm is filled completely with a light-staining, secretory product called **mucus**. This pushes the nucleus to the base of the cytoplasm. Lumens of these acini are larger than serous.
- **Seromucous cells**: Some salivary glands contain both serous and mucous acini in same **secretory** component. They are referred to as **seromucous cells**. In the submandibular glands, mucous acini are often capped by a crescent or moon-shaped cap of serous cells over them called a **serous demilunes of Giannuzzi**. The serous cells of a demilune drain into the lumen of the acinus through fine canaliculi passing through the intervals between mucous cells.
- **Myoepithelial cells (basket cells)**: Myoepithelial cells are contractile, their contraction helping to squeeze out secretion from secretory or conducting portion of the gland. They are present in relation to acini, intercalated, intralobular and extralobular ducts. They are located between the basal lamina and acinar or ductal cells. They contain actin and myosin filaments.

Conducting part

The secretory elements lead into a series of ducts through which their secretions are poured into the oral cavity. In sections through salivary glands, we see a large number of closely packed acini with ducts scattered between them. These elements are supported by the connective tissue that also divides the glands into lobules and forms capsules around them. Blood vessels, lymphatics, and nerves run in the connective tissue that may at places contain some adipose tissue.

- ❖ **Duct system**: The ducts are highly branched and range from very small intercalated ducts to very large terminal ducts. Secretions produced in acini pass along a system of ducts, different parts of which have differing structure.
- ❖ The smallest ducts are called **intercalated ducts** to which secretory acini are attached. These are lined by cuboidal or flattened cells.
- ❖ Many intercalated ducts join to form **striated ducts**, and they are lined by cuboidal to low columnar cells. They are so called because the basal parts of the cells show vertical striations.
- ❖ Striated ducts join with each other and form intralobular ducts of increasing caliber. Ducts arising from lobules unite to form **interlobular ducts**, which in turn forms **intralobar** and **interlobar ducts**. The **interlobular** are lined by simple columnar epithelium. Terminal part toward oral cavity gets lined by nonkeratinized stratified squamous epithelium.

Innervation of Salivary Glands

Secretion by salivary glands is under hormonal as well as neural control.

- ❖ A local hormone **plasmakinin** formed by secretory cells influences vasodilation.
- ❖ Salivary glands are innervated by autonomic nerves, both parasympathetic (cholinergic) and sympathetic (adrenergic). Parasympathetic nerves travel to secretory elements along ducts, while sympathetic nerves travel along arteries. Synaptic contacts between nerve terminals and effector cells form **neuroeffector junctions**.

Two types of junction, **epilemmal** and **hypolemmal**, are present.

1. At **epilemmal junctions**, the nerve terminal is separated from the secretory or effector cell by the basal lamina.
2. At **hypolemmal junctions**, the nerve terminal pierces the basal lamina and comes into direct contact with the effector cell.

Nerve impulses reaching one effector cell spread to others through intercellular contacts. Classically, salivary secretion has been attributed to parasympathetic stimulation. While this is true, it is believed that sympathetic nerves can also excite secretion either directly, or by vasodilation. Autonomic nerves not only stimulate secretion, but also appear to determine its viscosity and other characteristics. Autonomic nerve terminals are also seen on myoepithelial cells and on cells lining the ducts of salivary glands. The latter probably influence the reabsorption of sodium by cells lining the ducts. Salivary glands are sensitive to pain, and must therefore have a sensory innervation as well.

Parotid Salivary Gland (Plate 12.1)

❖ Parotid gland, the large serous salivary gland, located in the parotid region. Its excretory duct is called Stensen's duct, opens at vestibule of mouth into a small elevation on the mucosal surface of the cheek opposite the second upper molar tooth.

❖ It is compound tubuloacinar or racemose gland.

❖ The parotid gland is covered by a capsule from which arise numerous interlobular connective tissue septa that subdivide the gland into lobes and lobules. Blood vessels and interlobular excretory ducts are located in the connective tissue septa.

❖ Each lobule is made up of a cluster of secretory cells that form the serous acini. The cells of acini are pyramid shaped with spherical nuclei located at the base of the slightly basophilic cytoplasm. At high power, small secretory granules occupy the cell apices of the serous acini.

❖ The acini are surrounded by thin, contractile myoepithelial cells located between the basement membrane and acinar cells.

❖ The lobules may contain numerous adipose cells.

❖ The secretions of the acini flow to narrow channels called the intercalated that are lined by a simple squamous or low cuboidal epithelium.

❖ The secretion drains into larger striated ducts having larger lumens lined by simple columnar cells with basal striations. Striated ducts are large and conspicuous in parotid gland. The striations are formed by deep infolding of the basal cell membrane. Longitudinally oriented, elongated mitochondria are enclosed in between the infoldings. They empty their product into the intralobular excretory ducts which in turn drain into interlobular ducts located in the connective tissue septa.

❖ The lumen of ducts become progressively wider, and the epithelium get taller as they increase in size. The epithelium changes from columnar to pseudostratified or even stratified columnar in large lobar ducts close to their termination.

Submandibular Gland (Plates 12.2 and 12.3)

❖ It is a mixed gland, containing both serous and mucous acini, with serous acini predominating.

❖ The submandibular salivary gland is also a compound tubuloacinar gland.

❖ The serous acini have smaller, darker-stained pyramidal cells, spherical basal nuclei, and apical secretory granules. The mucous acini are larger with wide lumen exhibiting more variation in size and shape. The mucous cells are columnar with pale or almost colorless cytoplasm. The nuclei are flattened and pressed against the base of the cell membrane.

❖ The serous demilunes are dispersed among the acini. The mucous acini have a cap of serous cells that are thought to secrete into the highly convoluted intercellular space between the mucous cells.

❖ The thin, contractile myoepithelial cells are seen around serous, mucous acini, and intercalated ducts.

❖ The duct system of the submandibular gland is similar to that of the parotid gland.

Cells of Salivary Glands (Figs. 12.1 to 12.3)

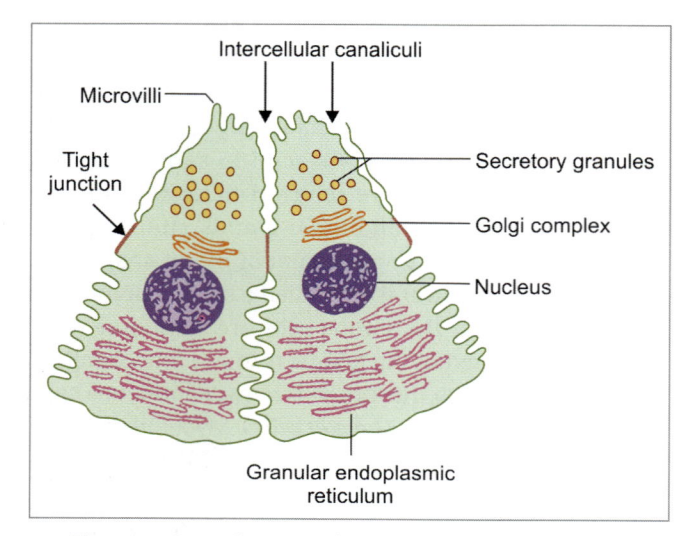

Fig. 12.1: Some features of serous cell in a salivary gland (schematic representation).

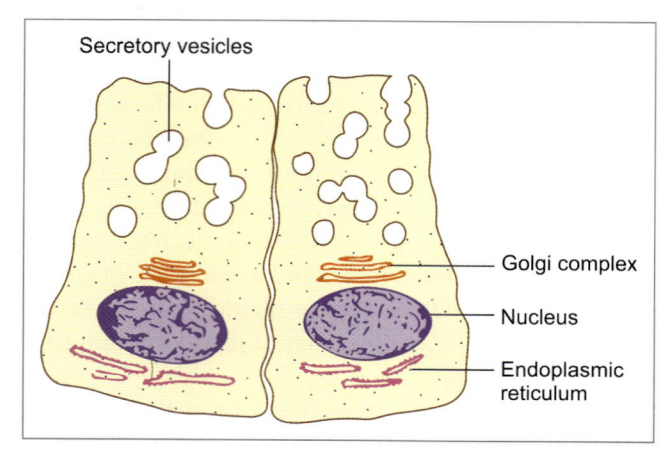

Fig. 12.2: Some features of mucous cells in salivary glands (schematic representation).

CHAPTER 12: Salivary Glands

Plate 12.1: Parotid gland

Parotid gland: (A) As seen in drawing; (B) Photomicrograph.

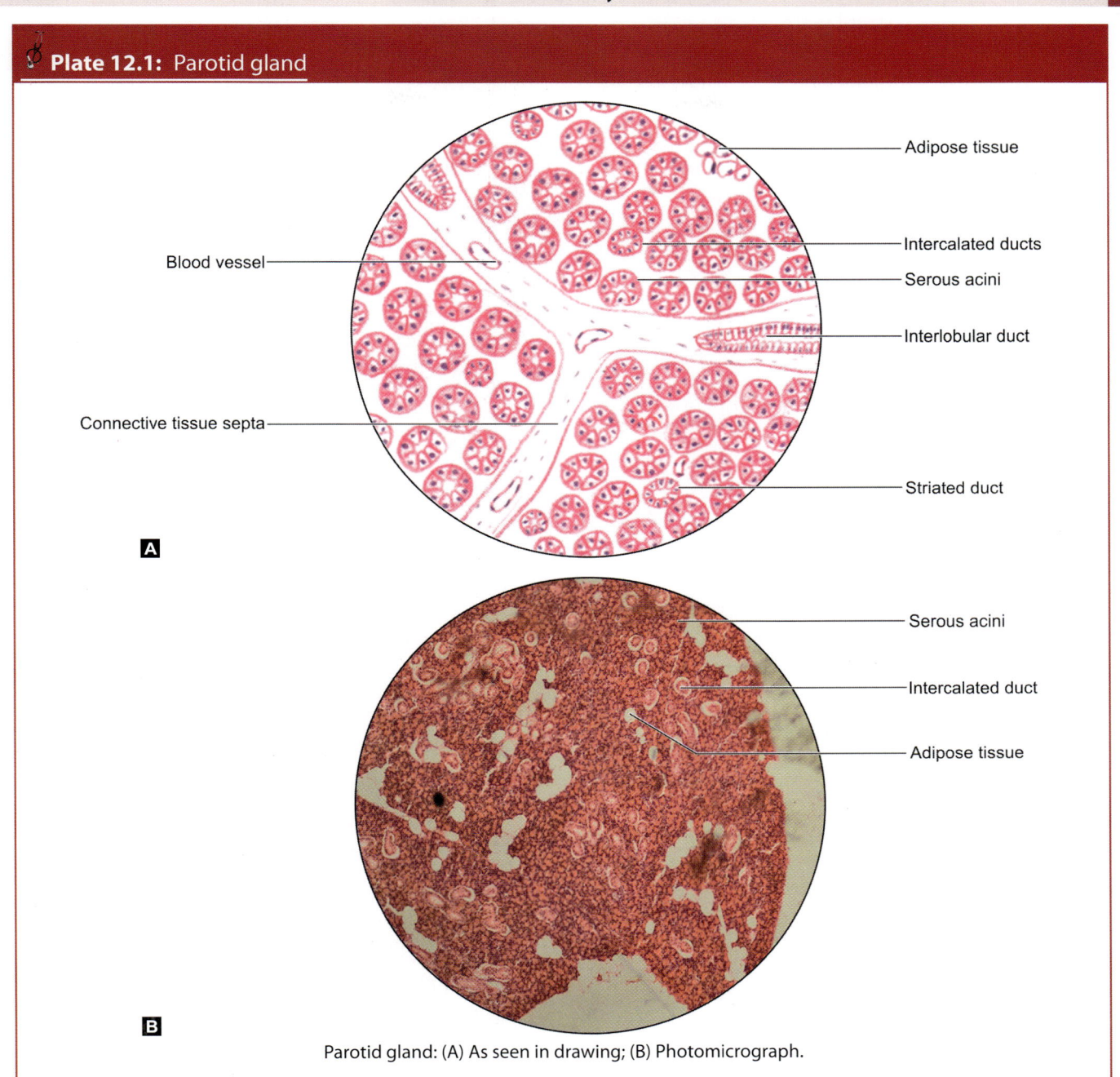

Points of identification
The parotid gland is a serous salivary gland. The characteristic features are:
- Only serous acini are present which contain basophilic zymogen granules and are darkly stained
- Intercalated and striated (intralobular) ducts are seen
- Interlobular duct can be seen
- It also contains adipocytes.

Plate 12.2: Submandibular gland (Low magnification)

Labels (A, drawing):
- Intercalated duct
- Serous demilune
- Interlobular connective tissue septa
- Blood vessel
- Intralobular duct
- Interlobular duct
- Serous acini
- Mucous acini

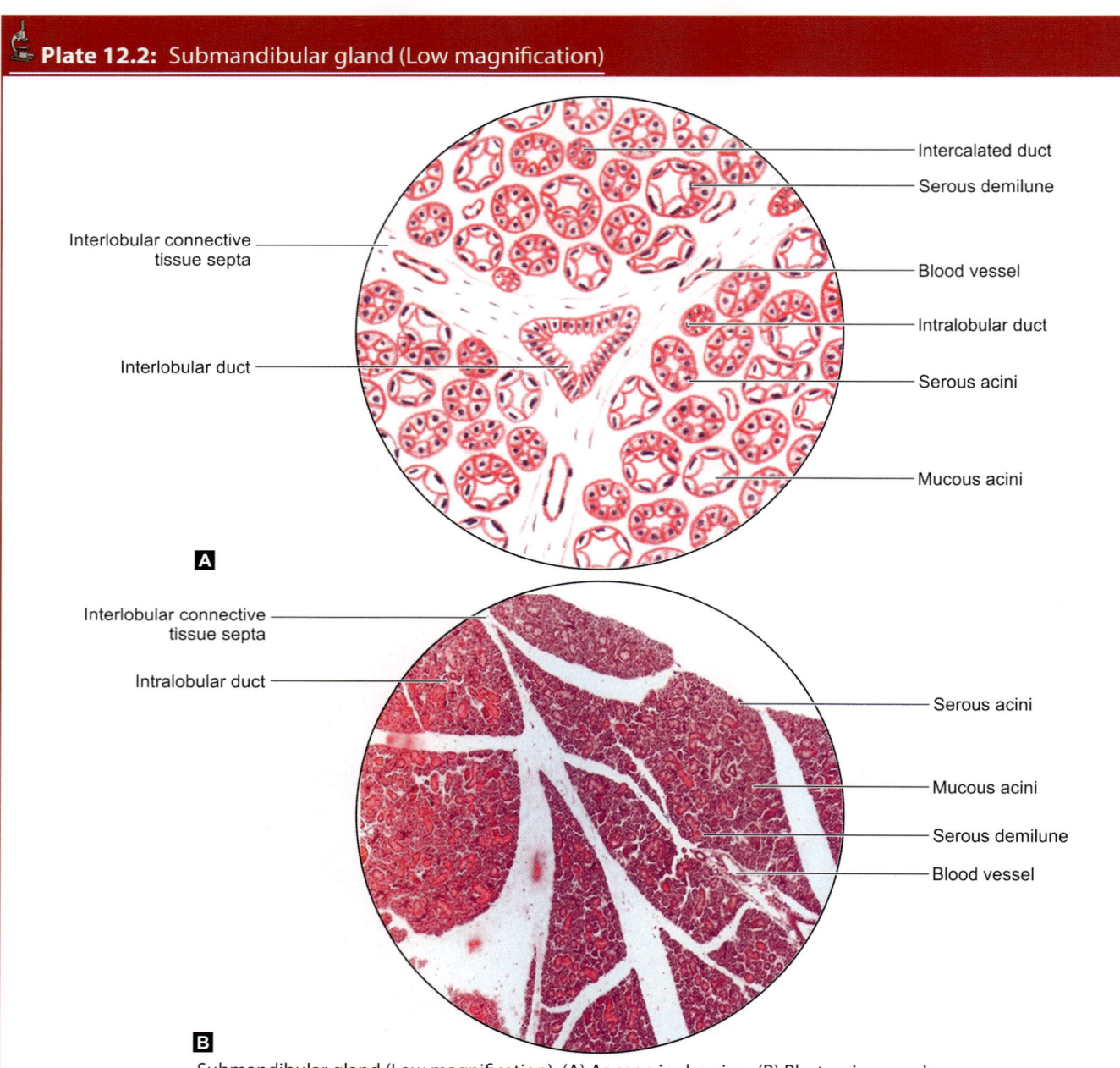

Labels (B, photomicrograph):
- Interlobular connective tissue septa
- Intralobular duct
- Serous acini
- Mucous acini
- Serous demilune
- Blood vessel

Submandibular gland (Low magnification): (A) As seen in drawing; (B) Photomicrograph.

Points of identification
- The submandibular gland is a mixed salivary gland, predominantly serous with a few mucous acini
- Serous cells are frequently located at the periphery of mucous acini in the form of a crescent and called as demilunes
- Striated ducts are more prominent than those in parotid gland.

CHAPTER 12: Salivary Glands

Plate 12.3: Submandibular gland (High magnification)

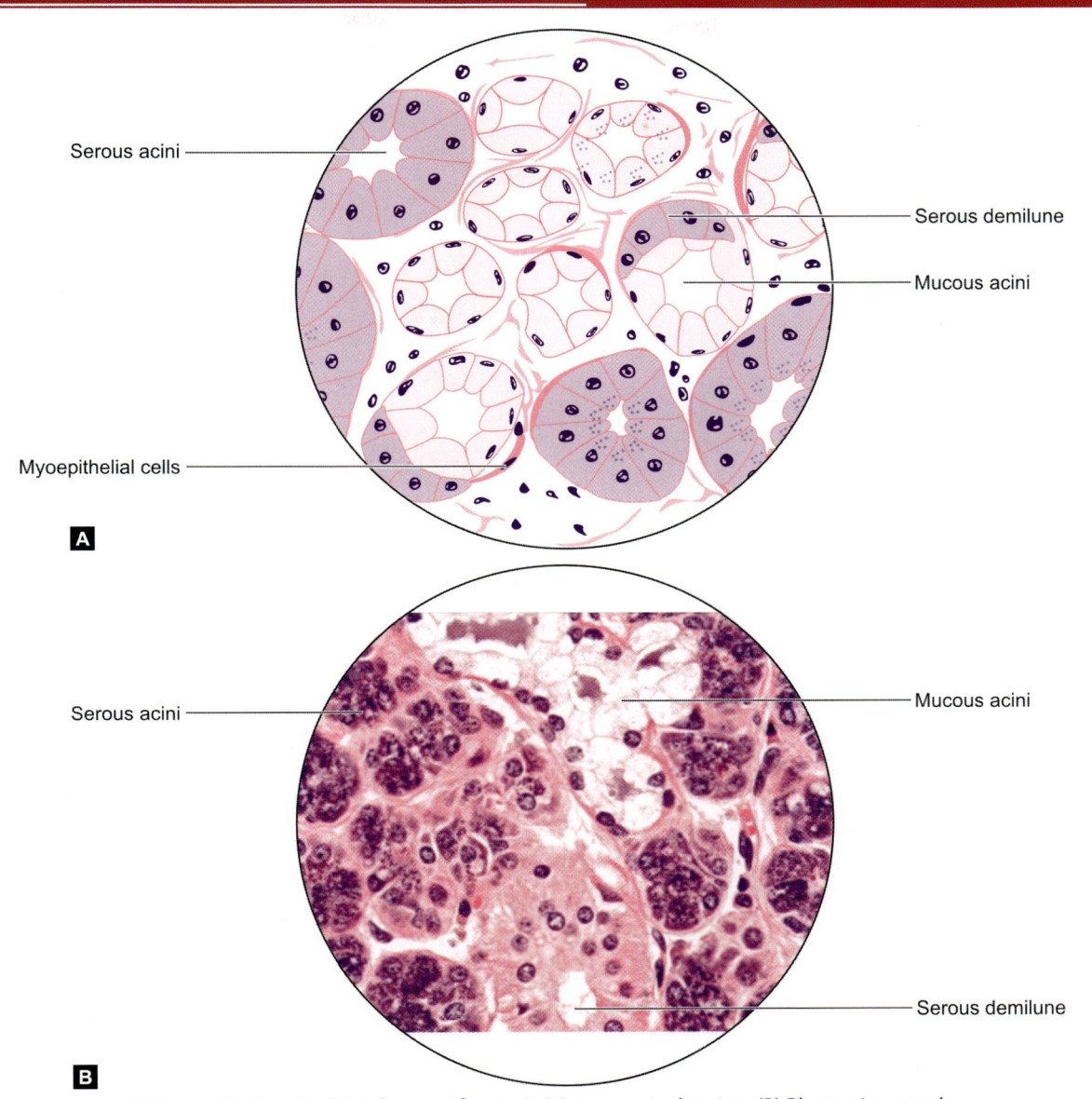

Serous acini
Serous demilune
Mucous acini
Myoepithelial cells

A

Serous acini
Mucous acini
Serous demilune

B

Submandibular gland (High magnification): (A) As seen in drawing; (B) Photomicrograph.

Points of identification
- In the high power view the serous and mucous acini can be identified by their staining reaction, and shape and position of nucleus
- The serous acini are darkly stained and have rounded nucleus placed near the center of the cell
- The mucous acini are lightly stained with flat nucleus placed toward the basement membrane
- The mucous acini are often associated with darkly stained crescentic patch of serous cells called serous demilune.

Plate 12.4: Sublingual salivary gland

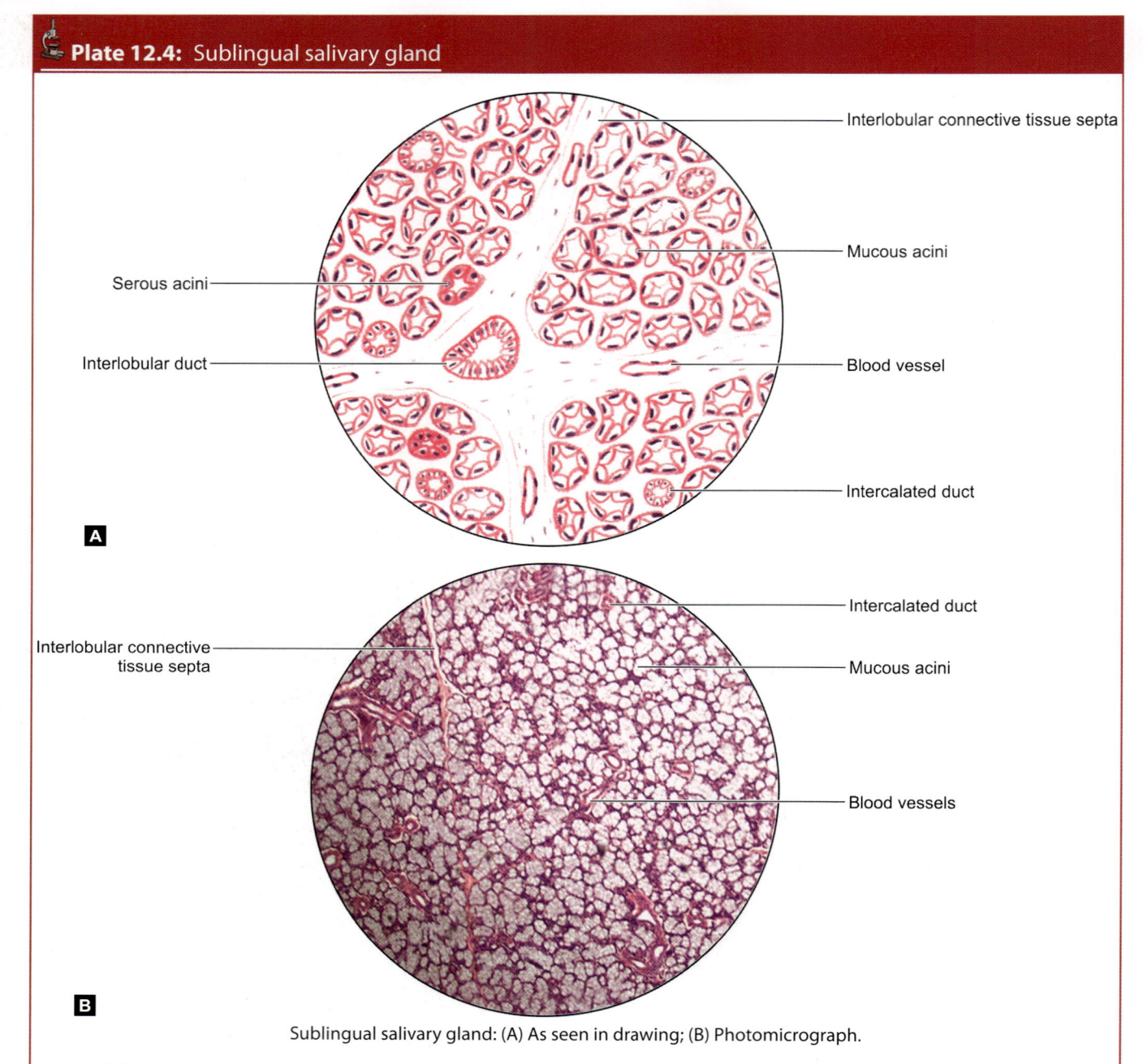

Sublingual salivary gland: (A) As seen in drawing; (B) Photomicrograph.

Labels in (A): Interlobular connective tissue septa; Mucous acini; Serous acini; Interlobular duct; Blood vessel; Intercalated duct.

Labels in (B): Intercalated duct; Mucous acini; Interlobular connective tissue septa; Blood vessels.

Points of identification
- The sublingual gland is predominantly a mucous gland but few serous acini may also be seen
- Serous demilunes may be present.

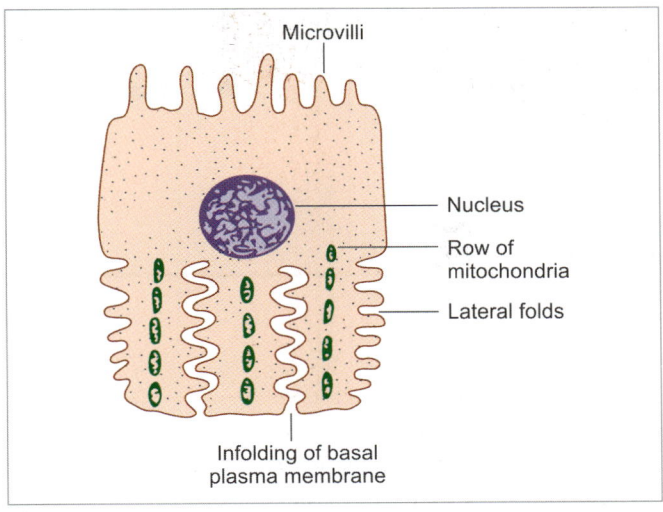

CHAPTER 12: Salivary Glands

Fig. 12.3: Electron microscopic structure of a cell from striated duct (schematic representation).

Sublingual Salivary Gland (Plate 12.4)

❖ It is also a compound, mixed tubuloacinar gland. Mucous acini are predominantly seen with few serous acini. The light-stained mucous acini are conspicuous in the section.

❖ In comparison with other salivary glands, the duct system of the sublingual gland is somewhat different. The intercalated ducts are short or absent, and not easily visualized in the section. In contrast, the nonstriated intralobular excretory ducts are more prevalent in the sublingual glands. The interlobular connective tissue septa are abundant in the sublingual compared to other two.

APPLIED HISTOLOGY

Tumors of salivary glands are common in the major salivary glands. Majority of them are benign and originate in the parotid gland (pleomorphic adenoma).

MULTIPLE CHOICE QUESTIONS

1. About 60% of the saliva is secreted in oral cavity by_____.
   a. Parotid
   b. Submandibular
   c. Sublingual
   d. Lingual
2. Nuhn's glands are located in the region of:
   a. Buccal
   b. Palatal
   c. Lingual
   d. Labial
3. Salivary gland is unique in that, its secretion is controlled by:
   a. Hormones
   b. Nerves
   c. Chemicals
   d. All of the above
4. Sublingual gland is ____ type of gland.
   a. Serous
   b. Mucous
   c. Mixed
   d. None of the above
5. Which of the following is correct about serous glands?
   a. They are specialized for the synthesis, storage, and secretion of proteins
   b. They contain secretory granules in the apical cytoplasm, and the secretion of granule content occurs by exocytosis
   c. Serous cells are pyramidal in shape
   d. All of the above
6. Serous demilunes are seen in the gland of:
   a. Pancreas
   b. Submandibular
   c. Liver
   d. Gastric
7. Identify this: 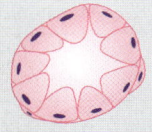
   a. Serous acini
   b. Mucous acini
   c. Serous demilunes
   d. Intercalated duct

Answers

1. b 2. c 3. d 4. b 5. d 6. b 7. b

CHAPTER 13

Placenta and Umbilical Cord

Learning objectives

To study the:
- Structure and functions of placenta
- Components and formation of placenta
- Placental circulation and barrier
- Microscopic structure
- Applied histology
- Umbilical cord

IDENTIFICATION POINTS

Placenta	Umbilical cord
☐ Section of tertiary villi of various sizes and shapes are seen ☐ Intervillous space containing maternal blood ☐ Anchoring villi, floating villi are seen ☐ Section of tertiary villi has core of mesoderm surrounded by cytotrophoblast and syncytiotrophoblast.	☐ Amnion lining the section of cord is made of simple squamous, cuboidal epithelium ☐ Two umbilical arteries and one umbilical vein are seen ☐ *Wharton's jelly*—mucoid connective tissue is seen.

PLACENTA

INTRODUCTION

Placenta is a fetomaternal organ. It connects growing fetus to the wall of gravid uterus. It is a disk-shaped organ and weighs 500 g. It has two surfaces—(1) An irregular maternal surface that is divided into 15–20 small lobules called maternal cotyledons and (2) A smooth fetal surface covered with amnion. The umbilical cord is attached at or near the center of this surface (Fig. 13.1).

FUNCTIONS

a. **Nutrition**: It maintains nutrition of the fetus through blood vessels that travel in the umbilical cord. It has several functions that facilitate growth of the fetus. It acts as a temporary organ that allows transport of oxygen and nutrients from the mother to the developing fetus.
b. **Excretion**: It eliminates carbon dioxide and waste products like urea from fetus into the maternal circulation.
c. **Immunological barrier**: Maternal immunoglobulin protects fetus against some infections.
d. **Barrier function**: It acts as a selective barrier allowing transfer of substances that facilitate growth and development of embryo. It prevents entry of harmful substances including certain drugs, viruses, and toxins.
e. **Hormone production**: Placenta synthesizes several hormones. The progesterone secreted helps to maintain the pregnancy after 4th month and estrogens secreted promotes uterine growth, development of mammary gland.

COMPONENTS

It is a disk-shaped organ having structural components of fetal and maternal origins.

The maternal component is contributed by decidua and fetal component by chorion.

Decidua

❖ The uterine endometrium is called decidua after the attachment (implantation) of fertilized embryo (blastocyst) to it (Fig. 13.2).

CHAPTER 13: Placenta and Umbilical Cord

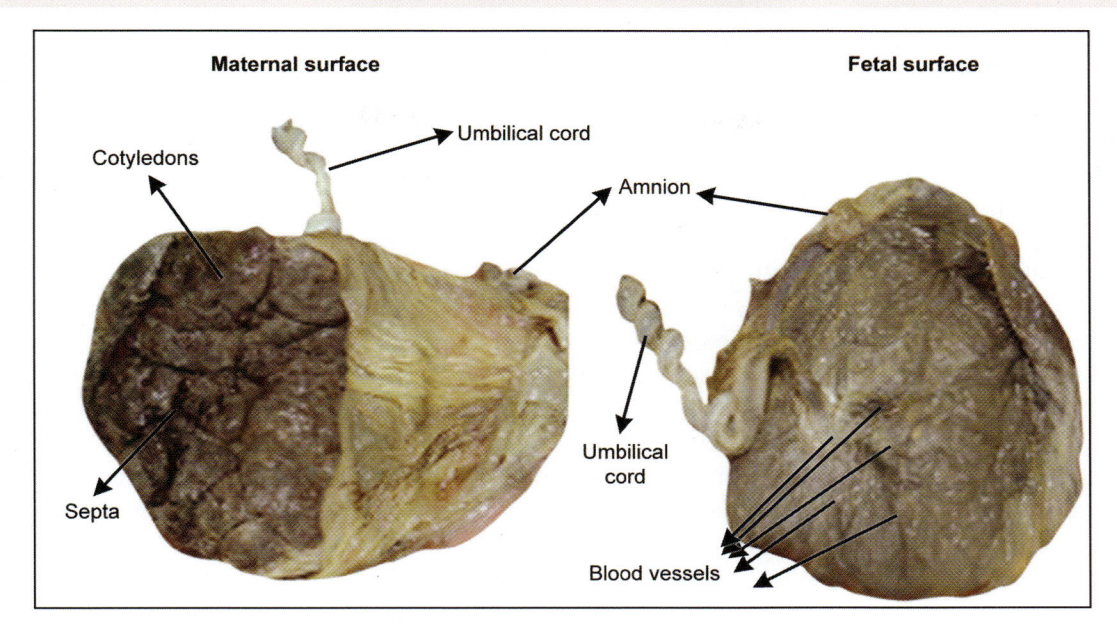

Fig. 13.1: Maternal and fetal surfaces of placenta showing maternal cotyledons and attachment of umbilical cord.

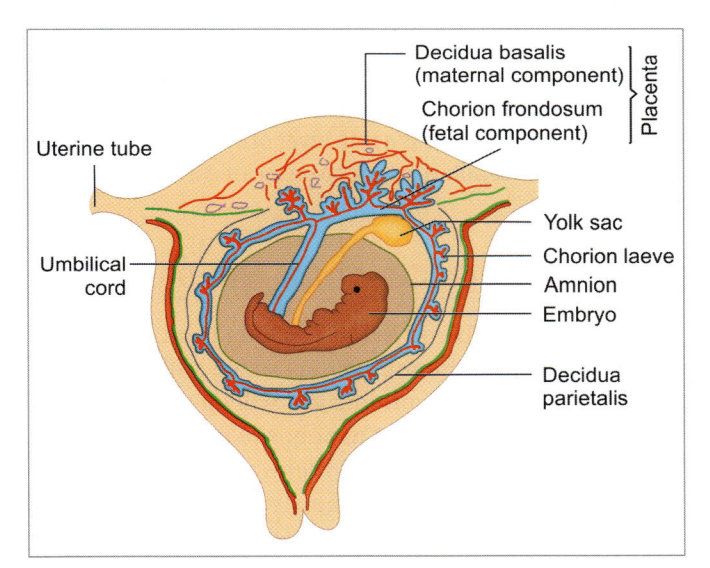

Fig. 13.2: Implantation and growing embryo in the wall of uterus.

- *Parts of decidua*: The endometrium (decidua) that contributes for placenta is called decidua and its parts are:
    - *Decidua basalis*: Part contributing for placenta
    - *Decidua capsularis*: Part surrounding embryo
    - *Decidua parietalis*: Part lining the cavity of uterus.

Chorion and Trophoblast

- The fertilized ovum undergoes series of cleavage divisions increasing the number of cells (blastomeres) that get reorganized into peripheral trophoblast and inner embryoblast. The embryoblast gives rise to the embryo.

- The trophoblast along with adjacent extraembryonic mesoderm contributes to the formation of chorion all around the developing embryo. Later blood vessels develop in the extraembryonic mesoderm forming chorionic vessels.
- That part of chorion coming in contact with decidua basalis is called chorion frondosum whereas the part in contact with decidua capsularis is called chorion laeve (Fig. 13.2).
- *Parts of chorion*:
    - *Chorion frondosum*: Contributes for fetal component of placenta
    - *Chorion laeve*: Covers the decidua capsularis.
- The trophoblast presents outer layer of syncytiotrophoblast and an inner layer of cytotrophoblast. The syncytiotrophoblast contains number of cell layers without cellular outlines. The cytotrophoblast consists of single layer of cuboidal cells.

FORMATION OF PLACENTA

- The maternal part of placenta is contributed by decidua basalis of endometrium that sends septa dividing it into 15–20 maternal cotyledons.
- The fetal part is contributed by chorion frondosum that is seen as a plate called **chorionic plate**. From the chorionic plate, 40–60 extensions fetal cotyledons arise and extend toward the maternal part called **decidua basalis**.

- Each extension is called **stem villus/truncus chorii** that shows ramifications into number of branches (ramus chorii, ramuli chorii) like the branches of a tree. Their terminal ramifications are called **chorionic villi** (Fig. 13.3).
- Villi attached to decidua basalis are called **anchoring villi**. Villi in the intervillous spaces bathed by maternal blood are called **floating villi**. The structural components of chorionic villous differs at different stages of embryonic development are of three types. The primary villi have innermost cytotrophoblast surrounded by Syncytiotrophoblast, while secondary villi have in addition a central core extraembryonic mesoderm; tertiary villi have three layers–an outer trophoblast (cyto and syncytio), middle layer of extraembryonic mesoderm with central core of chorionic vessels.
- The villi are separated by irregular spaces called **intervillous spaces**.

MICROSCOPIC STRUCTURE

- Microscopic structure of placenta at term present cut sections of tertiary villi of different sizes and shapes with maternal blood cells in between villi (Plate 13.1).
- If a section contains chorionic plate and amniotic membrane, extraembryonic mesoderm with blood vessels can be identified.
- Each villous has a central core of mesoderm with fetal capillaries lined with simple squamous epithelium and containing nucleated fetal red blood cell (RBC). In addition, macrophages (Hofbauer cells) and fibroblasts are present in the mesodermal core. It is covered with thin layer of intensely stained syncytiotrophoblast and discontinuously arranged cytotrophoblast (Fig. 13.4). Because of the disappearance of cytotrophoblast and thinning of syncytiotrophoblast, the fetal capillaries move toward the periphery thereby reducing the thickness of placental barrier.
- In **early placenta** at low magnification, a large numbers of villi projecting into the lacunae filled with maternal blood are seen; some villi show evidence of branching. Higher magnification shows a core of primitive mesenchyme invested by an inner layer of cytotrophoblast cells and an outer syncytiotrophoblast layer (Fig. 13.4).
- The **term placenta** at low magnification shows a huge numbers of villi cut in various planes and varying in diameter from large main stem villi to very small terminal branch villi. The villous pattern get highly developed and extensive branched as the placenta enlarges. Term placenta also shows the syncytial knots formed by syncytiotrophoblast nuclei that are aggregated together in clusters leaving zones of thin cytoplasm devoid of nuclei between.
- The proximity of blood in fetal capillaries to maternal blood reduces. There is a thin layer of syncytiotrophoblast only and the capillaries tend to be located in the periphery of the villi.

PLACENTAL CIRCULATION AND BARRIER

The circulation of blood in the placenta is unique in that maternal blood in the intervillous space and fetal blood in fetal capillaries of chorionic villi will be traversing side by side without mixing and in opposite directions. Yet the exchange takes place between the two circulations by the process of diffusion across the structural components forming the villi known as **blood placental barrier**.

Blood Placental Barrier

The tissues intervening between maternal and fetal blood constitutes the barrier. The exchange of gases, nutrients, and waste products occurs across this barrier. The thickness of the barrier reduces with progression of pregnancy to facilitate the increased efficiency of transport across the membrane to growing fetus.

At Early Pregnancy

Structures constituting the barrier from maternal to fetal blood are as follows:

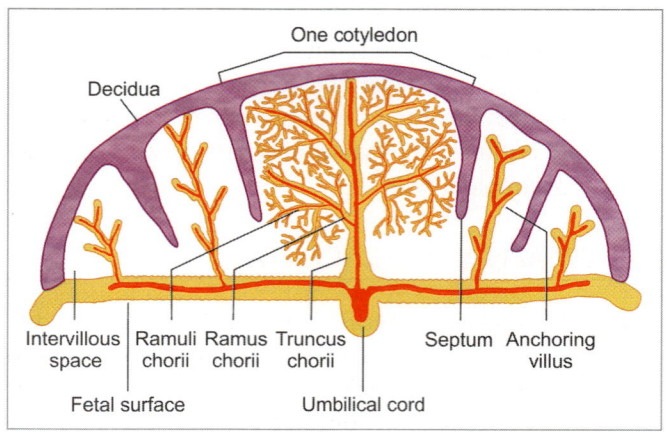

Fig. 13.3: Figure showing maternal and fetal components of placenta and cotyledons. Ramifications of fetal cotyledons are: Anchoring villi, truncus chorii, ramus chorii, ramuli chorii, floating villi in intervillous space.

CHAPTER 13: Placenta and Umbilical Cord

Plate 13.1: Placenta (Low magnification)

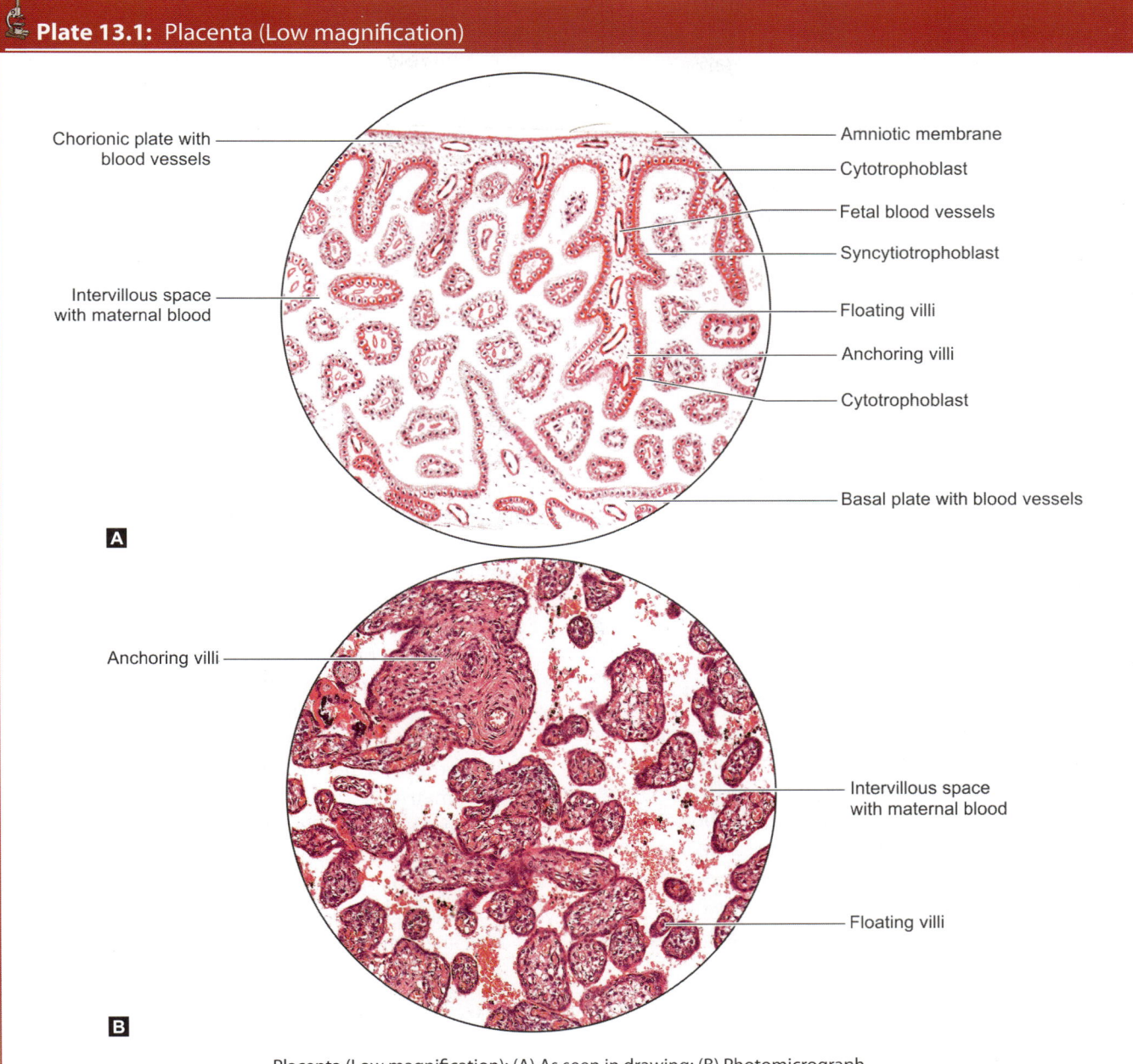

Placenta (Low magnification): (A) As seen in drawing; (B) Photomicrograph.

Points of identification
- Tertiary villi of various size and shapes seen
- Inter villous space containing maternal blood
- Truncus chorii, ramus chorii, ramuli chorii and floating villi in intervillous space seen
- Section of tertiary villi has core of mesoderm surrounded by cyto- and syncytiotrophoblast.

- Endothelium of fetal blood vessels and its basement membrane
- Mesoderm
- Cytotrophoblast and its basement membrane
- Syncytiotrophoblast.

At Term
Barrier gets thinner and improves the efficiency of exchange.
- Cytotrophoblast disappears
- Syncytiotrophoblast becomes thinner

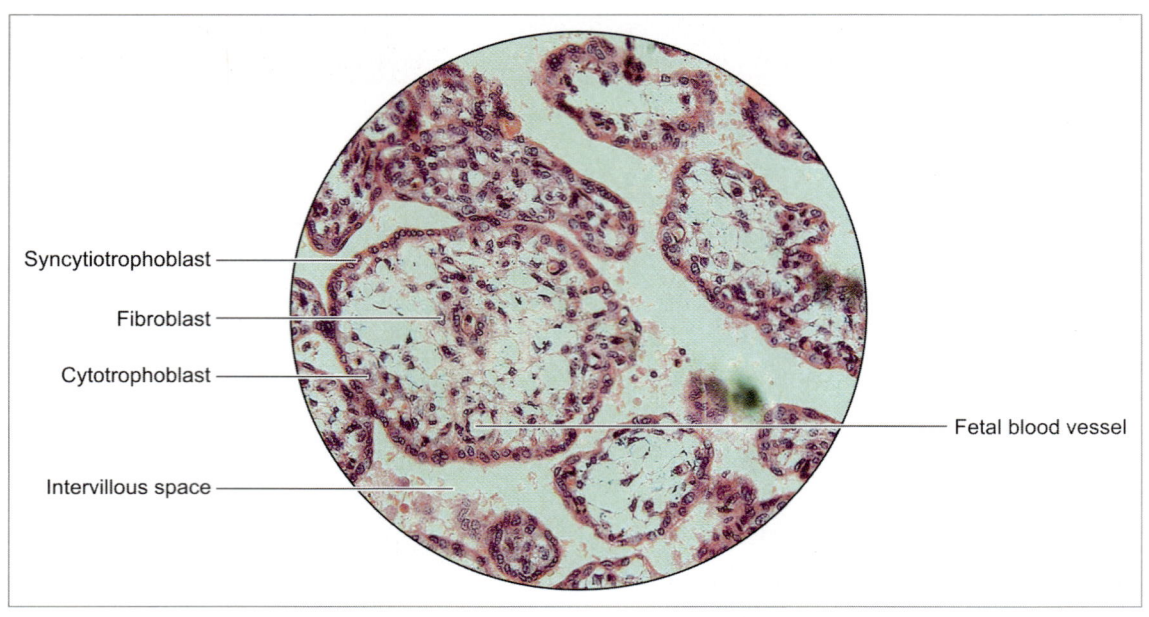

Fig. 13.4: Photomicrograph of sections of floating tertiary villi at high magnification.

- Connective tissue core gets edematous
- Fetal blood vessels move to periphery.

APPLIED HISTOLOGY

- **Abortions:** Initially corpus luteum of pregnancy secretes hormone progesterone and continues pregnancy. Once placenta is formed it takes over the function to maintain pregnancy. Any derangement during switch over might cause termination of pregnancy, hence abortion.
- **Placental insufficiency:** Placenta is essential for growth of the fetus and any abnormality hamper growth and development. Early pregnancy changes can lead to reduction in growth of the fetus, termed 'intrauterine growth restriction'(IUGR) several medical conditions can lead to placental insufficiency and IUGR: Maternal malnutrition, diabetes, twin or triplet pregnancies, pre-eclampsia or eclampsia, infections and abnormal implantation of the placenta in the uterus.
- **Structural placental abnormalities:**
  - *Placenta accreta:* The placenta attaches too deeply into the uterine wall but does not penetrate the myometrium.
  - *Placenta increta:* Placental villi penetrate deep into the muscular layer of the myometrium.
  - *Placenta percreta:* Penetrates through the entire uterine wall and attaches to another organ such as the bladder, rectum, intestines, or large blood vessels.

UMBILICAL CORD

INTRODUCTION

Umbilical cord is a tubular structure that connects developing fetus with placenta. This helps to conduit oxygen and nutrients from mother and takes away the fetal waste products.

- At birth, one end of the cord is attached to the anterior abdominal wall of the fetus and other end at fetal surface of placenta. The folding of embryo leads to formation of connecting stalk. It gets surrounded by a sleeve of amnion thus, forming umbilical cord.
- At full term, it is around 50 cm in length. But the length may vary. It is twisted to forming knots which may be due to movements of the fetus.

Microscopic Section of Umbilical Cord (Fig. 13.5)

- The cross-section of umbilical cord shows a covering of single-layered amnion which is simple cuboidal epithelium.
- It is filled with a gelatinous or mucous connective tissue, called as Wharton's jelly. This stroma supports the blood vessels and is derived from primary mesoderm. The

CHAPTER 13: Placenta and Umbilical Cord

ground substance is made up of primarily hyaluronic acid and chondroitin sulfate with a low abundance of collagen or reticular fibers.
- The mucoid connective tissue consists of a wide-meshed network of long, stretched fibrocytes made up of many interconnecting cell processes. They are stellate and spindle-like mesenchymal cells (indistinguishable from resting fibroblasts).
- The gelatinous tissue is embedded with a single umbilical vein and the two umbilical arteries. The umbilical arteries have thick muscular walls with double-layered muscular walls without an elastic layer. They carry deoxygenated blood from the fetus to the placenta. Umbilical veins deliver oxygenated blood from the placenta to the fetus. It has a thick layer of circular smooth muscle unlike adult veins that characteristically show thick longitudinal layer. In early pregnancy, umbilical veins are two in number but later right umbilical vein disappears.
- The remnant of allantois may be seen in the center.

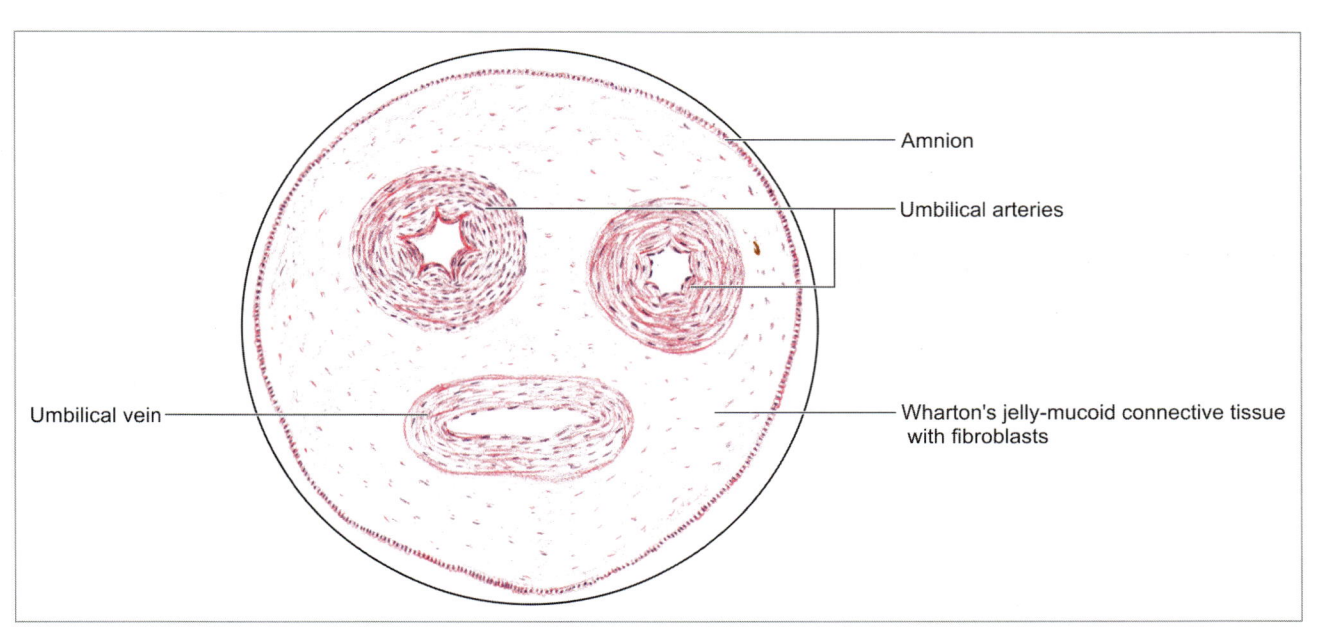

Fig. 13.5: Photomicrograph of umbilical cord.

MULTIPLE CHOICE QUESTIONS

1. The following feature is found in a primary placental villus:
   a. Cytotrophoblast cells filling the central core of a villus
   b. Fetal capillaries
   c. Mesodermal core
   d. Outer covering of syncytiotrophoblast
2. The portion of the decidua where the placenta is to be formed:
   a. Decidua basalis   b. Decidua capsularis
   c. Decidua parietalis   d. All of the above
3. Human placenta is:
   a. Epitheliochorial   b. Hemoendothelial
   c. Hemochorial   d. Syndesmochorial
4. Intervillous space contains:
   a. Maternal blood   b. Fetal blood
   c. Amniotic fluid   d. Cerebrospinal fluid
5. The connective tissue in umbilical cord is:
   a. Sclerous   b. Fluid
   c. Mucoid   d. Loose

Answers
   1. a   2. a   3. c   4. a   5. c

CHAPTER 14

Respiratory System

Learning objectives

To study the:
- Structure of nasal cavity, pharynx
- Structure of larynx (epiglottis)
- Structure of bronchial tree
- Lung—composition, microscopic structures, alveoli
- Applied histology

IDENTIFICATION POINTS

Epiglottis	*Trachea*	*Lung*
☐ Lined by pseudostratified ciliated columnar epithelium ☐ Lamina propria with serous and mucous glands ☐ Central core of elastic tissue.	☐ Pseudostratified ciliated columnar epithelium with goblet cells ☐ Lamina propria ☐ Submucosa with serous and mucous glands ☐ Presence of hyaline cartilage and trachealis muscle.	☐ Presence of alveolar ducts ☐ Alveolar sac lined by simple squamous epithelium ☐ Presence of intrapulmonary bronchus with varying amount of islands cartilage and smooth muscles ☐ Respiratory bronchioles with simple cuboidal epithelial lining lacking cilia and goblet cells.

INTRODUCTION

The respiratory system consists of:
- Conducting part that includes the nasal cavities, the pharynx, the trachea, the bronchi, and their intrapulmonary continuations, responsible for providing passage of air and conditioning the inspired air.
- Respiratory part that includes the lungs is involved in the exchange of oxygen and carbon dioxide between blood and inspired air.

COMMON FEATURES OF AIR PASSAGES

- Their walls have a skeletal framework made up of bone, cartilage, and connective tissue, which keeps the passages always patent.
- Smooth muscle present in the walls of the trachea and bronchi enables some alterations in the size of the lumen.
- The interior of the passages is lined over most of its extent by pseudostratified, ciliated, and columnar epithelium.
- The epithelium is kept moist by the secretions of numerous serous glands.
- Numerous goblet cells and mucous glands cover the epithelium with a protective mucoid secretion that serves to trap dust particles present in inhaled air.
- This mucous (along with the dust particles in it) is constantly moved toward the pharynx by the action of cilia.
- When excessive mucous accumulates, it is brought out by coughing, or is swallowed.
- Deep to the mucosa, there are numerous blood vessels that serve to warm the inspired air.

NASAL CAVITIES

- The nasal cavity is the beginning of the respiratory system.
- These are paired chambers separated by septum.
- It extends from the nostrils in front to the posterior nasal apertures behind.
- Each nasal cavity is a hollow organ composed of bone, cartilage, and connective tissue covered by mucous membrane.

Histologically, the wall of each half of the nasal cavity is divisible into three distinct regions.
1. Vestibule
2. Olfactory mucosa
3. Respiratory mucosa.

CHAPTER 14: Respiratory System

Vestibule
- It is the anterior dilated part of the nasal cavity.
- The *vestibule* is lined by skin continuous with that on the exterior of the nose.
- Hair and sebaceous glands are present.

Olfactory Mucosa
- Apart from their respiratory function, the nasal cavities serve as end organs for smell.
- Receptors for smell are located in the *olfactory mucosa* which is confined to a relatively small area on the superior nasal concha, and on the adjoining part of the nasal septum.
- Olfactory mucosa is yellow in color, in contrast to the pink color of the respiratory mucosa.
- It consists of a lining epithelium and a lamina propria.
- The *olfactory epithelium* is pseudostratified epithelium made of olfactory cells, sustentacular cells, and basal cells.

Respiratory Mucosa
The rest of the wall of each half of the nasal cavity is covered by *respiratory mucosa* lined by pseudostratified ciliated columnar epithelium. In the epithelium, the following cells are present (Fig. 14.1):
- *Ciliated cells* are the columnar cells with cilia on their free surfaces and are the most abundant cell type.
- *Goblet cells* (flask-shaped cells) scattered in the epithelium produce mucous.
- *Nonciliated columnar cells* with microvilli on the free surface probably secrete a serous fluid that keeps the mucosa moist.
- *Basal cells* lying near the basal lamina help to replace those lost cells.

Lamina Propria
The lamina propria of nasal mucosa contains lymphocytes, plasma cells, macrophages, a few neutrophils, and eosinophils. Eosinophils increase greatly in number in persons suffering from allergic rhinitis.

PHARYNX
- The pharynx consists of nasal, oral, and laryngeal parts.
- The nasal part is purely respiratory in function, but the oral and laryngeal parts are more intimately concerned with the alimentary system.
- The wall of the pharynx is fibromuscular.
- In the nasopharynx, the epithelial lining is ciliated columnar, or pseudostratified ciliated columnar. The inferior surface of the soft palate and over the oropharynx and laryngopharynx, the epithelium is stratified squamous.
- Subepithelial aggregations of lymphoid tissue are present on the posterior wall of the nasopharynx, and around the orifices of the auditory tubes, forming the nasopharyngeal and tubal tonsils.
- Numerous mucous glands are present in the submucosa, including that of the soft palate.

LARYNX
- Larynx is a specialized organ responsible for the production of voice. It houses the vocal cords. The wall of the larynx has a complex structure made up of a number of cartilages, membranes, and muscles.
- The epithelium lining the mucous membrane of the larynx is predominantly pseudostratified ciliated columnar, but in some parts that come in contact with swallowed food, the epithelium is lined by stratified squamous (anterior surface and upper part of the posterior surface of epiglottis, and the upper parts of the aryepiglottic folds, vocal folds).
- Numerous goblet cells and subepithelial mucous glands provide a mucous covering to the epithelium.

Cartilages of the Larynx
The larynx has a cartilaginous framework which is made of nine cartilages (three paired and three unpaired) that are connected to each other by membranes and ligaments

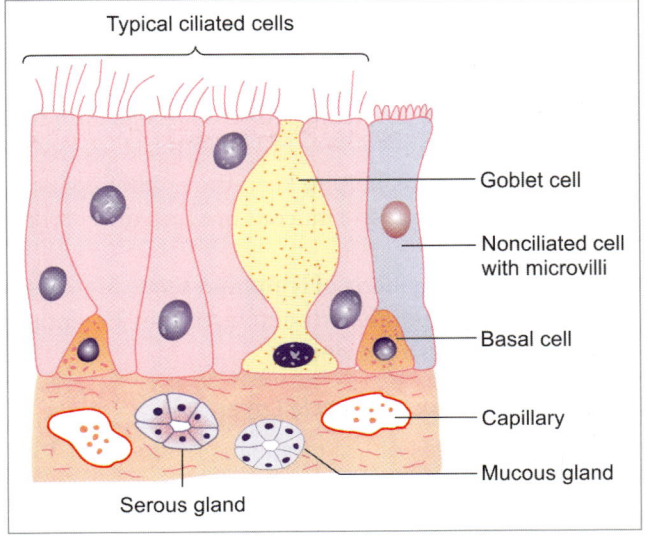

Fig. 14.1: Structure of respiratory part of nasal mucosa (schematic representation).

(Fig. 14.2). The cartilages are either hyaline or elastic in nature. These are as follows:
- ❖ *Hyaline cartilages*:
  - Thyroid (unpaired)
  - Cricoid (unpaired)
  - Arytenoid (paired).
- ❖ *Elastic cartilages*:
  - Epiglottis (unpaired)
  - Cuneiform (paired)
  - Corniculate (paired).

With advancing age, calcification may occur in hyaline cartilage, but not in elastic cartilage.

Epiglottis
- ❖ The epiglottis has a central core of elastic cartilage.
- ❖ Overlying the cartilage, there is mucous membrane.
- ❖ The greater part of the mucous membrane is lined by stratified squamous epithelium (nonkeratinizing).
- ❖ The mucous membrane over the lower part of the posterior surface of the epiglottis is lined by pseudostratified ciliated columnar epithelium. Some taste buds are present in the epithelium of the epiglottis.
- ❖ Numerous glands, predominantly mucous, are present in the mucosa deep to the epithelium. Some of them lie in depressions present on the epiglottic cartilage (Plate 14.1).

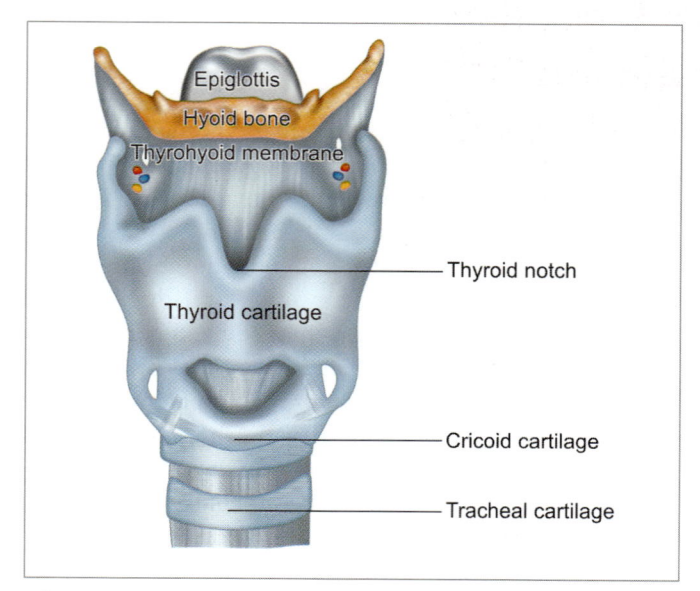

Fig. 14.2: Anterior view of the larynx (schematic representation).

TRACHEA AND PRINCIPAL BRONCHI

Trachea
- ❖ Trachea extends from the lower border of cricoid cartilage (C6) to its level of bifurcation (T4) into right and left bronchi.
- ❖ The trachea is a fibroelastic cartilaginous tube. The trachea consists of four layers (Plate 14.2).

Mucosa
- ❖ Mucosa of the tracheal lumen is lined by pseudostratified ciliated columnar epithelium. It also contains goblet cells, brush cells, small granule cell, and basal cells that lie next to the basement membrane. Numerous lymphocytes are seen in deeper parts of the epithelium.
- ❖ Cells: (a) **Ciliated cells**—the most numerous extending through the full thickness of the epithelium. They create mucociliary current to remove the inhaled dust particles, (b) **Brush cells**—they are columnar cells that bear blunt microvilli, (c) **Small granule cells (Kulchitsky cells)**—they are like enteroendocrine cells of gastrointestinal tract (GIT), secrete catecholamine, serotonin, etc., (d) **Mucous cells**—they are similar in appearance to intestinal goblet interspersed among the ciliated cells and also extend through the full thickness of the epithelium, and (e) **Basal cells**—reserve cells.
- ❖ Basement membrane is thick.
- ❖ Lamina propria contains lymphocytes, eosinophils, plasma cells, and fibroblasts with diffuse and nodular lymphatic aggregation[bronchus-associated lymphoid tissue (BALT)].

Submucosa
- ❖ The subepithelial connective tissue contains numerous elastic fibers.
- ❖ Submucosal glands help to keep the epithelium moist and provide a covering of mucous in which dust particles get caught.
- ❖ Numerous aggregations of lymphoid tissue are present in the subepithelial connective tissue. Eosinophil leukocytes are also present.

Cartilage and Smooth Muscle Layer
- ❖ The skeletal basis of the trachea is made up of 16–20 tracheal cartilages.

CHAPTER 14: Respiratory System

Plate 14.1: Epiglottis

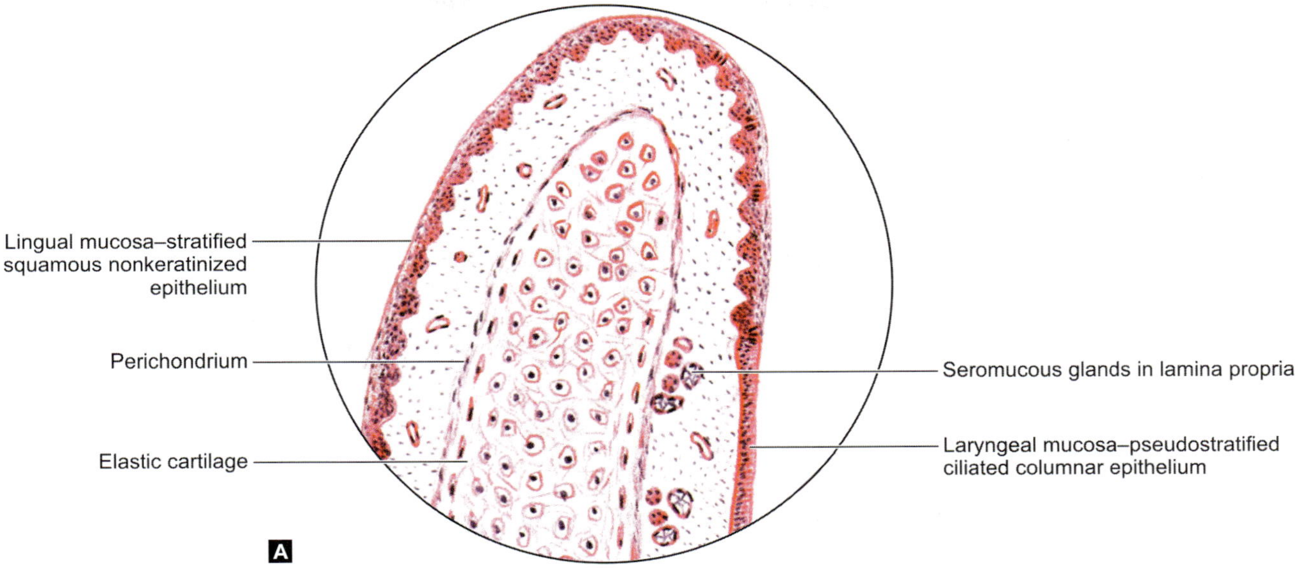

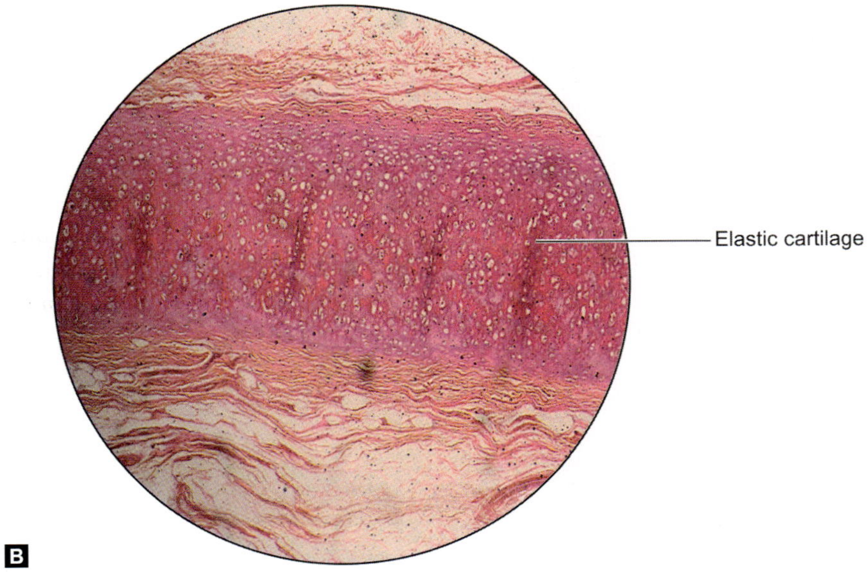

Labels (A):
- Lingual mucosa–stratified squamous nonkeratinized epithelium
- Perichondrium
- Elastic cartilage
- Seromucous glands in lamina propria
- Laryngeal mucosa–pseudostratified ciliated columnar epithelium

Labels (B):
- Elastic cartilage

Epiglottis: (A) As seen in drawing; (B) Photomicrograph.

Points of identification
- Lined by pseudostratified ciliated columnar epithelium
- Lamina propria with serous and mucous glands
- Central core of elastic tissue.

Textbook of Human Histology

Plate 14.2: Trachea

Trachea: (A) As seen in drawing; (B) Photomicrograph.

Points of identification
- Pseudostratified ciliated columnar epithelium with goblet cells
- Lamina propria
- Submucosa with serous and mucous glands
- Presence of hyaline cartilage and trachealis muscle.

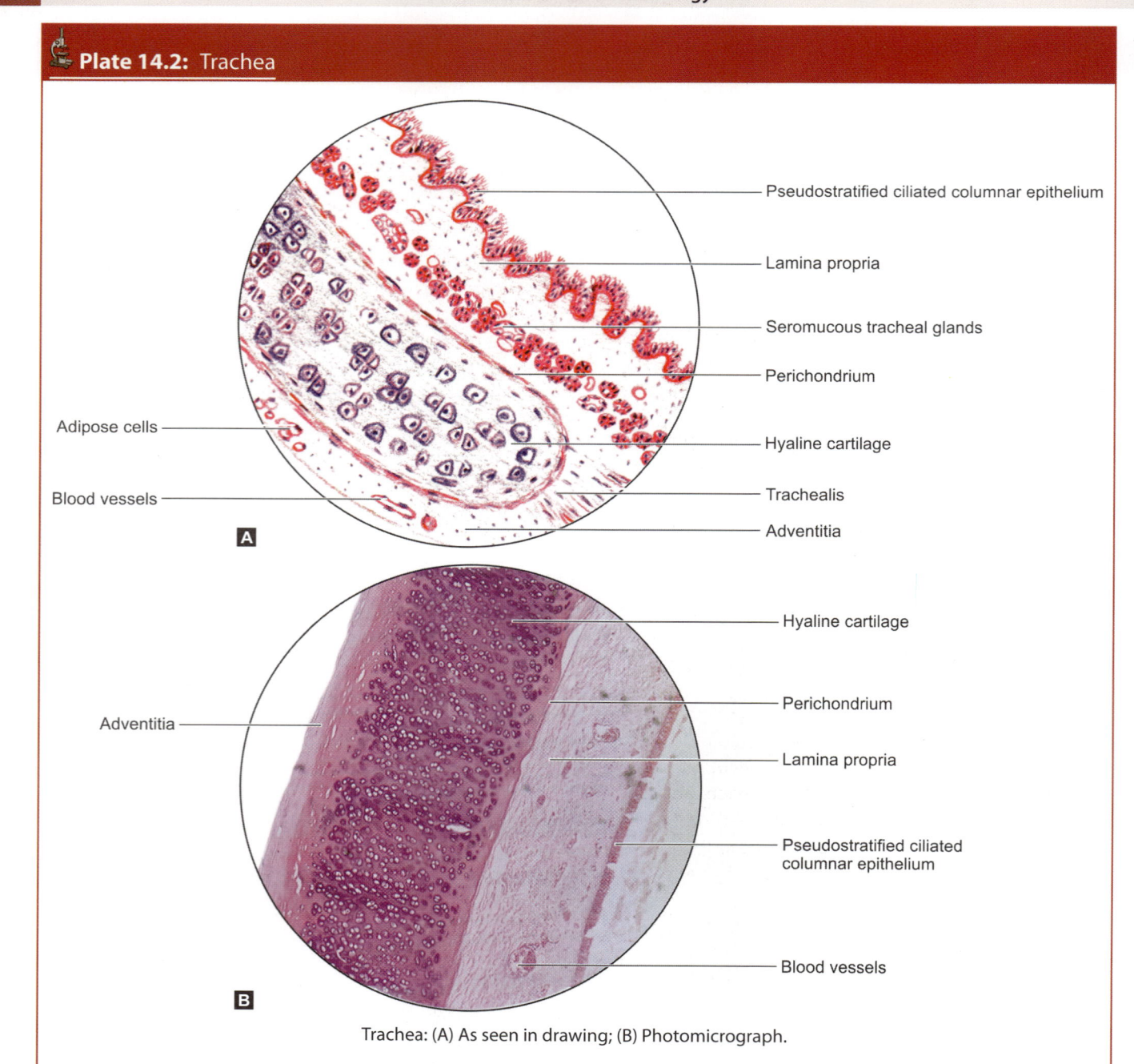

- ❖ Each of these is a C-shaped mass of hyaline cartilage.
- ❖ The open end of the "C" is directed posteriorly. The gaps between the cartilage ends, present on the posterior aspect, are filled in by smooth muscle and fibrous tissue.
- ❖ The intervals between the cartilages are filled by fibrous tissue that becomes continuous with the perichondrium covering the cartilages.
- ❖ The connective tissue in the wall of the trachea contains many elastic fibers.

Adventitia

It is made of fibroelastic connective tissue containing blood vessels and nerves.

Principal Bronchi

The trachea divides at the level of T4 into right and left principal bronchi (primary or main bronchi). They have a structure similar to that of the trachea.

LUNGS

The lungs are the principal respiratory organs that are situated on either side of mediastinum in the thoracic cavity. They are covered by visceral pleura. Structure of the lung includes the structure of intrapulmonary bronchial tree and alveoli.

Intrapulmonary Passages

- ❖ On entering the lung, the principal bronchus divides into secondary, or *lobar bronchi* (one for each lobe).
- ❖ Each lobar bronchus divides into tertiary, or *segmental bronchi* (one for each segment of the lobe).
- ❖ The segmental bronchi divide into smaller and smaller bronchi, which ultimately end in *bronchioles*.
- ❖ The lung substance is divided into numerous lobules each of which receives a *lobular bronchiole*.
- ❖ The lobular bronchiole gives off a number of *terminal bronchioles* (Fig. 14.3). As indicated by their name, the terminal bronchioles represent the most distal parts of the conducting passage.
- ❖ Each terminal bronchiole ends by dividing into *respiratory bronchioles*. These are so called because they are partly respiratory in function as some air sacs (*see* below) arise from them.
- ❖ Each respiratory bronchiole ends by dividing into a few *alveolar ducts*. Each alveolar duct ends in a passage, the *atrium*, which leads into a number of rounded *alveolar sacs*.
- ❖ Each alveolar sac is studded with a number of air sacs or *alveoli*. The alveoli are blind sacs having very thin walls through which oxygen passes from air into blood, and carbon dioxide passes from blood into air.

The structure of the larger intrapulmonary bronchi is similar to that of the trachea. As these bronchi divide into smaller ones, the following changes in structure are observed:

- ❖ The cartilages in the walls of the bronchi become irregular in shape and are progressively smaller.
- ❖ Cartilage is absent in the walls of bronchioles. This is the criterion that distinguishes a bronchiole from a bronchus.
- ❖ The amount of muscle in the bronchial wall increases as the bronchi become smaller. The presence of muscle in the walls of bronchi is of considerable clinical significance. Spasm of this muscle constricts the bronchi and can cause difficulty in breathing.

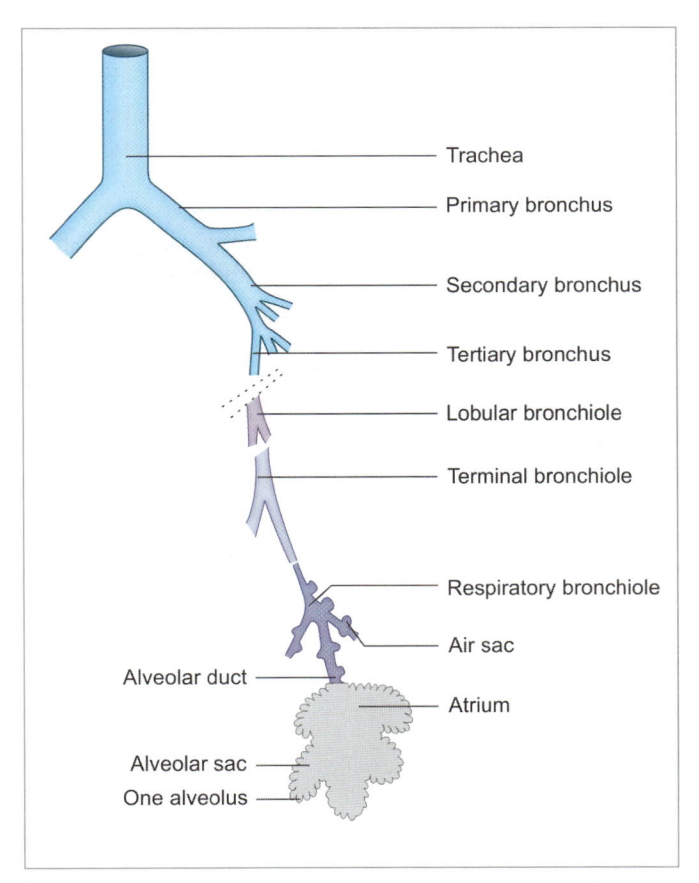

Fig. 14.3: Some terms used to describe the terminal ramifications of the bronchial tree (schematic representation).

- Subepithelial lymphoid tissue increases in quantity as bronchi become smaller. Glands become fewer and are absent in the walls of bronchioles.
- The trachea and larger bronchi are lined by pseudostratified ciliated columnar epithelium. As the bronchi become smaller, the epithelium first becomes simple ciliated columnar, then nonciliated columnar, and finally cuboidal (in respiratory bronchioles). The cells contain lysosomes and numerous mitochondria.
- Apart from typical ciliated columnar cells, various other types of cells are to be seen in the epithelium lining the air passages. They are goblet cells, nonciliated serous cells, basal cells, **cells of Clara** (nonciliated cells of terminal bronchiole) whose secretion reduces surface tension, and cells similar to diffuse endocrine cells of the gut (Figs. 14.4A to G).

The differences between bronchus and bronchioles are given in Table 14.1.

Alveoli

There are about 200 million alveoli in a normal lung. The total area of the alveolar surface of each lung is extensive. It has been estimated to be about 75 m². The total capillary surface area available for gaseous exchanges is about 125 m².

Structure of Alveolar Wall

- Each alveolus has a very thin wall. The wall is lined by simple squamous epithelium resting on the basement membrane (Plate 14.3).
- Deep to the basement membrane, there is a layer of delicate connective tissue through which pulmonary capillaries run. These capillaries have the usual endothelial lining that rests on a basement membrane.
- The barrier between air and blood is made up of the epithelial cells and their basement membrane, by endothelial cells and their basement membrane, and by intervening connective tissue. At many places, the two basement membranes fuse greatly reducing the thickness of the barrier.
- The endothelial cells lining the alveolar capillaries are remarkable for their extreme thinness.
- With the electron microscopy (EM), they are seen to have numerous projections extending into the capillary lumen. These projections greatly increase the surface of the cell membrane that is exposed to blood and is, therefore, available for the exchange of gases.
- At many places, the basement membrane of the endothelium fuses with that of the alveolar epithelium greatly reducing the thickness of the barrier between blood and air in alveoli.

Table 14.1: Differences between bronchus and bronchiole.

Characteristics	Bronchus	Bronchiole
Diameter	Larger diameter (more than 1 mm)	Smaller diameter (less than 1 mm)
Lining epithelium	Pseudostratified ciliated columnar epithelium with goblet cells	❑ *Large-sized bronchioles*: Simple columnar cells with few cilia and few goblet cells ❑ *Small-sized bronchioles*: Simple columnar or simple cuboidal cells with no cilia or no goblet cells
Smooth muscle layer	Present between mucosa and cartilage layer	Smooth muscles and elastic fibers form a well-defined layer beneath mucosa
Cartilage	Present in irregular patches	Absent
Glands in submucosa	Both serous and mucous acini present between cartilage and muscle layer	Absent

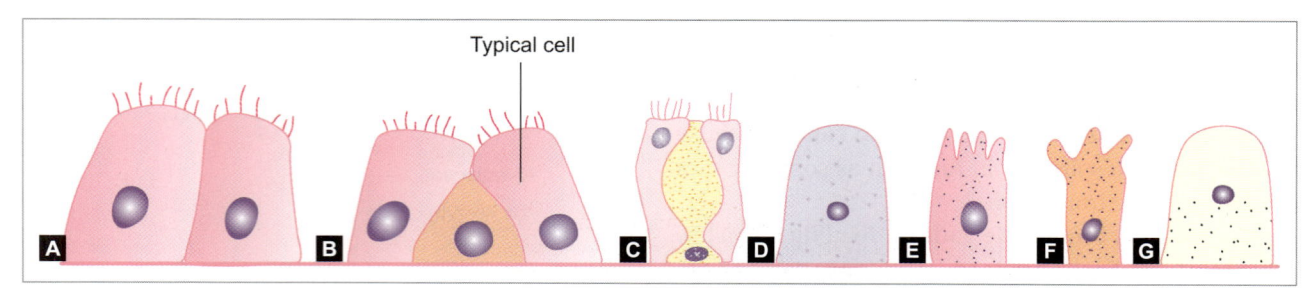

Figs. 14.4A to G: Various types of cells to be seen lining the respiratory passages: (A) Typical ciliated columnar; (B) Basal; (C) Goblet; (D) Serous; (E) Brush; (F) Clara; (G) Argyrophil (schematic representation).

CHAPTER 14: Respiratory System

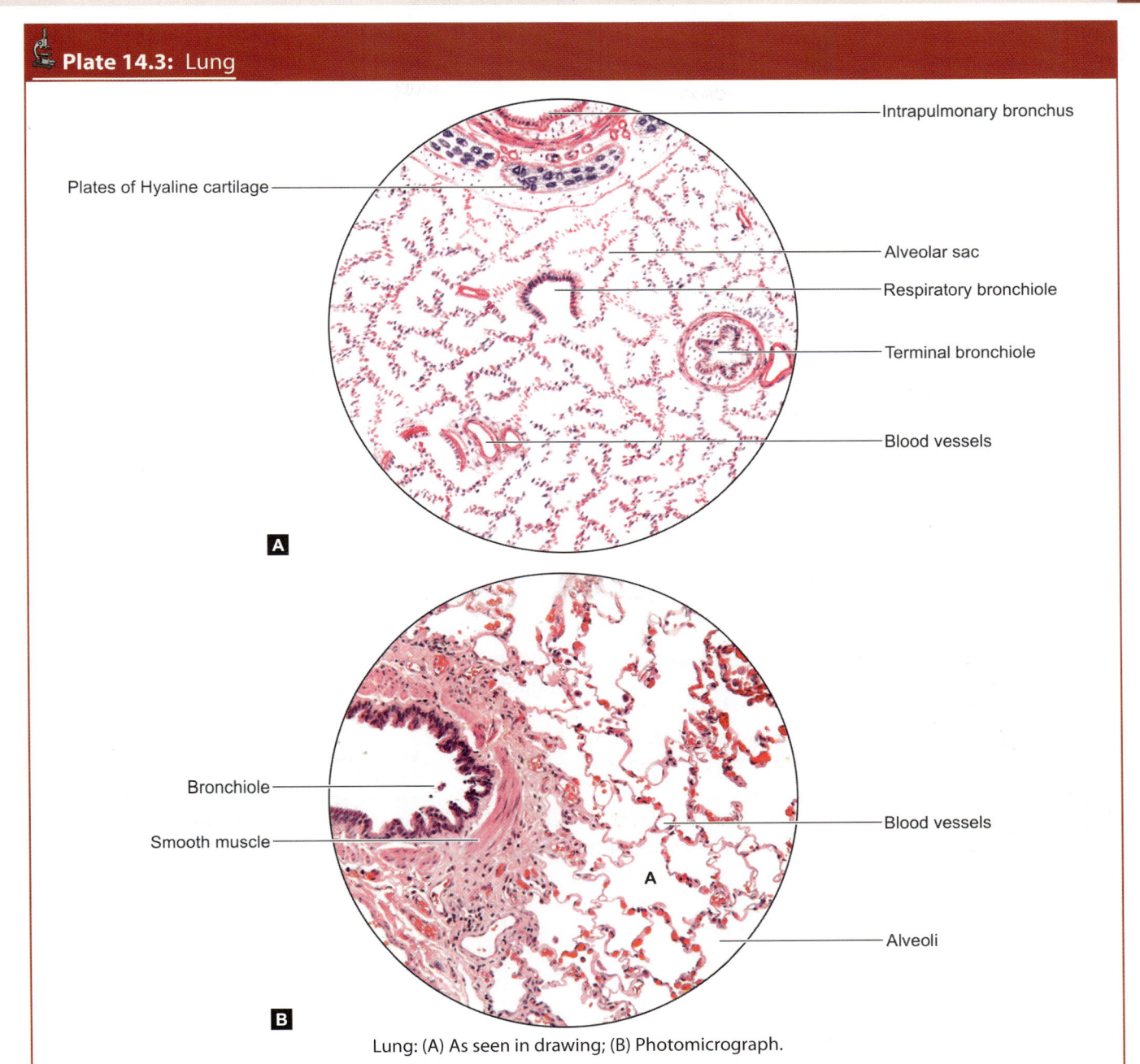

Plate 14.3: Lung

Lung: (A) As seen in drawing; (B) Photomicrograph.

Courtesy (B): Ivan Damjanov. Atlas of Histopathology, 1st edition. New Delhi: Jaypee Brothers Medical Publishers (P) Ltd; 2012. p. 37.

Points of identification
- Presence of alveolar ducts
- Alveolar sac lined by simple squamous epithelium
- Presence of intrapulmonary bronchus with varying amount of islands cartilage and smooth muscles
- Respiratory bronchioles with simple cuboidal epithelial lining lacking cilia and goblet cells.

Pneumocytes

Electron microscopy studies have shown that the cells forming the lining epithelium of alveoli (**pneumocytes**) are of various types (Fig. 14.5).

- The most numerous (lines 90% of the alveolar surface) cells are simple squamous cells called **type I alveolar epithelial cells**. Except in the region of the nucleus, these cells are reduced to a very thin layer (0.05–0.2 μm).
- Scattered in the epithelial lining, there are rounded secretory cells bearing microvilli on their free surfaces. These are designated as **type II alveolar epithelial cells** (Figs. 14.5 and 14.6). Their cytoplasm contains secretory granules (**multilamellar bodies**). These cells secrete **pulmonary surfactant** that reduces surface tension and prevents collapse of the alveolus during expiration. Surfactant contains phospholipids, proteins, and glycosaminoglycans produced in type II cells (a similar fluid is believed to be produced by the cells of Clara present in bronchial passages). Type II cells may multiply to replace damaged type I cells.
- **Type III alveolar cells**, or **brush cells**, of doubtful function, have also been described.

Different types of cells present in the respiratory system are summarized in Flowchart 14.1.

Connective Tissue

- The connective tissue framework of alveolus contains collagen fibers and numerous elastic fibers continuous with those of bronchioles.
- Fibroblasts, histiocytes, mast cells, lymphocytes, and plasma cells may be present. Pericytes are present in relation to capillaries.
- Alveolar macrophages which swallow dust particles are called as **dust cells**. In congestive heart failure (in which pulmonary capillaries become overloaded with blood), these macrophages phagocytose erythrocytes that escape from capillaries. The cells, therefore, acquire a brick red color and are then called **heart failure cells**. Macrophages also remove excessive surfactant and secrete several enzymes.

Pleura

The pleura is lined by flat mesothelial cells that are supported by loose connective tissue rich in elastic fibers, blood vessels, nerves, and lymphatics. There is considerable adipose tissue under parietal pleura.

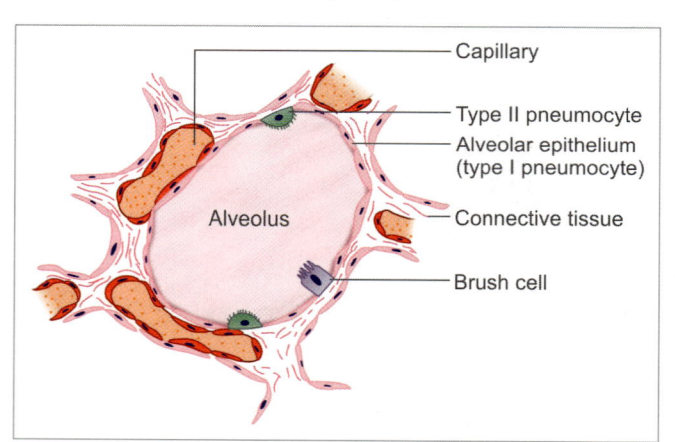

Fig. 14.5: Some cells to be seen in relation to an alveolus (schematic representation).

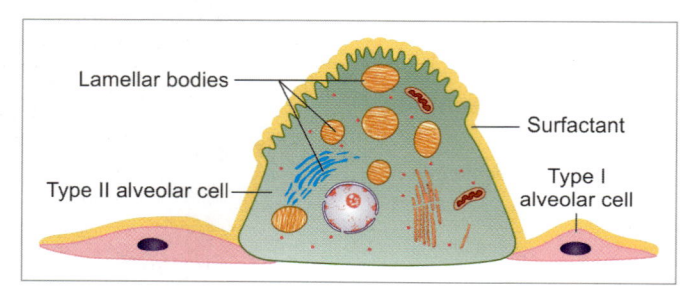

Fig. 14.6: Type II pneumocytes (schematic representation).

Flowchart 14.1: Different types of cells of respiratory system.

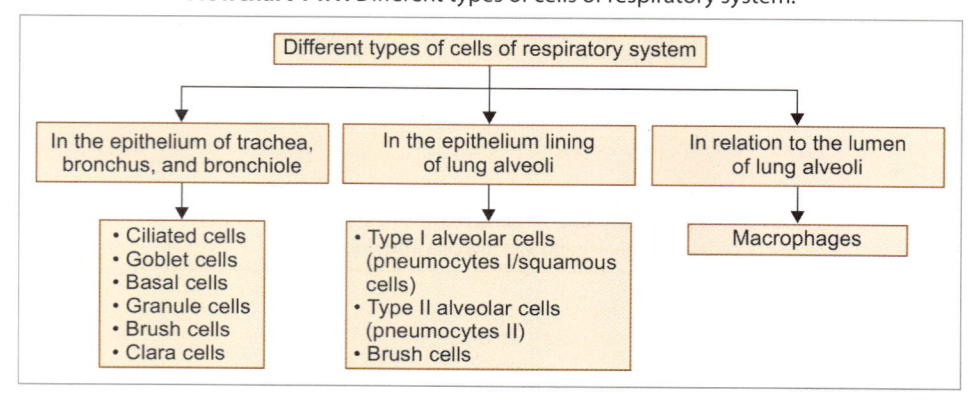

Different types of cells of respiratory system

- In the epithelium of trachea, bronchus, and bronchiole
  - Ciliated cells
  - Goblet cells
  - Basal cells
  - Granule cells
  - Brush cells
  - Clara cells
- In the epithelium lining of lung alveoli
  - Type I alveolar cells (pneumocytes I/squamous cells)
  - Type II alveolar cells (pneumocytes II)
  - Brush cells
- In relation to the lumen of lung alveoli
  - Macrophages

CHAPTER 14: Respiratory System

Added Information

Olfactory epithelium
- The *olfactory epithelium* is pseudostratified. It is much thicker than the epithelium lining the respiratory mucosa (about 100 μm). Within the epithelium, there is a superficial zone of clear cytoplasm below which there are several rows of nuclei (Fig. 14.7).
- Using special methods, **three types of cells** can be recognized in the epithelium (Fig. 14.8):
  1. *Olfactory cells* are modified neurons. Each cell has a central part containing a rounded nucleus. Two processes, distal and proximal, arise from this central part. The distal process (representing the dendrite) passes toward the surface of the olfactory epithelium. It ends in a thickening (called the *rod* or *knob*) from which a number of nonmotile olfactory cilia arise and project into a layer of fluid covering the epithelium. The proximal process of each olfactory cell represents the axon. It passes into the subjacent connective tissue where it forms one fiber of the olfactory nerve.
  2. The *sustentacular cells* support the olfactory cells. Their nuclei are oval and lie near the free surface of the epithelium. The free surface of each cell bears numerous microvilli (embedded in overlying mucous).

Contd...

Contd...

The cytoplasm contains yellow pigment (lipofuscin) that gives olfactory mucosa its yellow color. In addition to their supporting function, sustentacular cells may be phagocytic, and the pigment in them may represent remnants of phagocytosed olfactory cells.

  3. The *basal cells* lie deep in the epithelium and do not reach the luminal surface. They divide to form new olfactory cells to replace the dead cells. Some basal cells have a supporting function too.

Note:
- In vertebrates, olfactory cells are unique in being the only neurons that have cell bodies located in an epithelium.
- Olfactory cells are believed to have a short life. Dead olfactory cells are replaced by new cells produced by the division of basal cells. This is the only example of regeneration of neurons in mammals.

Lamina propria
The lamina propria, lying deep to the olfactory epithelium, consists of connective tissue within which blood capillaries, lymphatic capillaries, and olfactory nerve bundles are present. It also contains serous glands (of Bowman), the secretions of which constantly "wash" the surface of the olfactory epithelium. This fluid may help in transferring smell carrying substances from air to receptors on olfactory cells.

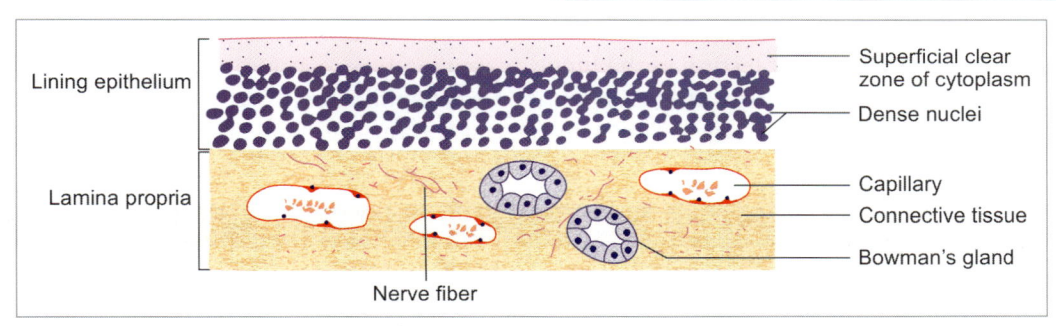

Fig. 14.7: Olfactory mucosa seen in section stained by routine methods (schematic representation).

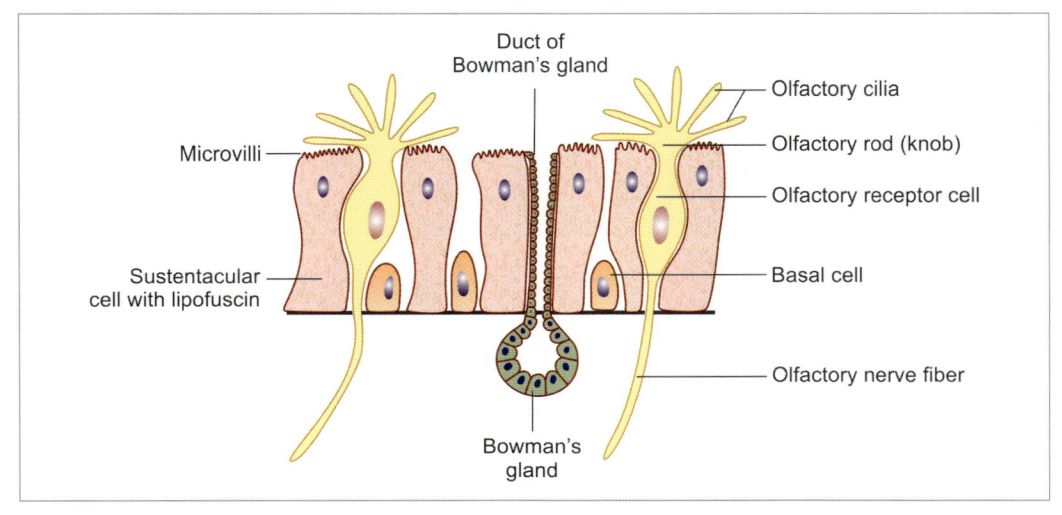

Fig. 14.8: Cells to be seen in olfactory epithelium (schematic representation).

APPLIED HISTOLOGY

- **Acute laryngitis:** This may occur as a part of the upper or lower respiratory tract infection. Atmospheric pollutants, such as cigarette smoke, exhaust fumes, industrial and domestic smoke, etc. predispose the larynx to acute bacterial and viral infections. Streptococci and *Haemophilus influenzae* cause acute epiglottitis which may be life-threatening.
- **Chronic laryngitis:** Chronic laryngitis may occur from the repeated attacks of acute inflammation, excessive smoking, chronic alcoholism, or vocal abuse. The surface is granular due to swollen mucous glands. There may be extensive squamous metaplasia due to heavy smoking, chronic bronchitis, and atmospheric pollution.
- **Acute respiratory distress syndrome (ARDS)** is a severe, at times life-threatening, form of progressive respiratory insufficiency which involves pulmonary tissues diffusely, i.e. involvement of the alveolar epithelium, alveolar lumina, and interstitial tissue. ARDS exists in two forms: (1) neonatal type and (2) adult type. Both have the common morphological feature of the formation of the hyaline membrane in the alveoli, and hence, it is also termed as hyaline membrane disease (HMD).
- **Bacterial pneumonia:** Bacterial infection of the lung parenchyma is the most common cause of pneumonia or consolidation of one or both the lungs. Two types of acute bacterial pneumonias are distinguished—(1) lobar pneumonia and (2) broncho (lobular) pneumonia, each with distinct etiologic agent and morphologic changes.
- **Chronic bronchitis** is a common condition defined clinically as persistent cough with expectoration on most days for at least 3 months of the year for 2 or more consecutive years. The cough is caused by the oversecretion of mucous. In spite of its name, chronic inflammation of the bronchi is not a prominent feature. The condition is more common in middle-aged males than females.
- **Asthma** is a disease of airways that is characterized by increased responsiveness of the tracheobronchial tree to a variety of stimuli, resulting in widespread spasmodic narrowing of the air passages which may be relieved spontaneously or by therapy. Asthma is an episodic disease manifested clinically by paroxysms of dyspnea, cough, and wheezing. However, a severe and unremitting form of the disease termed status asthmaticus may prove fatal.
- **Immotile cilia syndrome** that includes Kartagener's syndrome (bronchiectasis, situs inversus, and sinusitis) is characterized by ultrastructural changes in the microtubules causing immotility of cilia of the respiratory tract epithelium, sperms, and other cells. Males in this syndrome are often infertile.

MULTIPLE CHOICE QUESTIONS

1. Lining epithelium of alveoli is:
   a. Simple columnar
   b. Simple squamous
   c. Simple cuboidal
   d. Pseudostratified columnar
2. Surfactant is secreted by:
   a. Goblet cells
   b. Type I pneumocytes
   c. Type II pneumocytes
   d. Clara cells
3. Function of dust cells is:
   a. Phagocytosis
   b. Secretion of surfactant
   c. Exchange of gases
   d. Absorption
4. Skeletal framework of epiglottis is formed by:
   a. Elastic cartilage
   b. Hyaline cartilage
   c. White fibrocartilage cartilage
   d. Reticular tissue

Answers
1. b   2. c   3. a   4. a

CHAPTER 15

Digestive System: Oral Cavity and Related Structures

Learning objectives

To study the:
- Oral cavity
- Structure of lip
- Tooth:
  - General structure
- Structure of enamel
- Structure and types of dentin
- Structure of cementum and pulp
- Structure of tongue:
- Mucous membrane
- Structure and types of papillae
- Structure of taste bud
- Applied histology

IDENTIFICATION POINTS

Lip	Tooth	Tongue
☐ Presence of mucocutaneous junction	☐ Presence of enamel and dentin	☐ Mucous membrane showing numerous papillae
☐ Subepithelial connective tissue containing serous and mucous glands.	☐ Pulp cavity lined by odontoblasts	☐ Presence of taste buds
	☐ Presence of granular layer of Tomes	☐ Serous glands of von Ebner
	☐ Apical foramen at the apex of the root.	☐ Central core formed by skeletal muscles.

INTRODUCTION

The abdominal part of the alimentary canal (consisting of the stomach and intestines) is often referred to as the **gastrointestinal tract**. Closely related to the alimentary canal, there are several accessory organs that form part of the alimentary system. These include the structures of the oral cavity (lips, teeth, tongue, and salivary glands), liver, and pancreas.

The oral cavity is divided into a **vestibule** and the **oral cavity proper**. The vestibule is the space between the lips, cheeks, and teeth. The oral cavity proper lies behind the teeth and is bounded by the hard and soft palates above, the tongue and the floor of the mouth below, and the oropharynx posteriorly.

ORAL CAVITY

- The wall of the oral cavity is made up partly of bone (jaws and hard palate), and partly of muscle and connective tissue (lips, cheeks, soft palate, and floor of mouth).
- These structures are lined by mucous membrane which is lined by **stratified squamous epithelium** that rests on connective tissue, similar to that of the dermis. The epithelium differs from that on the skin in that it is not keratinized (exception—gums).
- Deep to the epithelium, there lies lamina propria containing vessels and nerves.
- Papillae of connective tissue (similar to dermal papillae) extend into the epithelium. The size of these papillae varies considerably from region to region.
- Over the alveolar processes (where the mucosa forms the gums), and over the hard palate, the mucous membrane is closely adherent to underlying periosteum. Elsewhere, it is connected to underlying structures by dense reticular layer. In the cheeks, this connective tissue contains many elastic fibers and much fat (especially in children).

LIPS

- Lips are fleshy folds which on the "external" surface are lined by skin, and on "internal" surface are lined by mucous membrane.
- The substance of each lip (upper or lower) is predominantly muscular (skeletal muscle) (Fig. 15.1).
- The upper and lower lips close along the red margin which represents the **mucocutaneous junction**. There

178   Textbook of Human Histology

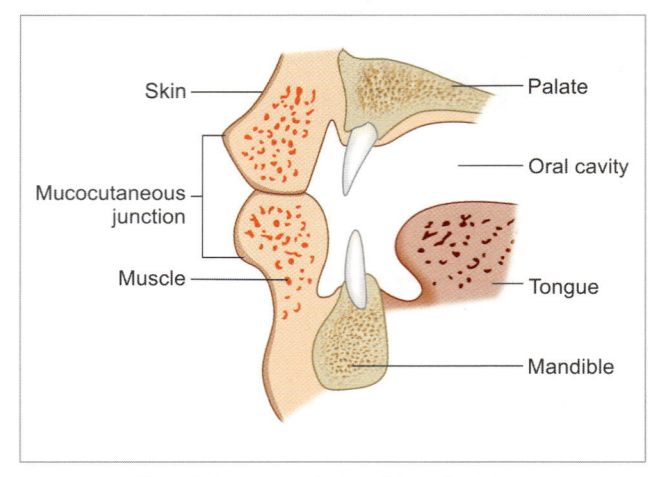

Fig. 15.1: Some relationships of the lips (schematic representation).

is a transitional zone between the skin and mucous membrane referred as the **vermilion**, because of its pink color in fair-skinned individuals. This part meets the skin along a distinct edge.

- The "external" surface of the lip is lined by true skin in which hair follicles and sebaceous glands can be seen.
- The mucous membrane is lined by **stratified squamous nonkeratinized epithelium** (Plate 15.1). This epithelium is much thicker than that lining the skin (especially in infants). The epithelium has a well-marked finger-like projections **rete ridge system** that extends into underlying connective tissue and anchors the epithelium to underlying connective tissue. A similar arrangement is seen in the mucosa over the palate. This arrangement helps to withstand friction.
- Beneath the epithelium, the mucosa has a layer of connective tissue (corresponding to the dermis), and a deeper layer of loose connective tissue. The latter contains numerous mucous glands, sebaceous glands (not associated with hair follicles). Their secretions prevent dryness and cracking of the exposed part of the mucosa.

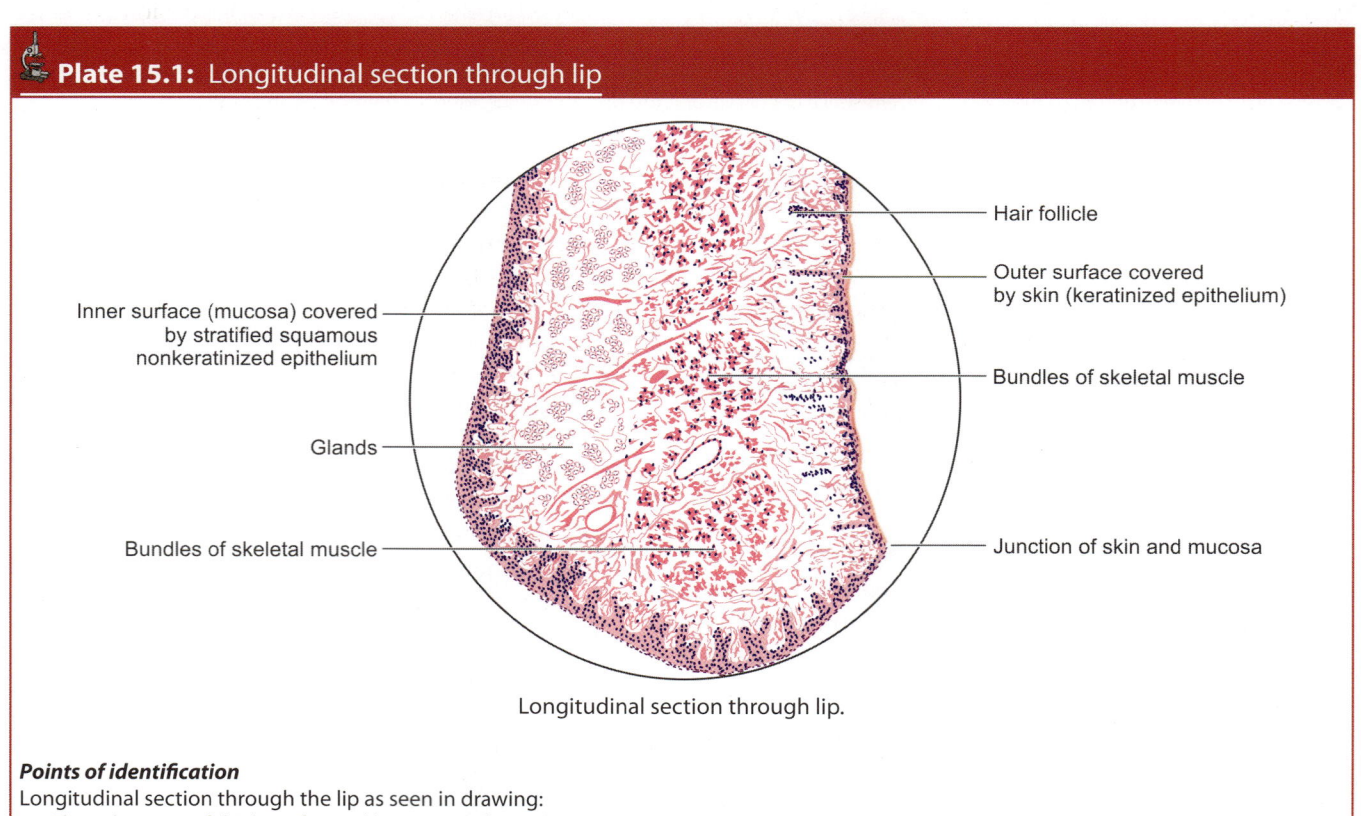

Plate 15.1: Longitudinal section through lip

Longitudinal section through lip.

Points of identification
Longitudinal section through the lip as seen in drawing:
- The substance of the lip is formed by a mass of muscle
- Each lip has an "external" surface covered by skin and an "internal" surface lined by mucous membrane
- There is a transitional zone between the skin and mucous membrane known as vermilion border.

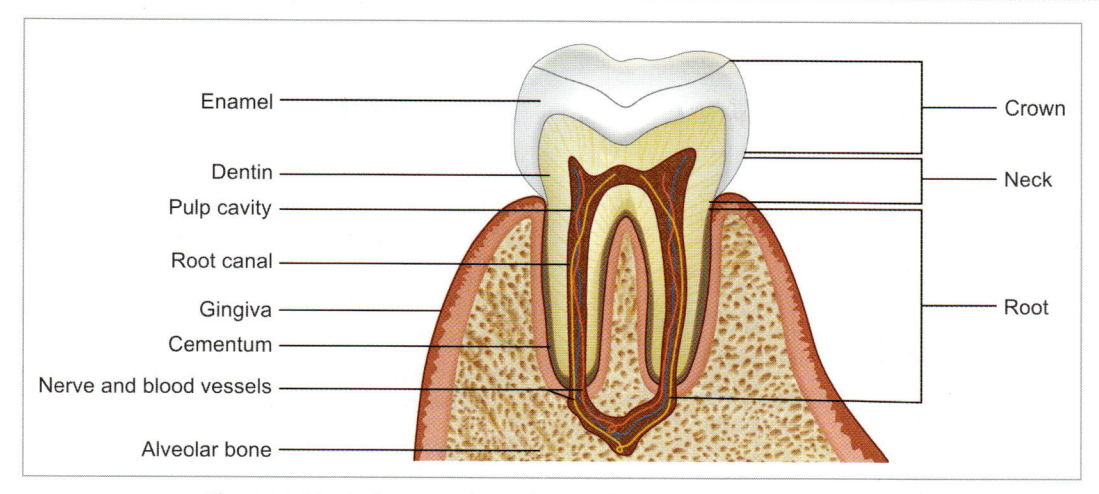

CHAPTER 15: Digestive System: Oral Cavity and Related Structures

Fig. 15.2: Vertical section through a tooth (schematic representation).

TEETH

General Structure

A tooth consists of an "upper" part, the ***crown***, which is seen in the mouth, and of one or more ***roots*** which are embedded in sockets in the jaw bone (mandible or maxilla). It is composed of three calcified tissues, namely: ***enamel***, ***dentin***, and the ***pulp*** (Figs. 15.2 and 15.3).

- The greater part of the tooth is formed by a bone-like material called ***dentin***.
- Within the dentin, there is a ***pulp canal*** (or ***pulp cavity***) that contains a mass of cells, blood vessels, and nerves that constitute the ***pulp***. The blood vessels and nerves enter the pulp canal through the ***apical foramen*** (Fig. 15.3) which is located at the apex of the root.
- In the region of the crown, the dentin is covered by a much harder white material called the ***enamel***.
- Over the root, the dentin is covered by a thin layer of ***cementum***. The cementum is united to the wall of the bony socket in the jaw by a layer of fibrous tissue called the ***periodontal ligament***.

Enamel

- Enamel is the hardest material in the body. It is made up almost entirely (96%) of inorganic salts.
- These salts are mainly in the form of complex crystals of hydroxyapatite (as in bone). The crystals contain calcium phosphate and calcium carbonate. Some salts are also present in amorphous form. The crystals of hydroxyapatite are arranged in the form of rod-shaped ***prisms***, which run from the deep surface of the enamel (in contact with dentin) to its superficial (or free) surface.
- Prisms are separated by ***interprismatic material***. Structure of prism and interprismatic material is same but they differ in their appearance due to difference in the orientation of hydroxyapatite crystals in them. The most superficial part of the enamel is devoid of prisms.
- During development, enamel is laid down in the form of layers. When seen in section, these layers can be distinguished as they are separated by lines running more or less parallel to the surface of the enamel. These lines are called the ***incremental lines*** or the ***lines of Retzius*** (Fig. 15.4).
- In some teeth, in which enamel formation takes place partly before birth and partly after birth (e.g. in milk teeth), one of the incremental lines is particularly marked. It represents the junction of enamel formed before birth with that formed after birth, and is called the ***neonatal line***.

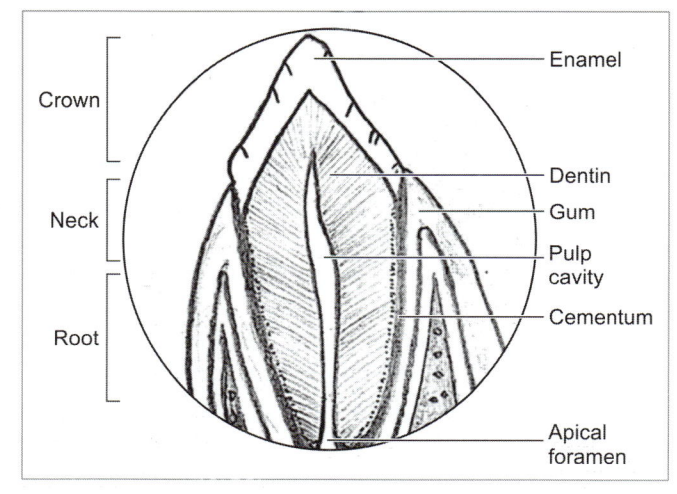

Fig. 15.3: Dried bone as seen in drawing.

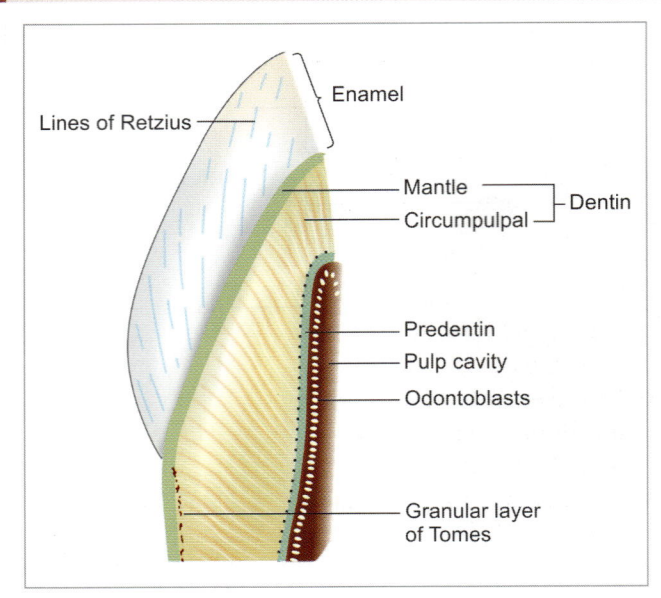

Fig. 15.4: Part of a tooth to show some features of the structure of enamel and dentin (schematic representation).

- At places, the enamel is penetrated by extraneous material. Projections entering the enamel from the dentin-enamel junction are called *enamel tufts*, and projections entering it from the free surface are called *enamel lamellae* (because of their shape). Dentinal tubules (*see* below) may extend into the enamel forming *enamel spindles*.

Dentin

Structure and composition

- Dentin is a hard material having several similarities to bone. It is made up basically of calcified ground substance (glycosaminoglycans) in which there are numerous collagen fibers (type 1).
- The calcium salts are mainly in the form of hydroxyapatite. Amorphous salts are also present.
- The inorganic salts account for 70% of the weight of dentin.
- Like bone, dentin is laid down in layers that are parallel to the pulp cavity. The layers may be separated by less mineralized tissue that forms the incremental lines of Von Ebner.
- Dentin is permeated by numerous fine canaliculi that pass radially from the pulp cavity toward the enamel (or toward cement). These are the dentinal tubules. The tubules may branch especially near the enamel-dentin junction. Dentinal tubules extend into the enamel as enamel spindles.
- The ground substance of dentin is more dense (than elsewhere) immediately around the dentinal tubules, and forms the *peritubular dentin* or the *dentinal sheath* (of Neumann).
- Each dentinal tubule contains a protoplasmic process arising from cells called *odontoblasts* that line the pulp cavity. These protoplasmic processes are called the *fibers of Tomes*.
- Near the surface of the root of the tooth (i.e. just deep to the cementum), the dentin contains minute spaces that give a granular appearance. This is the *granular layer of Tomes*.

Types of dentin

1. *Predentin*: Unmineralized dentin at the junction of dentin and the pulp cavity.
2. *Mantle dentin*: Dentin near the enamel-dentin junction is less mineralized (than elsewhere).
3. *Circumpulpal dentin*: Main part of dentin, i.e. between predentin and mantle dentin (Fig. 15.4).
4. *Primary dentin*: Dentin formed before eruption of the tooth.
5. *Secondary dentin*: Dentin formed after eruption of the tooth.

Cementum

- Cementum is the portion of tooth which covers the dentin at the root of tooth and is the site where periodontal ligament is attached. In old people, cementum may be lost, exposing the dentin.
- Cementum is similar to bone in morphology and composition and may be regarded as a layer of true bone that covers the root of the tooth.
- Toward the apex of the tooth, the cementum contains lacunae and canaliculi as in bone. The lacunae are occupied by cells similar to osteocytes (*cementocytes*). Some parts of cementum are acellular.
- Cementum is covered by a fibrous membrane called the *periodontal membrane* (or ligament). This membrane may be regarded as the periosteum of the cementum.
- Collagen fibers from this membrane extend into the cementum, and also into the alveolar bone (forming the socket in which the root lies) as fibers of Sharpey.
- The periodontal membrane fixes the tooth in its socket. It contains numerous nerve endings that provide sensory information.

Pulp

- Dental pulp lies inner to dentin and occupies the pulp cavity and root canal.

CHAPTER 15: Digestive System: Oral Cavity and Related Structures

- The dental pulp is made up of very loose connective tissue resembling embryonic mesenchyme (mucoid tissue).
- The ground substance is gelatinous and abundant. In it, there are many spindle-shaped and star-shaped cells.
- Delicate collagen fibers, numerous blood vessels, lymphatics, and nerve fibers are present. The nerve fibers are partly sensory and partly sympathetic.

TONGUE

- The tongue is a conical muscular organ lies in the floor of the oral cavity.
- It has a dorsal surface that is free, and a ventral surface that is free anteriorly, but is attached to the floor of the oral cavity posteriorly.
- The dorsal and ventral surfaces become continuous at the lateral margins, and at the tip (or apex) of the tongue.
- Near its posterior end, the dorsum of the tongue is marked by a V-shaped groove called the *sulcus terminalis* (Fig. 15.5).
- The apex of the "V" points backward and is marked by a depression called the *foramen cecum*.
- The limbs of the sulcus terminalis run forward and laterally. The sulcus terminalis divides the tongue into a larger (two-thirds) anterior, or oral part, and a smaller (one-third) posterior, or pharyngeal part.
- The substance of the tongue is made up chiefly of **skeletal muscle supported by connective tissue** (Plate 15.2). The muscle is arranged in bundles that run in vertical, transverse, and longitudinal directions. This arrangement of muscle permits intricate movements of the tongue associated with the chewing and swallowing of food, and those necessary for speech. The substance of the tongue is divided into right and left halves by a connective tissue septum.
- The surface of the tongue is covered by mucous membrane.

Mucous Membrane

- Mucous membrane of tongue is lined by **stratified squamous epithelium**. The epithelium is supported by a layer of connective tissue.
- On the ventral surface, the mucous membrane resembles that lining the rest of the oral cavity, and the epithelium is not keratinized.
- The mucous membrane covering the dorsum of the tongue is different over the anterior and posterior parts.
- Anterior part of the dorsal surface shows numerous projections called papillae.
- The mucous membrane of the posterior (pharyngeal) part of the dorsum of the tongue is devoid of papillae but bears numerous rounded elevations (lingual tonsil). Mucous membrane is separated from the underlying muscles by submucous coat which contains serous and mucous glands, aggregation of lymphatic follicles called **lingual tonsil**. Each lymphatic follicle is aggregation of lymphocytes with central recess, to which the ductules of mucous glands open.

Papillae

Each papilla consists of a lining epithelium and a core of connective tissue. The epithelium over the papillae is partially keratinized (parakeratinized). The papillae are of four types (Figs. 15.6A to D):

- *Filiform papillae*: They are the most numerous papillae present on the anterior two-thirds of the tongue. They lie in rows parallel to sulcus terminalis and transversely oriented toward the apex. They are small and conical in shape. The epithelium at the tips of these papillae is keratinized, thus makes the surface rough and helps to grasp the food particles. They lack taste buds.
- *Fungiform papillae*: These are larger mushroom-shaped reddish papillae, with rounded summits and narrower bases present at the apex of the tongue and along its lateral margins. Fungiform papillae bear taste buds (described below). In contrast to the filiform papillae, the epithelium on fungiform papillae is not keratinized.
- *Circumvallate papillae*: These are the largest papillae of the tongue about 8–12 in number. They are arranged in

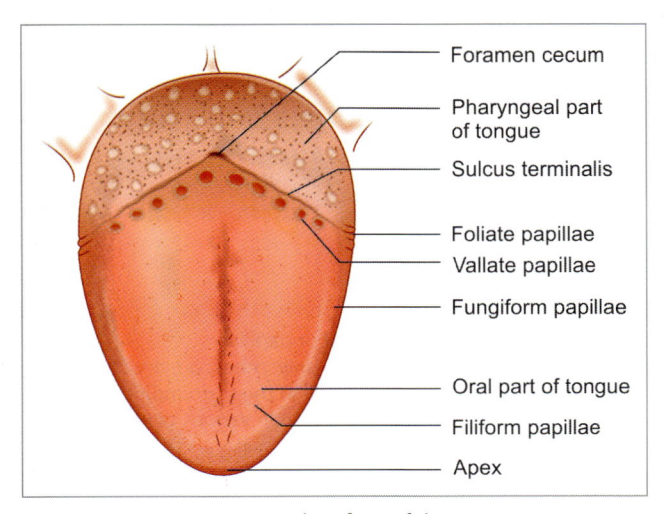

Fig. 15.5: Dorsal surface of the tongue (schematic representation).

Plate 15.2: Tongue: Anterior part

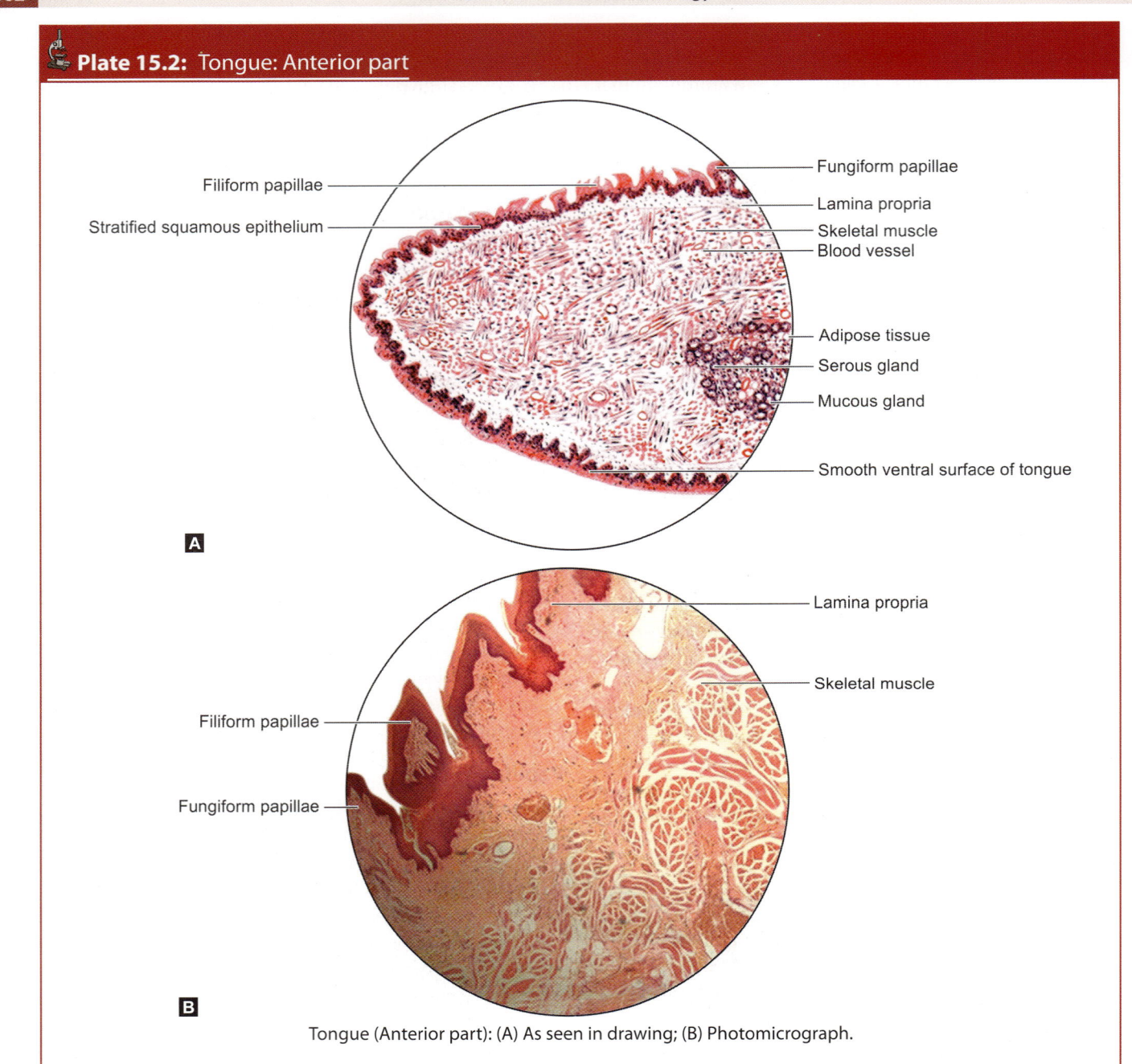

Tongue (Anterior part): (A) As seen in drawing; (B) Photomicrograph.

Points of identification
- The tongue is covered on both surfaces by stratified squamous epithelium (nonkeratinized)
- The ventral surface of the tongue is smooth, but on the dorsum the surface shows numerous projections or papillae
- Each papilla has a core of connective tissue covered by epithelium. Some papillae are pointed (filiform), while others are broad at the top (fungiform). A third type of papilla is circumvallate, the top of this papilla is broad and lies at the same level as the surrounding mucosa
- The main mass of the tongue is formed by skeletal muscle seen below the lamina propria. Muscle fibers run in various directions so that some are cut longitudinally and some transversely
- Numerous serous and mucous glands are present amongst the muscle fibers.

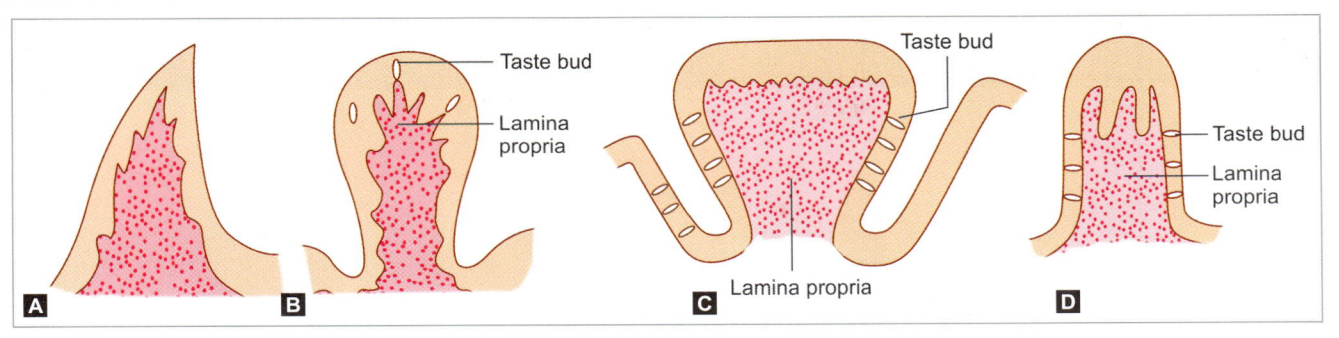

Figs. 15.6A to D: Papillae: (A) Filiform; (B) Fungiform; (C) Circumvallate; (D) Foliate (schematic representation).

a row just anterior and parallel to the sulcus terminalis. When viewed from the surface, each papilla is seen to have a circular top demarcated from the rest of the mucosa by a groove (Figs. 15.6A to D and Plate 15.3). Taste buds are present on the inner and outer walls of the groove trench and the floor receives the opening of ducts on serous glands. The secretion of serous glands makes the food soluble and also flushes it and thereby helps in the stimulation of taste buds in the groove.

❖ **Foliate papillae**: These are three to five vertical folds of mucous membrane occasionally present in man, along the posterior part of lateral margin of the tongue. They contain taste buds. The folate papillae are more prominent in rabbits.

Mucous and Serous Glands of Tongue

❖ Numerous mucous and serous glands (of Von Ebner) are present in the connective tissue deep to the epithelium of the tongue.
❖ Mucous glands are most numerous in the pharyngeal part, in relation to the masses of lymphoid tissue. They open into recesses of mucosa that dip into the masses of lymphoid tissue.
❖ The serous glands are present mainly in relation to circumvallate papillae, and open into the furrows surrounding the papillae.
❖ The largest glands in the tongue are present on the ventral aspect of the apex. They contain both mucous and serous acini and are referred to as the **anterior lingual glands of Blandin and Nuhn**.
❖ Numerous serous and mucous glands are present among the muscle fibers.

Taste Buds

Taste buds are present in relation to circumvallate papillae, fungiform papillae, and foliate papillae. Taste buds are also present on the soft palate, the epiglottis, the palatoglossal arches, and the posterior wall of the oropharynx.

❖ In H&E staining, they are pale staining oval structures which extend through the entire thickness of the epithelium.
❖ Each bud has a small cavity that opens to the surface through a **gustatory pore**. The cavity is filled by a material rich in polysaccharides.
❖ They are made up of modified epithelial cells (Fig. 15.7). The cells are elongated and are vertically orientated; those toward the periphery being curved like crescents (Fig. 15.8).
❖ Each cell has a central broader part containing the nucleus and tapering ends.
❖ The cells are of two basic types—*receptor cells/gustatory cells/neuroepithelial cells* and *supporting cells/sustentacular cells*.
❖ Gustatory cells are chemoreceptors, present in the central portion of the taste bud. They are spindle-shaped with large spherical nucleus. They form basal synapse with special afferent nerves of the tongue.
❖ Supporting cells are barrel-shaped cells, usually present toward the periphery, and form an envelope for the taste bud.
❖ The average life of cells is about 10 days.

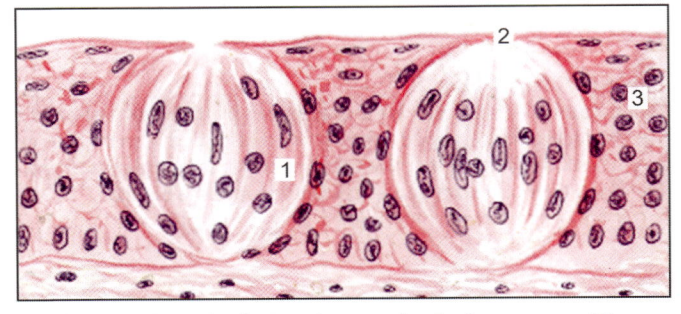

Fig. 15.7: Taste buds. 1—elongated cells; 2—pore; and 3—stratified squamous epithelium (schematic representation).

Plate 15.3: Vallate papilla

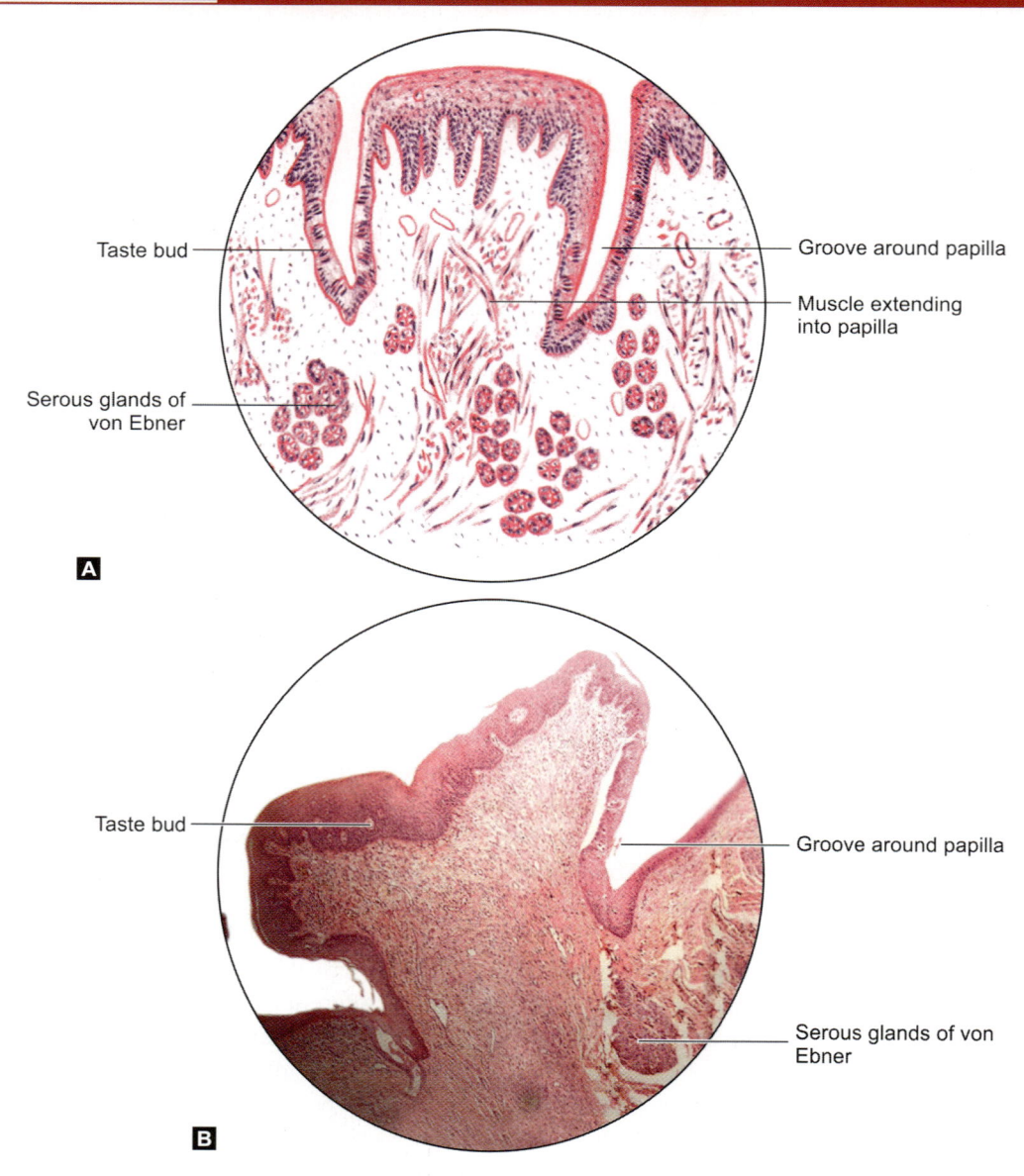

Vallate papilla: (A) As seen in drawing; (B) Photomicrograph.

Points of identification
- Circumvallate papillae are characterized by their dome-shaped structure lined by stratified squamous epithelium
- Numerous oval-shaped lightly stained taste buds can be seen on the lateral wall of the papillae
- The underlying connective tissue contains serous glands of von Ebner
- Skeletal muscle can be seen extending into the papillae.

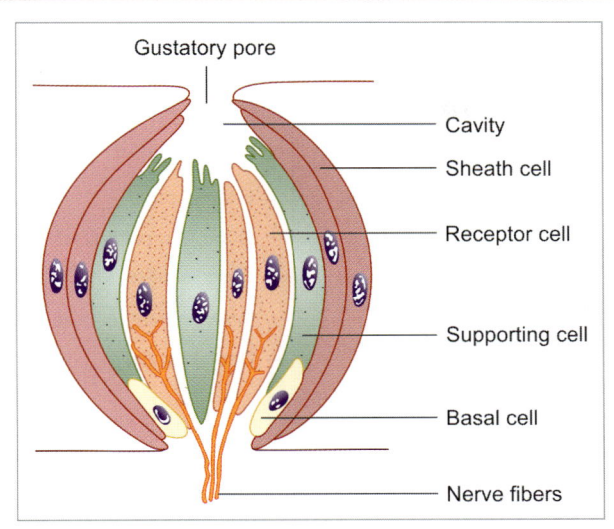

Fig. 15.8: Arrangement of cells in a taste bud (schematic representation).

APPLIED HISTOLOGY

Lips
- ❖ *Fordyce's granules*: Fordyce's granules are symmetric, small, light yellow macular spots on the lips and buccal mucosa, and represent collections of sebaceous glands.
- ❖ *Pyogenic granuloma*: This is an elevated, bright red swelling of variable size occurring on the lips, tongue, buccal mucosa, and gingiva. It is a vasoproliferative inflammatory lesion. **Pregnancy tumor** is a variant of pyogenic granuloma.
- ❖ *Cheilitis*: Inflammation of lips.

Tooth
- ❖ *Dental caries*: The most common disease of dental tissues, causing destruction of the calcified tissues of the teeth. Caries occurs chiefly in the areas of pits and fissures, mainly of the molars and premolars, where food retention occurs, and in the cervical part of the tooth.
- ❖ *Pulpitis*: It refers to the inflammation of the pulp. It may be acute, which is accompanied by severe pain and requires immediate intervention, or it may be chronic, where the pulp is exposed widely. It may protrude through the cavity forming polyp of the pulp.

Tongue
- ❖ *Fissured tongue*: It is a genetically-determined condition characterized by numerous small furrows or grooves on the dorsum of the tongue.
- ❖ *Hairy tongue*: In this condition, the filiform papillae are hypertrophied and elongated. These "hairs" (papillae) are stained black, brown, or yellowish-white by food, tobacco, oxidizing agents, or by oral flora.
- ❖ *Glossitis* refers to inflammation of tongue.
- ❖ *Bald tongue/atrophic glossitis*: Tongue without papillae, usually seen in nutritional deficiencies.
- ❖ *Geographic tongue*: It appears as patches on the tongue without papillae.

FURTHER READING

Oral Mucosa
It can be divided into three parts—masticatory mucosa, lining mucosa, and specialized mucosa.
- ❖ *Masticatory mucosa*: It lines the gum and hard palate which has keratinized (lacks stratum lucidum) and parakeratinized epithelium (superficial cells retain nuclei).
- ❖ *Specialized mucosa*: That presents on the dorsal surface of tongue which contains taste buds.
- ❖ *Lining mucosa*: The rest of the oral cavity has lining mucosa. It has fewer anchoring papillae so that it can adjust to the movement of underlying structures.

Stages in Tooth Development
- ❖ Each tooth may be regarded as a highly modified form of the stratified squamous epithelium covering the developing jaw (alveolar process).
- ❖ A thickening of epithelium grows downward into the underlying connective tissue and enlarges to form an **enamel organ** (Figs. 15.9A to D).
  - ■ *Bud stage (Fig. 15.9A)*: The enamel organ resembles a small bud, which is surrounded by the condensation of ectomesenchymal cells. In this stage, the enamel organ is made up of peripherally located low columnar cells and centrally located polygonal cells.
  - ■ *Cap stage (Fig. 15.9B)*: The enamel organ then proliferates to form a cap over the central condensation of ectomesenchymal cells which is called the dental papilla. The dental papilla and the dental sac become well-defined. Three layers are differentiated from the enamel organ are as follows:
    1. Inner dental/inner enamel epithelium
    2. Stellate reticulum
    3. Outer dental/outer enamel epithelium.
  - ■ *Early bell stage (Fig. 15.9C)*: The enamel organ resembles bell shape as a result of deepening of the undersurface of the epithelial cap. A cell layer forms in between the inner dental epithelium and stellate reticulum called the **stratum intermedium**.

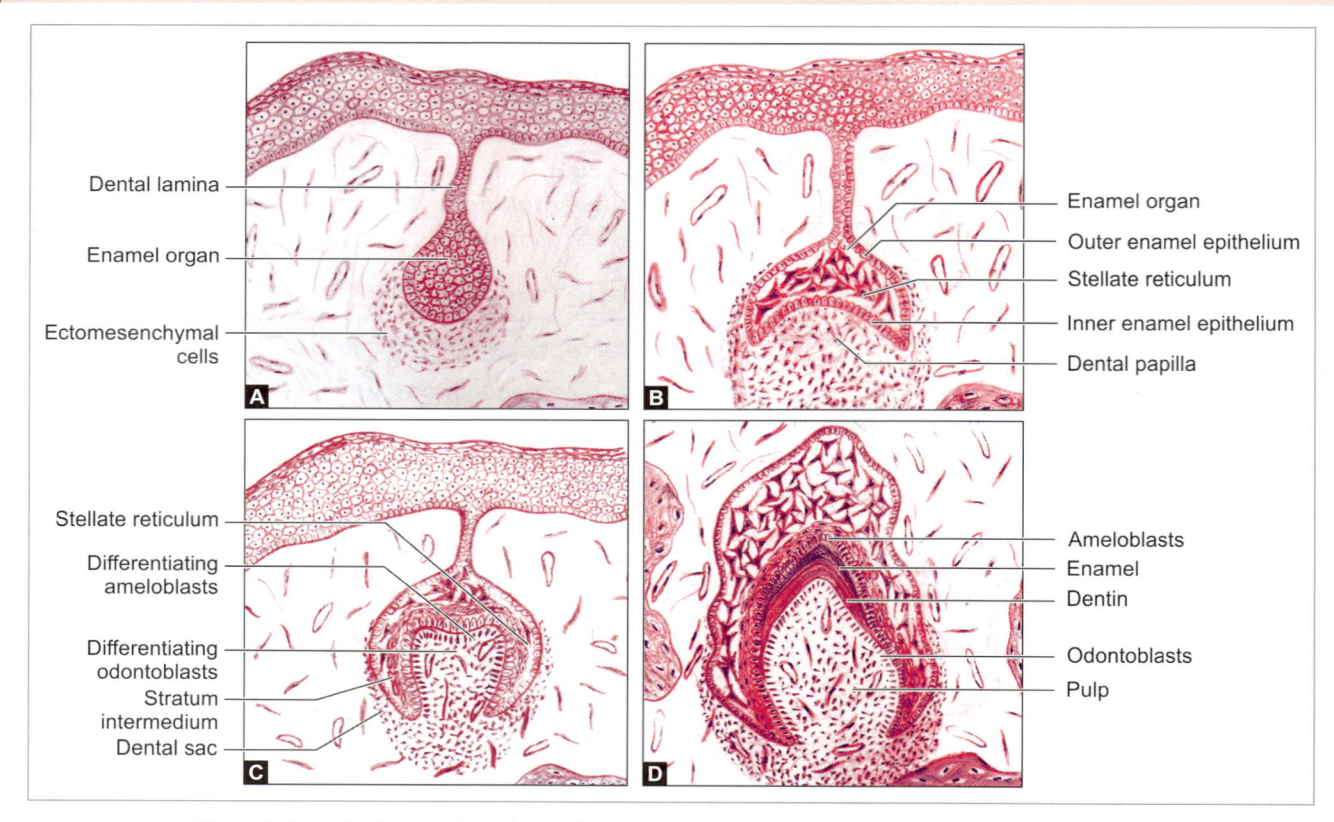

Figs. 15.9A to D: Stages of tooth development: (A) Bud stage; (B) Cap stage; (C) Early bell stage; (D) Advance bell stage (schematic representation).

The inner dental epithelium differentiates into tall columnar cells called the **ameloblasts**. The peripheral cells of the dental papilla differentiate into **odontoblasts**.

Under the organizing influence of inner dental epithelium, ameloblasts form enamel and odontoblasts produce dentin.

- *Advanced bell stage (Fig. 15.8D)*: In this stage, apposition of dental hard tissues occurs. Odontoblasts are dentin forming cells; ameloblasts are enamel forming cells. A layer of predentin is secreted by the odontoblasts. Both ameloblasts and odontoblasts behave in a way very similar to that of osteoblasts and lay down layer upon layer of enamel, or of dentin. The deposition of enamel and dentin continues until the crown formation is complete.

The formation of layers of enamel and dentin results in separation of ameloblasts and odontoblasts. The original line at which enamel and dentin formation begins is known as the enamel-dentin junction. At last, ameloblasts come to line the external aspect of the enamel. The odontoblasts persist as a lining for the pulp cavity.

When examined by EM, both ameloblasts and odontoblasts show the features typical of actively secreting cells. They have prominent Golgi complexes and abundant rough ER. The apical part of each cell is prolonged into a process. In the case of odontoblasts, the process runs into the proximal part of a dentinal tubule. In ameloblasts, the projection is called **Tomes process**. This process contains numerous microtubules and many secretory vesicles. Other smaller processes are present near the base of Tomes process. The organic matrix of enamel is released mainly by Tomes process, which also appears to be responsible for forming prisms of enamel.

Root Formation

Root formation is carried out by **Hertwig's epithelial root sheath** which is formed by the cervical portion of the enamel organ. It molds the shape of the roots and initiates radicular dentin formation.

The root sheath encloses the dental pulp except at apical portion. The rim of root sheath, the **epithelial diaphragm** surrounds the **primary apical foramen**. The root apex remains wide open until about 2 to 3 years after the eruption of the tooth, when the root development is completed.

MULTIPLE CHOICE QUESTIONS

1. Vermilion border of lip refers to:
   a. Inner border of lip
   b. Outer border of lip
   c. Mucocutaneous junction
   d. Angle of mouth
2. Papilla devoid of taste buds is:
   a. Circumvallate
   b. Filiform
   c. Fungiform
   d. Foliate
3. Cell which forms dentin is:
   a. Ameloblast
   b. Odontoblast
   c. Osteocyte
   d. Osteoblast
4. Dentin at the dentoenamel junction is called:
   a. Predentin
   b. Mantle dentin
   c. Circumpulpal dentin
   d. Primary dentin
5. Hardest material in the body is:
   a. Dentin
   b. Enamel
   c. Cementum
   d. Pulp tissue
6. Granular layer of Tomes is seen in:
   a. Dentin
   b. Enamel
   c. Cementum
   d. Pulp tissue
7. Structure which covers the dentin at the root is:
   a. Crown
   b. Enamel
   c. Cementum
   d. Pulp tissue

Answers
1. c   2. b   3. b   4. b   5. b   6. a   7. c

CHAPTER 16

Digestive System: General Plan of Gastrointestinal Tract, Stomach and Intestines

Learning objectives

To study the:
- General structure of GIT
- Layers of GIT with detailed structure
- Structure of esophagus
- Layers, cells, and functions of stomach
- Structure of small intestine: Duodenum, jejunum, ileum
- Differences between duodenum, jejunum, and ileum
- Structure of colon and vermiform appendix
- Structure of rectum and anal canal
- Applied histology

IDENTIFICATION POINTS

Esophagus
- Four layers of gastrointestinal tract (GIT): Mucosa, submucosa, muscularis externa, adventitia seen
- Lining epithelium is stratified squamous nonkeratinized epithelium
- Submucosa is studded with mucus-secreting esophageal glands.

Stomach (Fundus)
- Presence of four layers—mucosa, submucosa, muscularis externa, and serosa
- Shallow gastric pits occupying superficial one-fourth or less of the mucosa
- Presence of gastric glands in the mucosa
- Gastric glands with numerous oxyntic cells which give beaded appearance.

Stomach (Pylorus)
- Presence of four layers—mucosa, submucosa, muscularis externa, and serosa
- Deep gastric pits occupying two-third of the depth of the mucosa
- Presence of pyloric glands (mucous glands) in the mucosa that are simple/branched tubular glands which are coiled.

Duodenum
- Wall made up of four layers
- Mucosa—presence of numerous broad villi, lined by simple columnar epithelium with microvilli and goblet cells
- Presence of submucous Brunner's gland.

Jejunum
- Wall made up of four layers
- Mucosa—presence of numerous tall slender villi, lined by simple columnar epithelium with microvilli and goblet cells
- Absence of submucous Brunner's gland.

Ileum
- Wall made up of four layers
- Mucosa—presence of short, small fewer villi, lined by simple columnar epithelium with microvilli and numerous goblet cells
- Absence of submucous Brunner's gland.

Colon
- Wall made up of four layers
- Mucosa—absence of villi, lined by simple columnar epithelium with numerous goblet cells
- Lymphatic follicles dispersed in the lamina propria
- Presence of *Taenia coli*, appendices epiploicae.

Vermiform appendix
- Wall made up of four layers
- Mucosa—absence of villi, lined by simple columnar epithelium with numerous goblet cells
- Submucosa packed with numerous lymphatic follicles, extending into lamina propria
- Absence of *Taenia coli*, appendices epiploicae.

■ INTRODUCTION

❖ The gastrointestinal tract (GIT) or alimentary canal is a long muscular tube that begins at the oral cavity and ends in the anus.

❖ Different parts of the tract are specialized to perform different functions, and hence structural modifications are seen in various parts of the GIT.

❖ The esophagus and anal canal are merely transport passages.

❖ The part of the alimentary canal from the stomach to the rectum is the proper digestive tract, responsible for digestion and absorption of food.

❖ Reabsorption of secreted fluids is an important function of the large intestine.

CHAPTER 16: Digestive System: General Plan of Gastrointestinal Tract, Stomach and Intestines

GENERAL STRUCTURE OF GIT

- ❖ The structure of the alimentary canal, from the esophagus up to the anal canal, shows several features that are common to all these parts.
- ❖ From the upper end of the esophagus up to the lower end of the anal canal, the alimentary canal has the form of a fibromuscular tube.
- ❖ The wall of the tube is made up of the following layers (from inner to outer side) (Fig. 16.1):
  - The innermost layer is the **mucous membrane** that is made up of:
    - ♦ A lining epithelium
    - ♦ A layer of connective tissue, the *lamina propria*, that supports the epithelium
    - ♦ A thin layer of smooth muscle called the *muscularis mucosae*.
  - The mucous membrane rests on a layer of loose areolar tissue called the **submucosa**.
  - Thick layer of muscle **muscularis externa** that surrounds the submucosa.
  - Covering the muscularis externa, there is a **serous layer** or an **adventitial layer**.
    Primarily, it is the mucosa in which changes are seen in the alimentary tract; the other layers remain almost the same.

Mucosa

A. *Lining Epithelium*
- The lining epithelium is columnar all over the gut; except in the esophagus, and in the lower part of the anal canal, where it is stratified squamous.
- This stratified squamous epithelium has a **protective** function in these structures.
- The cells of the columnar epithelium are either absorptive or secretory.

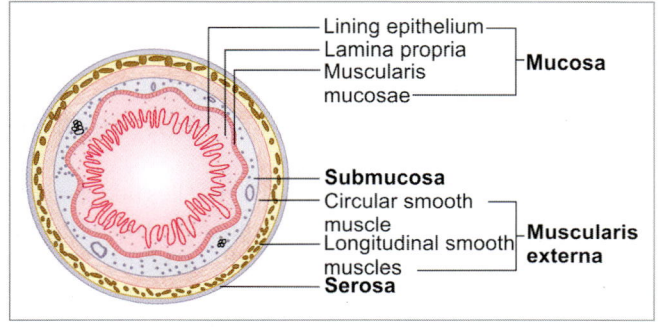

Fig. 16.1: Layers of the gut (schematic representation).

- The epithelium of the gut presents an extensive **absorptive** surface. The factors contributing to the increase in the surface are as follows:
  - ♦ The presence of **numerous folds** involving the entire thickness of the mucous membrane. These folds can be seen by naked eye. The submucosa extends into the folds (Plica circularis of small intestine).
  - ♦ At numerous places the epithelium dips into the lamina propria forming **crypts**.
  - ♦ In the **small intestine**, the mucosa bears numerous finger-like processes that project into the lumen. These processes are called *villi*. Each villus has a surface lining of epithelium and a core formed by an extension of the connective tissue of the lamina propria. The luminal surfaces of the epithelial cells bear numerous **microvilli.**
- The epithelium of the gut also performs a very important **secretory** function. The secretory cells are arranged in the form of numerous glands as follows:
  - ♦ Some glands are **unicellular**, the secretory cells being scattered among the cells of the lining epithelium.
  - ♦ In some organs, the epithelium dips into the lamina propria forming **simple tubular glands** (These are the crypts referred to above).
  - ♦ In other structures (e.g. in the esophagus, duodenum) there are **compound tubuloalveolar glands** lying in the submucosa. They open into the lumen of the gut through ducts traversing the mucosa.
  - ♦ Finally, there are **glands**—salivary glands, pancreas, and liver that form distinct organs lying outside the gut wall. They pour their secretions into the lumen of the gut through large ducts (in this respect, these glands are similar to the salivary glands). The liver and pancreas, and most of the salivary glands, are derivatives of the epithelial lining of the gut. Embryologically, this epithelium is derived from endoderm.

B. *Lamina Propria*
- The lamina propria is made up of collagen and reticular fibers embedded in a glycosaminoglycan matrix. Some fibroblasts, blood capillaries, lymph vessels, and nerves are seen in this layer.
- In the small intestine, the lamina propria forms the core of each villus. It surrounds and supports glandular elements and the overlying epithelium.

- Mucosal glands also extend into lamina propria of the gut and are readily seen in certain organs like esophagus and anal canal. They mainly lubricate the mucosa and protect it from chemical injury.
- Prominent aggregations of lymphoid tissue (as well as scattered lymphocytes) are present in the lamina propria. Some of this lymphoid tissue extends into the submucosa and is called as gut-associated lymphoid tissue (GALT).

C. **Muscularis Mucosae**
- This is a thin layer of smooth muscle that separates the connective tissue of the lamina propria from the submucosa.
- It consists of an *inner layer* in which the muscle fibers are arranged *circularly* (around the lumen) and an *outer layer* in which the muscle fibers run *longitudinally*.
- The muscularis mucosa extends into mucosal folds, but not into villi.
- Contractions of the muscularis mucosae are important for the local mixing of intestinal contents and also facilitate absorption and secretion.

Submucosa

- This layer made up of dense irregular connective tissue connects the mucosa to the muscularis externa.
- Numerous blood vessels, lymphatics, and nerve fibers traverse the submucosa.
- Smaller branches of larger blood vessels enter the mucous membrane, muscularis externa, and serosa.
- Submucosal plexus of unmyelinated nerve fibers and ganglion cells constitute **Meissner's plexus** in this layer.
- In addition, at certain regions, submucosa contains mucous glands (esophagus and proximal part of duodenum).

Muscularis Externa

- Over the greater part of the gut, the muscularis externa consists of smooth muscle. *The exceptions are the upper part of the esophagus and anal canal where this layer contains striated muscle fibers.*
- The muscle layer consists (typically) of an *inner layer of circular layer* and an *outer longitudinal layer* of smooth muscle fibers.
- Both layers actually consist of spirally arranged fasciculi, the turns of the spiral being compact in the circular layer, and elongated in the longitudinal layer.
- The arrangement of muscle fibers shows some variation from region to region. In the stomach, an additional oblique layer is present. In the colon, the longitudinal fibers are gathered to form prominent bundles called the *taenia coli*.
- Localized thickenings of circular muscle fibers form *sphincters* that can occlude the lumen of the gut. For example, the *pyloric sphincter* is present around the pyloric end of the stomach, and the *internal anal sphincter* surrounds the anal canal. A functional sphincter is seen at the junction of the esophagus with the stomach. A valvular arrangement at the ileocaecal junction (ileocaecal valve) prevents regurgitation of cecal contents into the ileum.
- Thin layer of connective tissue is present between the two muscle layers. It contains plexus of nerves called **Myenteric plexus/Auerbach's plexus**. It also contains blood vessels and lymphatics.
- Contraction of muscles in this layer helps in mixing and propulsion of luminal contents by slow rhythmic movement called **Peristalsis**.

Serous or Adventitia

- Outermost layer of the gut, covering the muscle coat.
- It is a serous membrane lined by simple squamous epithelium called **mesothelium** and minimal amount of connective tissue. This layer is nothing but visceral peritoneum that covers most parts of the gastrointestinal tract and extends over the abdominal wall to form parietal peritoneum.
- Large blood vessels, lymphatics, and nerve trunk traverse through serosa.
- In some places where a peritoneal covering is absent (e.g. thoracic part of the esophagus, duodenum, etc.) the muscle coat is covered by an adventitia made up of connective tissue only.

Nerve Plexuses

The gut is richly innervated by autonomic nervous system (enteric nervous system). The nerve fibers form two distinct plexus:
1. The **submucosal plexus of Meissner**, that lies in the submucosa (near its junction with the circular muscle layer) has only parasympathetic fibers which are secretomotor.
2. The **myenteric plexus of Auerbach**, that lies between the circular and longitudinal coats of muscularis externa has both sympathetic and parasympathetic fibers but only cell bodies of parasympathetic neurons.

These plexus are both under intrinsic and extrinsic control. Nerve fibers in these plexuses are both afferent and efferent.

CHAPTER 16: Digestive System: General Plan of Gastrointestinal Tract, Stomach and Intestines

ESOPHAGUS

- The esophagus is a long muscular tube beginning at the end of cricoid cartilage and opens into the cardiac end of stomach.
- It conducts chewed food (bolus) and liquids to stomach.
- Its length is about 25 cm.

Microscopic Features

The wall of esophagus (Plate 16.1) has the usual four layers viz., mucosa, submucosa, muscularis externa, and an external adventitia. The esophagus does not have a serous covering except over a short length near its lower end.

Mucosa

- The mucous membrane of the esophagus shows several longitudinal folds that disappear when the tube is distended.
- The mucosa is lined by **stratified squamous nonkeratinized epithelium**. Occasionally melanocytes and endocrine cells are encountered.
- Finger-like processes (or papillae) of the connective tissue of the lamina propria project into the epithelial layer (just like dermal papillae). This helps to prevent separation of epithelium from underlying connective tissue.
- At the upper and lower ends of the esophagus, some tubuloalveolar mucous glands are present in the lamina propria which are called as esophageal cardiac glands.
- The muscularis mucosae are made of longitudinally oriented smooth muscle fibers which are thick in the upper end of the esophagus and help in swallowing.

Submucosa

- The only special feature of the submucosa is the presence of **compound tubuloalveolar mucous glands** called esophageal glands proper, more concentrated in the upper half of the esophagus. They help to lubricate the luminal wall.
- Small aggregations of lymphoid tissue may be present in the submucosa, especially near the lower end. Some plasma cells and macrophages are also present.

Muscularis Externa

- Consists of inner circular and outer longitudinal layer of smooth muscle fibers. But in the upper third of the esophagus, it is made of only skeletal muscle fibers.
- In the middle third, it is a combination of both smooth muscle and skeletal muscle fibers.
- In the lower third, it is made up of only smooth muscle fibers like the rest of the GIT.
- Myenteric plexus is present between outer and inner muscular layer which produces peristalsis by stimulating muscularis externa.

Adventitia

- The muscle layer of the esophagus is surrounded by dense fibrous tissue that forms an adventitial coat for the esophagus.
- The lowest part of the esophagus is intra-abdominal and has a covering of peritoneum.

> **Added Information**
>
> The circular muscle fibers present at the lower end of the esophagus could possibly act as a sphincter guarding the cardioesophageal junction. However, the circular muscle is not thicker here than elsewhere in the esophagus, and its role as a sphincter is not generally accepted. However, a **physiological sphincter** does appear to exist. The anatomical factors that could account for this sphincteric action are not agreed upon.

STOMACH

- Stomach is a hollow muscular organ that receives food bolus from esophagus.
- The food passes through the esophagus and enters the stomach where it is converted into a thick paste known as **chyme**.
- Anatomically, stomach is divided into four regions: (1) *cardia*, (2) *fundus*, (3) *body*, and (4) *pylorus* (Fig. 16.2).
- Histologically fundus and body of stomach have a similar structure.

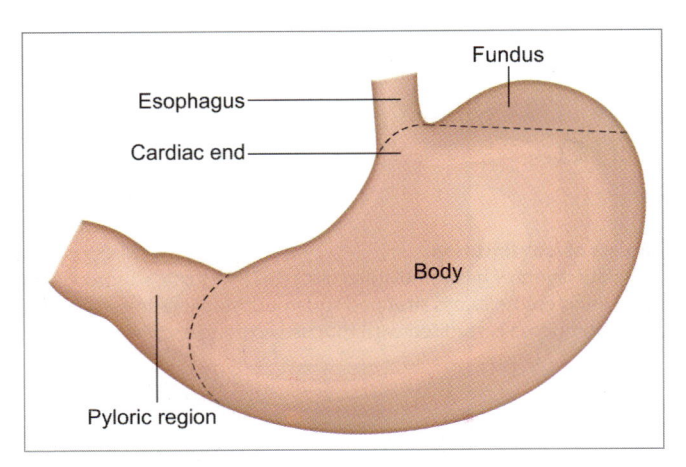

Fig. 16.2: Anatomical regions of stomach (schematic representation).

Plate 16.1: Esophagus

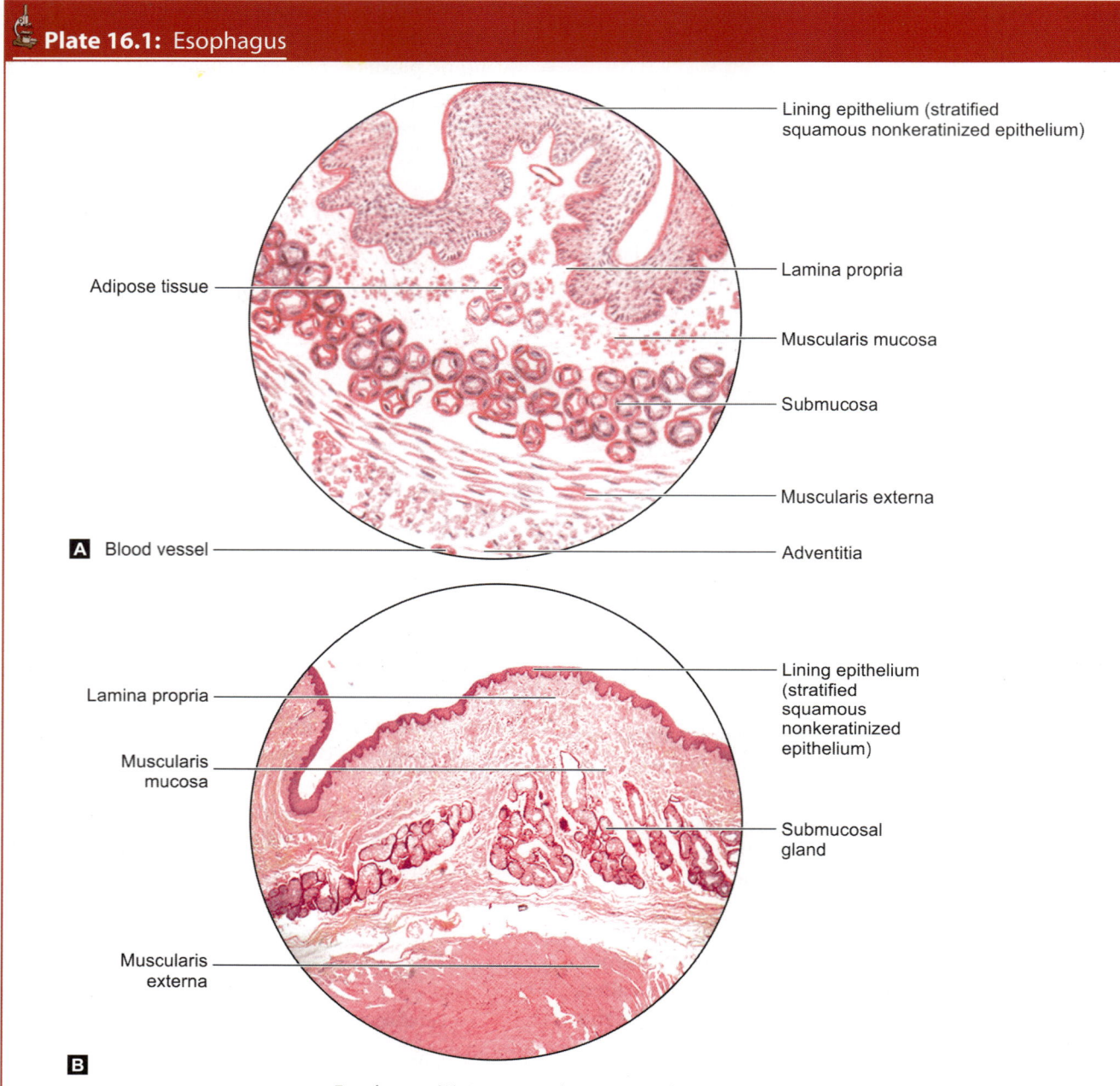

Esophagus: (A) As seen in drawing; (B) Photomicrograph.

Points of identification
- Four layers of gastrointestinal tract (GIT): Mucosa, submucosa, muscularis externa, adventitia seen
- Lining epithelium is stratified squamous nonkeratinized epithelium
- Submucosa is studded with mucus-secreting esophageal glands.

Functions

- It acts as temporary reservoir of food.
- Secretes copious amount of mucous, so that prevents autodigestion of the tissues.
- Helps in digestion of proteins.
- Acidic environment of stomach provides protection against microbes.
- Intrinsic factor secreted in the stomach aids in absorption of vitamin B_{12}.

Microscopic Features

The wall of the stomach has the four basic layers, (Plates 16.2 and 16.3 and Table 16.1) from within outward they are: (1) mucous membrane, (2) submucosa, (3) muscularis externa, and (4) serosa.

Mucous Membrane

- As seen with the naked eye, (Fig. 16.3) the mucous membrane is thick, soft, and velvety, presents numerous vertical folds (or *rugae*) that disappear when the stomach is distended.
- Mucous membrane consists of lining epithelium, supported by lamina propria and muscularis mucosa.

Lining epithelium

- The surface and gastric pits are lined by **simple columnar epithelium** resting on basement membrane.
- They are mucus-secreting cells with apical large mucin granules which are usually removed during processing of tissues so that the cells look empty (or vacuolated).
- Mucus secreted by cells of the lining epithelium protects the gastric mucosa against acid and enzymes produced by the mucosa itself.

- At numerous places, the lining epithelium dips into the lamina propria and forms numerous depressions called **gastric pits** (Fig. 16.3). Deep to the gastric pits, the mucous membrane is packed with numerous **gastric glands**. Depending on their presence in different regions of stomach, these glands are of three types: *(1) Gastric (fundic), (2) cardiac, and (3) pyloric.*

Gastric glands

The main gastric glands are present over most of the stomach except in the pyloric region and in a small area near the cardiac end. Though they are synonymously called as fundic glands, they are also present in the body of the stomach.

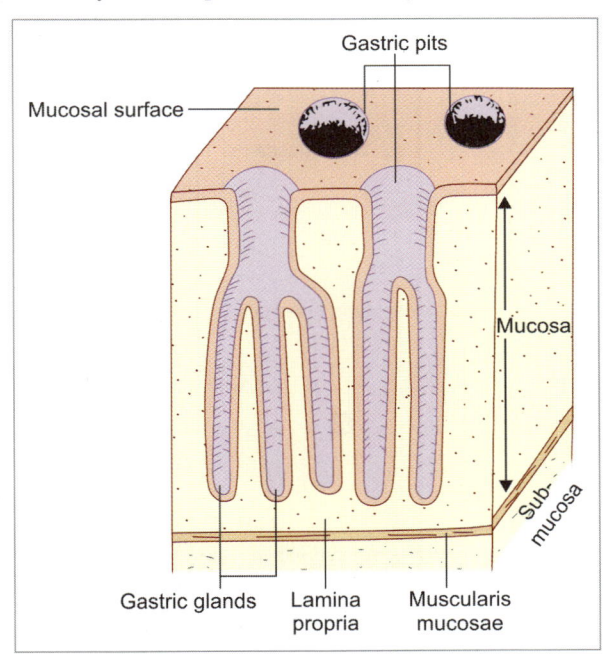

Fig. 16.3: Basic structure of the mucous membrane of the stomach (schematic representation).

Table 16.1: Salient features of each region of stomach.		
Cardia	**Fundus and body**	**Pylorus**
Shallow gastric pits	Shallow gastric pits occupying superficial one-fourth or less of the mucosa	Deep gastric pits occupying two-thirds of the depth of the mucosa
Presence of cardiac glands (mucous secreting glands) in the mucosa	Presence of gastric glands in the mucosa	Presence of pyloric glands in the mucosa
Cardiac glands are either simple tubular, or compound tubuloalveolar	Gastric glands are simple or branched tubular glands. They secrete enzymes and hydrochloric acid	Pyloric glands (mucous glands) are simple or branched tubular glands that are coiled
Change of epithelium from stratified squamous of the esophagus to simple columnar epithelium in stomach	Epithelium is simple columnar	Epithelium is simple columnar. Circular muscle layer is thick and is called as pyloric sphincter

Plate 16.2: Stomach (Fundus)

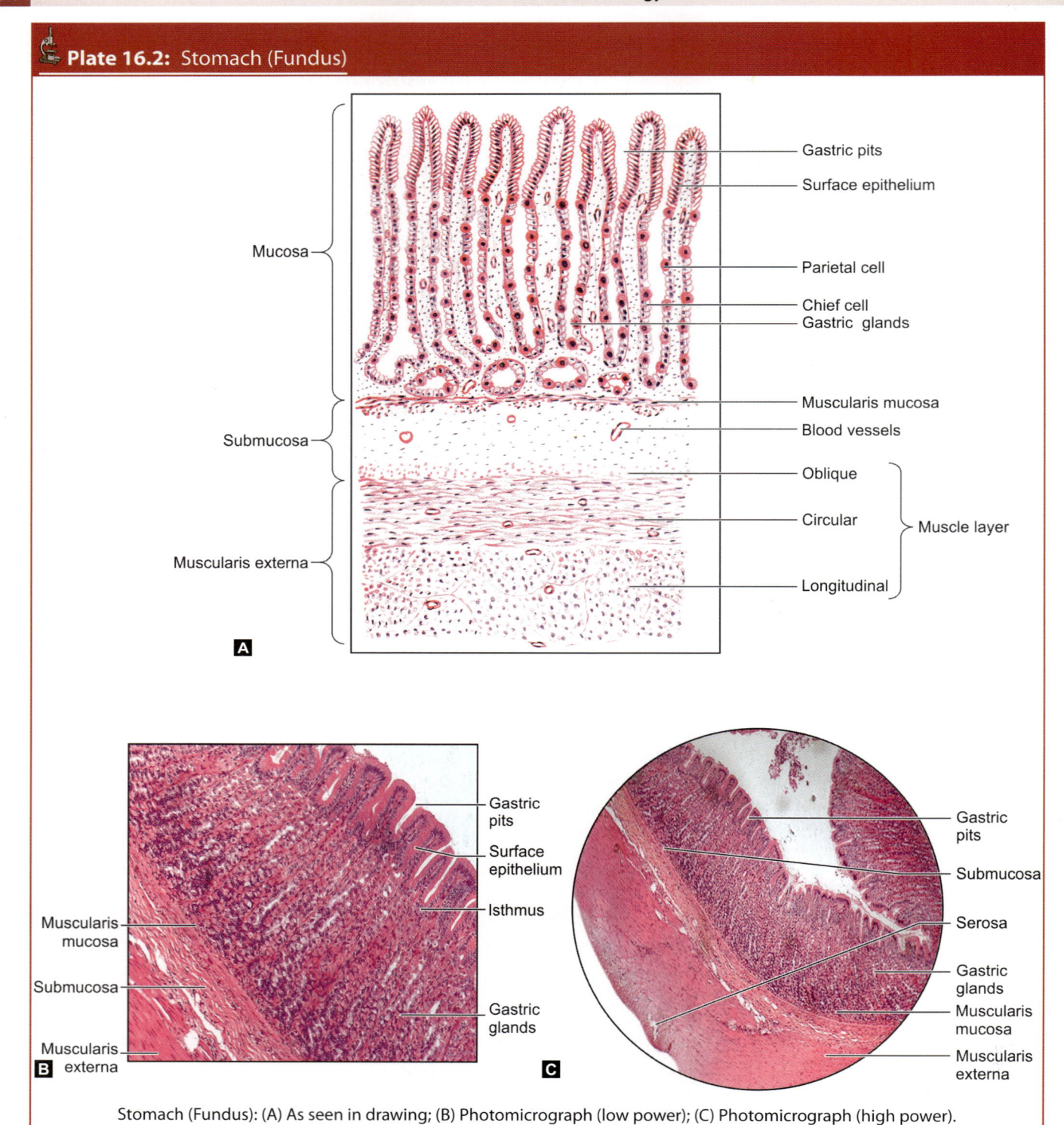

Stomach (Fundus): (A) As seen in drawing; (B) Photomicrograph (low power); (C) Photomicrograph (high power).

Points of identification
- Presence of four layers—mucosa, submucosa, muscularis externa, and serosa
- Shallow gastric pits occupying superficial one-fourth or less of the mucosa
- Presence of gastric glands in the mucosa
- Gastric glands with numerous oxyntic cells which give beaded appearance.

CHAPTER 16: Digestive System: General Plan of Gastrointestinal Tract, Stomach and Intestines

Plate 16.3: Stomach (Pylorus)

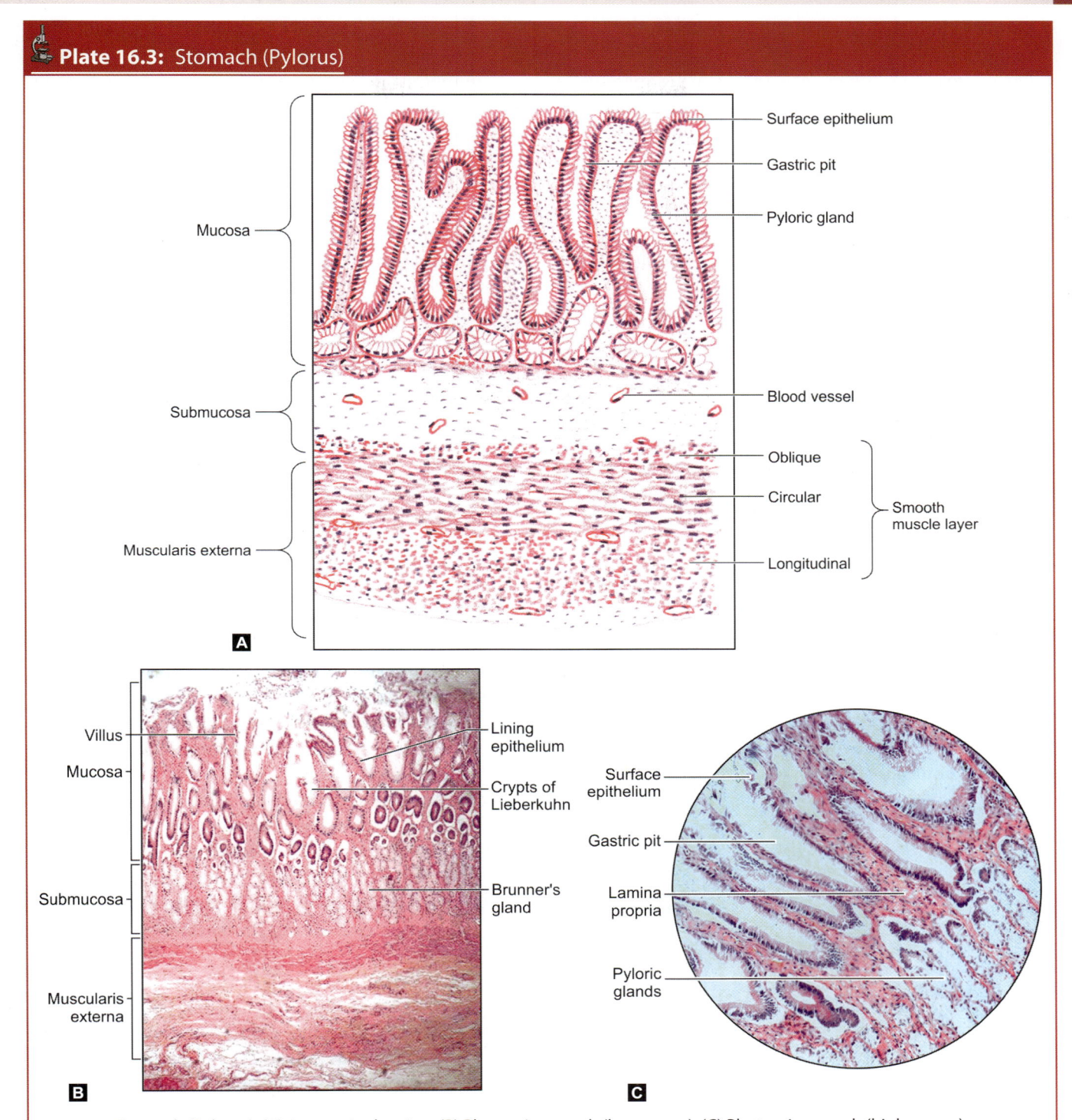

Stomach (Pylorus): (A) As seen in drawing; (B) Photomicrograph (low power); (C) Photomicrograph (high power).

Points of identification
- Presence of four layers—mucosa, submucosa, muscularis externa, and serosa
- Deep gastric pits occupying two-thirds of the depth of the mucosa
- Presence of pyloric glands (mucous glands) in the mucosa that are simple/branched tubular glands which are coiled.

❖ Simple or branched tubular glands that lie at right angles to the mucosal surface.
❖ Open into gastric pits, each pit receiving the openings of several glands. Here the gastric pits occupy the superficial one-fourth or less of the mucosa, the remaining thickness being closely packed with gastric glands.

The following types of cells are present in the epithelium lining the glands.

1. *Chief cells/peptic cells/zymogen cells*
   - They are most numerous cells particularly in the basal parts of the glands.
   - The cells are cuboidal or low columnar. Their cytoplasm is basophilic.
   - With special methods, the chief cells are seen to contain prominent secretory granules in the apical parts of their cytoplasm. The granules contain pepsinogen that is a precursor of pepsin.
   - With the EM, the cytoplasm is seen to contain abundant rough endoplasmic reticulum and a prominent Golgi complex. The luminal surfaces of the cells bear small irregular microvilli.
   - Chief cells secrete the digestive enzymes of the stomach including pepsin. Pepsin is produced by action of gastric acid on pepsinogen. Pepsin breaks down proteins into small peptides. It is mainly through the action of pepsin that solid food is liquefied.

2. *Oxyntic cells/parietal cells*
   - They are large, ovoid or polyhedral, with a large central nucleus (Fig. 16.4).
   - They are present singly, sandwiched between peptic cells and basement membrane. They are more numerous in the upper half of the gland than in its lower half.
   - They are called oxyntic cells because they stain strongly with eosin.
   - They are called parietal cells as they lie against the basement membrane, and often bulge outward (into the lamina propria) creating a beaded appearance.
   - The EM shows that each parietal cell has a narrow apical part that reaches the lumen of the gland. The apical cell membrane shows several invaginations into the cytoplasm, producing tortuous intracellular canaliculi that communicate with the glandular lumen. The walls of the canaliculi bear microvilli that project into the canaliculi. The cytoplasm (in the intervals between the canaliculi) is packed with mitochondria. The mitochondria are responsible for the granular appearance and eosinophilia of the cytoplasm (seen with the light microscope). Secretory granules are not present.
   - Oxyntic cells secrete hydrochloric acid. They also produce an *intrinsic factor of Castle* (a glycoprotein) that combines with vitamin B_{12} (present in ingested food and constituting an *extrinsic factor*) to form a complex necessary for normal formation of erythrocytes.

3. *Mucous neck cells*
   - They are large cells with a clear cytoplasm found near the upper end (or "neck") of the glands, also called *mucous neck cells*.
   - The nucleus is flattened and is pushed to the base of the cell by accumulated mucous.
   - The supranuclear part of the cell contains prominent granules. The chemical structure of the mucus secreted by these cells is different from that secreted by mucous cells lining the surface of the gastric mucosa.

4. *Endocrine cells*
   - Near the basal parts of the gastric glands there are *endocrine cells* that contain membrane bound neurosecretory granules.
   - As the granules stain with silver salts, these have been called *argentaffin cells* in the past.
   - These cells are flattened. They do not reach the lumen, but lie between the chief cells and the basement membrane.
   - These cells probably secrete the hormone *gastrin*. Some of the cells can be shown to contain serotonin (5HT).

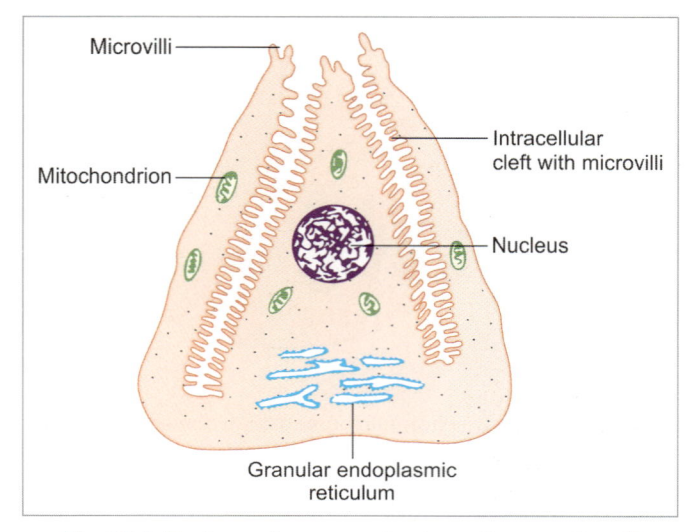

Fig. 16.4: Electron microscope structure of an oxyntic cell (schematic representation).

5. **Stem cells**
   - Some undifferentiated cells (stem cells) that multiply to replace other cells are also present.
   - They increase in number when the gastric epithelium is damaged (for example, when there is a gastric ulcer), and play an important role in healing.

Cardiac glands
- These are confined to a small area (cardia) near the opening of the esophagus.
- In this region, the mucosa is relatively thin.
- Gastric pits are shallow (as in the body of the stomach).
- The cardiac glands are either simple tubular, or compound tubule-alveolar.
- They are mainly mucus-secreting. An occasional oxyntic or peptic cell may be present.

Pyloric glands
- In the pyloric region of the stomach, the gastric pits are deep and occupy two-thirds of the depth of the mucosa.
- The pyloric glands that open into these pits are short and occupy the deeper one-third of the mucosa.
- They are simple or branched tubular glands that are coiled.
- The glands are lined by mucus-secreting cells. Occasional oxyntic and argentaffin cells may be present.
- In addition to other substances, pyloric glands secrete the hormone gastrin.

Lamina propria
- The lamina propria is relatively scanty.
- Made of reticular fibers and other connective tissue cells.
- Occasional aggregations of lymphoid tissue are present in it.

Muscularis mucosae
- The muscularis mucosae of the stomach is thin.
- Apart from the usual circular (inner) and longitudinal (outer) layers, an additional circular layer may be present outside the longitudinal layer.
- The smooth muscle helps in the expulsion of the secretion of gastric glands.

Submucosa
Consists of loose areolar tissue with blood vessels, lymphatics, and nerve plexus.

Muscularis Externa
- The muscularis externa of the stomach is well-developed.
- Made of three layers: (1) inner oblique, (2) middle circular, and (3) longitudinal layer.
- The appearance of the layers in sections is, however, highly variable depending upon the part of the stomach sectioned.
- Longitudinal layer covers the entire organ and is more thick along the curvatures. At the pyloric end, it forms two strata: (1) superficial and (2) deep. Superficial layer is continuous with the corresponding layer of duodenum, whereas deep layer forms dilator component of pyloric sphincter. This layer helps in expulsion of gastric contents into duodenum.
- The circular fibers are greatly thickened at the pylorus where they form the pyloric sphincter (sphincteric component). This layer retains the gastric content in situ till completion of digestion. Unlike the longitudinal layer, it is not continuous with that of duodenum.
- Both circular and longitudinal layer are continuous with corresponding muscle of esophagus but does not form any anatomical sphincter.
- Oblique layer covers the fundus and the body. Has inverted "U" shaped loop of smooth muscle fibers covering the adjoining surfaces. Along the lesser curvature it forms free margin, contraction of which makes the cardioesophageal angle more acute, thereby prevents regurgitation of gastric contents into esophagus.
- Between the layers of muscles there exists, myenteric/Aurebach's plexus of nerves.

Serosa
Gastric serosa is derived from peritoneum and is continuous with the parietal peritoneum of abdominal cavity via greater omentum and visceral peritoneum of liver via lesser omentum. But the lesser curvature, greater curvature, and bare area of stomach are devoid of serosa.

SMALL INTESTINE

Introduction
The small intestine is a tube about 5 m long. It is divided into three parts.

In the craniocaudal sequence, these are:
- **Duodenum** (about 25 cm long)
- **Jejunum** (about 2 m long)
- **Ileum** (about 3 m long).

Small intestine is the principal site for absorption of products of digestion. It also secretes some hormones through enteroendocrine cells. Complete digestion of ingested food occurs in small intestine.

Structure (Table 16.2)

- The wall of the small intestine is made up of the four layers: (1) mucosa, (2) submucosa, (3) muscularis externa, and (4) serosa (Fig. 16.5).
- The serosal and muscular layers correspond exactly to the general structure of alimentary canal.
- The submucosa is also typical except in the duodenum, where it contains the **glands of Brunner**.
- The mucous membrane exhibits several special features that are discussed below.

Table 16.2: Distinguishing features of duodenum, jejunum, and ileum (Plates 16.4 to 16.6).

Duodenum	Jejunum	Ileum
Lumen—wider, wall—thicker	Lumen—wider, wall—thicker	Lumen—narrow, wall—thinner
Large, thick circular folds in the lumen	Large, thick circular folds in the lumen	Small, few circular folds in the lumen
Numerous broad villi	Numerous tall villi	Only few, short and slender villi
Mucus-secreting Duodenal glands or glands of Brunner	Very few Peyer patches extending into submucosa—only in the distal part	Numerous Peyer's patches extending into mucosa

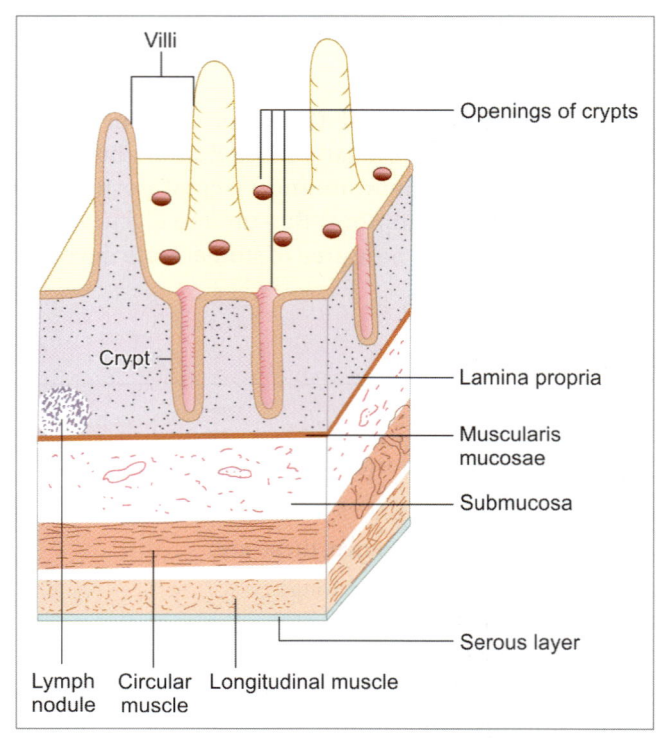

Fig. 16.5: Basic structure of the small intestine (schematic representation).

Mucous Membrane

Mucous membrane is made up of lining epithelium resting on basement membrane, lamina propria, and muscularis mucosa. The surface area of the mucous membrane of the small intestine is extensive (to allow adequate absorption of food). This is achieved by the following features.

- The considerable length of the intestine.
- The presence of numerous circular folds (**plicae circularis**) in the mucosa.
- The presence of numerous finger-like processes, or **villi**, that project from the surface of the mucosa into the lumen.
- The presence of numerous depressions or **crypts** that invade the lamina propria.
- The presence of microvilli on the luminal surfaces of the cells lining the mucosa.

1. *Circular folds:*
   - They are permanent circular folds, called the **Valves of Kerckring**. The folds are large and readily seen with the naked eye. Sometimes they may be semilunar or spiral.
   - Each fold is made up of all layers of the mucosa (lining epithelium, lamina propria, and muscularis mucosae). The submucosa also extends into the folds (Fig. 16.6).
   - They are absent in the first 1 or 2 inches of the duodenum. They are prominent in the rest of the

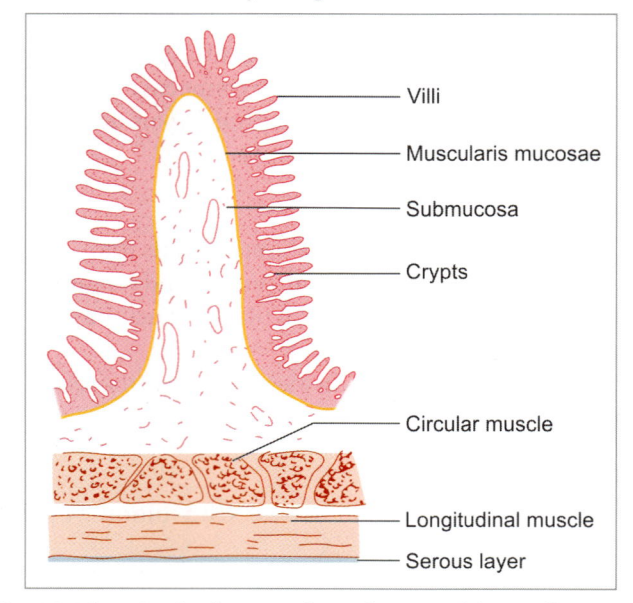

Fig. 16.6: Longitudinal section through a part of the small intestine seen at a very low magnification to show a circular mucosal fold (schematic representation). Note the submucosa extending into the mucosal fold.

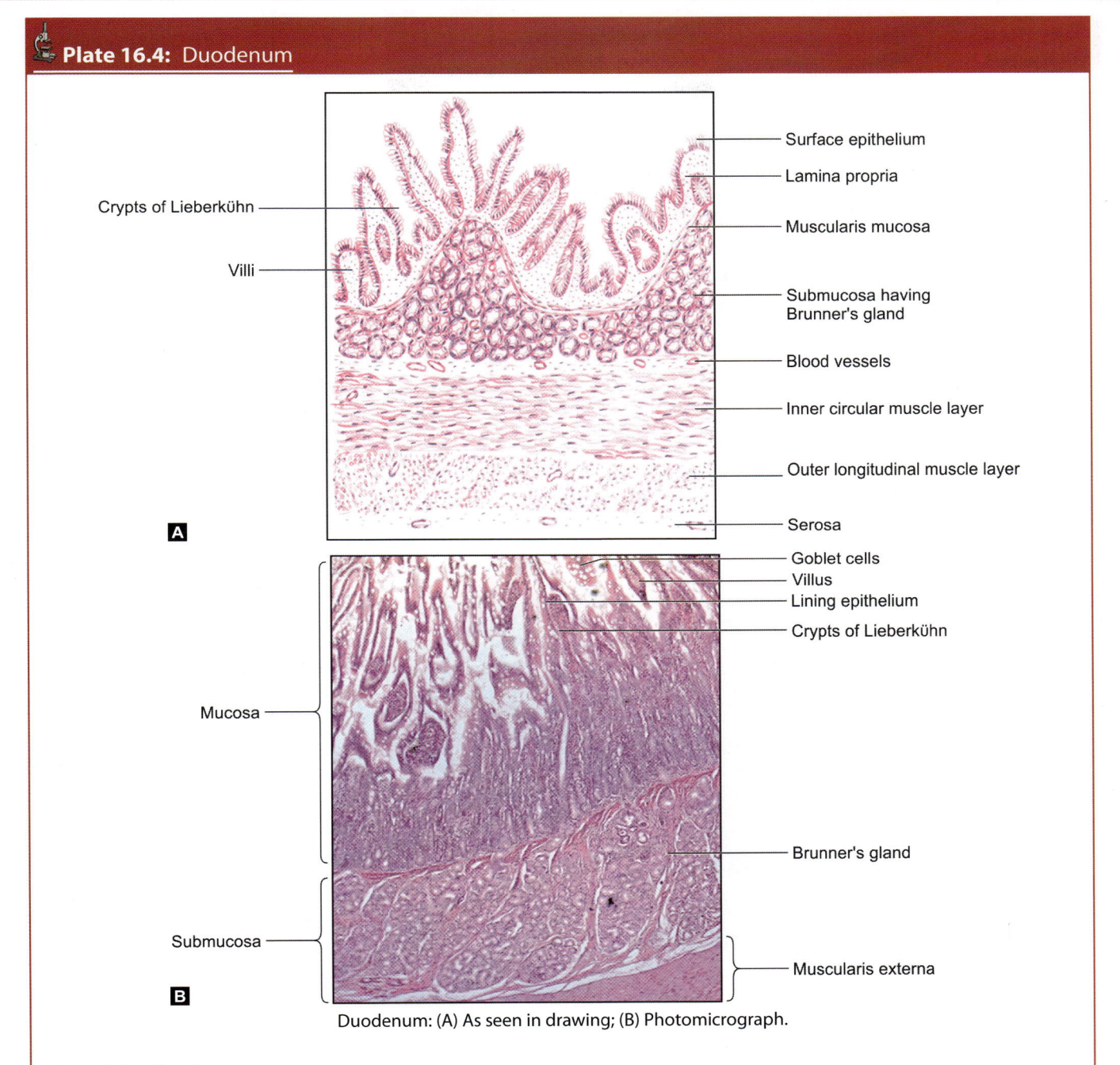

CHAPTER 16: Digestive System: General Plan of Gastrointestinal Tract, Stomach and Intestines

Plate 16.4: Duodenum

Duodenum: (A) As seen in drawing; (B) Photomicrograph.

Points of identification
- Wall made up of four layers
- Mucosa—presence of numerous broad villi, lined by simple columnar epithelium with microvilli and goblet cells
- Presence of submucous Brunner's gland.

Textbook of Human Histology

Plate 16.5: Jejunum

Labels (A, drawing):
- Mucosa
  - Villus
  - Lining epithelium
  - Lamina propria
  - Goblet cell
- Submucosa
  - Muscularis mucosa
- Muscularis externa
  - Inner circular
  - Outer longitudinal
  - Smooth muscle layer

Labels (B, photomicrograph):
- Crypts of Lieberkühn
- Lining epithelium
- Villus
- Submucosa

Jejunum: (A) As seen in drawing; (B) Photomicrograph.

Points of identification
- Wall made up of four layers
- Mucosa—presence of numerous tall slender villi, lined by simple columnar epithelium with microvilli and goblet cells
- Absence of submucous Brunner's gland.

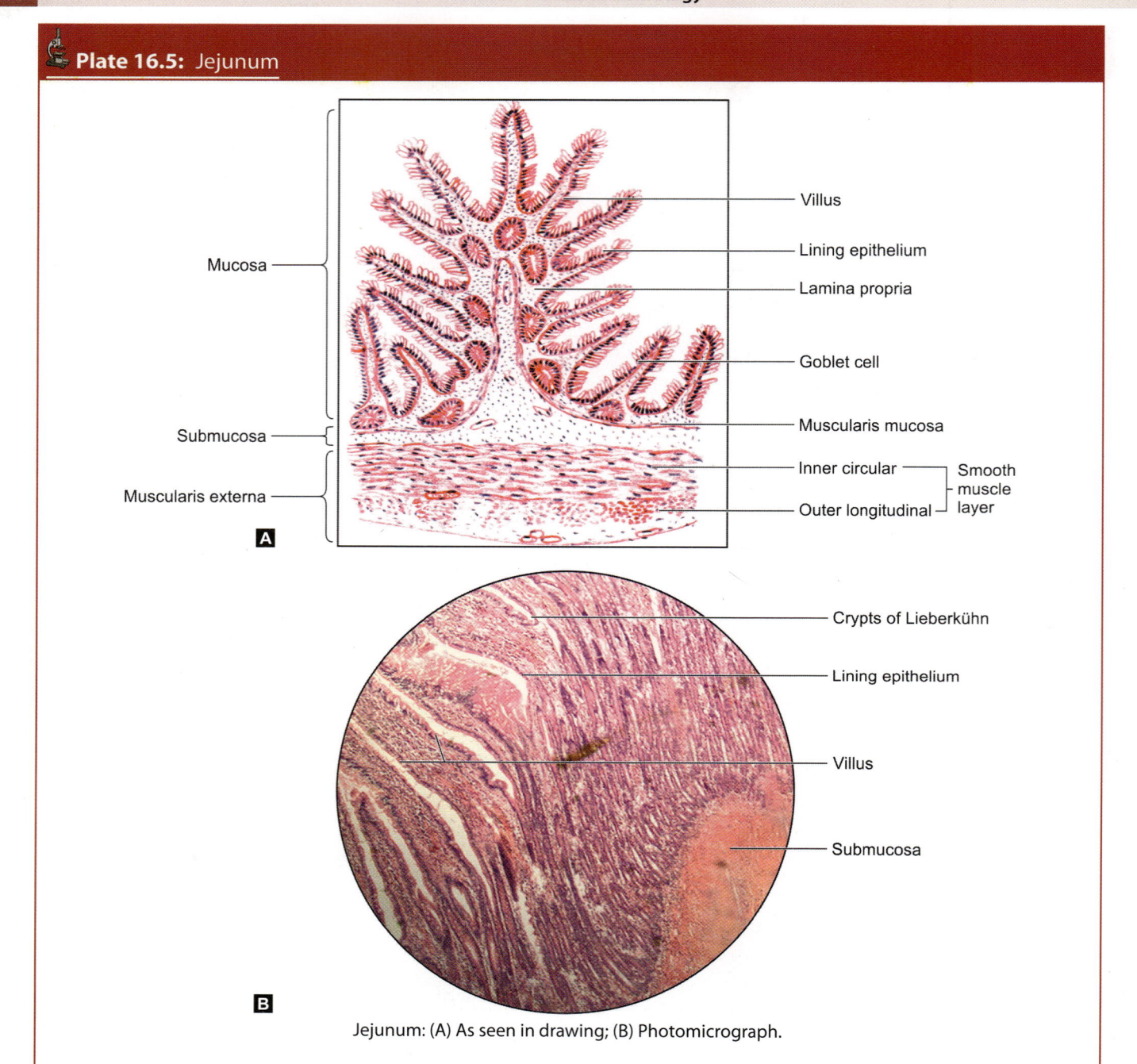

CHAPTER 16: Digestive System: General Plan of Gastrointestinal Tract, Stomach and Intestines 201

Plate 16.6: Ileum

A — Labels: Mucosa, Submucosa, Muscularis externa; Lining epithelium, Villus, Goblet cell, Lamina propria, Peyer's patch, Muscularis mucosa, Inner circular, Outer longitudinal (Muscle layer)

B — Labels: Lining epithelium with goblet cell, Villus, Peyer's patches

Ileum: (A) As seen in drawing; (B) Photomicrograph.

Points of identification
- Wall made up of four layers
- Mucosa—presence of short, small fewer villi, lined by simple columnar epithelium with microvilli and numerous goblet cells
- Absence of submucous Brunner's gland.

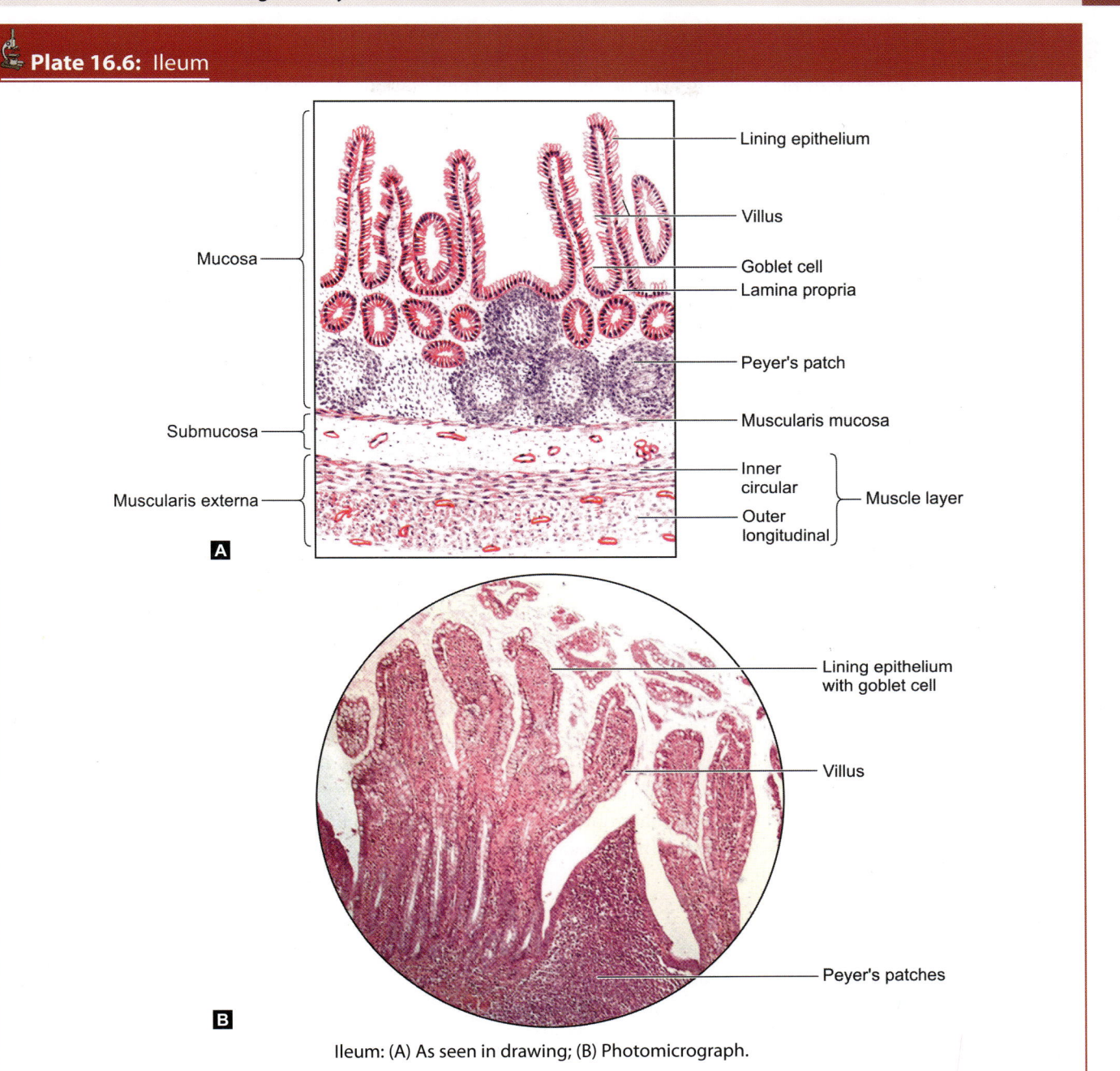

duodenum, and in the whole of the jejunum. The folds gradually become fewer and less marked in the ileum. The terminal parts of the ileum have no such folds.
- Apart from adding considerably to the surface area of the mucous membrane, the circular folds tend to slow down the passage of contents through the small intestine thus facilitating absorption.

2. *Villi:*
   - The villi are, typically, finger-like projections consisting of a core of reticular tissue covered by a surface epithelium (Fig. 16.6).
   - The connective tissue core contains numerous blood capillaries forming a plexus.
   - The endothelium lining the capillaries is fenestrated thus allowing rapid absorption of nutrients into the blood.
   - Each villus contains a central lymphatic vessel called a lacteal. Lymphatic capillary is blind toward the tip and ends in a plexus of lymphatic vessels present in the lamina propria. They are concerned with fat absorption. Occasionally, the lacteal may be double.
   - Some muscle fibers derived from the muscularis mucosae extend into the villus core and surround the lacteal.
   - Lamina propria contains reticular fibers and other connective tissue cells. Plasma cells of lamina propria provide surface immunity by secreting IgA.

3. *Crypts:* The crypts (of Lieberkühn) are tubular invaginations of the epithelium into the lamina propria. They are simple tubular **intestinal glands** which open between the bases of adjacent villi.

Epithelial Lining

❖ The epithelium lining the luminal surface (villi, and areas intervening between them) is mainly columnar, specialized for absorption. The tall columnar cells are called **enterocytes**. Scattered amongst the columnar cells there are mucus-secreting goblet cells.

❖ The cells lining the crypts (intestinal glands) are predominantly undifferentiated. These cells multiply to give rise to absorptive columnar cells and to goblet cells.

❖ Near the bases of the crypts there are **Paneth cells** that secrete enzymes. Endocrine cells (bearing membrane bound granules filled with various neuroactive peptides) are also present.

Cells of small intestine
❖ **Absorptive columnar cells**
   - Each cell has an oval nucleus located in its lower part. When seen with the light microscope the luminal surface of the cell appears to be thickened and to have striations in it, perpendicular to the surface (Fig. 16.7).
   - This *striated border* is made up of microvilli arranged in a very regular manner as seen through electron microscope. The presence of microvilli greatly increases the absorptive surface of the cell.
   - Each microvillus has a wall of plasma membrane containing fine filaments. These filaments extend into the apical part of the cell where they become continuous with a plexus of similar filaments and form **terminal web**. The surface of each microvillus is covered by a layer of fine fibrils and mucous (*glycocalyx*).
   - The plasma membrane on the lateral sides of absorptive cells shows folds that interdigitate with those of adjoining cells. Adjacent cells are united by typical junctional complexes and by scattered desmosomes. Intercellular canals may be present between adjacent cells. The cytoplasm of absorptive cells contains the usual organelles, including lysosomes and smooth ER. These cells are responsible for absorption of amino acids, carbohydrates, and lipids present in digested food.

❖ **Goblet cells**
   - Each goblet cell has an expanded upper part that is distended with mucin granules (Figs. 16.8 and 16.9).
   - The nucleus is flattened and is situated near the base of the cell.

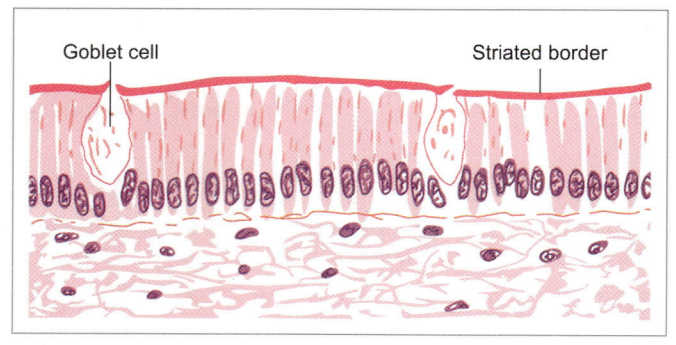

Fig. 16.7: Cells of small intestine (schematic representation).

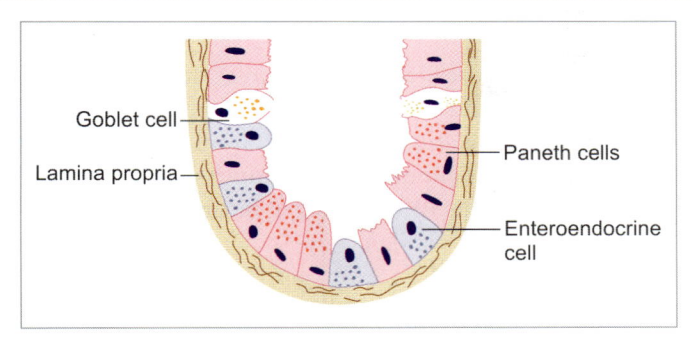

CHAPTER 16: Digestive System: General Plan of Gastrointestinal Tract, Stomach and Intestines

Fig. 16.8: Columnar epithelium lining the small intestine. Note the striated border and some goblet cells (schematic representation).

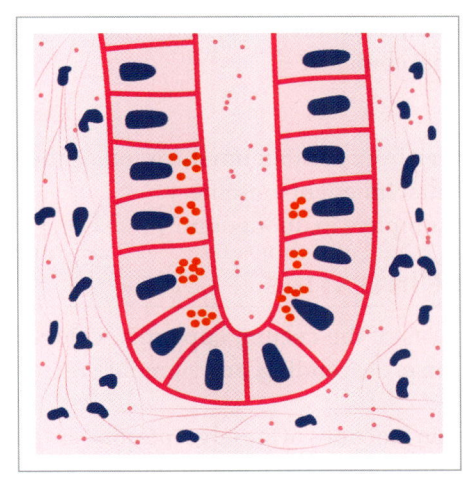

Fig. 16.9: High power view of an intestinal crypt showing Paneth cells with red staining supranuclear granules (schematic representation).
Courtesy: Dr V Subhadra Devi, SVIMS-SPMC (W), Tirupati.

- Goblet cells are mucus-secreting cells. In consonance with their secretory function, these cells have a prominent Golgi complex and abundant rough endoplasmic reticulum toward the basal region.
- The luminal surface of the cell bears some irregular microvilli.
- In routine hematoxylin and eosin (H&E) staining, the apical part of goblet cells appears pale, as the mucin granules are washed out during preparations. It stains brightly with the PAS technique.
- Mucous cells increase in number as we pass down the small intestine, being few in the duodenum and most numerous in the terminal ileum.

❖ **Undifferentiated cells**
- These are columnar cells present in the walls of intestinal crypts. They are similar to absorptive cells, but their microvilli and terminal webs are not so well developed. The cytoplasm contains secretory granules.
- Undifferentiated cells proliferate actively by mitosis. The newly formed cells migrate upward from the crypt to reach the walls of villi.
- Here they differentiate either into typical absorptive cells, or into goblet cells. These cells migrate toward the tips of the villi where they are shed off. In this way, the epithelial lining is being constantly replaced, each cell having a life of only a few days.
- The term "*intermediate cells*" has been applied to differentiating stem cells that show features intermediate between those of stem cells and fully differentiated cells.

❖ **Paneth cells (zymogen cells)**
- These cells are found only in the deeper parts of intestinal crypts.
- They contain prominent eosinophilic secretory granules (Figs. 16.8 and 16.9).
- With the EM, Paneth cells are seen to contain considerable Golgi apparatus, rough endoplasmic reticulum, and other organelles.
- They are known to produce lysozyme that destroys bacteria. They may also produce other enzymes.

❖ **Endocrine cells**
- Cells containing membrane-bound vesicles filled with neuroactive substances are present in the epithelial lining of the small intestine.
- They are most numerous near the lower ends of crypts. As the granules in them stain with silver salts, these cells have, in the past, been termed argentaffin cells (Fig. 16.10).

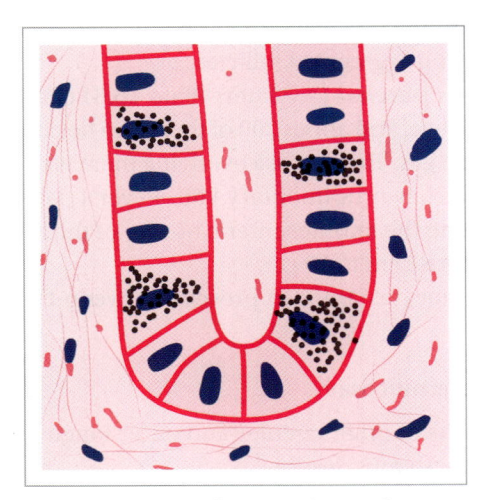

Fig. 16.10: High power view of intestinal crypt showing argentaffin cell with black staining granules that are mostly infranuclear (schematic representation).
Courtesy: Dr V Subhadra Devi, SVIMS-SPMC (W), Tirupati.

- Some of them also give a positive chromaffin reaction, so also called **enterochromaffin cells**. With the introduction of immunohistochemical techniques, it has now been demonstrated that these cells are of various functional types, and contain many amines having an endocrine function.
❖ **M cells**
  - They are epithelial cells lying on the Peyer's patch or large lymphatic aggregation.
  - They possess microfolds instead of microvilli, through which they engulf the microbes gaining access to the lumen.
  - In the form of vesicles, these microbes are transported to the basolateral surface to the vicinity of T lymphocytes in the intercellular space, hence stimulating the GALT. Hence they are also called as antigen-transporting cells.

Lamina propria

Made of meshwork of reticular fibers; is thickly populated with lymphatic aggregations, lymphocytes, plasma cells and other components of immune system apart from connective tissue associated fibroblasts, eosinophils, leukocytes, macrophages, and mast cells.
❖ Solitary and aggregated lymphatic follicles (Peyer's patches) are present in the lamina propria of the small intestine constituting GALT. The solitary follicles become more numerous, and the aggregated follicles larger, in proceeding caudally along the small intestine. They are most prominent in the terminal ileum (Plate 16.6). Their lymphoid tissue may occasionally extend into the submucosa. Villi are few or missing in the mucosa overlying aggregated follicles.
❖ **Peyer's patches** (*see* later; Plate 16.6) can be seen by naked eye, and about 200 of them can be counted in the human gut. The mucosa overlying them is devoid of villi or may have rudimentary villi. Peyer's patches always lie along the antimesenteric border of the intestine and measure 2 cm to 10 cm.
❖ Lymphocytes are also present between the epithelial cells.

Muscularis mucosae

❖ Consists of inner circular and outer longitudinal layers of smooth muscles.
❖ Few fibers extend to the mucosa and help in the movement of villi and expulsion of secretions from the intestinal glands.

Submucosa

❖ Consists of loose areolar tissue containing blood vessels, lymphatics, and nerve plexus (Meissner's plexus).
❖ Submucosal glands of Brunner are the characteristic feature of duodenum. They are branched tubular glands, secreting mucus which is rich in bicarbonate ions.

Muscularis Externa

❖ Made of inner circular and outer longitudinal layer.
❖ Contains myenteric plexus between these two layers.
❖ Inner circular mainly concerned with segmentation movement (local mixing of chime). Peristalsis involves coordinated contraction of both layers for propulsion of intestinal contents.

Serosa

❖ Is derived from peritoneum surrounding the tube except at the attachment of mesentery.
❖ It is incomplete in duodenum.

LARGE INTESTINE

❖ It consists of the cecum, appendix, colon (ascending, transverse, descending, and sigmoid), rectum, and anal canal.
❖ The main functions of the large intestine are absorption of water and conversion of the liquid, undigested material into solid feces.
❖ It harbors some nonpathogenic bacteria that produce vitamin B_{12} necessary for hemopoiesis and vitamin K required for coagulation of blood.

Colon

The structure of the colon conforms to the general description of the structure of the gut by having four layers from inside to outside—mucosa, submucosa, muscularis externa, and serosa (Table 16.3 and Plate 16.7).

Mucous Membrane

❖ The mucous membrane of the colon shows numerous crescent-shaped folds but **Villi** are **absent**.
❖ The mucosa shows numerous closely arranged tubular glands or crypts similar to those in the small intestine.
❖ The mucosal surface and the glands are lined by an epithelium made up predominantly of columnar cells. Their main function is to absorb excess water and electrolytes from intestinal contents.
❖ Numerous goblet cells are present, their number increasing in proceeding caudally. The mucous secreted

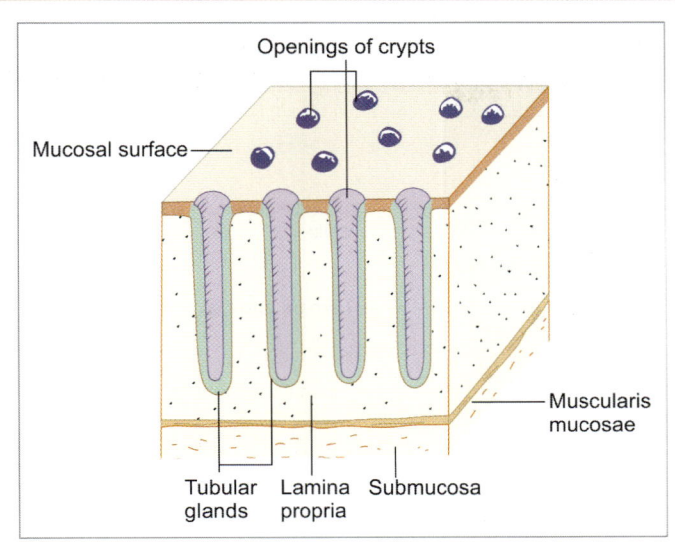

CHAPTER 16: Digestive System: General Plan of Gastrointestinal Tract, Stomach and Intestines

Fig. 16.11: Basic features of the structure of the mucous membrane of the large intestine (schematic representation).

Table 16.3: Differences between small intestine and large intestine.

Small intestine	Large intestine
Narrow lumen	Wider lumen
Villi present in the mucosa	Villi absent in the mucosa
Crypts of Lieberkühn contains columnar, goblet, and Paneth cells	Long and numerous crypts containing predominantly goblet cells. Paneth cells absent
Numerous Peyer patches in the ileum along antimesenteric border	Lymphatic follicles dispersed along different parts
Taenia coli, sacculations, and appendices epiploicae are absent	Taenia coli, sacculations, and appendices epiploicae are present

by them serves as a lubricant that facilitates the passage of semisolid contents through the colon.
- Some endocrine cells and stem cells are seen but Paneth cells are absent.
- The epithelium overlying solitary lymphatic follicles (present in the lamina propria) contains M-cells similar to those described in the small intestine. Scattered cells bearing tufts of long microvilli are also seen. They are probably sensory cells.
- Lamina propria is made up of thick coat of collagen fibers present between the basal lamina of epithelium and venous plexus. It helps in regulation of water and electrolyte absorption.

Submucosa

The submucosa often contains fat cells. Some cells that contain PAS-positive granules, termed ***muciphages***, are also present. These are most numerous in the rectum.

Muscularis Externa

- The longitudinal layer of muscle is unusual. Most of the fibers in it are collected to form three thick bands, the ***Taenia coli*** (Fig. 16.12).
- A thin layer of longitudinal fibers is present in the intervals between the taenia. The taeniae are shorter in length than other layers of the wall of the colon. This results in the production of ***sacculations (Houstra coli)*** on the wall of the colon.

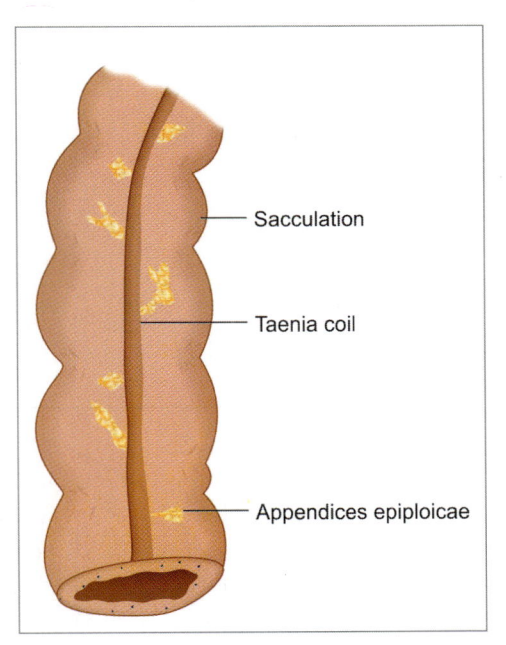

Fig. 16.12: Segment of the colon (schematic representation).

Serosa

The serous layer is missing over the posterior aspect of the ascending and descending colon. In many situations, the peritoneum forms small pouch-like processes that are filled with fat. These yellow masses are called the ***appendices epiploicae***.

Vermiform Appendix (Plate 16.8)

Appendix is a finger-like extension from the cecum. It is the narrowest part of the gut. From inside to outside, it is made up of—mucosa, submucosa, muscularis externa, and serosa.

Plate 16.7: Colon

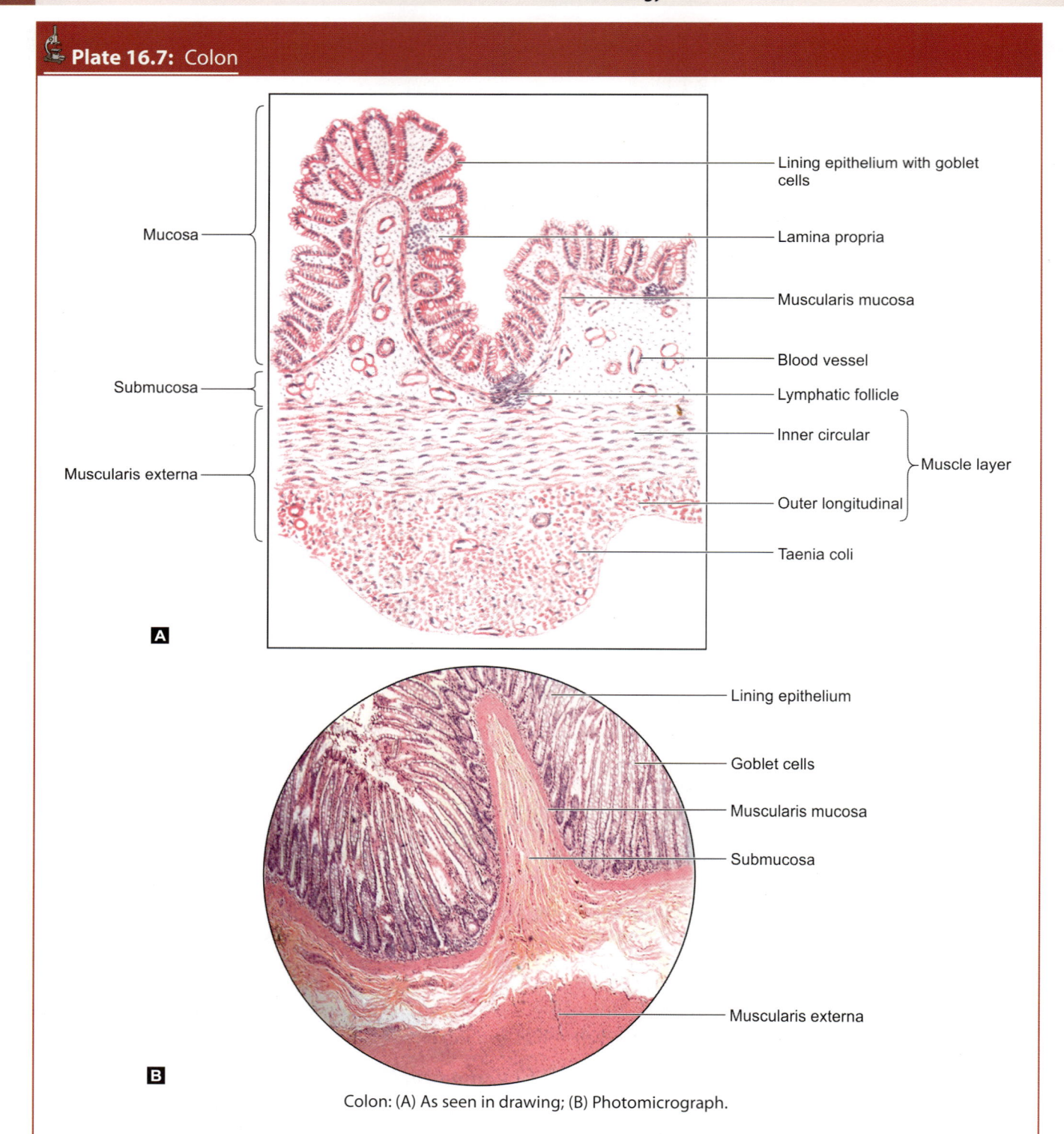

Colon: (A) As seen in drawing; (B) Photomicrograph.

Points of identification
- Wall made up of four layers
- Mucosa—absence of villi, lined by simple columnar epithelium with numerous goblet cells
- Lymphatic follicles dispersed in the lamina propria
- Presence of *taenia coli*, appendices epiploicae.

CHAPTER 16: Digestive System: General Plan of Gastrointestinal Tract, Stomach and Intestines

Plate 16.8: Vermiform appendix

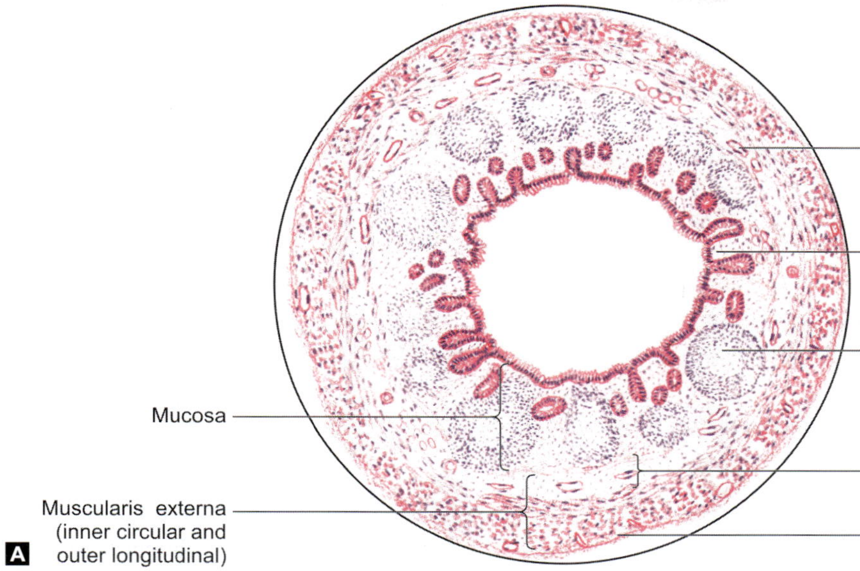

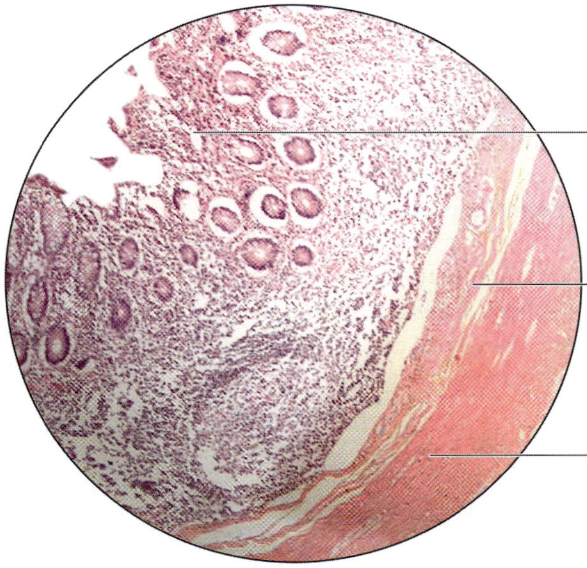

Vermiform appendix: (A) As seen in drawing; (B) Photomicrograph.

Points of identification
- Wall made up of four layers
- Mucosa—absence of villi, lined by simple columnar epithelium with numerous goblet cells
- Submucosa packed with numerous lymphatic follicles, extending into lamina propria
- Absence of taenia coli, appendices epiploicae.

- **Mucous membrane:** Is devoid of villi, poorly formed crypts. **Epithelium is** lined by simple columnar cells, numerous goblet cells, and occasional enterochromaffin cells. Epithelium rests on basement membrane, supported by **lamina propria and muscularis mucosae**.
- **Submucosa:** Contains loose areolar tissue and abundant lymphatic follicles. The lymphoid tissue is not present at birth. It gradually increases and is best seen in children about 10 years old. Subsequently, there is progressive reduction in quantity of lymphoid tissue. Hence, it is also called *abdominal tonsil*.
- **Muscularis externa:** Consists of inner circular and outer longitudinal layers of smooth muscle. At places the muscle coat is deficient and is called as *hiatus muscularis*. *Taenia coli* are absent.
- **Serosa**: Derived from peritoneum covers the entire organ except at the attachment of mesoappendix.

Rectum

The structure of the rectum is similar to that of the colon except for the following:
- Mucous membrane has temporary (longitudinal) and permanent (horizontal) folds.
- Permanent folds/Houston's valves are semilunar in shape, made of mucosa, submucosa, and thickened circular muscle coat.
- A continuous coat of longitudinal muscle is present. There are no taenia coli.
- Peritoneum covers the front and sides of the upper one-third of the rectum; and only the front of the middle third. The rest of the rectum is devoid of a serous covering.
- There are no appendices epiploicae.

Anal Canal

The anal canal is about 4 cm long. The upper 3 cm are lined by mucous membrane and the lower 1 cm by skin (Fig. 16.13).

Mucosa

- The mucous membrane of the upper 15 mm of the canal is lined by columnar epithelium. The mucous membrane of this part shows 6 to 12 longitudinal folds that are called the **anal columns**. The lower ends of the anal columns are united to each other by short transverse folds called the **anal valves**. The anal valves together form a transverse line that runs all around the anal canal, this is the **pectinate/dentate line**. Above each anal valve there is a depression called the **anal sinus**. Mucus-secreting anal glands open into each sinus.

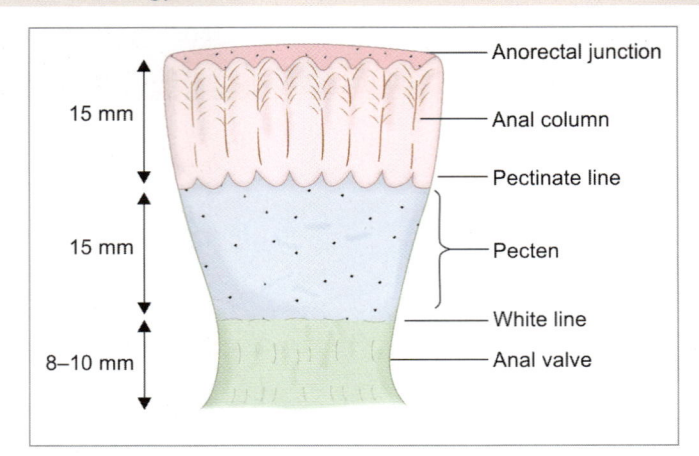

Fig. 16.13: Some features in the interior of the anal canal (schematic representation).

- The mucous membrane of the next 15 mm of the rectum is lined by nonkeratinized stratified squamous epithelium. This region does not have anal columns. The mucosa has a bluish appearance because of the presence of a dense venous plexus between it and the muscle coat. This region is called the **pecten** or **transitional zone**. The lower limit of the pecten forms the **white line of Hilton**.
- The lowest 8 to 10 mm of the anal canal are lined by true skin in which hair follicles, sebaceous glands, and sweat glands (circumanal) are present.

Submucosa

- Prominent venous plexuses are present in the submucosa of the anal canal.
- The internal hemorrhoidal plexus lies above the level of the pectinate line, while the external hemorrhoidal plexus lies near the lower end of the canal.
- Anal glands also extend into the submucosa.

Muscularis Externa

- The anal canal is surrounded by circular and longitudinal layers of muscle continuous with those of the rectum. The circular muscle is thickened to form the **internal anal sphincter**.
- Outside the layer of smooth muscle, there is the **external anal sphincter** that is made up of striated muscle.

APPLIED HISTOLOGY

Esophagus

- Mucous glands near the gastric end of esophagus help to protect the regurgitated gastric content which causes heartburn. If the condition persists for longer

time it can cause gastroesophageal reflux disease (GERD).
- One of the common causes of GERD is abnormal relaxation of lower esophageal sphincter.
- **Barrett's esophagus:** This is a condition in which, following reflux esophagitis, stratified squamous epithelium of the lower esophagus is replaced by columnar epithelium (columnar metaplasia). The condition is seen more commonly in later age and is caused by factors producing gastroesophageal reflux disease.
- **Achalasia (cardiospasm):** Achalasia of the esophagus is a neuromuscular dysfunction due to which the cardiac sphincter fails to relax during swallowing and results in progressive dysphagia and dilatation of the esophagus (megaesophagus).

Stomach

- **Gastritis:** The term "gastritis" is commonly employed for any clinical condition with upper abdominal discomfort like indigestion or dyspepsia in which the specific clinical signs and radiological abnormalities are absent. The condition is of great importance due to its relationship with peptic ulcer and gastric cancer.
- Certain clinical conditions (like autoimmune disorders) can cause achlorhydria, where there is absence of HCl due to damaged gastric mucosa. **Achlorhydria** can in turn lead to vitamin B_{12} deficiency due to lack of intrinsic factor.
- **Gastric ulcer:** Gastric ulcer may occur due to damage to the gastric mucosa barrier. It is most common along the lesser curvature and pyloric antrum. Food-pain pattern, vomiting, significant weight loss, and deep tenderness in the midline in epigastrium are the main presentations.
- **Zollinger–Ellison syndrome:** Caused by excessive secretion of gastrin by enter enteroendocrine cells, which in turn continuously stimulate parietal cells to secret HCl thus causing gastric and duodenal ulcers.

Small Intestine

- **Crohn's disease or regional enteritis** is an idiopathic chronic ulcerative inflammatory bowel disease, characterized by transmural, non-caseating granulomatous inflammation, affecting most commonly the segment of terminal ileum and/or colon, though any part of the gastrointestinal tract may be involved.
- **Celiac sprue** is the most important cause of primary malabsorption occurring in temperate climates. The condition is characterized by significant loss of villi in the small intestine and thence diminished absorptive surface area. The condition occurs in two forms:
  1. Childhood form, seen in infants and children and is commonly referred to as coeliac disease.
  2. Adult form, seen in adolescents and early adult life and used to be called idiopathic steatorrhea.

> **Added Information**
>
> **Endocrine cells of the gut**
> - The lining epithelium of the stomach, and of the small and large intestines, contains scattered cells that have an endocrine function. These were recognized by early workers because of the presence, in them, of infranuclear granules that blackened with silver salts. They were, therefore, termed **argentaffin** cells.
> - The granules also show a positive chromaffin reaction and have, therefore, also been called **enterochromaffin** cells.
> - More recently, by the use of immunohistochemical methods, several other biologically active substances (amines or polypeptides) have been located in these cells.
> - Many of these substances are also found in the nervous system where they function as neurotransmitters.
> - They also act as hormones. This action is either local on neighboring cells (paracrine effect); or on cells at distant sites (through the bloodstream).
> - Very similar cells are also to be seen in the pancreas. All these cells are now grouped together under the term **gastroenteropancreatic endocrine system**.
> - Some features of this system are similar to those of amine-producing cells in other organs. All these are included under the term APUD cell system.

Colon and Rectum

- **Ulcerative colitis** is an idiopathic form of acute and chronic ulcero-inflammatory colitis affecting chiefly the mucosa and submucosa of the rectum and descending colon, though sometimes it may involve the entire length of the large bowel.
- Acute inflammation of the appendix, **acute appendicitis**, is the most common acute abdominal condition confronting the surgeon. The condition is seen more commonly in older children and young adults, and is uncommon at the extremes of age. The disease is seen more frequently in the West and in affluent societies which may be due to variation in diet—a diet with low bulk or cellulose and high protein intake more often causes appendicitis.
- Hemorrhoids or piles are the varicosities of the hemorrhoidal veins. They are called "internal piles" if dilatation is of superior hemorrhoidal plexus covered over by mucous membrane, and "external piles" if they involve inferior hemorrhoidal plexus covered over by the

skin. They are common lesions in elderly and pregnant women. They commonly result from increased venous pressure.

Some of the cell types recognized, and their secretory products are given in the Table 16.4.

Table 16.4: Different types of endocrine cells in the gut and in the pancreas.

Cell type	Secretory products	Stomach	Small intestine	Large intestine	Pancreas
D_1	Vasoactive intestinal polypeptide	+	+	+	+
D	Somatostatin	+	+		+
EC_1	5HT + Substance P		+	+	
L	Enteroglucagon		+	+	
G	Gastric encephalin	+	+		
EC_2	5HT + Motilin		+		
S	Secretin		+		
I	Cholecystokinin pancreozymin		+		
K	Gastric inhibitory peptide		+		
N	Neurokinin		+		
ECn	5HT + Unknown	+			
B	Insulin				+
A	Glucagon	?	?		+
PP	Pancreatic polypeptide		?		+

MULTIPLE CHOICE QUESTIONS

1. Toughest layer of esophagus is:
   a. Mucosa   b. Submucosa
   c. Muscularis externa   d. Adventitia
2. Lining epithelium of esophagus is:
   a. Simple squamous epithelium
   b. Transitional epithelium
   c. Pseudostratified epithelium
   d. Stratified squamous nonkeratinized epithelium
3. Mucous glands of esophagus are found in:
   a. Lining epithelium   b. Submucosa
   c. Muscularis externa   d. Adventitia
4. Nerve plexus of muscularis externa is called as:
   a. Meissner's plexus   b. Aurebach's plexus
   c. Barrett's plexus   d. Brachial plexus
5. Brunner's gland are found in the mucosa of:
   a. Stomach   b. Colon
   c. Duodenum   d. Esophagus
6. Following cells are found in small intestine, *except*:
   a. Stem cells   b. Goblet cells
   c. Neck cells   d. Paneth cells
7. Cells which give beaded cells to the mucosa of the stomach are:
   a. Stem cells   b. Chief cells
   c. Neck cells   d. Parietal cells
8. Peyer's patches are characteristic feature of:
   a. Stomach   b. Colon
   c. Ileum   d. Esophagus

Answers
1. c   2. d   3. b   4. b   5. c   6. c   7. d   8. c

CHAPTER 17

Hepatobiliary System and Pancreas

Learning objectives

To study the:
- Structure and function of liver
- Bile
- Structure of gallbladder
- Structure of pancreas
- Differences between serous salivary gland and pancreas
- Applied histology

IDENTIFICATION POINTS

Liver	Gallbladder	Pancreas
❏ Central vein surrounded by hexagonal plate of hepatocytes ❏ Presence of portal triad consisting of arteriole branch of hepatic artery, bile ductule, and venule branch of portal vein ❏ Hepatic sinusoids between the hepatocytes.	❏ Wall made up of three layers—mucosa, fibromuscular layer, and serosa ❏ Mucosa showing honeycombed appearance, lined by simple tall columnar epithelium with striated border.	❏ Presence of serous acini, lined by pyramidal cells with basal rounded nucleus ❏ Presence of islets of Langerhans ❏ Presence of lightly stained squamous—centroacinar cells.

■ INTRODUCTION

The hepatobiliary system comprises of liver, gallbladder, and extrahepatic ducts.

■ LIVER

- Liver is the largest gland of the body situated mainly in the right hypochondrium, below the right dome of diaphragm in the abdomen.
- The liver may be regarded as a modified exocrine gland.
- The functions are:
  - Metabolism of carbohydrates, proteins, and fats.
  - Synthesis of plasma proteins, fibrinogen, and prothrombin, and the regulation of blood glucose and lipids.
  - Storage of glucose (as glycogen), lipids, vitamin A, metabolism of vitamin D, and processing of vitamin K.
  - Storage and metabolism of iron, degradation of various substances (including drugs and alcohol).
  - Removal of bile pigments and their excretion through bile.
  - Modification of thyroxine, growth hormone; degradation of insulin and glucagon.
  - During fetal life, the liver is the center for hemopoiesis.
  - The macrophage cells (of Kupffer) lining the sinusoids of the liver have a role similar to that of other cells of the mononuclear phagocyte system. They are of particular importance as they are the first cells of this system that come in contact with materials absorbed through the gut. They also remove damaged erythrocytes from blood.
- **Blood supply of liver**: Liver has dual blood supply from portal vein (venous blood) and hepatic artery. Around 70% of nutrition is provided by portal vein which carries blood from gut, pancreas, and spleen containing absorbed substances, destroyed blood cells, and secretions of pancreas and intestinal cells. Remaining 30% of nutrition is conveyed by hepatic artery. Both the vessels enter the liver at porta hepatis, where the bile duct and lymphatics leave the organ. Hence, blood and bile travel in opposite direction within the parenchyma. Within the organ, the branches of hepatic artery and portal vein supply the liver

sinusoids. Sinusoids drain into hepatic venule (central vein). Central veins of adjacent lobules unite to form interlobular veins. Finally, blood from the liver is drained into inferior vena cava via hepatic veins.

- **Macroscopic structure of liver**: The liver is covered by a thin layer of connective tissue capsule called Glisson's capsule. This connective tissue extends into the liver substance through the portal canals (portal triads) and surrounds them. The liver substance is divisible into large lobes, each of which consists of numerous lobules (Plate 17.1).

Microscopic Features

The liver is an accessory gland of gastrointestinal system made up of stroma and parenchyma.

- **Stroma**: It is formed by extensions from Glisson's capsule. Blood vessels, nerves, lymphatic vessels, and bile ducts travel within the connective tissue stroma. It branches extensively and divides the parenchyma into basic structural units called *classical liver lobule*.
- **Parenchyma**: Consists of organized plates of hepatocytes, which in the adult are normally one cell thick and are separated by sinusoidal capillaries.
- **Hepatic sinusoids**: They are present between the hepatic laminae and also between the cords of hepatocytes. They are fenestrated sinusoids lined by endothelial cells and Kupffer cells. Adjacent sinusoids communicate thereby maintains optimal intersinusoidal pressure by acting as vascular pressure. Blood from the sinusoids open into a central vein that occupies the center of the lobule. Hence, hepatic sinusoids work in centripetal direction. Finally, central vein drains into hepatic veins (which leave the liver to end in the inferior vena cava).

Liver Lobules

The parenchyma of liver is divided into units based on three ways:

- **Classical/hepatic lobules**:
  - Hepatic lobules are hexagonal in shape with 1 mm width (Fig. 17.1).
  - Lobules are surrounded by scanty connective tissue (in humans). Central axis of the lobule is occupied by central vein (tributary of hepatic vein).
  - From the central vein, cords of hepatocytes radiate outward as plates/sheets of cells called hepatic laminae. Each lamina is one cell thick, cells within the laminae branch and anastomose. About 20 hepatocytes are present in each lamina.

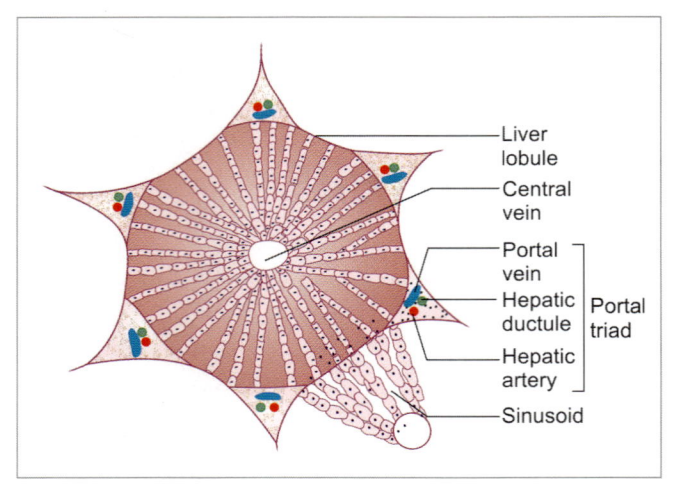

Fig. 17.1: Classic liver lobule (schematic representation).

- Hepatocytes are separated by spaces, known as hepatic lacunae which are occupied by hepatic sinusoids. Hepatocytes are bathed in the sinusoidal blood.
- At the periphery, the adjacent hepatic laminae join and form limiting plate which overlies on portal canals.
- Limiting plates have perforations through which the terminal branches of venules open into sinusoid. Branches of hepatic artery either join the branches of venules or directly open into the sinusoid.
- In some animals, e.g. pig, the classic lobule can be easily recognized because of well-differentiated, relatively thick layers of connective tissue forming structural units. But in humans due to scanty connective tissue around the portal canals, hepatocytes are continuous with adjacent laminae. Hence, hepatic lobules may not be considered as structural/functional units but an independent venous unit drained by particular central vein.
- **Portal canal**: These are angular intervals at the periphery of each lobule, filled by connective tissue. Each "canal" contains: A radicle of portal vein, hepatic arteriole, and interlobular bile duct. These three structures collectively form a **portal triad** (Fig. 17.2).
- Blood from the branch of the portal vein, and from the branch of the hepatic artery, enters the sinusoids at the periphery of the lobule and passes toward its center. Blood vessels and hepatic ducts present in portal canals are surrounded by a narrow interval

CHAPTER 17: Hepatobiliary System and Pancreas

Plate 17.1: Liver (Panoramic view)

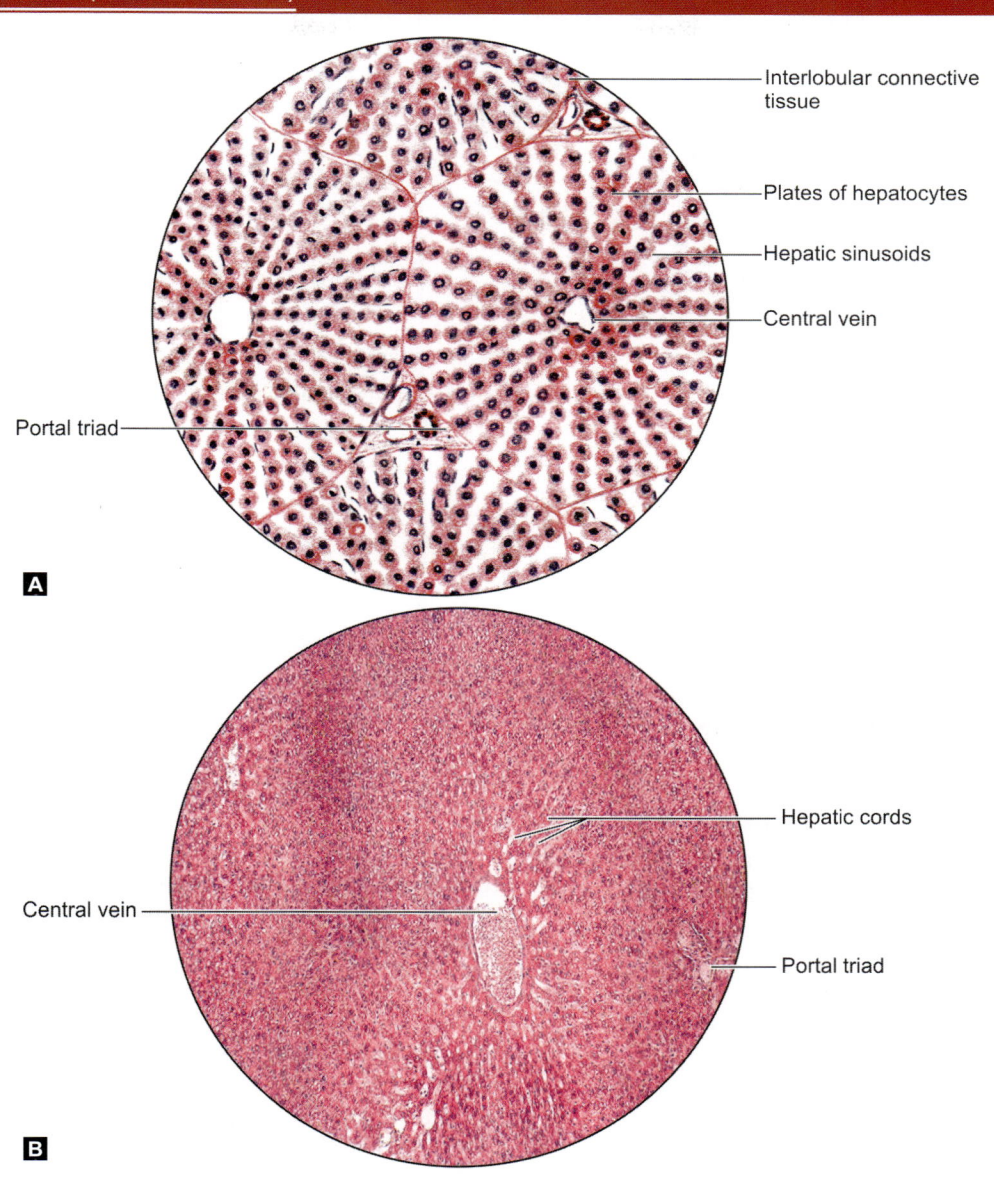

Liver (Panoramic view): (A) As seen in drawing; (B) Photomicrograph.

Points of identification
- The panoramic view of liver shows many hexagonal areas called hepatic lobules. The lobules are partially separated by connective tissue
- Each lobule has a small round space in the center. This is the central vein
- A number of broad irregular cords of cells seem to pass from this vein to the periphery of the lobule. These cords are made up of polygonal liver cells—hepatocytes
- Along the periphery of the lobules, there are angular intervals filled by connective tissue
- Each such area contains a branch of the portal vein, a branch of the hepatic artery, and an interlobular bile duct
- These three constitute a portal triad.

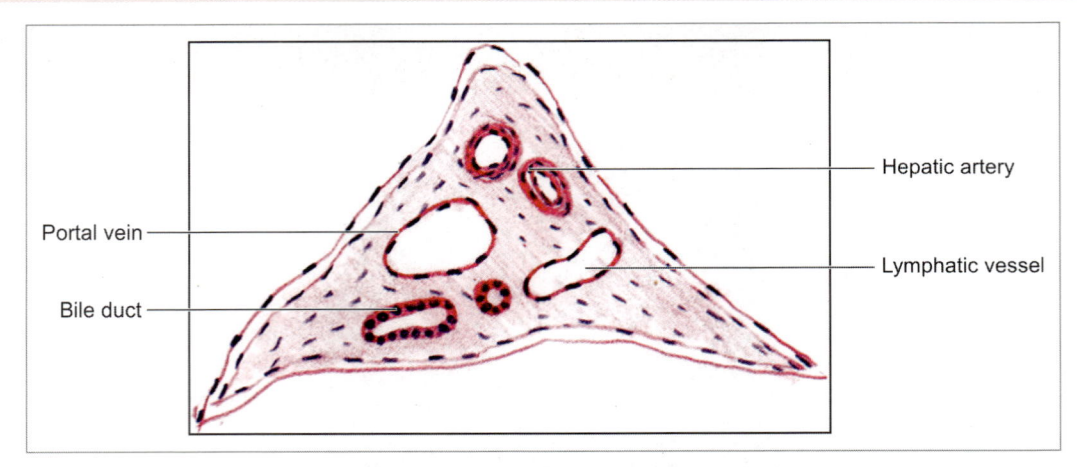

Fig. 17.2: Portal triad (schematic representation).

called **the *space of Mall***. Lymphatics of liver begin in this space as blind radicles.

- **Portal lobule**:
  - They are triangular territory of liver tissue with portal triad at center and central vein at each corner of the triangle (Fig. 17.3).
  - It is called the **nutritional lobule** of the liver, obtained by joining the central vein of three adjacent hepatic lobules.
- **Portal acinus**:
  - It is a diamond-shaped smaller unit of liver tissue supplied by one hepatic arteriole (Fig. 17.4) running along the line of junction of two hepatic lobules. Two central veins lie at the ends of the acinus. They are functional unit of liver.
  - The long axis of the acinus is formed by joining two central veins and short by joining adjacent portal triads.
  - According to the gradient of blood supply, acinus can be divided into three zones—inner zone/zone 1 (around the hepatic arteriole, hence well oxygenated), intermediate zone/zone 2 (moderately oxygenated), and outer zone/zone 3 (least oxygenated). Hence, cells in zone 1 are the first to get not only oxygen, nutrients but also toxins from the sinusoidal blood. Hence, show morphologic changes after bile duct occlusion early. They are last to perish if circulation is impaired and the first to regenerate. Zone 3, on the other hand, is first to show ischemic necrosis on reduced perfusion and also fat accumulation.

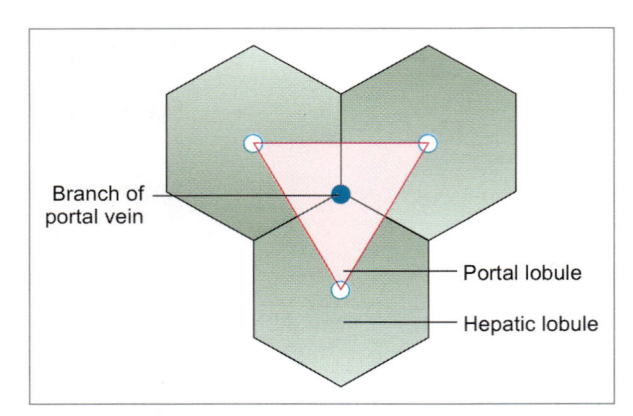

Fig. 17.3: Scheme to show the concept of portal lobules (pink). Hepatic lobules are shaded green. Note that the portal lobule is made up of parts of three hepatic lobules.

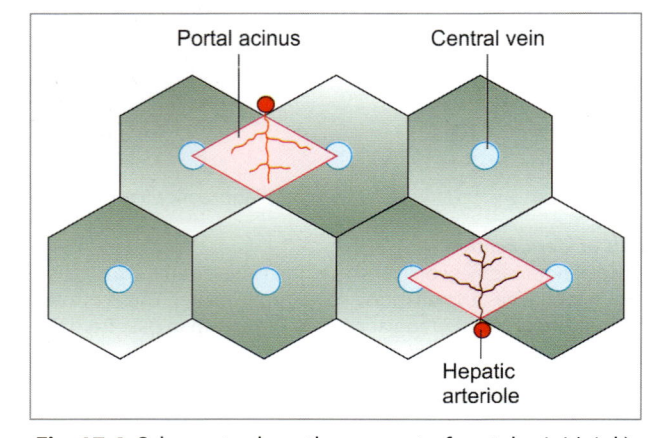

Fig. 17.4: Scheme to show the concept of portal acini (pink).

They are the last to be affected by toxic substances and bile stasis.

Biliary Duct System

- Canaliculi are merely spaces present between plasma membranes of adjacent liver cells into which bile secreted by liver cells is poured.
- At the periphery of a lobule, the canaliculi become continuous with delicate intralobular ductules, which in turn become continuous with larger interlobular ductules of portal triads. Hence, bile canaliculi functions in centrifugal direction.
- The interlobular ductules are lined by cuboidal epithelium. Some smooth muscle is present in the walls of larger ducts.

Cells of Liver

- **Hepatocytes**:
  - Hepatocyte is a large cell with a round open faced nucleus, with prominent nucleoli (Plate 17.2).
  - The cytoplasm of liver cells contains numerous mitochondria, abundant rough and smooth endoplasmic reticulum, a well-developed Golgi complex, lysosomes, and vacuoles containing various enzymes. Numerous free ribosomes are present. These features are to be correlated with the high metabolic activity of liver cells.
  - Stored glycogen, lipids, and iron (as crystals of ferritin and hemosiderin) are usually present.
  - Glycogen is often present in relation to smooth endoplasmic reticulum. Many hepatocytes show two nuclei, or a single polyploid nucleus.
  - Liver cells are arranged in the form of anastomosing plates, one cell thick, separated by sinusoids (Fig. 17.5). In this way, each liver cell has a sinusoid on two sides.
  - The surface of a hepatocyte can show three kinds of specialization (Figs. 17.6 and 17.7):
    - **Sinusoidal surface**: The cell surfaces adjoining sinusoids bear microvilli that project into the space of Disse. The cell surface here also shows many coated pits that are concerned with exocytosis. Both these features help in active transfer of materials from sinusoids to hepatocytes, and vice versa. About 70% of the surface of hepatocytes is of this type.
    - **Canalicular surface**: Areas of cell membrane bear longitudinal depressions that are opposed to similar depressions on neighboring hepatocytes and form the wall of a bile canaliculus. Irregular microvilli project into the canaliculus. On either side of the canaliculus, the cell membranes of adjoining cells are united by junctional complexes and forms blood-bile barrier, which prevents escaping of bile into intercellular space. About 15% of the hepatocyte surface is canalicular.
    - **Intercellular surface**: These are areas of cell surface where adjacent hepatocytes are united to each other just as in typical cells. Communicating junctions allow exchanges between the cells. About 15% of the hepatocyte surface is intercellular.
  - **Space of Disse**: The surface of the liver cell is separated from the endothelial lining of the

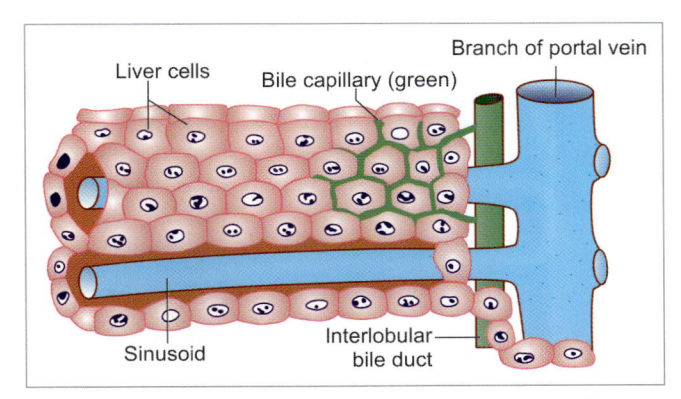

Fig. 17.5: Relationship of bile capillaries to liver cells (schematic representation).

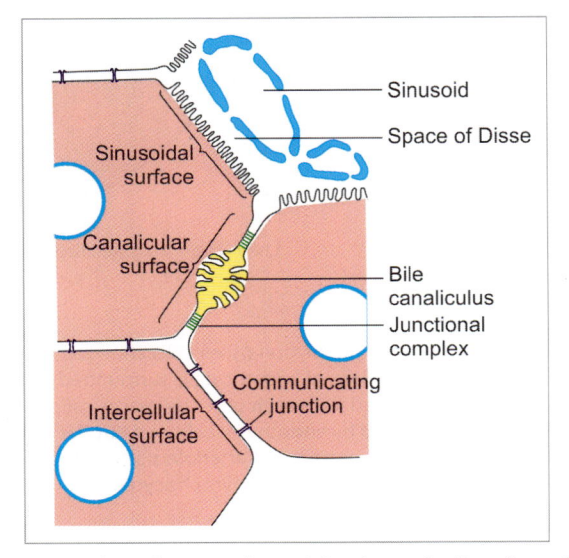

Fig. 17.6: Three functional specializations of cell surface of a hepatocyte (schematic representation).

Plate 17.2: Liver (High magnification)

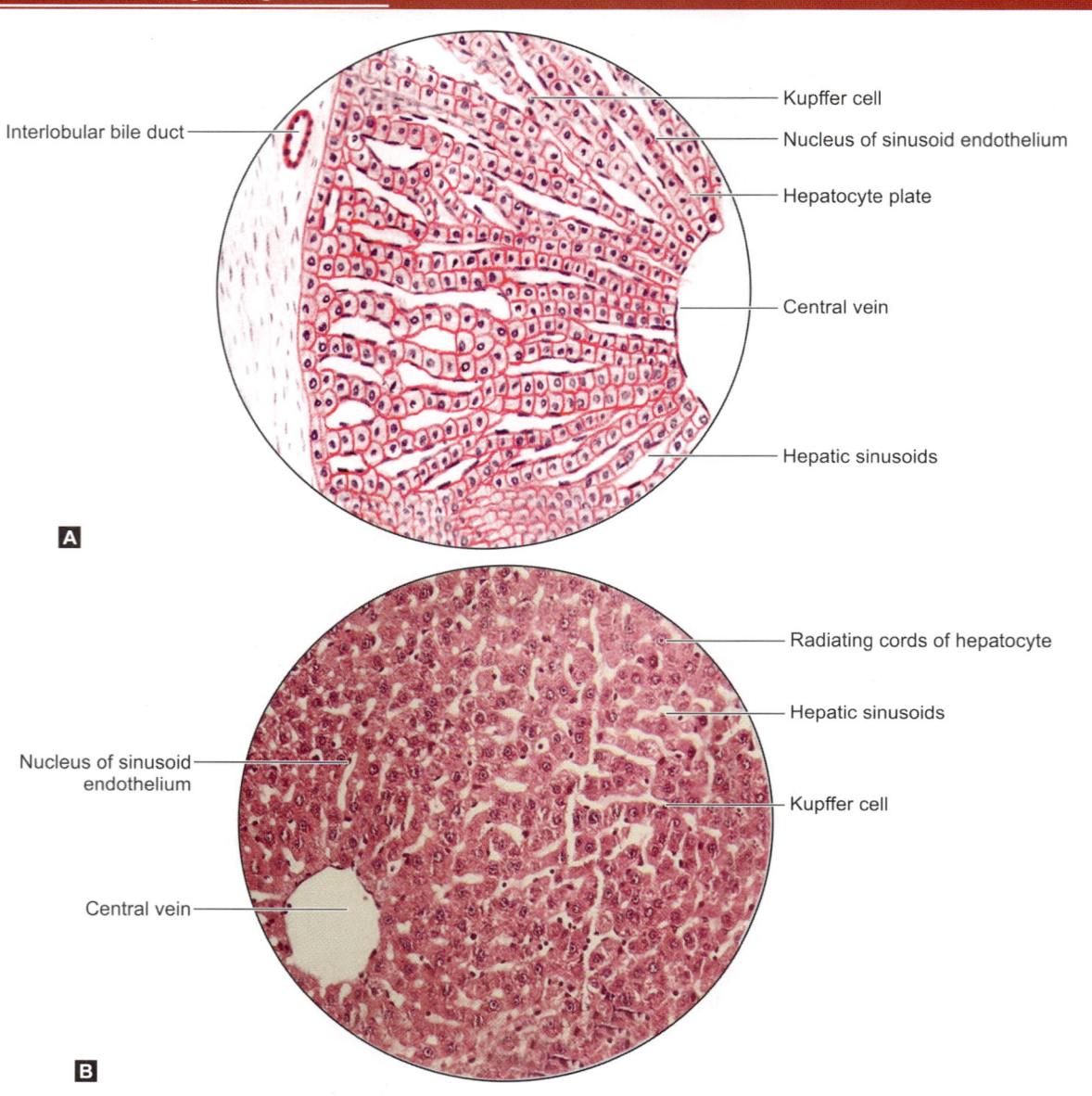

Liver (High magnification): (A) As seen in drawing; (B) Photomicrograph.

Points of identification
On high magnification:
- The lobule is made up of polygonal liver cells arranged in the form of radiating cords
- The central round nucleus of hepatocyte is surrounded by abundant pink cytoplasm
- The cords are separated from each other by spaces called sinusoids
- The sinusoids are lined by endothelial cells and Kupffer cells (macrophage cells)
- Each portal tract contains a hepatic arteriole, portal venule, and one or two interlobular bile ducts. Normally, these structures are surrounded by fibroconnective tissue and a few lymphocytes.

CHAPTER 17: Hepatobiliary System and Pancreas

sinusoid by a narrow perisinusoidal space (of Disse) (Fig. 17.8). Microvilli of the liver cells extend into this space and lie intimately related to circulating blood. Some fat cells and Ito cells are also seen in this space. They are intralobular, in contrast to **space of Mall**, which are interlobular. The portal triad is bordered by the outermost hepatocytes of the lobule (Fig. 17.2). A small space between the connective tissue stroma and hepatocytes at the edges of triad is called the periportal space or **space of Mall**. The lymph is thought to be originated from this space.

- **Kupffer cells**:
  - They are star-/stellate-shaped cells, found lining the walls of hepatic sinusoids.
  - Derived from bone marrow, they belong to mononuclear phagocyte system (MPS), hence clears the cellular debris and microbes from the blood.
  - Recent studies have confirmed their role in final breakdown of senile and damaged RBCs.
- **Ito cells**:
  - They are also stellate-shaped, present in the perisinusoidal space of Disse.
  - They are the primary storehouse of vitamin A.
  - It helps in remodeling of extracellular matrix during recovery from liver damage.
  - Under pathological conditions, they differentiate into myofibroblasts and synthesize collagen.

Bile

- The exocrine secretion of the liver cells is called bile. Bile is poured out from liver cells into very delicate bile canaliculi that are present in intimate relationship to the cells.
- From the canaliculi, bile drains into progressively larger ducts that end in the bile duct. This duct conveys bile into the duodenum where bile plays a role in digestion of fat.

EXTRAHEPATIC BILIARY APPARATUS

The extrahepatic biliary apparatus consists of the gallbladder and the extrahepatic bile ducts.

Gallbladder

- Gallbladder is a blind muscular sac situated on the visceral surface of liver in the fossa on inferior surface.
- The gallbladder stores and concentrates bile.
- This bile is discharged into the duodenum through cystic duct, which joins common hepatic duct to form common bile duct when required.

Microscopic Structure

The wall of the gallbladder is made up of: (a) Inner mucous membrane, (b) Middle fibromuscular coat, and (c) Outer serous layer that cover part of the organ (Plate 17.3).

Mucous membrane

- Mucous membrane is thrown into numerous folds, which gives the surface *honeycomb* appearance.
- The mucous membrane of the gallbladder is lined by simple tall columnar epithelium with microvilli showing striated border.
- Do not contain goblet cells in contrast to small intestine.
- Mucosa contains lamina propria, which lacks the mucosal glands and lymphatic vessels.
- Muscularis mucosa and submucosa are absent.
- Sometimes, deep mucosal diverticula can extend into the muscularis externa and they are called as

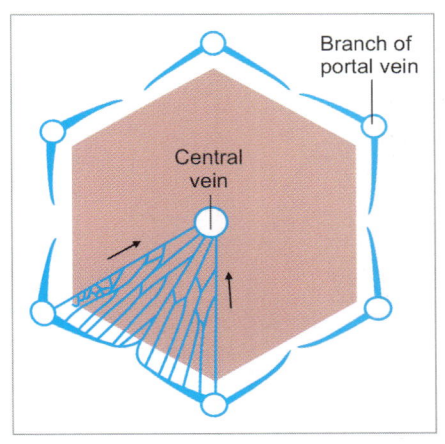

Fig. 17.7: Scheme to show the presence of several branches of the portal vein around a hepatic lobule. The manner in that they open into sinusoids is shown. The intervals between the sinusoids are occupied by liver cells (schematic representation).

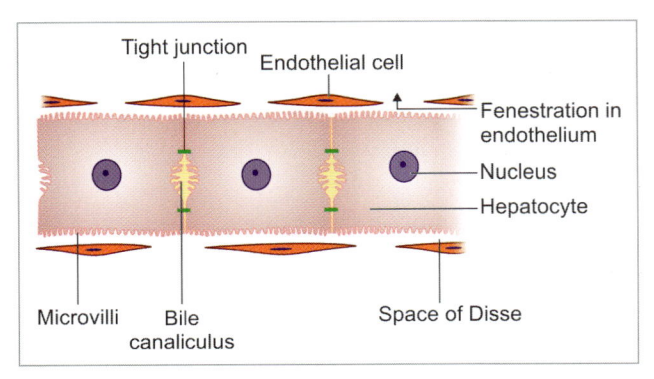

Fig. 17.8: Space of Disse and bile canaliculus (schematic representation).

Plate 17.3: Gallbladder

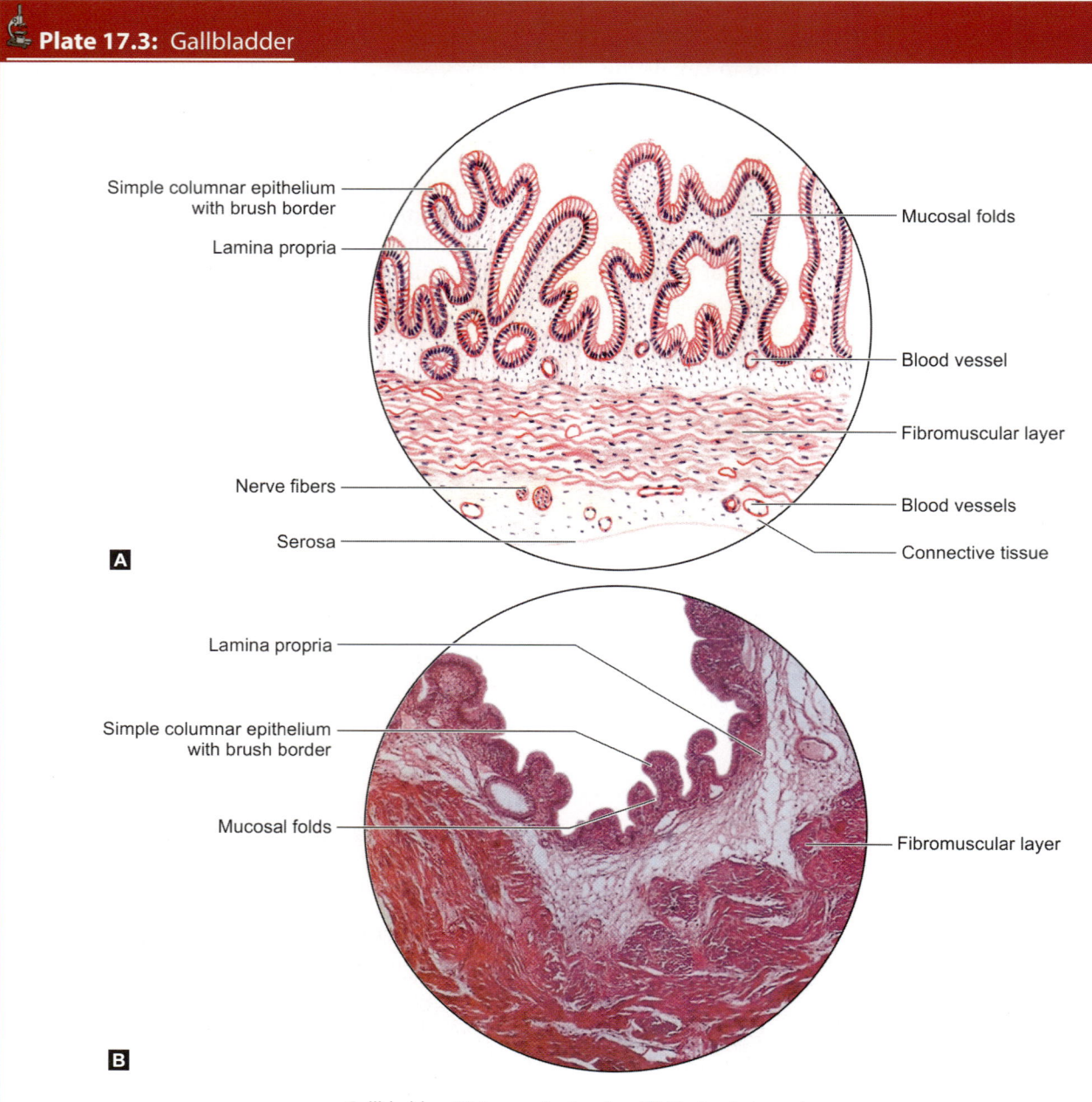

Gallbladder: (A) As seen in drawing; (B) Photomicrograph.

Points of identification
- The mucous membrane is lined by tall columnar cells with striated border
- The mucosa is highly folded and some of the folds might look-like villi
- Crypts may be found in lamina propria
- Submucosa is absent
- The muscle coat is poorly developed with numerous connective tissue fibers interspersed among muscle. This is called as fibromuscular coat
- A serous covering lined by flattened mesothelium is seen.

Note: Gallbladder can be differentiated from small intestine by absence of villi, goblet cells, submucosa, and proper muscularis externa.

CHAPTER 17: Hepatobiliary System and Pancreas

Rokitansky–Aschoff sinuses. If present, they may contribute as risk factor for stone formation and infection.

Fibromuscular coat

- Muscularis externa is made up of mainly connective tissue (collagen and elastic fibers) with some amount of smooth muscle.
- Smooth muscle fibers are arranged in random direction.

Serosa

- The serosal layer has a lining of mesothelium (peritoneum) resting on connective tissue.
- This layer also contains large blood vessels, lymphatic network, and nerve plexus along with elastic fibers and adipose tissue.
- The fundus and lower surface of body of gallbladder is covered by serosa, whereas the upper surface is attached to the fossa for gallbladder by means of connective tissue (adventitia).

Extrahepatic Ducts

These are the right, left, and common hepatic ducts; the cystic duct; and the bile duct. All of them have a common structure. They have a mucosa surrounded by a wall made up of connective tissue, in which some smooth muscle may be present. The mucosa is lined by a tall columnar epithelium with a striated border.

Hepatopancreatic Duct

- At its lower end, the bile duct is joined by the main pancreatic duct, the two usually forming a common hepatopancreatic duct (or ampulla) that opens into the duodenum at the summit of the major duodenal papilla.
- The mucosa of the hepatopancreatic duct is highly folded. These folds are believed to constitute a valvular mechanism that prevents duodenal contents from entering the bile and pancreatic ducts.
- **Sphincter of Oddi**:
  - Well-developed smooth muscle is present in the region of the lower end of the bile duct. This muscle forms the *sphincter of Oddi*.
  - From a functional point of view, this sphincter consists of three separate parts. The *sphincter choledochus* surrounds the lower end of the bile duct. It is always present, and its contraction is responsible for filling of the gallbladder. A less developed *sphincter pancreaticus* surrounds the terminal part of the main pancreatic duct (Fig. 17.9). A third sphincter surrounds the hepatopancreatic duct (or ampulla) and often forms a ring round the lower ends of both the bile and pancreatic ducts. This is the *sphincter ampullae*.
  - The sphincter ampullae and the sphincter pancreaticus are often missing.

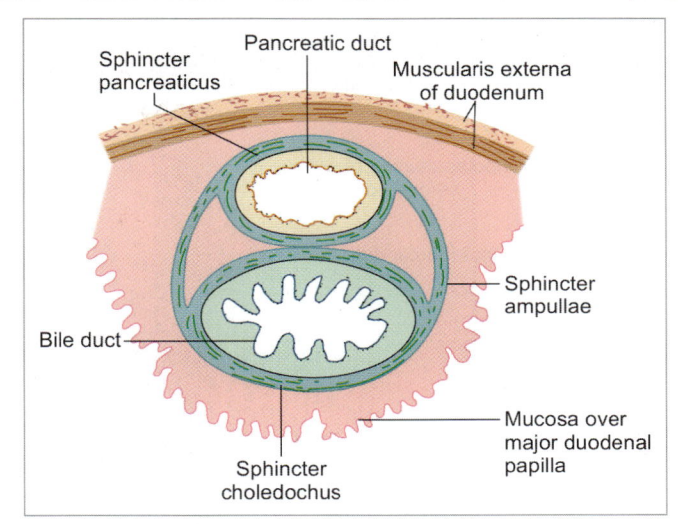

Fig. 17.9: Section through the major duodenal papilla to show the components of the sphincter of Oddi (schematic representation).

PANCREAS

- Pancreas is a retroperitoneal organ, extends from the concavity of the duodenum to the hilum of the spleen.
- It is a gland that is partly exocrine, and partly endocrine, the main bulk of the gland being constituted by its exocrine part (Plate 17.4).
- The exocrine pancreas secretes enzymes that play a very important role in the digestion of carbohydrates, proteins, and fats. After digestion and absorption through the gut, these products are carried to the liver through the portal vein.
- The endocrine pancreas produces two very important hormones, **insulin**, and **glucagon**. These two hormones are also carried through the portal vein to the liver where they have a profound influence on the metabolism of carbohydrates, proteins, and fats.
- The functions of the exocrine and endocrine parts of the pancreas are, thus, linked. The linkage between the two parts is also seen in their common embryonic derivation from the endodermal lining of the gut.

Exocrine Pancreas

The exocrine pancreas is in the form of *compound tubuloalveolar serous gland*. Its general structure is very similar to that of parotid gland.

Plate 17.4: Pancreas

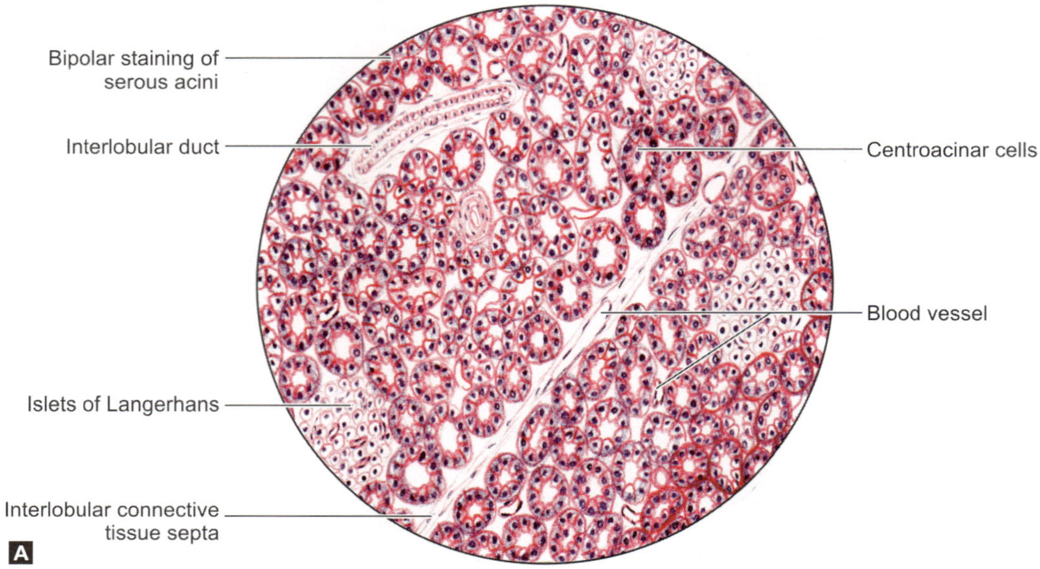

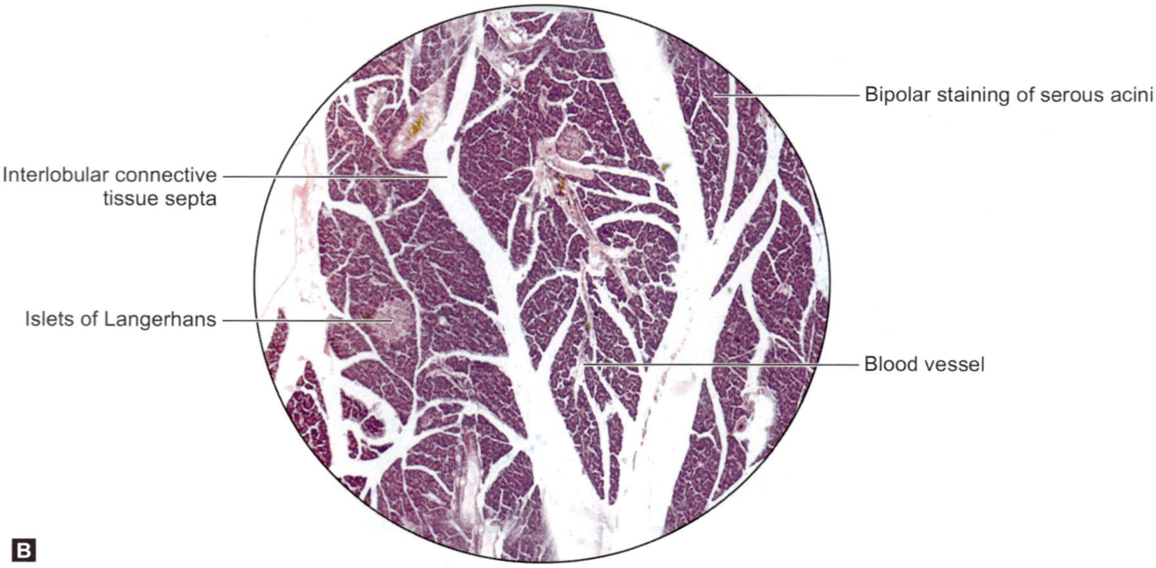

Pancreas: (A) As seen in drawing; (B) Photomicrograph.

Points of identification
- Made up of serous acini
- The cells forming the acini of the pancreas are highly basophilic (bluish staining). The lumen of the acinus is very small
- Some acini may show pale staining (centroacinar cell) in the center
- Among the acini, some ducts are seen
- The ducts have a distinct lumen, lined by cuboidal epithelium
- At some places, the acini are separated by areas where we see aggregations of cells quite different from those of the acini
- These aggregations form the pancreatic islets: pale staining cells arranged as groups, surrounded by blood vessels
- In the photomicrograph, an interlobular duct lined by cuboidal epithelium is surrounded by lobules of acinar cells which have small basal nuclei and granular eosinophilic or slightly basophilic cytoplasm. Islets of Langerhans appear as groups of small cells with lightly stained cytoplasm.

CHAPTER 17: Hepatobiliary System and Pancreas

- **Capsule**: A delicate capsule surrounds the pancreas. Septa extend from the capsule into the gland and divide it into lobules. Each lobule consists of ramified ducts ending in numerous alveoli/acini.
- **Pancreatic acini**: The secretory elements of the exocrine pancreas are long and tubular (but they are usually described as acini as they appear rounded or oval in sections). Their lumen is small (Fig. 17.10) and they have following cells:

  Secretory cells:
  - The cells lining the alveoli are pyramidal in shape.
  - They have spherical nuclei located toward basal region.
  - With hematoxylin and eosin staining, the cytoplasm is highly basophilic (blue) particularly in the basal part as the basal region is packed with rough endoplasmic reticulum and shows striations. Even the spherical nucleus is located toward the basement membrane.
  - With suitable fixation and staining, numerous secretory (or zymogen) granules can be demonstrated in the apical part of cytoplasm. These granules are eosinophilic. They decrease considerably after the cell has poured out its secretion.

  Centroacinar cells:
  - The junction between the alveoli and intercalated ducts is lined by cuboidal cells called *centroacinar cells*.
  - They are called so because they appear to be located near the center of the acinus.
  - Actually these cells belong to the intercalated ducts that are invaginated into the secretory elements.

  Some cell bodies of autonomic neurons and undifferentiated cells are also present in relation to the secretory elements.

- **Duct system**:
  - Secretions produced in the acini are poured into *intercalated ducts* (also called *intralobular ducts*).
  - These ducts are lined by flattened pale-stained epithelium and are invaginated deeply into the secretory elements (Fig. 17.10). As a result of this invagination, the intercalated ducts are not conspicuous in sections.
  - From the intercalated ducts, the secretions pass into larger, *interlobular ducts*. These are lined by low columnar cells, endocrine and occasional goblet cells.
  - They finally pass into the duodenum through the *main pancreatic duct* and the *accessory pancreatic duct*.
  - The cells lining the pancreatic ducts control the bicarbonate and water content of pancreatic secretion. These actions are under hormonal and neural control.
  - The walls of the larger ducts are formed mainly of fibrous tissue. They are lined by a columnar epithelium.
  - The terminal part of the main pancreatic duct is surrounded by a sphincter. A similar sphincter may also be present around the terminal part of the accessory pancreatic duct.

Endocrine Pancreas

- The endocrine pancreas is in the form of numerous rounded collections of cells that are embedded within the exocrine part.
- These collections of polyhedral cells are called **the pancreatic islets, or the islets of Langerhans**. The human pancreas has about one million islets. They are most numerous in the tail of the pancreas.
- Each islet is separated from the surrounding alveoli by a thin layer of reticular tissue.
- The islets are very richly supplied with blood through a dense capillary plexus. The intervals between the capillaries are occupied by cells arranged in groups or as cords.
- In ordinary preparations stained with H and E, all the cells appear similar, but with the use of special procedures, three main types of cells can be distinguished.

Alpha Cells (A-Cells)

- In islets of the human pancreas, the alpha cells (or A-cells) tend to be arranged toward the periphery (or cortex) of the islets.
- They form about 20% of the islet cells. They contain smaller granules that stain brightly with acid fuchsin. They do not stain with aldehyde fuchsin.
- When seen with electron microscopy, the granules of alpha cells (A2) appear to be round or ovoid with high electron density.
- The alpha cells secrete the hormone glucagon.

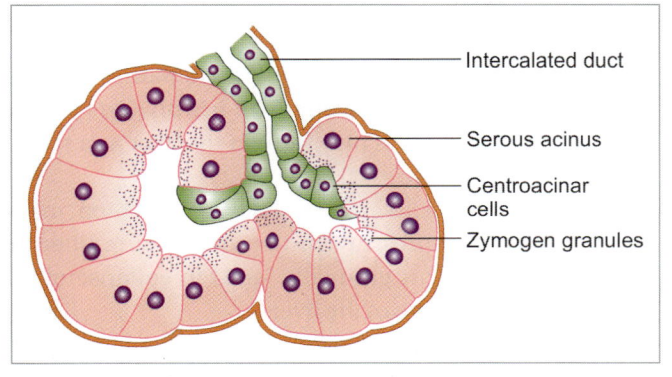

Fig. 17.10: Pancreatic serous acinus.

Beta Cells (B-Cells)

* The beta cells (or B-cells) tend to lie near the center (or medulla) of the islet.
* About 70% of the cells of islet are of this type. The beta cells contain granules (larger than alpha cells) that can be stained with aldehyde fuchsin.
* When seen with electron microscopy, the granules of beta cells are fewer, larger, and of less electron density than those of alpha cells.
* The beta cells secrete the hormone insulin.

Delta Cells (D-Cells)

* Delta cells (or D-cells), like alpha cells, are also peripherally placed.
* The delta cells (also called type III cells) stain black with silver salts (i.e. they are argyrophile).
* They resemble alpha cells in having granules that stain with acid fuchsin, and are, therefore, sometimes called A1 cells in distinction to the glucagon producing cells that are designated A2. The two can be distinguished by the fact that A2 cells are not argyrophile.
* When seen with electron microscopy, the granules of delta cells (A1) appear to be round or ovoid with low electron density.
* The delta cells probably produce the hormones gastrin and somatostatin. Somatostatin inhibits the secretion of glucagon by alpha cells, and (to a lesser extent) that of insulin by beta cells. Pancreatic islets are richly innervated by autonomic nerves. Noradrenaline and acetylcholine released at nerve endings influence secretion by islet cells.

DIFFERENCES BETWEEN SEROUS SALIVARY GLAND AND PANCREAS (TABLE 17.1)

Table 17.1: Differences between serous salivary gland and pancreas.

Serous salivary gland	Pancreas
Contains only exocrine part	Contains both exocrine and endocrine parts
Islets of Langerhans are absent	Islets of Langerhans are present
Striated ducts are present	Striated ducts are present
Centroacinar cells are absent	Centroacinar cells are present within the acini
Myoepithelial cells are seen between the basement membrane and acinar cells	Myoepithelial cells are absent

Added Information

> The secretory cells produce two types of secretion: One of these is watery and rich in bicarbonate. Bicarbonate is probably added to pancreatic secretion by cells lining the ducts. It helps to neutralize the acid contents entering the duodenum from the stomach. Production of this secretion is stimulated mainly by the hormone *secretin* liberated by the duodenal mucosa. The other secretion is thicker and contains numerous enzymes (including trypsinogen, chymotrypsinogen, amylase, lipases, etc.). The production of this secretion is stimulated mainly by the hormone cholecystokinin (pancreozymin) liberated by endocrine cells in the duodenal mucosa.
> Secretion by cells of the exocrine pancreas and the composition of the secretion are influenced by several other amines produced either in the gastrointestinal mucosa or in pancreatic islets (these include gastrin, vasoactive intestinal polypeptide, and pancreatic polypeptide). Secretion is also influenced by autonomic nerves, mainly parasympathetic.
> The enzymes are synthesized in the rough endoplasmic reticulum. From here, they pass to the Golgi complex where they are surrounded by membranes, and are released into the cytoplasm as secretory granules.
> The granules move to the luminal surface of the cell where the secretions are poured out by exocytosis.
> Within the cell, the enzymes are in an inactive form. They become active only after mixing with duodenal contents. Activation is influenced by enzymes present in the epithelium lining the duodenum.
> Apart from the three main types of cells described earlier, some other types are also present in the islets of Langerhans. These are the PP cells containing pancreatic polypeptide (and located mainly in the head and neck of the pancreas), and D1 cells (or type IV cells) probably containing vasoactive intestinal polypeptide (or a similar amine).
> A few cells secreting serotonin, motilin, and substance P are also present. Hence, in the cellular mass of islets, two zones are noted. Homocellular medulla in the center containing mainly beta cells and heterocellular cortex containing mixture of alpha, delta, and PP cells.

APPLIED HISTOLOGY

Liver

* Inflammation in the liver is called hepatitis. It is frequently caused by viruses (viral hepatitis), and by a protozoan parasite **Entamoeba histolytica** (amebic hepatitis). An abscess may form in the liver as a sequel of amebic hepatitis.
* Cirrhosis of the liver is a disease in which many hepatocytes are destroyed, the areas being filled by fibrous tissue. This gradually leads to collapse of the normal architecture of the liver.
* Fish liver oils (e.g. cod liver oil) are important nutritional sources of vitamin A.

CHAPTER 17: Hepatobiliary System and Pancreas

- Hepatocytes have lifespan of about 5 months. Also, they are capable of considerable regeneration when liver substance is damaged due to hepatotoxic processes, disease, or surgery.
- One effect of cirrhosis of the liver is to disrupt the flow of blood (reduction of vascular sponge) through the liver sinusoids. As a result of increased resistance to blood flow, there is increased blood pressure in the portal circulation (**portal hypertension**). In portal hypertension, anastomoses between the portal and systemic veins dilate to form varices (e.g. at the lower end of the esophagus). Rupture of these varices can result in fatal bleeding.
- When a large number of hepatocytes are destroyed, this leads to liver failure. Hepatic failure may be acute or chronic. Accumulation of waste products in blood (due to lack of detoxification by the liver) ultimately leads to unconsciousness (**hepatic coma**) and death.

Gallbladder

- Inflammation of the gallbladder is called cholecystitis.
- Stones may form in the gallbladder (gallstones; cholelithiasis). A gallstone passing through the bile duct can cause severe pain. This pain is biliary colic. In such cases, surgical removal of the gallbladder may be necessary (cholecystectomy).
- Blockage of the bile duct (by inflammation, by a gallstone, or by carcinoma) leads to accumulation of bile in the biliary duct system, and within the bile capillaries.
- As pressure in the passages increases, bile passes into blood leading to jaundice. The sclera, the skin, and the nails appear to be yellow in color, and bile salts and pigments are excreted in urine. Jaundice occurring as a result of such obstruction is called obstructive jaundice. Jaundice is seen in the absence of obstruction in cases of hepatitis.

Pancreas

- **Acute pancreatitis**: Acute pancreatitis is an acute inflammation of the pancreas presenting clinically with "acute abdomen". The condition occurs in adults between the age of 40 years and 70 years and is more common in females than in males. The onset of acute pancreatitis is sudden, occurring after a bout of alcohol or a heavy meal. Characteristically, there is elevation of *serum amylase* level within the first 24 hours and elevated serum lipase level after 3–4 days.
- **Chronic pancreatitis**: Chronic pancreatitis or *chronic relapsing pancreatitis* is the progressive destruction of the pancreas due to repeated mild and subclinical attacks of acute pancreatitis. Most patients present with recurrent attacks of severe abdominal pain at intervals of months to years. Weight loss and jaundice are often associated.
- Diabetes mellitus is due to insulin resistance or decreased secretion of insulin by beta cells.

MULTIPLE CHOICE QUESTIONS

1. Epithelial cells that line the biliary tree are:
    a. Hepatocytes
    b. Ito cells
    c. Cholangiocytes
    d. Kupffer cells
2. Macrophages in the liver are:
    a. Hepatocytes
    b. Ito cells
    c. Cholangiocytes
    d. Kupffer cells
3. Most proximal tributary of biliary tree is called:
    a. Canal of Cloquet
    b. Canal of Nuck
    c. Canal of Hering
    d. Canal of Schlemm
4. Cells which store vitamin A in liver are:
    a. Hepatocytes
    b. Ito cells
    c. Cholangiocytes
    d. Kupffer cells
5. Structural and functional unit of liver are:
    a. Hepatic lobule
    b. Portal triad
    c. Liver acinus
    d. Portal lobule
6. Gallbladder is devoid of:
    a. Mucosa
    b. Submucosa
    c. Lamina propria
    d. Serosa
7. Lining epithelium of the gallbladder is:
    a. Simple squamous
    b. Simple columnar
    c. Simple cuboidal
    d. Pseudostratified ciliated columnar
8. Centroacinar cells are:
    a. Simple squamous
    b. Simple columnar
    c. Simple cuboidal
    d. Pseudostratified ciliated columnar
9. All the following cells are the members of pancreatic islets, except:
    a. Alpha cells
    b. Beta cells
    c. Delta cells
    d. Gamma cells

Answers
1. c   2. d   3. c   4. b   5. c   6. b   7. b   8. a   9. d

CHAPTER 18

Urinary System

Learning objectives

To study the:
- Microscopic structure of kidney
- Structure of nephron
- Structure of juxtaglomerular apparatus
- Structure of ureters
- Structure of urinary bladder
- Applied histology

IDENTIFICATION POINTS

Kidney	Ureters	Urinary bladder
☐ Presence of cortex and medulla	☐ Star-shaped lumen is seen	☐ Wall is made up of mucous, muscular, and adventitia layers
☐ Medullary rays are seen in the cortex	☐ Wall is made up of mucous, muscular, and serous layers	☐ Mucosa is thrown into folds
☐ Number of glomerulus is seen	☐ It is lined by transitional epithelium	☐ It is lined by transitional epithelium
☐ Cut section of proximal convoluted tubule (PCT) lined by columnar epithelium is seen	☐ It has inner longitudinal and outer circular layer of smooth muscles.	☐ It has inner and outer longitudinal and middle circular layer of smooth muscle.
☐ Cut section of distal convoluted tubule (DCT), loop of Henle, and ducts are seen.		

INTRODUCTION

The urinary organs are:
- A pair of kidneys
- A pair of ureters
- The urinary bladder
- The urethra.

FUNCTIONS

- The urinary organs are responsible for the production, storage, and passing of urine.
- Toxic byproducts of metabolism are removed from blood through urine by kidney. These include urea and creatinine that are end products of protein metabolism.
- Many drugs, or their breakdown products, are also excreted in urine.
- Conserves salts, glucose, proteins, and water.
- Kidneys help to regulate blood pressure, hemodynamics, and the acid-base balance of the body.
- Urine production, and the control of its composition, is exclusively the function of the kidneys. The urinary bladder is responsible for storage of urine until it is voided. The ureter and urethra are simple passages for transport of urine.

Note: In diseased conditions, urine can contain glucose as in diabetes mellitus, or proteins in kidney disease, the excretion of which is normally prevented.

KIDNEYS

- Kidneys are bean-shaped organs situated retroperitoneally on the posterior abdominal wall.
- The kidney is invested by thin adhering capsule consisting of dense irregular collagen fibers.

Macroscopic Structure

On coronal section, the kidney consists of an outer **cortex** and an inner **medulla**. Cortex appears dark brown and granular and medulla contains 8–12 pyramidal-shaped pale striated region called renal pyramids.

Medulla

- Medulla is made up of 8–10 triangular areas of renal tissue called the **renal pyramids** which are striated, pale,

CHAPTER 18: Urinary System

and conical structure (Fig. 18.1). Each pyramid has a base directed toward the cortex; and an apex or papilla that is directed toward the renal pelvis, and fits into a minor calyx.
* Pyramids show striations that pass radially toward the apex. Striations are caused by series of U-shaped loops of Henle, collecting tubules, and ducts of Bellini and arteriolae recti and venae recti.

Cortex

The renal cortex consists of the following:
* Cortex is granular in appearance and consists of *renal columns* and *cortical arches*.
* Tissue lying between the bases of the pyramids and the surface of the kidney is called the *cortical arches* or *cortical lobules*.
* Cortical arches show light and dark striations. The light lines are called *medullary rays.* Medullary ray is a conical mass, the apex is directed toward the surface of the kidney and the base is continuous with the striations of the pyramid. Each ray is made up of collecting tubules and ducts of Bellini (Plate 18.1).
* Tissue lying between adjacent pyramids is called the *renal columns*.
* One pyramid is surrounded by a "shell" of cortex. The pyramid capped with cortex is known as the *lobe* of kidney.
* The area of the cortical arch bounded on each side by interlobular blood vessels with central medullary ray is known as the *lobule* of the kidney.

The kidney has a convex lateral margin; and a concavity on the medial side that is called the *hilum*. The hilum leads into a space called the *renal sinus*. The renal sinus is occupied by the upper expanded part of the ureter called the *renal pelvis*.

Within the renal sinus, the pelvis divides into two or three *major calyces* and each major calyx divides into a three to four *minor calyces* (Fig. 18.1). The dilated outer end of each minor calyx presents a cup-shaped depression to receive renal papillae. The renal papilla is the location where the renal pyramids in the medulla empty urine into the minor calyx.

Microscopic Structure

* The kidney is composed of 1–4 million closely packed uriniferous tubules.
* Each uriniferous tubule consists of a secreting part which develops from metanephric blastema called the *nephron* and collecting part which develops from ureteric bud called a *collecting tubule and ducts of Bellini*.
* Urinary tubules are held together by scanty connective tissue. Blood vessels, lymphatics, and nerves lie in this connective tissue.

Nephron

* These are the structural and functional unit of kidney and there are about 1–4 million nephrons in each kidney. Length of nephron varies from 50 mm to 55 mm (Fig. 18.2).
* The nephron consists of a *renal corpuscle* (or *Malpighian corpuscle*) for filtration and a long *renal*

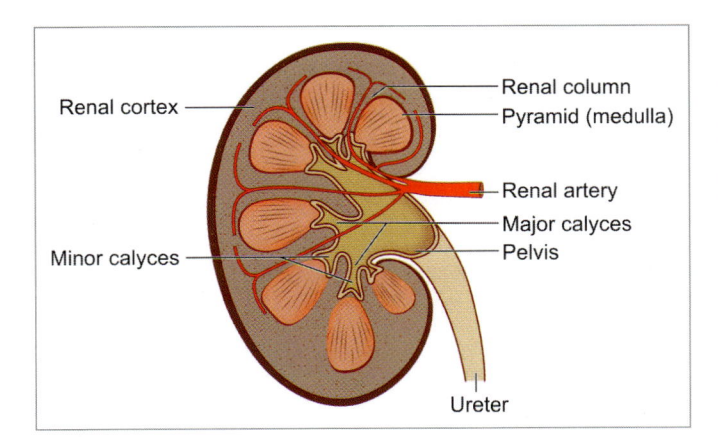

Fig. 18.1: Some features seen in a coronal section through the kidney (schematic representation).

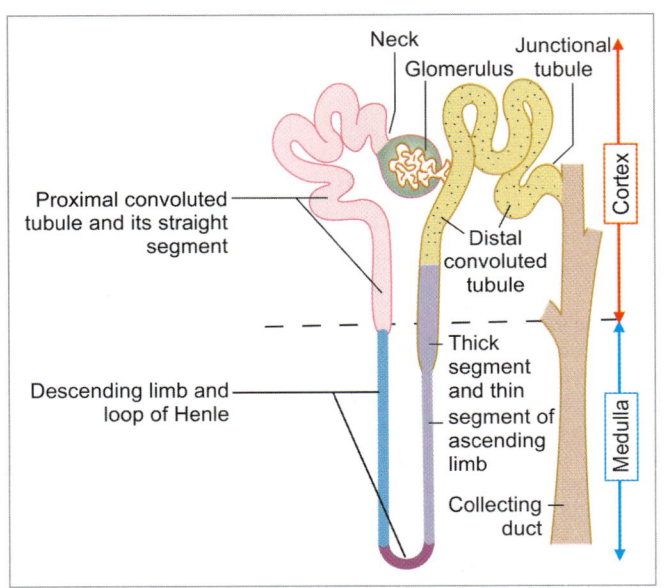

Fig. 18.2: Parts of a nephron. A collecting duct is also shown (schematic representation).

Plate 18.1: Kidney (Low magnification)

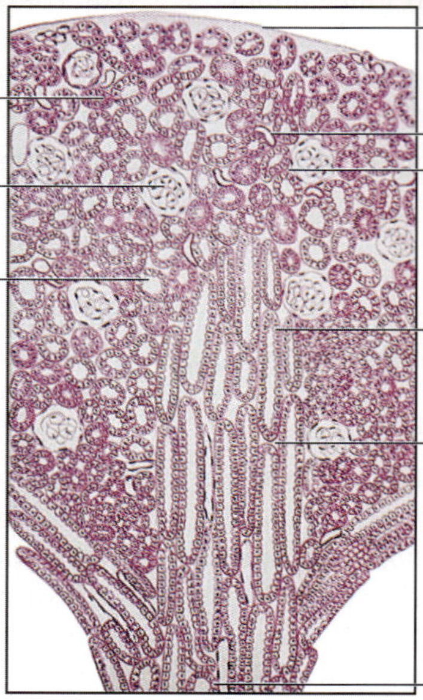

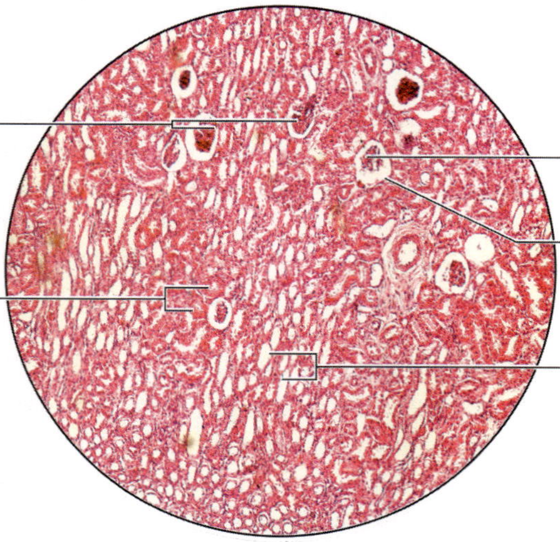

Kidney (Low magnification): (A) As seen in drawing; (B) Photomicrograph of cortex.
Courtesy (B): Balakrishna Shetty, Sweekritha H Poonja. HISTOLOGY Practical Manual, 4th edition. New Delhi: Jaypee Brothers Medical Publishers (P) Ltd; 2019. p. 108.

Points of identification
- The kidney is covered by a capsule
- Deep to the capsule there is the cortex
- Deep to the cortex there is the medulla of the kidney
- In the cortex we see circular structures called renal corpuscles surrounding which there are tubules cut in various shapes
- The dark pink stained tubules are parts of the proximal convoluted tubules (PCT): their lumen is small and indistinct. It is lined by cuboidal epithelium with brush border
- Lighter staining tubules, each with a distinct lumen, are the distal convoluted tubules (DCT). They are lined by simple cuboidal epithelium
- PCT are more in number than DCT
- In the medulla we see very light staining, elongated, parallel running tubules. These are collecting ducts and loop of Henle. Some of them extend into the cortex forming a medullary ray. The collecting ducts are lined by simple cuboidal epithelium and loop of Henle (thin segments) are lined by simple squamous epithelium
- Cut sections of blood vessels are seen both in the cortex and medulla.

Note: When we look at a section of the kidney we see that most of the area is filled with a very large number of tubules. These are of various shapes and have different types of epithelial lining. This fact by itself suggests that the tissue is the kidney.

CHAPTER 18: Urinary System

tubule for selective reabsorption. Renal tubule is made up of three parts:
1. The proximal convoluted tubule
2. Loop of Henle
3. The distal convoluted tubule.

❖ Renal corpuscles and the greater parts of the proximal and distal convoluted tubules are located in the cortex of the kidney. The loops of Henle and the collecting ducts lie in the medullary rays and in the substance of the pyramids.

❖ Two types of nephrons are found in the kidney. The *cortical/superficial* nephrons whose corpuscles located in the outer cortex and *juxtamedullary* nephrons whose corpuscles located in the inner cortex near medulla or corticomedullary junction and its tubular parts extend into the medulla.

Renal Corpuscle

❖ The renal corpuscle is also called a Malpighian body consists of a rounded tuft of blood capillaries called the **glomerulus** and a cup-like double-layered covering for the glomerulus called the **glomerular capsule/Bowman's capsule** (Fig. 18.3).

❖ The glomerular capsule represents the cup-shaped blind beginning of the renal tubule. Between the two layers of the capsule, there is a **urinary space** that is continuous with the lumen of the renal tubule.

Glomerulus

❖ The glomerulus is a lobulated tuft of anastomosing fenestrated capillaries formed by afferent and efferent arterioles, which project into the Bowman's capsule (Plate 18.2). Blood enters the tuft through an afferent arteriole and leaves it through an efferent arteriole.

❖ The afferent and efferent glomerular arterioles are approximated to each other to form the **vascular pole** of the renal corpuscle.

❖ Each lobule consists of a capillary loop which is suspended in the capsular space by a mesentery derived from visceral layer.

❖ Mesentery contains **mesangium** that is made up of mesangial cells surrounded by a noncellular mesangial matrix.

❖ Mesangial cells contain filaments similar to myosin and they bear angiotensin II receptors. It is believed that stimulation by angiotensin causes the fibrils to contract. This suggests that mesangial cells play a role in controlling blood flow through the glomerulus. Mesangial cells also play a role in phagocytosis, support to the glomerulus, and synthesize extracellular matrix.

❖ The mesangium becomes prominent in a disease called glomerulonephritis.

Glomerular Capsule/Bowman's Capsule

❖ It is the dilated blind end of the renal tubule which is invaginated by the glomerular plexus.

❖ The capsule is a double-layered cup consists of outer parietal and inner visceral layers. The two layers of which are separated by the urinary space.

❖ The parietal layer is lined by continuous flattened epithelium resting on basement membrane. The visceral layer is lined by discontinuous polyhedral cells known as podocytes.

❖ The urinary space becomes continuous with the lumen of the renal tubule at the **urinary pole** of the renal corpuscle and this pole lies opposite the vascular pole.

❖ The **podocytes** are so called because they possess foot-like processes. The podocytes are separated from the basement membrane by filtrate-filled spaces.

❖ The podocytes have numerous long tentacle like **major/primary** process that are parallel to the basement membrane. Each major has numerous **secondary processes** called **pedicels** (or end feet) that rest on the basal lamina. The cell body of the podocyte comes in contact with the basal lamina only through the pedicels (Fig. 18.4).

❖ The pedicels of adjacent podocytes interdigitate and form spaces called **filtration slits**. These slits are covered by a thin membrane called **slit diaphragm** through which the filtration takes place.

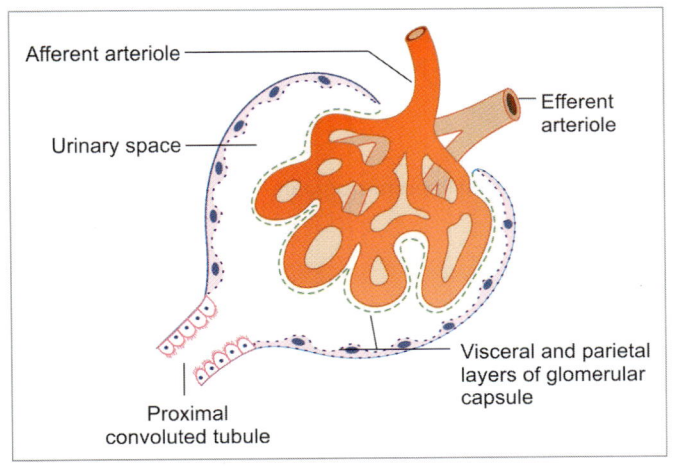

Fig. 18.3: Basic structure of a renal corpuscle (schematic representation).

228 Textbook of Human Histology

Plate 18.2: Renal cortex (High magnification)

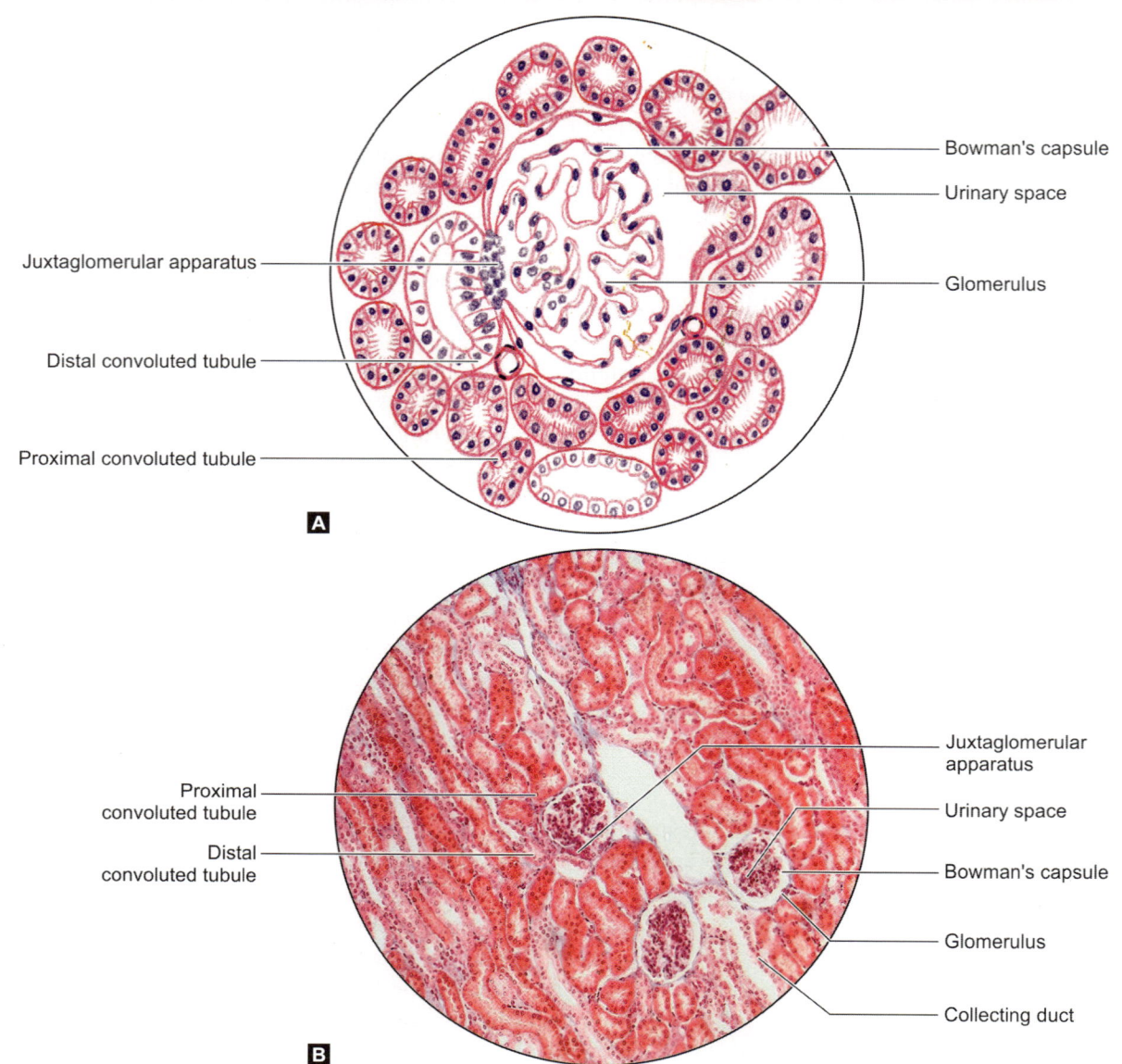

Labels in A: Bowman's capsule, Urinary space, Glomerulus, Juxtaglomerular apparatus, Distal convoluted tubule, Proximal convoluted tubule

A

Labels in B: Proximal convoluted tubule, Distal convoluted tubule, Juxtaglomerular apparatus, Urinary space, Bowman's capsule, Glomerulus, Collecting duct

B

Renal cortex (High magnification): (A) As seen in drawing; (B) Photomicrograph.

Points of identification
- In the high power view of renal cortex large renal corpuscles can be identified
- The renal corpuscle consists of a tuft of capillaries that form a rounded glomerulus, and an outer wall, the glomerular capsule (Bowman's capsule)
- A urinary space between the glomerulus and the capsule is seen
- Proximal convoluted tubules are dark staining. They are lined by cuboidal cells with a prominent brush border. Their lumen is indistinct
- Distal convoluted tubules are lighter staining. The cuboidal cells lining them do not have a brush border. Their lumen is distinct.

CHAPTER 18: Urinary System

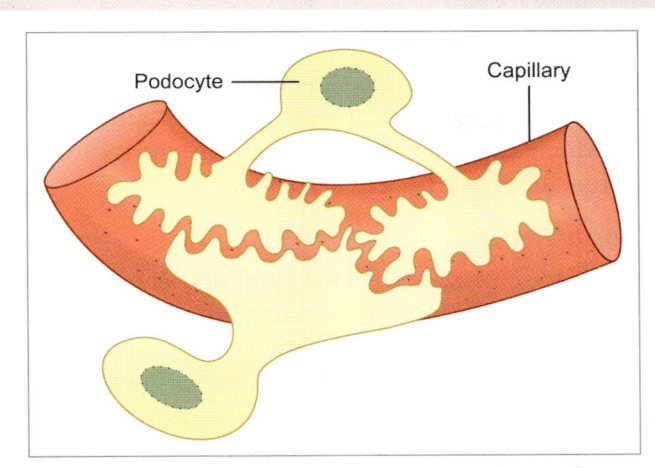

Fig. 18.4: Relationship of podocytes to a glomerular capillary.
Note that the entire surface of the capillary is covered by processes of podocytes, the bare areas being shown only for sake of clarity (schematic representation).

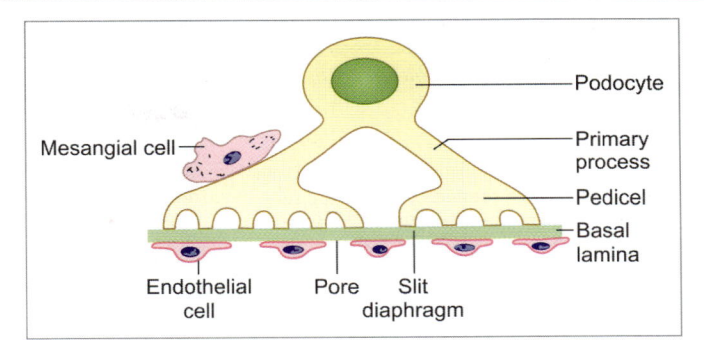

Fig. 18.5: Filtration slits (schematic representation).

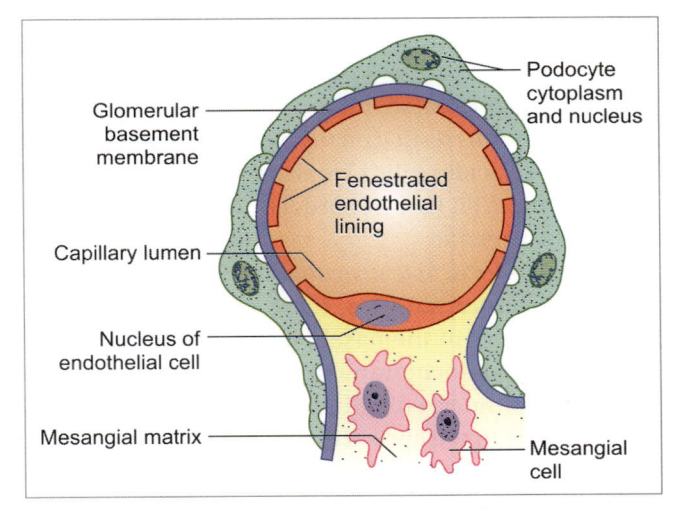

Fig. 18.6: Relationship of a glomerular capillary to podocytes, basement membrane, and mesangium (schematic representation).

Glomerular Basement Membrane

- As compared to typical membranes, the glomerular basement membrane is very thick (about 300 nm). The membrane acts as filtration barrier that separates urinary space from blood in the capillaries.
- It is made up of three layers. There is a central electron dense layer called *lamina densa*, and inner and outer electron lucent layers called *lamina rara interna* and *externa*.
- The lamina densa contains a network of collagen (type IV) fibrils, and thus acts as a physical barrier. The electron lucent layers contain the glycosaminoglycan heparan sulfate and bear the negative charges. The glomerular basement membrane is, therefore, both a physical barrier and an electrical barrier to the passage of large molecules.
- Glomerular basement membrane acts as an ultrafilter and allows filtration of water and simple solutes of blood plasma into capillary space. The glomerular filtrate consists of blood plasma without proteins, lipid droplets, and blood cells. Macromolecules greater than 4 nm cannot pass through the filtration slits (Fig. 18.5).
- As shown in Figure 18.6, the glomerular basement membrane and podocyte does not go all round a glomerular capillary and the gap is filled in by mesangium.
- ***Glomerular filtration barrier*** separates blood in the capillaries from urinary space. It is formed by fenestrated endothelium of capillaries, glomerular basement membrane, and pedicles of podocytes.

Renal Tubule

The renal tubule consists of the **PCT**, the ***loop of Henle*** consisting of a ***descending limb***, a ***loop***, and an ***ascending limb*** and the **DCT**, which ends by joining a collecting tubule.

Proximal Convoluted Tubule

- Urinary space continuous as PCT at the urinary pole. The ***PCTs*** are 40–60 μm in diameter with small lumen.
- The initial part of PCT is convoluted and present in the cortex and the terminal part is straight and descends into the medulla to become continuous with the descending limb of the loop of Henle (Table 18.1).
- The junction of the PCT with the glomerular capsule is narrow and is referred as the ***neck***. The ***neck*** is lined by simple squamous epithelium which continuous with that of the glomerular capsule.

Table 18.1: Comparison between PCT and DCT.

Proximal convoluted tubule	Distal convoluted tubule
Begins from the Bowman's capsule	Begins from ascending limb of loop of Henle
Lengthy so more number of PCT sections are seen in cortex of kidney	Shorter so less number of DCT are seen in cortex of kidney section
Continuous with loop of Henle	Continuous with collecting duct
Lined by cuboidal epithelium with microvilli	Lined by cuboidal epithelium without microvilli
Cytoplasm is more acidophilic	Cytoplasm is less acidophilic/basophilic
More convoluted	Less convoluted
Main function is reabsorption	Main function is secretion

- Proximal convoluted tubule is lined by cuboidal or low columnar cells resting on the basement membrane. The cells have acidophilic cytoplasm and apex of the cells have microvilli (brush border). The nuclei are central and euchromatic.
- *Electron microscopic structure*: The basal part of the cell shows a vertical striation. These striations are produced by infoldings of the basal plasma membrane and by numerous mitochondria that lie longitudinally in the cytoplasm intervening between the folds (Fig. 18.7). Only close to the apex, the cells are connected by tight junctions and rest of the surfaces they are separated by intercellular clefts (Plate 18.3).
- The presence of microvilli, and of the basal infoldings greatly increases the surface area available for transport.

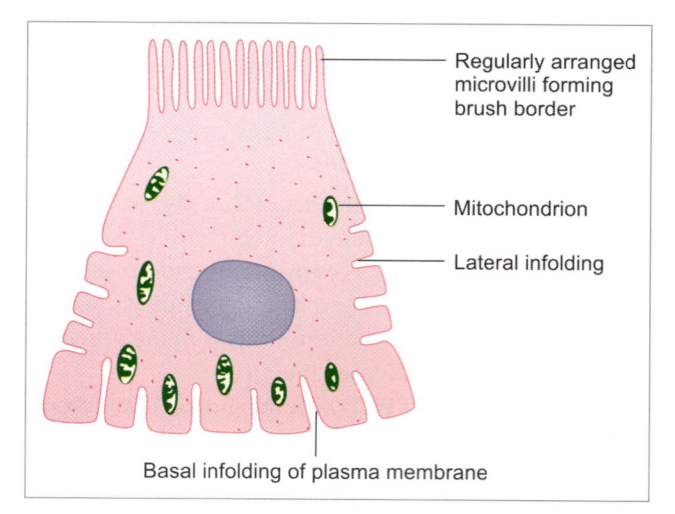

Fig. 18.7: Some features of the ultrastructure of a cell lining a proximal convoluted tubule (schematic representation).

Functions

- About 80% of the filtrate is reabsorbed by PCT.
- Active reabsorption of water, glucose, amino acids, sodium, calcium chloride, phosphate, and bicarbonate from the filtrate back to the blood.

Loop of Henle

- The loop of Henle is U-shaped and consists of the descending thin limb, the loop, and ascending thin limb. The descending limb enters the renal pyramid as a continuation of the proximal tubule. The loop of the juxtamedullary nephron reaches close to the apical zone of the pyramid and of the cortical nephrons reaches up to the basal zone of the pyramid. The ascending limb re-enters the cortex and reaches close to the vascular pole.
- The descending limb and the loop constitutes thin *segment* of the loop with a diameter of 15 μm. It is lined by a squamous epithelium resting on basement membrane.
- The ascending limb constitutes the thick *segment* of the loop of Henle with diameter of 30 μm in diameter. It is lined by cuboidal epithelium.
- The loops are surrounded by arteriolae rectae and venae rectae and the capillary between them. The loop of Henle is also called the *ansa nephroni*.
- With the electron microscopy (EM), the flat cells lining the thin segment of the loop of Henle show very few organelles indicating that the cells play only a passive role in ionic movements across them. In some areas, the lining epithelium may show short microvilli, and some basal and lateral infoldings.

Functions

- About 5% of the fluid is absorbed by loop of Henle.
- Ascending limb actively pumps out chloride and sodium ion passively into the tissue space.
- Descending limb diffuses water out and some chloride and sodium ion enters the loop.
- The loops of Henle maintain a graded osmolarity of the interstitial fluid of the pyramid. From apex to base of the pyramid, the interstitial fluid becomes successively hypertonic, isotonic, and hypotonic.

Distal Convoluted Tubule

- Distal convoluted tubule begins from the vascular pole of the nephron as a continuation of the ascending limb of loop of Henle and terminates in the collecting tubule.

CHAPTER 18: Urinary System

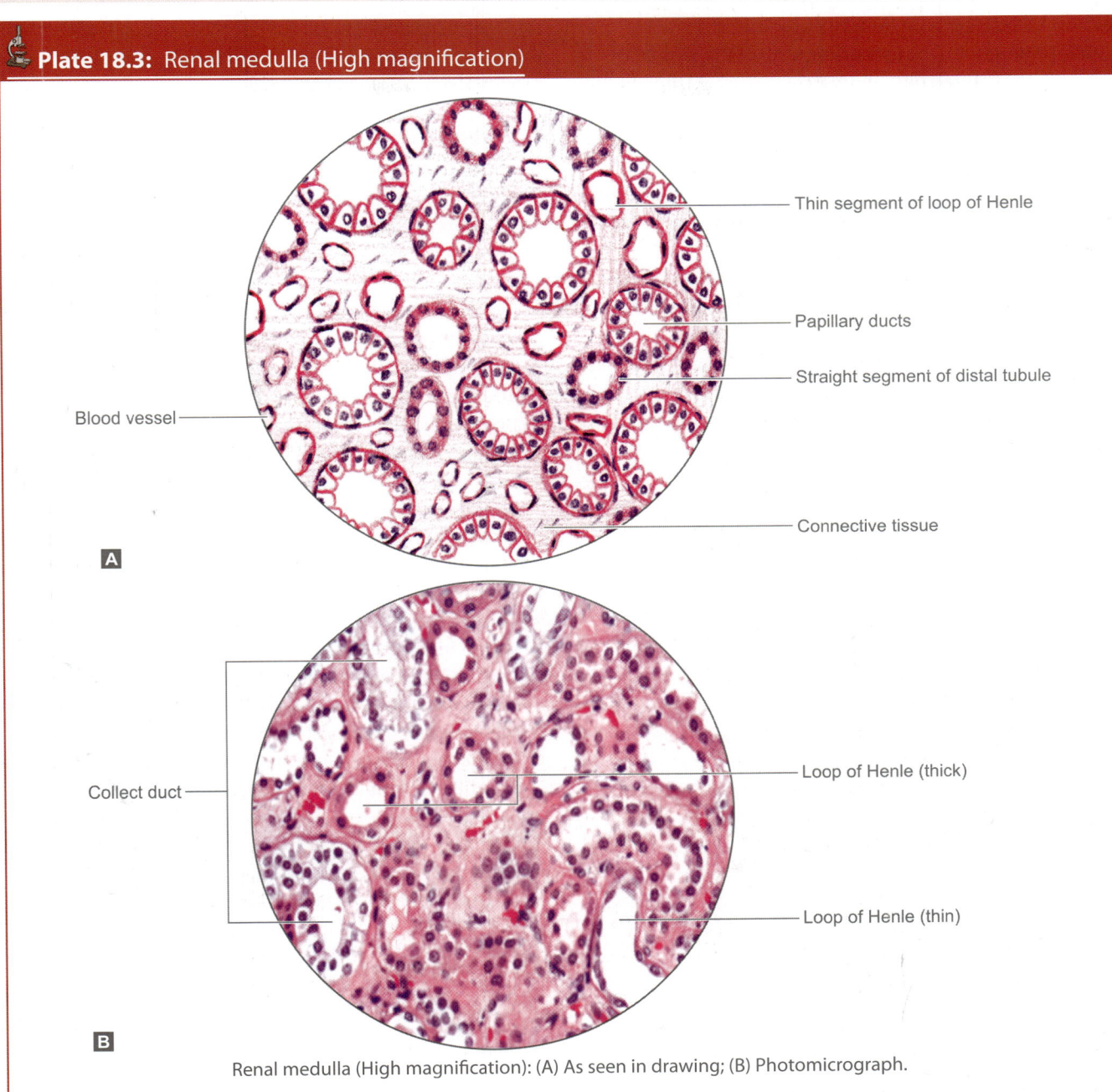

Plate 18.3: Renal medulla (High magnification)

Renal medulla (High magnification): (A) As seen in drawing; (B) Photomicrograph.

Points of identification
- A high power view of a part of the renal medulla shows a number of collecting ducts cut longitudinally or transversely
- They are lined by a cuboidal epithelium, the cells of which stain lightly. Cell boundaries are usually distinct. The lumen of the tubule is also distinct
- Sections of the thin segment of the loop of Henle are seen. They are lined by flattened cells, the walls being very similar in appearance to those of blood capillaries
- Sections through the thick segments of loops of Henle are seen. They are lined by cuboidal epithelium.

In the photomicrograph, collecting ducts and thick segments and thin segments of the loops of Henle can be identified.

- The distal convoluted tubule has a straight part continuous with the ascending limb of the loop of Henle, and a convoluted part lying in the cortex. At the junction between the two parts, the distal tubule lies very close to the vascular pole of the renal corpuscle of the nephron to which it belongs.
- The terminal part of the DCT is called the *junctional tubule* or *connecting tubule*, which joins the collecting duct.
- The distal convoluted tubules are 20–50 μm in diameter and lined by cuboidal epithelium without brush border.
- At the junction of the straight and convoluted parts of the DCTs, the cells show specializations that are described here in connection with the juxtaglomerular apparatus (Fig. 18.8).

Functions

- Active absorption of about 15% of water from the filtrate.
- Absorbs sodium ions in exchange of excretion of potassium ions. This is regulated by aldosterone.
- Distal tubule receives hypotonic fluid and it helps in acidification of urine and isotonic fluid enters collecting tubule.

Note: Students may be confused by somewhat different terminology used in some books. The straight part of the PCT is sometimes described as part of the loop of Henle, and is termed the *descending thick segment*, in distinction to the ascending thick segment. Some workers regard the thin segment alone to be the loop of Henle. They include the descending and ascending thick segments with the proximal and DCTs, respectively.

Collecting Tubule and Ducts

- The collecting tubules pass through the medullary rays, receive many junctional tubules and enter the pyramids as *ducts of Bellini*.
- Three are cortical, medullary, and papillary (ducts of Bellini) collecting tubules. Cortical collecting tubules are located in the medullary rays; medullary tubules are formed by the union of many cortical tubules.
- The smallest collecting tubules are 40–50 μm in diameter, and the largest as much as 200 μm.
- Both collecting tubule and ducts of Bellini are lined by a simple cuboidal epithelium.
- The walls of cortical and medullary collecting tubules are lined by two types of cells called **principal/clear cells** with very few organelles, a few microvilli, and some basal infoldings and some **dark cells** or **intercalated cells** with microvilli.
- The cells of the collecting ducts do not have microvilli or lateral infoldings of plasma membrane.
- Ducts of Bellini are surrounded by hypertonic tissue fluid of renal pyramids. Collecting tubules and ducts play a role in final concentration of urine.
- Collecting tubules and ducts convey and modify the ultrafiltrate from the nephron to the minor calyces.

> **Added Information**
>
> The only real barrier across which filtration occurs is the basal lamina or the glomerular basement membrane that is thickened at the filtration slits by the glomerular slit diaphragm. The efficacy of the barrier is greatly enhanced by the presence of a high negative charge in the basement membrane and in podocyte processes. Loss of this charge, in some diseases, leads to excessive leakage of protein through the barrier.

Juxtaglomerular Apparatus (Plate 18.2)

Juxtaglomerular apparatus is a specialized organ situated near the glomerulus of each nephron (juxta = near). The juxtaglomerular apparatus is formed by three different structures:

a. Macula densa of the DCT.
b. Juxtaglomerular cells of the afferent arteriole.
c. Lacis cells/extraglomerular mesangial cells/cells of polkissen.

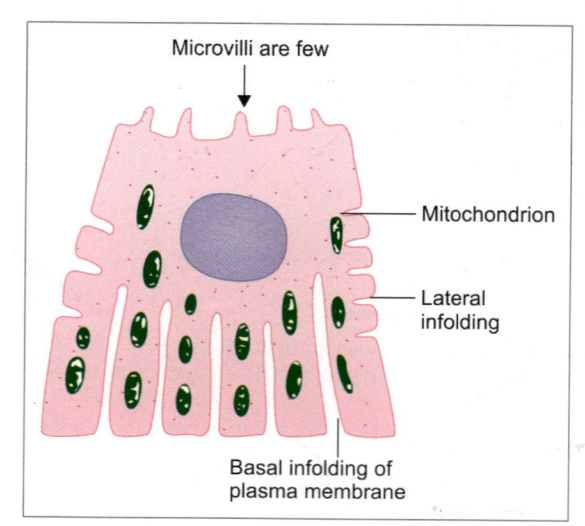

Fig. 18.8: Some features of ultrastructure of a cell lining a distal convoluted tubule (schematic representation).

Macula Densa

- These are the modified cells of DCT near afferent arteriole.
- The wall of the DCTs comes in close contact with the afferent arterioles where the basement membranes of the tubules disappear. Here the lining cells are densely packed together, and are columnar rather than cuboidal as in the rest of the tubule. These cells form the *macula densa*.
- The cells of the macula densa lie in close contact with the juxtaglomerular cells.
- The cells of the macula densa monitor the ionic constitution of the fluid passing across tubule and influence the release of renin by the juxtaglomerular cells.

Juxtaglomerular Cells (JG Cells)

- It is a modified smooth muscle cells located in the tunica media of afferent glomerular arterioles and are situated very close to the macula densa.
- A part of the DCT at the junction of its straight and convoluted parts lies close to the vascular pole of the renal corpuscle, between the afferent and efferent arterioles. In this region, the muscle cells in the wall of the afferent arteriole are modified and are large and rounded (epithelioid) with spherical nuclei. These are called *juxtaglomerular cells*.
- They are innervated by unmyelinated adrenergic nerve fibers.
- Juxtamedullary cells are regarded, by some, as highly modified myoepithelial cells as they contain contractile filaments in the cytoplasm.

Functions of juxtaglomerular cells

- It secretes an enzyme *renin*. The juxtaglomerular cells act as baroreceptors reacting to a fall in blood pressure by release of renin. Secretion of renin is also stimulated by low sodium blood levels and by sympathetic stimulation.
- Renin acts on a substance called *angiotensinogen* present in blood and converts it into *angiotensin I*. Angiotensin-converting enzyme (ACE) (present mainly in the lungs) converts angiotensin I into *angiotensin II*.
- Angiotensin II reduces the diameter of blood vessels and increases blood pressure. It also stimulates the secretion of aldosterone by the adrenal cortex, thus influencing the reabsorption of sodium ions by the DCTs and that of water through the collecting ducts. In this way, it helps to regulate plasma volume and blood pressure.

Note: In addition to renin, the kidney produces the hormone erythropoietin (which stimulates erythrocyte production). Some workers have claimed that erythropoietin is produced by juxtaglomerular cells, but the site of production of the hormone is uncertain.

Lacis Cells/Extraglomerular Mesangial Cells/Cells of Polkissen

These are polyhedral cluster of cells lie between the macula densa, afferent and efferent arterioles, and vascular pole of nephron. These cells are so called as they bear processes that form a lace-like network. The function of lacis cells is unknown.

Renal Blood Vessels

- At the hilum of the kidney, each renal artery divides into a number of *lobar arteries* one for each pyramid. Each lobar artery divides into two or more *interlobar arteries* that enter the tissue of the renal columns and run toward the surface of the kidney. At the base of the pyramids, the interlobar arteries divide dichotomously into *arcuate arteries which arch over the base of the pyramids* (Fig. 18.9).
- The arcuate arteries run at right angles to the parent interlobar arteries. They lie parallel to the renal surface at the junction of the pyramid and the cortex. They give off a series of *interlobular arteries* that run through the cortex at right angles to the renal surface to form subcapsular plexus. Each interlobular artery gives off a series of arterioles that enter glomeruli as *afferent arterioles*. Blood from these arterioles circulates through

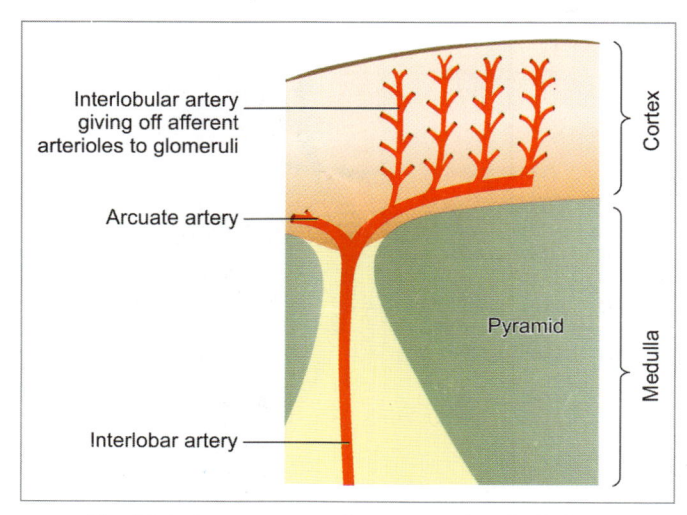

Fig. 18.9: Arrangement of arteries within the kidney (schematic representation).

glomerular capillaries that join to form **efferent arterioles** that emerge from glomeruli.

- Efferent arterioles arising from the **cortical glomeruli** divide into capillaries that surround the proximal and DCTs. These capillaries drain into **interlobular veins** and through them into **arcuate veins** and **interlobar veins**.
- Efferent arterioles arising from **juxtamedullary glomeruli** divide into 12–25 straight vessels that descend into the medulla. These are the **descending vasa recta** (Fig. 18.10). Side branches arising from the vasa recta join a capillary plexus that surrounds the descending and ascending limbs of the loop of Henle and also the collecting tubules. The capillary plexus consists predominantly of vessels running longitudinally along the tubules. It is drained by **ascending vasa recta** that run upward parallel to the descending vasa recta to reach the cortex and they drain into interlobular or arcuate veins.
- There are two sets of arterioles and capillaries intervene between the renal artery and vein. The first capillary system, present in glomeruli, is concerned exclusively with the removal of waste products from blood. It does not supply oxygen to renal tissues. An exchange of gases between blood and renal tissue is entirely through the second capillary system present around tubules.
- It has also been held that interlobular arteries divide the renal cortex into small lobules. Each lobule is defined as the region of cortex lying between two adjacent interlobular arteries. A medullary ray, containing a collecting duct, runs vertically through the middle of the lobule (midway between the two arteries) (Fig. 18.11). Glomeruli lie in a zone adjacent to the arteries while other parts of the nephron lie nearer the center of the lobule.

Renal Interstitium

The space between the tubules and blood vessels form the renal interstitium. It occupies a small volume in cortex but increases in medulla. It contains scanty amount of connective tissue with fibroblasts, interstitial dendritic cells, collagen fibers, and ground substances rich in proteoglycan. In medulla, the secreting interstitial cells are present and they help in the synthesis of prostaglandins and prostacyclins.

URETERS

- Ureters are muscular tubes that conduct urine from renal pelvis to the urinary bladder. Each ureter is about 3–4 mm in diameter and approximately 25–30 cm in length.
- The wall of the ureter has three layers:
  1. An inner mucous membrane
  2. A middle layer of smooth muscle
  3. *An outer fibrous coat*: Adventitia.

Fig. 18.10: Behavior of efferent arterioles of glomeruli in the superficial and deeper parts of the renal cortex (schematic representation).

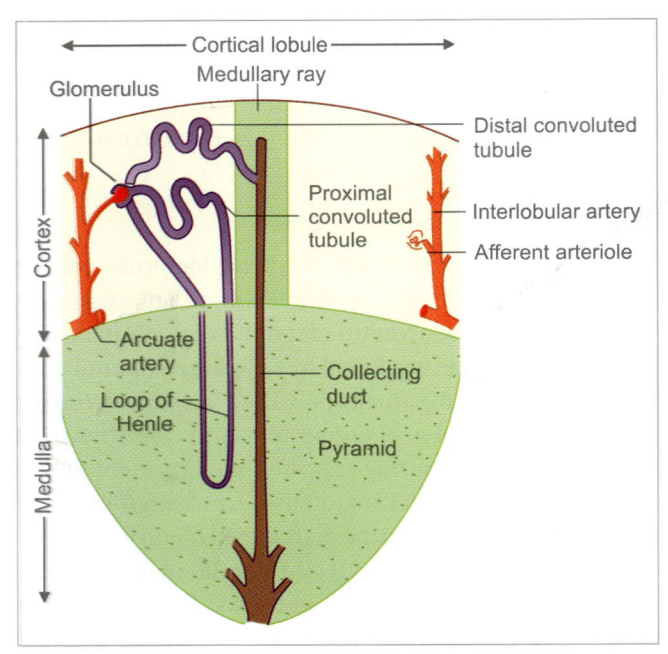

Fig. 18.11: The concept of cortical lobules (schematic representation).

Mucous Membrane

- The mucosa shows a number of longitudinal folds that give the lumen a star-shaped appearance in transverse section. The folds disappear when the ureter is distended.
- The mucous membrane has a lining of **transitional epithelium** that is four to five cells thick and an underlying dense, irregular connective tissue the **lamina propria**. The epithelium is separated from lamina propria by a basal lamina.

Muscle Coat

- The muscle coat is composed of two inseparable smooth muscle layers—(1) An inner longitudinal layer and (2) An outer circular layer. A third layer of longitudinal fibers is present outside the circular coat in the lower one-third of the ureter.
- Traced above the circular muscle surrounds the renal papillae and exerts milking action to squeeze urine from ducts to minor calyces. Traced below outer two layers are continuous with the detrusor muscle of bladder and inner longitudinal layer forms muscle of Bell.
- Muscle cells of the ureter intercommunicate with each other and form a syncytium. The waves of peristalsis pass downward through muscle and not depend on the nerve supply.

Adventitia

- Adventitia is the outer fibrous coat consisting of loose connective tissue. It contains numerous blood vessels, nerves, lymphatics, and some fat cells.
- At proximal and distal parts of the ureter, it blends with the capsule of the kidney and connective tissue of the urinary bladder wall, respectively (Plate 18.4).

> **Added Information**
>
> Reflux of urine from the urinary bladder into the ureters is prevented by the oblique path followed by the terminal part of the ureter, through the bladder wall. When the musculature of the bladder contracts this part of the ureter is compressed. This mechanism constitutes a physiological sphincter.

URINARY BLADDER

- Urinary bladder is a muscular bag, where urine is stored temporarily and is discharged periodically via urethra during micturition.
- The wall of the urinary bladder from inside outward consists of four layers—(1) Mucosa (2) Submucosa (3) Muscular layer (4) Outer serosa.

Mucous Membrane

- The mucous membrane is lined by transitional epithelium/urothelium which is urine proof, devoid of muscularis mucosae. Surface epithelium is polyhedral with abundant cytoplasm and prominent nuclei. Some nuclei have polyploid number of chromosomes. The cytoplasm of surface cells spread like umbrella to allow distension of the bladder without tension of individual cells, hence called **umbrella cells**.
- In the empty bladder, the mucous membrane is thrown into numerous folds that disappear when the bladder is distended.
- The lamina propria has superficial dense irregular and deeper loose connective tissue. It contains some mucous glands near the internal urethral orifice.
- When the bladder is distended, the lining epithelium becomes thinner due to the ability of the epithelial cells to change shape and shift over one another (Plate 18.5).

Note: Umbrella cells haave intercellular junctional complexes and surface their is covered by double lipid layer with uroplakins (integral membrane protein) together called Urothelial plaques. These plaques are discontinuous and termed as asymmetric unit membrane. This arrangement helps to protect underlying cells from cytotoxic and hypertonic effects of urine

Submucous Layer (Considered to be Lamina Propria of Mucous Layer)

It consists of loose areolar tissue all over the bladder except at the trigone where mucous membrane is adherent to the muscular layer.

Muscular Coat

- The muscle layer is thick and composed of three interlaced layers of smooth muscles. They are arranged as internal and external layers of longitudinal fibers and in between them there is a thicker layer of circular (or oblique) fibers.
- The muscle is called **detrusor muscle** and contraction of this muscle is responsible for emptying of the bladder.
- At the internal urethral orifice/neck of bladder, the circular fibers are thickened to form the **sphincter vesicae/internal sphincter muscle** in men.
- The external longitudinal layer continues to the muscle layer of prostate in men and to the external urethral meatus in women.

Serous Layer/Adventitia

- The serous layer is composed of dense irregular connective tissue. The superior surface of the bladder is

Plate 18.4: Ureter

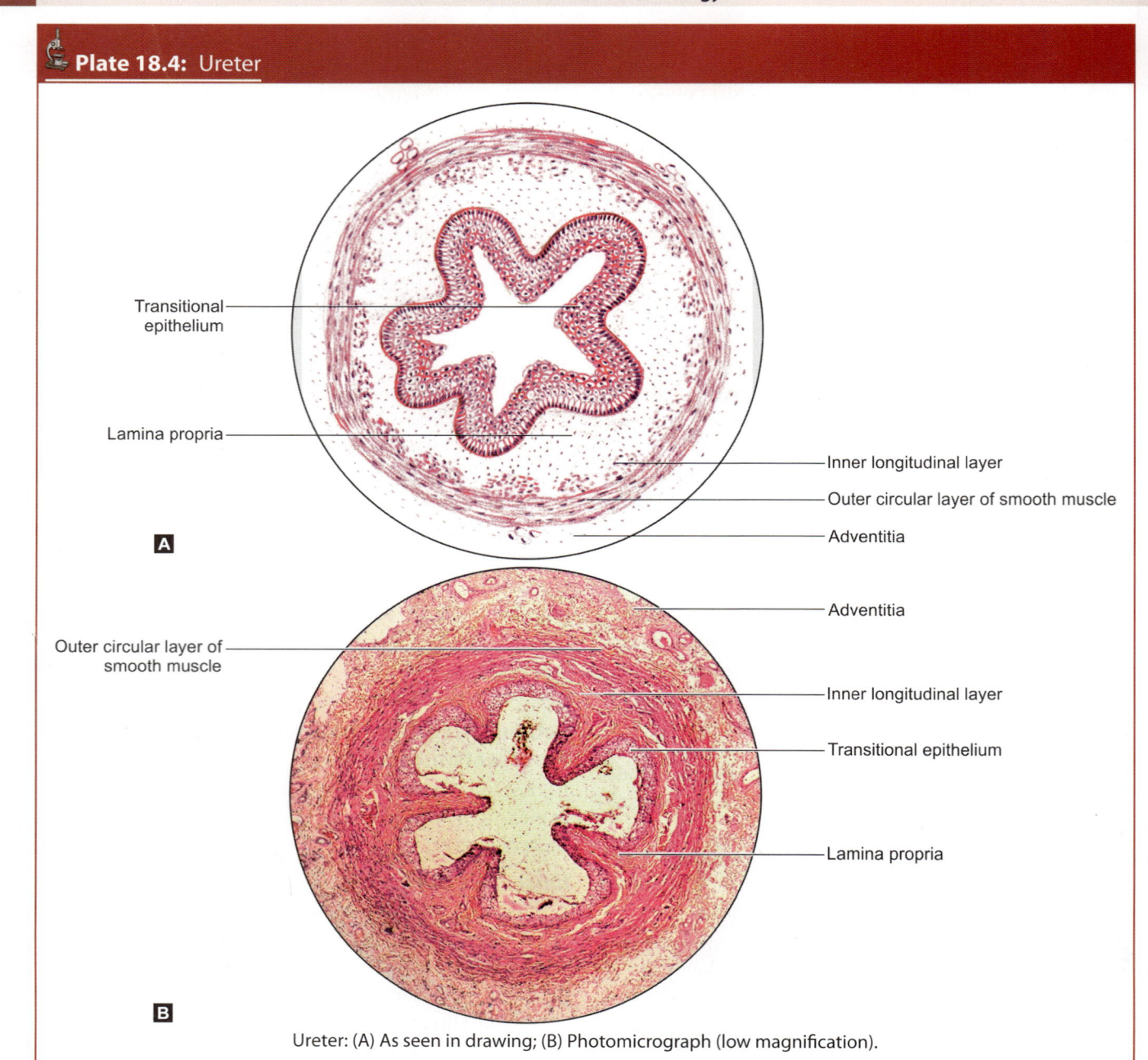

Ureter: (A) As seen in drawing; (B) Photomicrograph (low magnification).

Points of identification
- The ureter can be recognized because it is tubular and its mucous membrane is lined by transitional epithelium
- The epithelium rests on a layer of connective tissue (lamina propria)
- The mucosa shows folds that give the lumen a star-shaped appearance
- The muscle coat has an inner layer of longitudinal fibers and an outer layer of circular fibers. This arrangement is the reverse of that in the gut
- The muscle coat is surrounded by connective tissue–adventitia in which blood vessels and fat cells are present.

CHAPTER 18: Urinary System

Plate 18.5: Urinary bladder

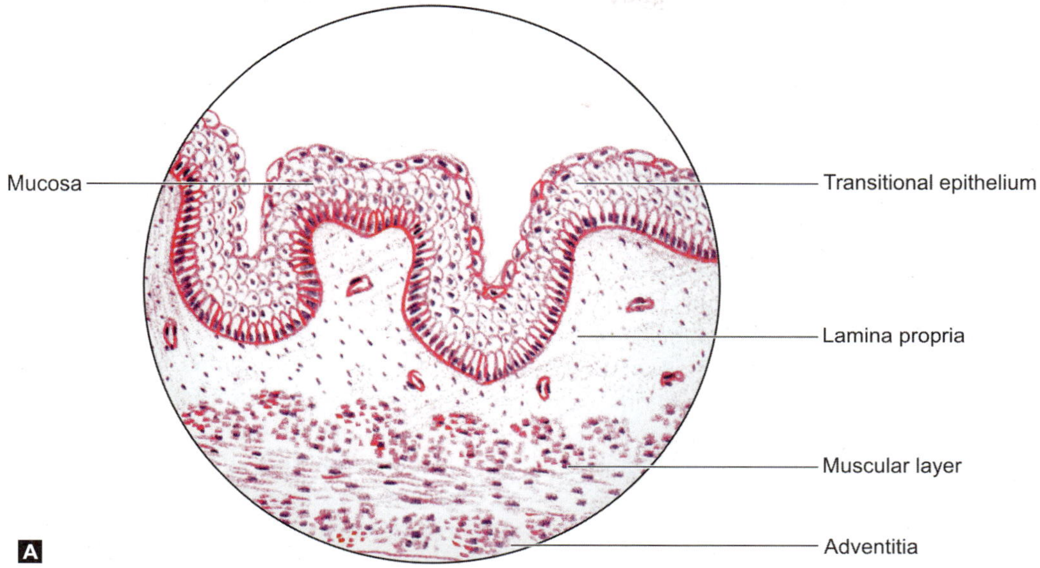

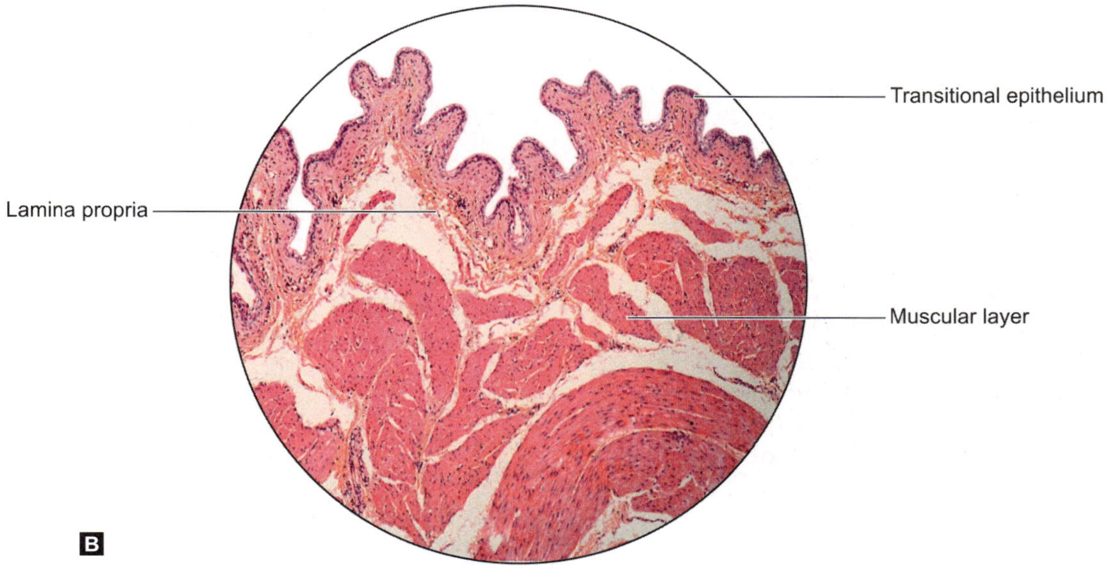

Urinary bladder: (A) As seen in drawing; (B) Photomicrograph.

Points of identification
- The urinary bladder is easily recognized because the mucous membrane is lined by transitional epithelium
- The epithelium rests on lamina propria
- The muscle layer is thick. It has inner and outer longitudinal layers between which there is a layer of circular or oblique fibers. The distinct muscle layers may not be distinguishable
- The outer surface is lined in parts by peritoneum (serosa) (not seen in the photomicrograph).

covered by mesothelium of peritoneum, forming serous layer.
* The inferior part of the bladder is covered with adventitia which is made of fibroelastic connective tissue carrying blood vessels, nerves, and lymphatics.

URETHRA

* Urethra is a tube that carries urine from bladder to the exterior. In males, semen also passes through the urethra. Although the male urethra is much longer than the female urethra, the structure of the two is the same.
* The wall of the urethra is composed from inside outward—mucous membrane, submucosa, and muscular layer.
* In male, the prostatic urethra is surrounded by prostatic tissue, and the penile urethra by erectile tissue of the corpus spongiosum.

Female Urethra

Mucous Membrane

* The mucous membrane consists of a lining epithelium that rests on connective tissue. The epithelium varies in different parts of the urethra.
* In female, it is lined by stratified squamous nonkeratinized epithelium along the length except near the bladder it is by transitional epithelium.
* In male, prostatic urethra is lined by transitional epithelium, membranous urethra by stratified columnar epithelium, spongy/penile urethra by stratified columnar interspersed with patches of pseudostratified columnar and stratified squamous nonkeratinized epithelia.
* The mucosa shows invaginations or recesses into which mucous glands open. **Littre's glands** are the mucous glands found along the entire length of the urethra and most abundant at the spongy part of the male urethra. Its secretion lubricates the epithelial lining of the urethra.

Submucosa

The submucosa consists of loose connective tissue.

Muscle Coat

* The muscle coat consists of an inner longitudinal layer and an outer circular layer of smooth muscle. This coat is better defined in the female urethra. In the male urethra, it is well-defined only in the membranous and prostatic parts, the penile part being surrounded by occasional fibers only.
* In addition to this smooth muscle, the membranous part of the male urethra, and the corresponding part of the female urethra are surrounded by striated muscle that forms the *external urethral sphincter*.

APPLIED HISTOLOGY

* Defects in the glomerular basement membrane are responsible for the nephrotic syndrome in which large amounts of protein are lost through urine. The regular arrangement of podocyte processes is also disorganized in this condition.
* The presence of albumin in the urine (**albuminuria**) is the result of increased permeability of the glomerular endothelium. Causes of albuminuria are hypertension, vascular injury, and bacterial infections.
* **Glomerulonephritis or Bright's disease** is the term used for diseases that primarily involve the renal glomeruli.
* **Nephrotic syndrome** is a constellation of features in different diseases having varying pathogenesis; it is characterized by findings of massive proteinuria, hypoalbuminemia, edema, hyperlipidemia, lipiduria, and hypercoagulability.
* **Hydronephrosis** is the term used for dilatation of renal pelvis and calyces due to partial or intermittent obstruction to the outflow of urine. Hydronephrosis develops if one or both the pelviureteric sphincters are incompetent, as otherwise there will be dilatation and hypertrophy of the urinary bladder but no hydronephrosis. Hydroureter nearly always accompanies hydronephrosis. Hydronephrosis may be unilateral or bilateral.
* **Ureterocele** is cystic dilatation of the terminal part of the ureter which lies within the bladder wall. The cystic dilatation lies beneath the bladder mucosa and can be visualized by cystoscopy.
* **Cystitis** is the inflammation of the urinary bladder. Cystitis is caused by a variety of bacterial and fungal infections. Cystitis, like urinary tract infection (UTI), is more common in females because of the shortness of urethra which is liable to fecal contamination and due to mechanical trauma during sexual intercourse.

CHAPTER 18: Urinary System

MULTIPLE CHOICE QUESTIONS

1. What makes the renal corpuscle?
   a. Bowman's capsule and glomerulus
   b. Bowman's capsule and tubules
   c. Glomerulus and tubules
   d. Bowman's capsule, glomerulus, and tubules
2. Renal corpuscles are found in:
   a. Cortex
   b. Medulla
   c. Both cortex and medulla
   d. Pyramid
3. Podocytes are the cells that lines the:
   a. Glomerulus
   b. Bowman's capsule
   c. Tubules
   d. Ducts
4. What is the function of the brush border on the proximal convoluted tubule?
   a. Decrease the surface area
   b. Secretion
   c. Motility
   d. Absorption
5. Renin is secreted by which cell?
   a. Macula densa
   b. Juxtaglomerular
   c. Interstitial
   d. Lacis
6. Ureter is lined by _____ epithelium.
   a. Squamous
   b. Stratified squamous
   c. Transitional
   d. Pseudostratified
7. Proximal convoluted tubule is lined by which epithelium?
   a. Squamous
   b. Cuboidal
   c. Columnar
   d. Transitional
8. Which hormone regulates the reabsorption of sodium and potassium ions at distal convoluted tubule?
   a. Aldosterone
   b. Angiotensin I
   c. Angiotensin II
   d. ACE
9. The ultrafiltrate leaving the thin ascending loop of Henle is _____ to plasma.
   a. Hypotonic
   b. Isotonic
   c. Hypertonic
   d. None of the above
10. Littre glands are present in:
    a. Kidney
    b. Ureter
    c. Bladder
    d. Urethra
11. Which is true regarding JG apparatus?
    a. JG cells are modified smooth cells of efferent arteriole
    b. Macula densa are modified cells of distal convoluted tubule near afferent arteriole
    c. Lacis cells are extraglomerular mesangial cells
    d. JG apparatus secretes angiotensin
12. Which of the following is mismatched?
    a. Visceral layer of Bowman's capsule—podocytes
    b. Parietal layer of Bowman's capsule—simple squamous epithelium
    c. Distal tubule cells—brush border
    d. Thin segment of Henle's loop—simple squamous epithelium
13. A small protein passes through the glomerular basement membrane into the glomerular filtrate. Cells of which of the following tissues would remove the protein from the filtrate?
    a. Visceral epithelium of the renal corpuscle
    b. Distal convoluted tubule
    c. Proximal convoluted tubule
    d. Parietal layer of the renal corpuscle
14. Ducts of Bellini opens into the:
    a. Renal tubules
    b. Minor calyces
    c. Major calyces
    d. Renal pelvis
15. Which of the following is false about renal column?
    a. It consists of cortical tissue
    b. Interlobular arteries pass through them
    c. It is located adjacent to the renal pyramids
    d. It is part of the medulla of the kidney
16. The tuft of capillaries in the renal corpuscle is called the:
    a. Glomerulus
    b. Calyx
    c. Renal pyramid
    d. Renal sinus
17. This part of the nephron extends into the medulla.
    a. Proximal convoluted tubule
    b. Loop of Henle
    c. Distal convoluted tubule
    d. Papillary duct
18. What is a renal pyramid and its overlying cortex called?
    a. Lobule
    b. Lobe
    c. Renal columns
    d. Medullary ray

Answers
| 1. a | 2. a | 3. b | 4. d | 5. b | 6. c | 7. c | 8. a | 9. b |
| 10. d | 11. c | 12. c | 13. c | 14. b | 15. b | 16. a | 17. b | 18. b |

CHAPTER 19

Central Nervous System: Spinal Cord, Cerebellar Cortex and Cerebral Cortex

Learning objectives

To study the:
- Structure of spinal cord
- Layers of cerebrum
- Cells of cerebrum
- Layers of cerebellum
- Neurons of cerebellum
- Applied histology

IDENTIFICATION POINTS

Spinal cord
- Presence of outer white and inner gray matter
- Gray matter consists of anterior horn and posterior horn
- Central canal is present in the gray commissure
- White matter consists of anterior, lateral, and posterior funiculi.

Cerebrum
- Presence of outer gray and inner white matter
- Cerebral cortex is made up of six laminae from superficial to deep: Plexiform, outer granula, outer pyramidal, inner granular, inner pyramidal, and pleomorphic layer
- Pyramidal, stellate, granule, cells of Martinotti, and horizontal cells of Cajal are present
- Pyramidal cells are present in almost all the layers.

Cerebellum
- Presence of outer gray and inner white matter
- Cerebellar cortex is made up of three layers from superficial to deep: molecular, Purkinje cell, and granular layer
- Purkinje, granule, Golgi, stellate, and basket cells are present
- Purkinje cells are flask shaped and present as a single stratum.

INTRODUCTION

- The central nervous system (CNS) consists of brain and spinal cord floating in cerebrospinal fluid. They are protected by the skull and vertebrae and is surrounded by meninges. The classification of nervous system is depicted in Flowchart 19.1.
- Section through CNS shows **gray and white** matter.
- **Gray matter** consists of the aggregation of cell bodies of neurons, dendrites, unmyelinated/initial part of axons, and neuroglial cells. Fibers within the gray matter are unmyelinated, and this causes these regions to appear gray.
- **White matter** consists predominantly of myelinated fibers along with some unmyelinated fibers and neuroglial cells. It is the reflection of light by myelin that gives this region its whitish appearance.
- Blood vessels are present in both gray and white matter.
- In the cerebrum and cerebellum, gray matter present on the surface forming **cerebral and cerebellar cortex**.

Deep to the cortex, there is white matter, but within the latter, several isolated masses of gray matter are present. Such aggregations of neuronal cell bodies embedded in white matter in the CNS are called **nuclei**.
- In the spinal cord and brainstem, the white matter is peripheral and the gray matter is central. It assumes a shape of H in the spinal cord.
- The axons arising from in one mass of gray matter terminate by synapsing with neurons in other masses of gray matter. Such axons connecting two or more masses of gray matter form bundles, and the aggregations of such fibers are called **tracts**. Larger collections of fibers are also referred to as **funiculi, fasciculi,** or **lemnisci**. Large bundles of fibers connecting the cerebral or cerebellar hemispheres to the brainstem are called **peduncles**.

SPINAL CORD

- The spinal cord is an elongated and cylindrical part of CNS and located within the upper two-thirds of the vertebral

CHAPTER 19: Central Nervous System: Spinal Cord, Cerebellar Cortex and Cerebral Cortex

Flowchart 19.1: Classification of nervous system.

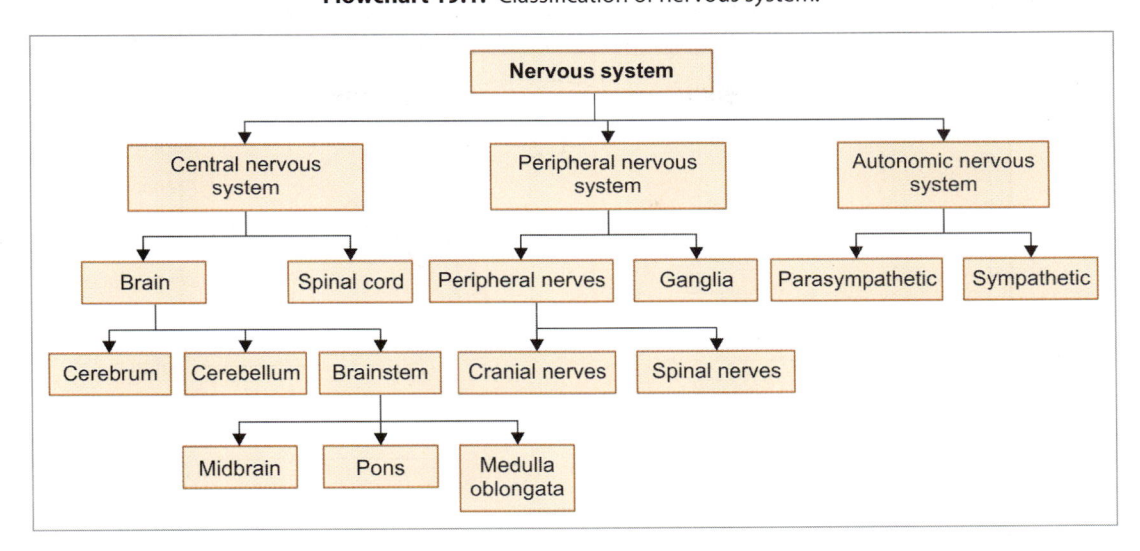

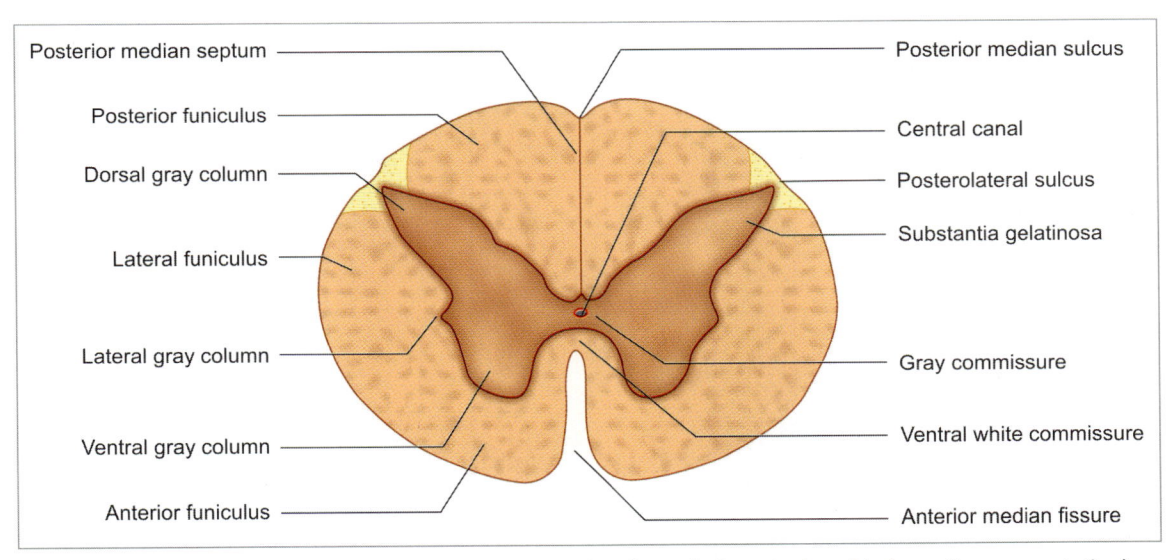

Fig. 19.1: Main features to be seen in a transverse section through the spinal cord (schematic representation).

canal. It is the continuation of medulla oblongata and ends as tapering/conical structure called the ***conus medullaris***. The conus is continuous and, below, with a fibrous cord called the ***filum terminale*** (modification of pia mater).

❖ It is surrounded by meninges: Outer dura, middle arachnoid, and inner pia mater. On cross-section, the spinal cord presents outer white and inner gray matter (Fig. 19.1 and Plate 19.1).

Gray Matter

❖ It consists of cell bodies of nerve cells, neuroglia, and blood vessels and arranged in H-shaped column (Plate 19.1).

❖ The gray matter presents a pair of larger anterior/ventral gray column called ***anterior/ventral horn*** and a narrow elongated posterior/dorsal gray column called ***posterior/dorsal horn***, an intermediate region intervenes between anterior and posterior horns, and a ***gray commissure*** connects the symmetrical halves of gray matter across the midline.

❖ Anterior gray column is broad and short and presents head and base. Posterior gray column is longer and narrower than the anterior column and consists of base, neck, head and apex ventrodorsally. Base is continuous with the intermediate region of gray matter.

Plate 19.1: Spinal cord

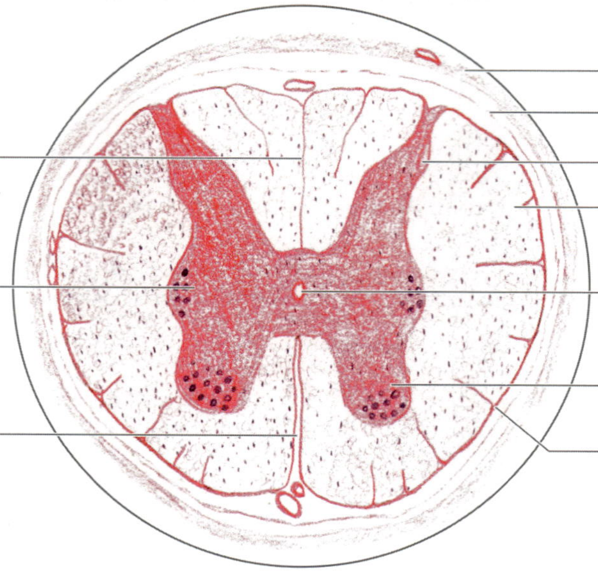

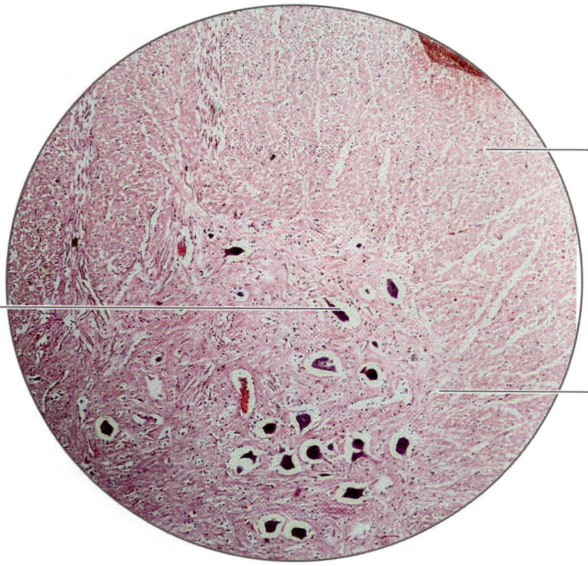

Spinal cord: (A) As seen in drawing; (B) Gray matter (photomicrograph).

Points of identification
- The spinal cord has a characteristic oval shape.
- It is made up of white matter (containing mainly of myelinated fibers), and gray matter (containing neurons and unmyelinated fibers).
- The gray matter lies toward the center and is surrounded all round by white matter.
- The gray matter consists of a centrally placed mass and projections (horns) that pass forwards and backwards.

CHAPTER 19: Central Nervous System: Spinal Cord, Cerebellar Cortex and Cerebral Cortex

- Intermediate region presents between the base of anterior and posterior horns. In thoracic and upper lumbar region of the spinal cord, it forms a small lateral projection from the base of anterior horn called as the *lateral gray column*.
- The *gray commissure* is traversed by the **central canal**, which contains cerebrospinal fluid and it is lined by ependyma. Central canal is continuous with fourth ventricle through the canal of medulla. Within the conus medullaris, the central canal is enlarged to form **terminal ventricle**. Central canal divides the gray commissure into ventral and dorsal parts.
- The cell bodies of neurons differ in size and in the prominence of Nissl substance in different regions of spinal gray matter. They are most prominent in the anterior gray column.

White Matter

- It consists of nerve fibers, neuroglia, and blood vessels. It occupies the periphery of H-shaped gray matter.
- It is divided into right and left halves by a deep **anterior median fissure** and posterior **median septum**. Each half of the white matter of the spinal cord is arranged into anterior, lateral, and posterior funiculi.
- *Anterior funiculus* extends on each side from anterior median fissure to the most lateral fibers of the ventral nerve roots, and it is medial and ventral to the anterior gray column. Anterior white commissure connects the anterior funiculi of both sides, and it is present in front of ventral gray commissure.
- *Lateral funiculus* intervenes between the emerging of the ventral roots of spinal nerves and posterolateral sulcus where dorsal nerve roots emerge and present lateral to and between the anterior and posterior gray columns. The anterior and lateral funiculi are collectively referred to as the *anterolateral funiculus*.
- *Posterior funiculus* extends on each side from the posterolateral sulcus to the posteromedian septum and presents medial to the dorsal gray matter.
- The white matter of the right and left halves of the spinal cord is continuous across the middle line through the *ventral white commissure* which lies anterior to the *gray commissure*. The white matter contains tracts (ascending or descending) that connect gray matter at different levels of the spinal cord. Some tracts ascend into (or descend from) the brainstem, the cerebellum, or the cerebral cortex. Details of such tracts are given in books of neuroanatomy.
- The cross-section of spinal cord varies depending on the region of spinal cord. The features detailed in Table 19.1.

CEREBRAL CORTEX

General Features

- Cerebral hemispheres are separated from each other by longitudinal fissure.
- A thin layer of gray matter present on the surface of the cerebrum forming the *cerebral cortex*. Cerebral hemisphere comprises a mantle of gray matter at the surface, white matter beneath the cortex, and some collections of subcortical gray matter masses in the white matter known as basal ganglia.
- Gray matter of the cerebral cortex contains the cell bodies of neurons along with their processes, neuroglia, and blood vessels. The neurons are of various sizes and shapes. They establish extremely intricate connections with each other and with axons reaching the cortex from other masses of gray matter.
- The cortex is subdivided into *allocortex/old cortex* which form about 10% of the cortex and *isocortex/neocortex* which comprises 90% of the cortex.

Table 19.1: Differences in cross-section of the spinal cord at different levels.

Content	Cervical	Thorax	Lumbar	Sacral
Gray matter	▫ More ▫ Ventral horn is bulbous and broad ▫ Lateral horn is absent	▫ Less ▫ Ventral and dorsal horns are slender ▫ Lateral horn is present	▫ More ▫ Ventral and dorsal horns are bulbous and broad ▫ Lateral horn is present in only upper two segments	▫ More ▫ Ventral and dorsal horns are bulbous and broad ▫ Lateral horn is absent
White matter (volume of white matter is progressively increasing from below upward)	Abundant	Abundant but less than cervical	Less	Least
Position of central canal	Ventral	Ventral	Central	Dorsal
Cross-section	Oval	Round and small	Oval but smaller than cervical	Round and very small

- For accommodation in the rigid cranial cavity, the cerebral cortex is folded into numerous *gyri* separated by *sulci*.

Structure of the Neocortex

- The neocortical gray matter thickness ranges from 1.5 mm to 4 mm, thick over gyri and thin over sulci.
- The cortical gray matter presents horizontal lamination and consists of six superimposed layers.

Neurons in the Cerebral Cortex

Cortical neurons vary in size, in the shape of their cell bodies, and in the lengths, branching patterns, and orientation of their processes (Fig. 19.2). Cortical neurons are of four basic types:
1. Pyramidal
2. Stellate/granule cells
3. Cells of Martinotti
4. Horizontal cells of Cajal.

Pyramidal Cells

- **Pyramidal cells** are about 5.5 billion in number, and it constitutes about two-thirds of all cortical neurons. Their cell bodies are pyramidal in shape, with the apex generally directed toward the surface of the cortex.
- A large apical dendrite arises from the apex and extends toward superficial layer of the cortex and divides horizontally. Numerous basal dendrites arise from basal angles and extend horizontally. All the dendrites are provided with numerous dendritic spines, which establish synaptic contacts with the projection fibers from other cortical neurons.
- The axon arises from the base of the pyramid and gives rise to efferent projection, association, or commissural fibers. The larger cell axons possess longer axons and form projection fibers to the basal ganglia, brainstem, or spinal cord. Small-sized cells provide association or commissural fibers. The collateral branches of the axons projects back the cortex and makes synapse with the stellate cells or other interneurons.
- Once committed to perform specific function, pyramidal cells do not change the modus operandi.

Stellate Neurons/Granule Cells

- The **stellate neurons** are relatively small and multipolar and belong to type II neurons. They form about one-third of the total neuronal population of the cortex.
- Their axons are short and end within the cortex. Their processes extend chiefly in a vertical direction within the cortex, but in some cases, they may be oriented horizontally.
- Dendrites make synapses with afferent projection fibers and with the collaterals of pyramidal axons. The axons of stellate cells form ascending and descending branches and establish synapses with the dendritic spines of pyramidal neurons or other interneurons.
- Fusiform cells are modified stellate neurons.

Cells of Martinotti

They are multipolar small neurons present in almost all layers of the cortex but more in sixth layer. They have smaller dendrites and elongated axons which run vertically outward to ramify in the superficial layer.

Horizontal Cells of Cajal

They are located in first layer. Their neurites extend tangentially and integrate numerous columnar units of cortex.

Lamina of Cerebral Cortex

- The cells of the cortex are arranged in horizontal lamination and also in vertical columns. Vertical columns are the functional units of the cortex, since within the columns pyramidal cells, stellate cells, and other interneurons communicate with one another by short synaptic loops resulting in large output.

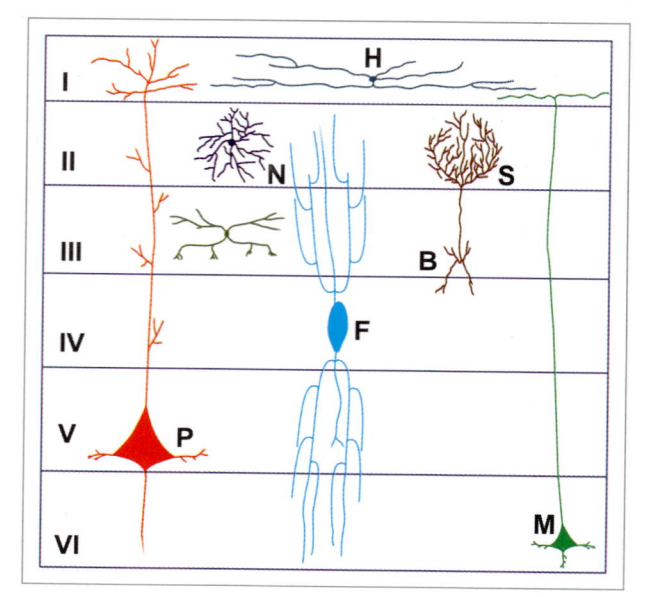

Fig. 19.2: Some of the cell types to be seen in the cerebral cortex (schematic representation). (B: basket cells; F: fusiform cells; H: horizontal cell of Cajal; M: cells of Martinotti; N: neuroglia form cell; P: pyramidal cell; S: stellate cell)

CHAPTER 19: Central Nervous System: Spinal Cord, Cerebellar Cortex and Cerebral Cortex

- Axon collaterals of pyramidal cells excite some interneurons of the column and inturn it discharge repeated excitatory impulses to the aforesaid pyramidal cells of that column. Simultaneously, the axon collaterals of pyramidal cells inhibit some other interneurons of the column and latter inhibit the pyramidal cells of the surrounding columns. The neuronal sharpening is achieved by a group of excited neurons in an inhibitory surround.

  The *horizontal lamination* (Fig. 19.3 and Plate 19.2) of the neocortex is arranged from outside inward, which is as follows:
  - *Lamina I*: Plexiform or molecular layer
  - *Lamina II*: External/outer granular layer
  - *Lamina III*: Outer pyramidal cell layer
  - *Lamina IV*: Internal/inner granular layer
  - *Lamina V*: Ganglionic layer/inner pyramidal layer
  - *Lamina VI*: Polymorphic/pleomorphic layer.

- The *plexiform layer* is made up predominantly of horizontal nerve fibers with the occasional horizontal cells of Cajal. Fibers are derived from apical dendrites of pyramidal cells, axons of stellate and Martinotti cells, and neuritis of horizontal cells of Cajal.

- *Outer granular layer* is packed with numerous stellate cells and small number of pyramidal cells.

- *Outer pyramidal layer* predominantly contains pyramidal cells and few stellate cells. Small-sized pyramidal cells lie in the superficial part and medium-sized cells in the deeper part of the layer.

- *Inner granular layer* densely packed with stellate cells with medium-sized pyramidal cells dispersed in irregular manner. Inner part of this layer is traversed by tangential fibers of the *outer band of Baillarger* more marked in **visual cortex** of occipital lobe, hence it is also called striate cortex.

- *Ganglionic/inner pyramidal layer* contains medium- and large-sized pyramidal cells. Large neurons called as *giant pyramidal cells of Betz* lie in the deeper zone of the layer. In neocortex, small pyramidal cells are located superficially; medium-sized cells in more deep, and large cells lie further deeply. Tangential fibers of *inner band of Baillarger* traverse at the outer part of this layer.

- **Polymorphic layer is the deepest layer** and contains multipolar neurons, which are probably modified pyramidal cells. *Cells of Martinotti* are more in this layer with axons run vertically to ramify in the molecular layer.

- In addition to the cell bodies of neurons, the cortex contains abundant nerve fibers. Many of these are vertically oriented. In addition to the vertical fibers, the cortex contains transversely running fibers called the *external band of Baillarger and internal band of Baillarger*.

- Most of the afferent fibers from the specific nuclei of thalamus make synapses in the laminae I–IV. Afferent projection fibers from other nuclei of thalamus and ascending reticular system terminate in all the layers of cortex. Laminae II and IV are concerned with sensory, laminae III and V with somatomotor or visceral motor activities. Laminae I and VI are for the association of sensory and motor behavior.

- Efferent projection fibers from pyramidal cells of fifth layer give rise to corticostriate, corticobulbar, corticopontine, and corticospinal fibers. Modified pyramidal cells of sixth layer give rise to corticothalamic fibers. Pyramidal cells of third layer give rise to association and commissural fibers.

Layer		Contents
Plexiform or molecular		Transverse fibers and some scattered neurons
External granular		Mainly stellate neurons
Pyramidal		Mainly pyramidal neurons; Some stellate cells and basket cells
Internal granular		Stellate neurons; Outer band of Baillarger
Ganglionic		Giant pyramidal cells; Inner band of Baillarger
Multiform or polymorphic		Neurons of various sizes and shapes; Merge with white matter

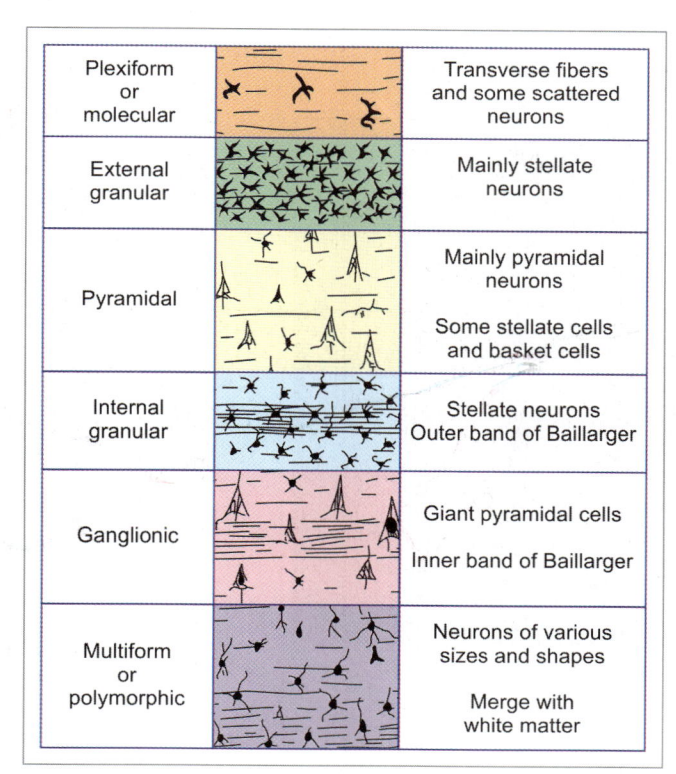

Fig. 19.3: Laminae of cerebral cortex (schematic representation).

Plate 19.2: Cerebral cortex

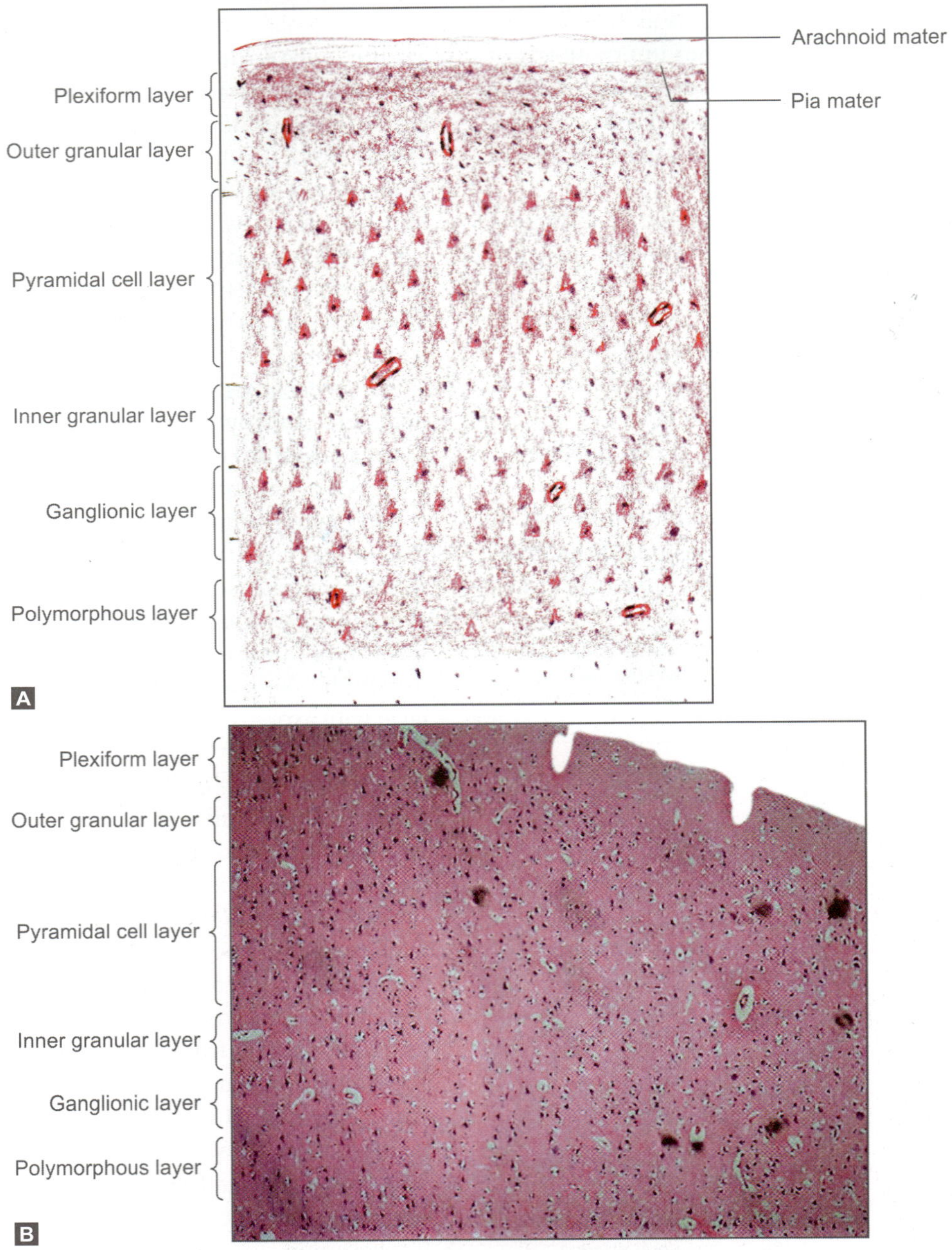

Cerebral cortex: (A) As seen in drawing; (B) Photomicrograph.

Points of identification
- A slide of cerebral cortex shows outer gray and inner white matter
- Multipolar neurons of various shapes are arranged in six layers in the gray matter
- Axons of these neurons are present in the white matter
- Neuroglia and blood vessels are present in gray and white matter.

CHAPTER 19: Central Nervous System: Spinal Cord, Cerebellar Cortex and Cerebral Cortex

> **Added Information**
>
> **Variations in Cortical Structure**
> - The structure of the cerebral cortex shows considerable variation from region to region, both in terms of thickness and in the prominence of the various laminae described above. Finer variations form the basis of the subdivisions into Brodmann's areas. These are as follows:
>   ◊ In the **agranular cortex**, the external and internal granular laminae are inconspicuous. This type of cortex is seen most typically in the precentral gyrus (area 4) and is, therefore, believed to be typical of "motor" areas. It is also seen in some other areas.
>   ◊ In the **granular cortex**, the granular layers are highly developed, while the pyramidal and ganglionic layers are poorly developed or absent. In the visual area, the external band of Baillarger is prominent and forms a white line that can be seen with the naked eye when the region is freshly cut across. This **stria of Gennari** gives the name **striate cortex** to the visual cortex.
>   ◊ Between the two extremes represented by the agranular and granular varieties of cortex, three intermediate types described are **frontal cortex**, **parietal cortex**, and **polar cortex**. The frontal type is nearest to the agranular cortex, the pyramidal cells being prominent, while the polar type is nearest to the granular cortex.

CEREBELLAR CORTEX

General Features

- The cerebellum lies in the posterior cranial fossa. The cerebellum has a superficial layer of gray matter, the *cerebellar cortex*, a medullary core of white matter, and four pairs of *cerebellar nuclei* embedded in the white matter.
- The cortex is thrown into numerous transverse folds called *folia* separated by *fissures*.
- The central core of each cerebellar hemisphere is formed by white matter which is continuous with the peduncles. The white matter of the two sides is connected by a thin lamina of fibers that are closely related to the fourth ventricle. The upper part of this lamina forms the superior medullary velum, and its inferior part forms the inferior medullary velum. Both of these take part in forming the roof of the fourth ventricle.
- The *cerebellar nuclei* are as follows (Fig. 19.4):
  - The **dentate nucleus** lies in the center of each cerebellar hemisphere. It is made up of a thin lamina of gray matter that is folded upon it so that it resembles a crumpled purse.
  - The **emboliform nucleus** lies on the medial side of the dentate nucleus.
  - The **globose nucleus** lies medial to the emboliform nucleus.
  - The **fastigial nucleus** lies close to the middle line in the anterior part of the superior vermis.

Structure of the Cerebellar Cortex

- The cerebellar cortex is entirely uniform in structure, and their neurons with processes are arranged in geometrical configuration.
- The cortex consists of three layers as follows (Plate 19.3 and Fig. 19.5):
  1. **Outer molecular layer**
  2. **Middle Purkinje cell layer**
  3. **Inner granular layer,** which rests on white matter.
- The neurons of the cerebellar cortex are of five main types. All of them are inhibitory except granule cells.
  1. **Purkinje cells**, forming the layer named after them
  2. **Granule cells**, forming the granular layer
  3. **Stellate cells**, present in molecular layer
  4. **Basket cells**, present in the molecular layer
  5. **Golgi cells**, present in the granular layer.

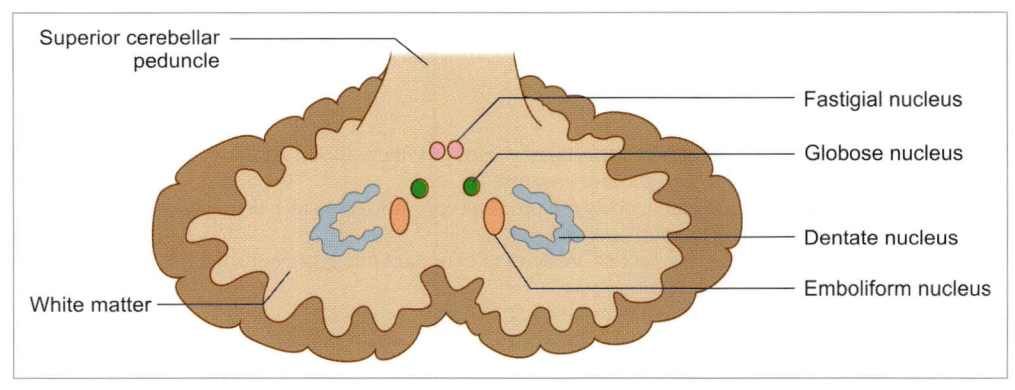

Fig. 19.4: Cerebellar nuclei (schematic representation).

Plate 19.3: Cerebellar cortex

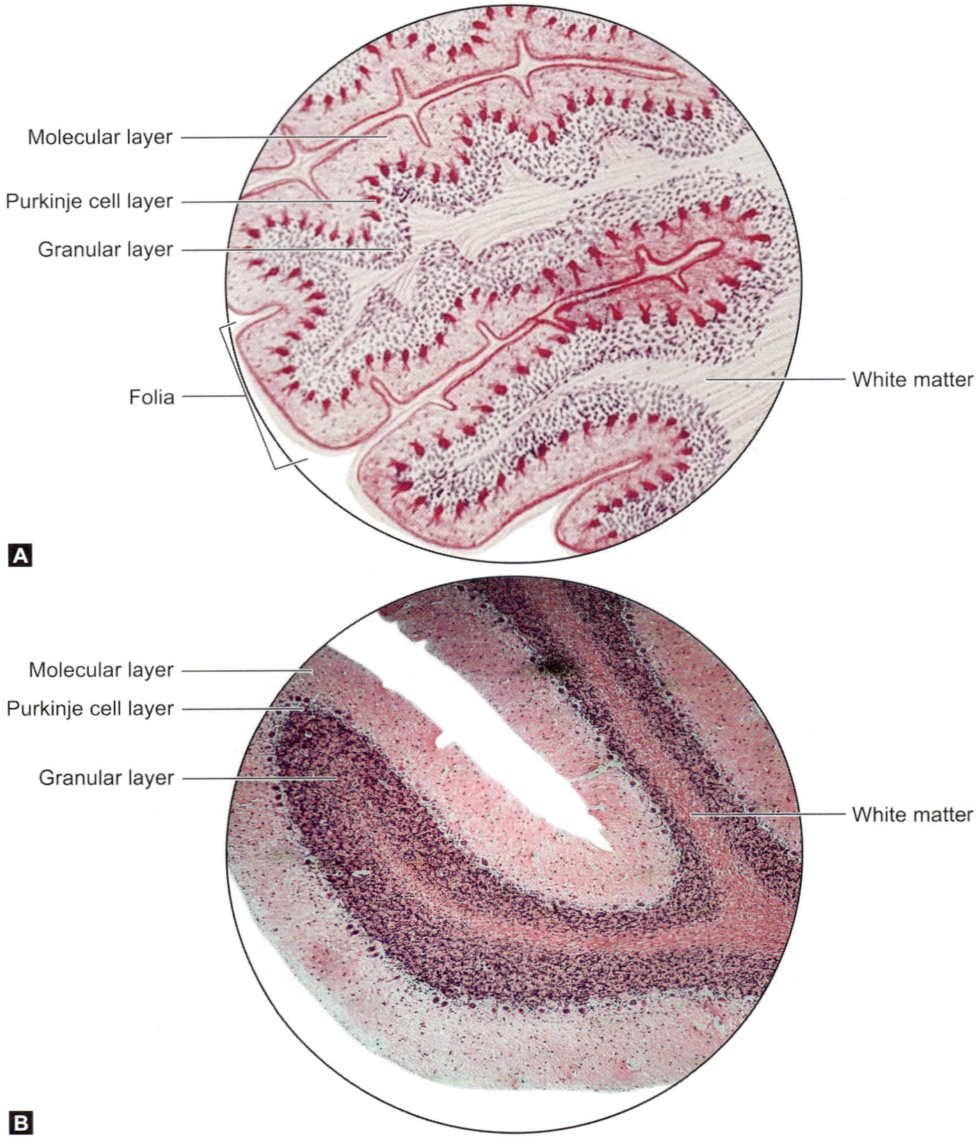

Cerebellar cortex: (A) As seen in drawing; (B) Photomicrograph.

Points of identification
- The section of cerebellum shows leaf-like folia
- The cortex is covered by pia mater which appears as a thin layer of collagen fibers. Blood vessels may be seen just beneath the pia mater
- Outer gray matter is arranged in three layers from without inwards:
  1. *Molecular layer*: Very few nuclei of neurons seen. Many cell processes present. Appears pale
  2. *Purkinje cell layer*: Single layer of big flask-shaped pink neurons
  3. *Granular cell layer*: Appears very dark blue because of presence of abundant nuclei of neurons
- Inner white matter shows axons which appear as pink fibers
- Nuclei of neuroglia are present both in gray and white matter.

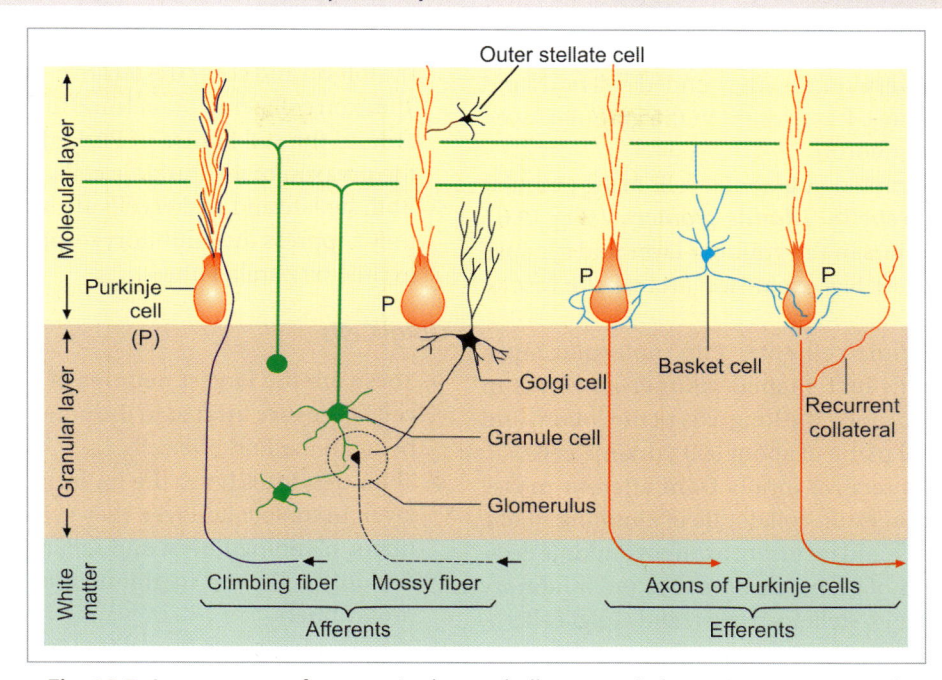

CHAPTER 19: Central Nervous System: Spinal Cord, Cerebellar Cortex and Cerebral Cortex

Fig. 19.5: Arrangement of neurons in the cerebellar cortex (schematic representation).

Molecular Layer

- The molecular layer is the superficial layer of the cortex and situated just below the pia mater.
- This layer predominantly consists of unmyelinated nerve fibers which are derived from the parallel fibers axons of the granule, stellate, and basket cells, sensory climbing fibers, dendrites of Purkinje, and Golgi cells. This layer stains light as it consists of few cells and more of nerve fibers.
- Two types of cells are found in this layer: (1) stellate cells (situated in the superficial part of the molecular layer) and (2) basket cells (situated in the deeper layer).

Purkinje Cell Layer

- The Purkinje cell layer contains flask-shaped cell bodies of Purkinje cells which are arranged as a single stratum.
- A dendrite arises from the "neck" of the "flask" and passes "upward" into the molecular layer, and axons make synaptic connections with the deep cerebellar nuclei.

Granular Layer

- It is the innermost layer and packed with cell bodies and dendrites of granule cells and a few Golgi cells with their processes and brush cells.
- It also contains sensory mossy fibers with their synaptic glomeruli. The granular layer stains deeply with hematoxylin as it is densely packed with granular cell.

Cells of Cerebellum

Purkinje Cells

- Cell bodies of Purkinje cells are large and flask shaped and present in the middle layer as a single stratum.
- The dendrites arise from the neck of the flask and pass upward into the molecular layer at right angles to the long axis of the cerebellar folium. Here it divides and subdivides to form an elaborate dendritic tree. First three orders of the dendritic tree are smooth, and subsequent branches are provided with spines for synaptic contacts.
- The axon arises from the bottom of the cell and passes downward through the granular layer to enter into the white matter and makes synaptic contact with deep cerebellar nuclei. The proximal part of unmyelinated axon makes synaptic contact with collaterals of basket cells. Recurrent collateral from Purkinje cells makes synapses with the stellate, basket, Golgi, and other Purkinje cells.
- Purkinje cells receive **input** from parallel fibers of granule cells, axons of stellate cells, axons of basket cells, climbing fibers, and recurrent axon collaterals of other Purkinje cells.
- Purkinje cells give **output** to deep cerebellar nuclei, lateral vestibular nucleus, stellate, basket, Golgi, and to other Purkinje cells through axon collaterals.
- They act as sole output neurons from the cerebellar cortex and exert inhibitory influence to the deep cerebellar and lateral vestibular nuclei.

Granule Cells

- Granule cells are very small with rounded cell body and four to five dendrites. It is present in the granular layer. It is the excitatory neuron.
- The spaces not occupied by granular cells in the granular layer are called **cerebellar islands/glomeruli** (Fig. 19.6).
- The dendrites radiate in the granular layer and synapse in glomeruli as claw-like expansion around the rosette of mossy fibers.
- The axons of granule cell enter into molecular layer, where it bifurcates in T-shaped manner and runs in opposite direction along the long axis of the folium and covers a territorial plane of about 500 Purkinje cells.
- The granule cells receive inputs from afferent mossy fibers through glomeruli, collaterals of climbing fibers, axons of Golgi cells, and recurrent axons of Purkinje cells.
- The parallel fibers of granule cells excite the inhibitory response of Purkinje, stellate, basket, and Golgi cells.

Outer Stellate Cells

- These cells are present in the molecular layer. Their cell bodies and processes lie at right angles to the long axis of folium.
- Their dendrites synapse with parallel fibers of granule cells and collateral climbing fibers, while their axons synapse with dendritic spine of Purkinje cells near their origin.

Basket Cells/Inner Stellate Cells

- These cells lie in the deeper part of the molecular layer, and their arrangements and connections are almost similar to stellate cells.
- Their dendrites ramify in the molecular layer and are intersected by parallel fibers with which they synapse. They also receive recurrent collaterals from Purkinje cells, climbing fibers, and mossy fibers.
- The axons of these cells pass at right angles to the axis of the folium and cover the territory of 10–12 Purkinje cells. The axon collaterals branch and form networks or baskets around the cell bodies of Purkinje cells and synapse at the preaxon of the Purkinje cells.
- Both stellate and basket cells are inhibitory neurons, and they suppress the inhibitory response of Purkinje cells if excited by parallel fibers.

Golgi Cells

- These are the largest neurons of cerebellar cortex. The cell bodies are located in the outer part of granular layer beneath the Purkinje cells.
- Their dendrites enter the molecular layer and granular layer. In molecular layer, they synapse with the parallel fibers, climbing fibers, and recurrent axon collateral of Purkinje cells, and in granular layer they synapse with mossy fibers.
- They receive inputs from parallel fibers and mossy fibers which excite the Golgi cells and recurrent axon collateral of Purkinje cells which inhibit the Golgi cells.
- They give output to dendrites of granule cells.
- Golgi cells are inhibitory neurons, and they diminish the excitability of granule cells.

Afferent Fibers Entering the Cerebellar Cortex

The afferent fibers to the cerebellar cortex are of two types, and they reach the cerebellum through peduncles: (1) Mossy fibers and (2) Climbing fibers, and both the fibers are excitatory.

Mossy Fibers

- All fibers entering the cerebellum other than olivocerebellar end as mossy fibers which synapse with many granule and few Golgi cells.
- Mossy fibers originate from the vestibular nuclei (vestibulocerebellar), pontine nuclei (pontocerebellar), and spinal cord (spinocerebellar) and terminate in the granular layer of the cortex within glomeruli.
- Each mossy fiber divides into 30–40 terminal swellings called the **rosette**, which forms the central component of glomeruli. A single rosette is surrounded by and makes synapses with the dendrites of 15 granule cells.
- A single mossy fiber activates about 450 granule cells, and their parallel fibers excite about 450–500 Purkinje cells (Fig. 19.6). Afferent inputs through mossy fibers pass through granule cells to reach the Purkinje cells.

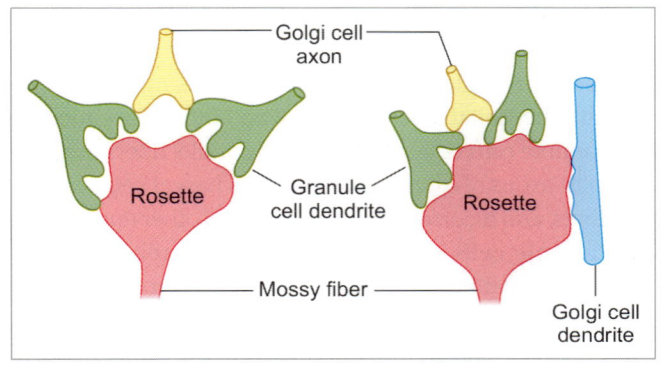

Fig. 19.6: Structure of cerebellar glomeruli. The outer capsule is not shown (schematic representation).

Climbing Fibers

- These fibers are derived mainly from the inferior olivary complex (Fig. 19.5). They pass through the granular and Purkinje cell layer to reach the molecular layer. Each climbing fiber exerts specific influence on one Purkinje cell.
- Each fiber provides collateral branches to synapse with the deep cerebellar nuclei and makes monosynaptic connections with the single Purkinje cells. In molecular layer the collaterals of climbing fibers synapse with all other types of neurons.

Efferent Fibers

- Efferent fibers of the cerebellar cortex are from Purkinje cells into deep cerebellar or vestibular nuclei. Axons of the Purkinje cells are inhibitory to cerebellar nuclei.
- The fibers from dentate, emboliform, and globose nuclei leave cerebellum through the superior cerebellar peduncle. The fibers from the fastigial nucleus leave the cerebellum through inferior cerebellar peduncle.

Glomerulus

Glomerulus is covered by Bergmann glia cells. It is composed of:
- A rosette of mossy fiber in the center forming presynaptic element
- Claw-like dendritic expansions of granule cells enveloping the rosette forming postsynaptic element
- Axon terminal of Golgi cells which come in contact with dendrites of granule cells as presynaptic element.

APPLIED HISTOLOGY

- **Parkinson's disease**: Slowly progressive neurologic disorder caused by the loss of dopamine-secreting cells in the substantia nigra and basal ganglia of the brain.
- **Cerebellar ataxia**: Purkinje cells in the cerebellar cortex are damaged leading to the development of poor coordination of voluntary movement.
- **Motor neuron disease**: A group of neurodegenerative disorders that selectively affect motor neurons, the cells which control voluntary muscles of the body.

Added Information

- The climbing fibers when stimulated directly facilitate the inhibitory function of Purkinje cells to the deep cerebellar nuclei, but at the same time stellate and basket cells are stimulated by the climbing fibers exert their inhibitory function on the same Purkinje cells. This type of alteration of response of Purkinje cells is called **feed forward inhibition**.
- When mossy fibers and granule cells are stimulated and the excitatory waves are conveyed by the parallel fibers to the Purkinje, stellate, basket, and Golgi cells results in feed forward inhibition. Inhibitory Golgi cells on facilitation suppresses the excitation of the granule cells, this type of alteration of excitatory influence of granule cells is called **feed backward inhibition**.
- When the sensory input to the cerebellum is excitatory, the output from the cerebellar cortex is inhibitory.
- The row of excited Purkinje cell is surrounded by the zones of inhibition at the periphery. This helps in neuronal sharpening.

MULTIPLE CHOICE QUESTIONS

1. All of the following are the components of gray matter; *except*:
    a. Cell bodies
    b. Myelinated nerve fiber
    c. Neuroglia
    d. Dendrites
2. Lateral horn is present in ____ segment of spinal cord.
    a. Cervical
    b. Thorax
    c. Lumbar
    d. Sacral
3. Which of the following is not a layer of cerebral cortex?
    a. External granular
    b. External pyramidal
    c. Plexiform
    d. Purkinje
4. Outer band of Baillarger is present in which layer of cerebral cortex?
    a. Outer pyramidal
    b. Outer granular
    c. Inner pyramidal
    d. Inner granular
5. Output neuron of cerebellar cortex is:
    a. Purkinje
    b. Stellate
    c. Granule
    d. Golgi
6. Cerebellar glomerulus is composed of all, *except*:
    a. Mossy fibers
    b. Climbing fibers
    c. Granule cells
    d. Golgi cells

Answers
1. b   2. b   3. d   4. d   5. a   6. b

CHAPTER 20

Male Reproductive System

Learning objectives

To study the:
- Structure of testis, seminiferous tubules, and Sertoli cells
- Spermatogenesis
- Structure of epididymis, vas deferens, and seminal vesicle
- Structure of prostate
- Applied histology

IDENTIFICATION POINTS

Testis	Epididymis	Vas deferens	Seminal vesicle	Prostate
❑ Surface is covered by visceral layer of tunica vaginalis ❑ Cut sections of seminiferous tubules are seen ❑ Wall of the each seminiferous lined by a generation of spermatogenic cells and supporting cells of Sertoli ❑ Between the tubules, fibrous connective tissue is present ❑ Interstitial cells of Leydig are present between the tubules.	❑ Cut sections of ductules are seen ❑ Ducts are lined by pseudostratified columnar epithelium with stereocilia ❑ Epithelium contains principal and basal cells ❑ Spermatozoa clumps are present in the ducts ❑ The ductules are surrounded by a thin circular coat of smooth muscle fibers.	❑ Wall is composed of three layers: (1) outer adventitia, (2) middle muscle, and (3) inner mucosal layer ❑ Mucosa is lined by simple columnar throughout and pseudostratified columnar epithelium at the distal end ❑ Lamina propria is seen ❑ Muscle layer consists of inner longitudinal muscle layer, middle circular muscle layer, and outer longitudinal muscle layer.	❑ The wall is composed of three layers: (1) outer adventitia, (2) middle muscle, and (3) inner mucosal layer ❑ Mucosal layer is highly folded ❑ Lined by pseudostratified columnar epithelium ❑ Muscle wall consists of inner circular and outer longitudinal layers ❑ Adventitial layer.	❑ Fibromuscular glandular tissue ❑ Glandular tissue is made up of numerous follicles of compound tubuloalveolar glands ❑ Follicles are lined by pseudostratified columnar epithelium.

INTRODUCTION

The male reproductive system consists of (Fig. 20.1):
- A pair of testis
- ***Genital ducts***: The epididymis, the ductus deferens, and ejaculatory ducts
- ***Accessory sex glands***: A pair of seminal vesicle, prostate, and a pair of bulbourethral glands
- Male urethra
- Penis.

The testes are responsible for the formation of male gametes called spermatozoa and synthesis and storage of testosterone. The glands secrete the noncellular portion of semen. Ducts deliver the semen to the female genital tract.

TESTIS

General Structure of Testis

- Each testis is about 4 cm long and is located in the scrotum and produces **spermatozoa** and **testosterone**. The adult testes are placed outside the body in scrotum for normal spermatogenesis as the temperature is 2–3°C less than the body temperature.
- Testis is surrounded by a capsule from outside inward: visceral layer of ***tunica vaginalis, tunica albuginea***, and ***tunica vasculosa***.

CHAPTER 20: Male Reproductive System

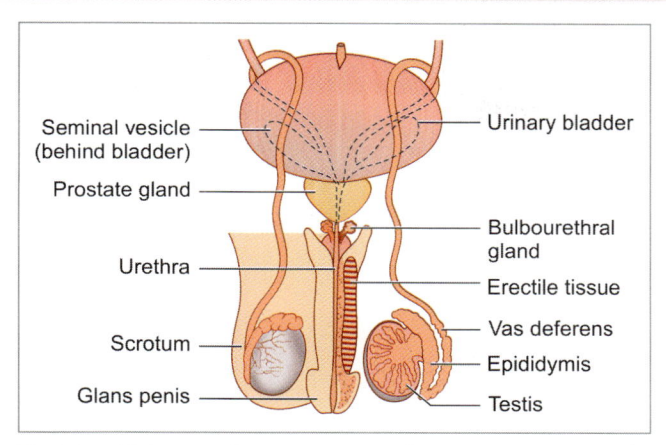

Fig. 20.1: Male reproductive system (schematic representation).

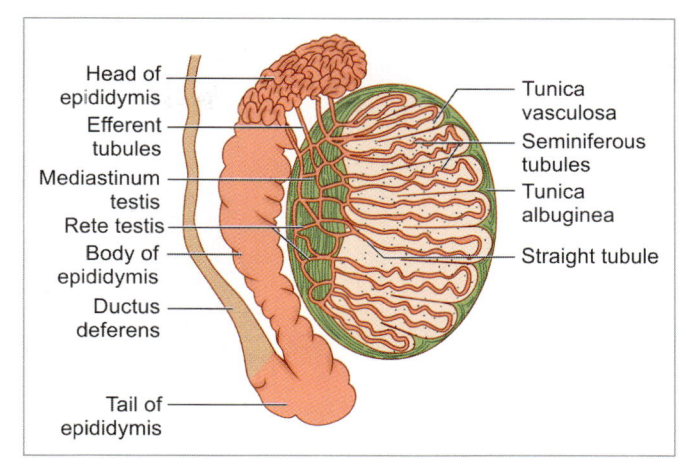

Fig. 20.2: Basic structure of the testis (schematic representation).

- Tunica albuginea is a thick fibrous membrane which covers the entire testis and projects into the interior from posterior border as an incomplete partition known as *mediastinum testis*. The visceral layer of tunica vaginalis covers the tunica albuginea, except in the region of the mediastinum testis.
- From the anterior surface of the mediastinum testis, numerous septa radiate and divide the substance of the testis into a number of lobules. About 200–300 lobules are present in each testis. Each lobule is roughly conical, the apex of the cone being directed toward the mediastinum testis.
- Individual lobule of the testis is lined by an aereolar and vascular membrane called *tunica vasculosa*.
- Each lobule contains two to three highly convoluted **seminiferous tubules**. Near the apex of the lobule, the seminiferous tubules lose their convolutions and join one another to form about 20–30 larger, **straight tubules** (or **tubuli recti**) (Fig. 20.2). These straight tubules enter the fibrous tissue of the mediastinum testis and unite to form a network called the **rete testis**.
- At the upper end the rete testis gives off 12–20 **efferent ductules** and enters into the head of the **epididymis**. This duct is highly coiled on itself and forms the body and tail of the epididymis. The head of the epididymis is made up of highly convoluted continuations of the efferent ductules. At the lower end of the head of the epididymis, these tubules join to form a single tube called the duct of the epididymis. The duct continuous as **ductus deferens** forms the tail of epididymis (Plate 20.1).

General Structure of Seminiferous Tubules

- Seminiferous tubules are highly convoluted structures present in each lobule of the testes. Each testis has about 200 lobules with one to three seminiferous tubules per lobule, and the total number of tubules is between 400 and 600.
- When stretched out, each tubule is 70–80 cm in length and has a diameter of about 150 μm. The combined length of all seminiferous tubules in one testis is between 300 mt and 900 mt.
- Within a lobule, the spaces between seminiferous tubules are filled by very loose connective tissue, containing blood vessels and lymphatics.
- Wall of the each seminiferous tubule is covered by fibrous connective tissue and lined by a generation of *spermatogenic cells and supporting cells of Sertoli*. The connective tissue and epithelium are separated by a basement membrane.

Details of cells lining a seminiferous tubule seen at a high magnification. Note that the cell boundaries are indistinct, and nuclei are prominent.

- The outermost row of nuclei belongs to sustentacular cells (Sertoli) and to spermatogonia; some of which are undergoing mitosis (note very dense nucleus of irregular shape).
- Passing inward toward the center of the tubule, we have large darkly staining nuclei of spermatocytes, and many smaller nuclei of spermatids.
- Toward the center of the tubule a number of developing spermatozoa are seen. The sperms are often found in clusters embedded in the cytoplasm of Sertoli cells.
- In the adult testis, sustentacular cells are less prominent than germ cells. They are more prominent than germ cells before puberty and in old age.

Plate 20.1: Testis (Low magnification)

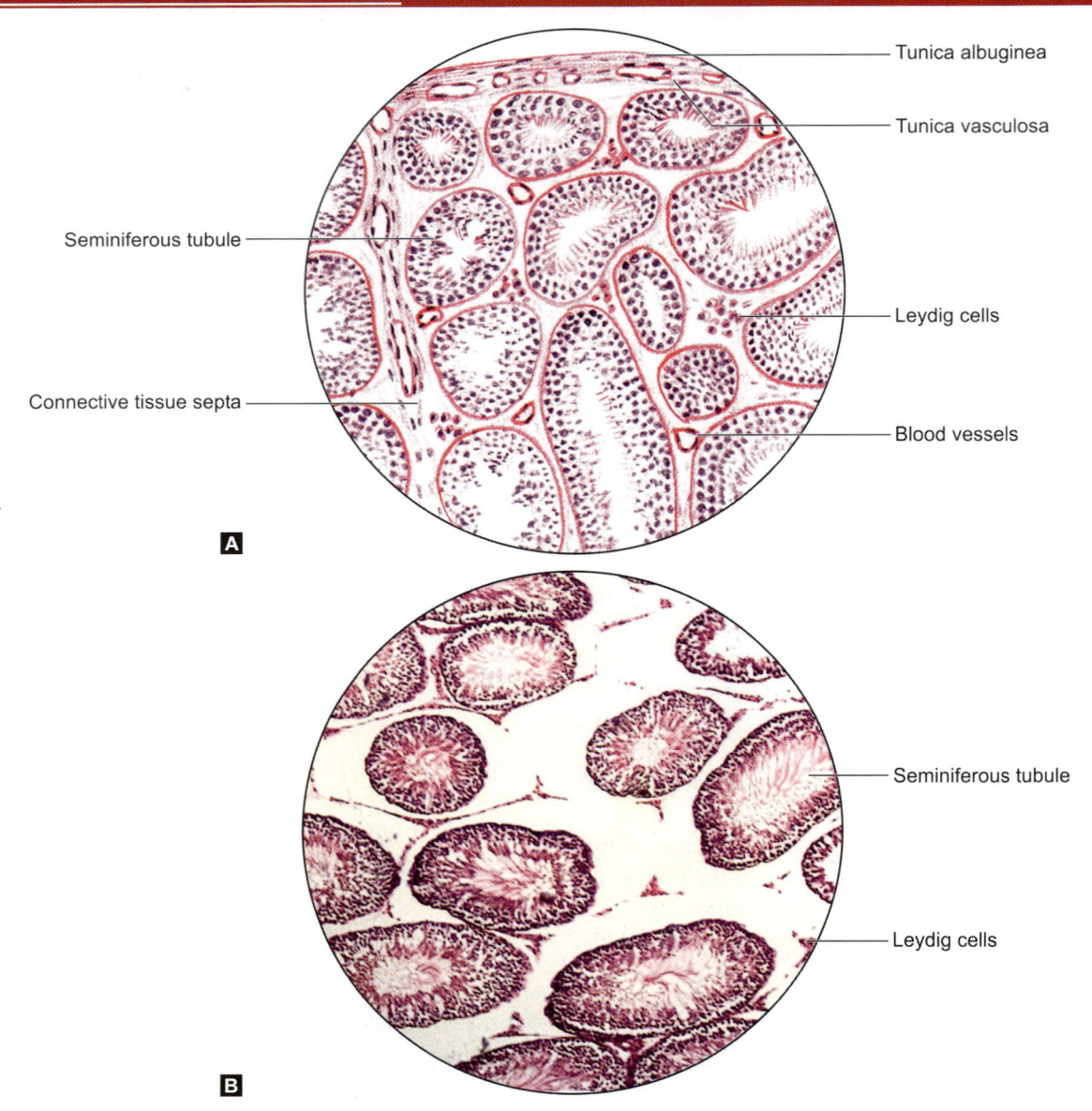

Testis (Low magnification): (A) As seen in drawing; (B) Photomicrograph.

Points of identification
The testis has an outer fibrous layer, the tunica albuginea deep to which:
- A number of seminiferous tubules cut in various directions are seen
- The tubules are separated by connective tissue, containing blood vessels and groups of interstitial cells of Leydig
- Each seminiferous tubule is lined by several layers of cells
- Cells are of two types:
    1. Spermatogenic cells which produce spermatozoa
    2. Sustentacular (Sertoli) cells which have a supportive function.

Note: The appearance of the cellular lining of the seminiferous tubules is characteristic and a student who has studied sections through them carefully (even at low magnification) is not likely to mistake the seminiferous tubules for anything else. The points to note are: (a) the many layers of cells; (b) the great variety in size and shape of the cells and of their nuclei; (c) the lack of a well-defined margin of the lumen; and (d) inconspicuous cell boundaries.

Spermatogenic Cells (Germ Cells)

- Spermatogenic cells represent the various stages of maturation of spermatozoa. They are arranged in developmentally higher order from the basal lamina to the lumen, namely spermatogonia, spermatocytes, spermatids, and spermatozoa (Plate 20.2). However, all types of cells are not seen in any one part of the seminiferous tubule at a given time.
- In a given segment of the tubule, there is a gradual change in the type of cells encountered. Over a period of time, waves of maturation of germ cells pass along the length of a seminiferous tubule, and this is referred to as spermatogenic cycle.

Sustentacular Cells or Cells of Sertoli

- These are tall, elongated columnar/pyramidal-shaped cells. It has basally located, oval nucleus with centrally placed prominent nucleolus. The base of each sustentacular cell rests on the basement membrane, spermatogonia being interposed among the sustentacular cells.
- The apex of the sustentacular cell reaches the lumen of the seminiferous tubule. Numerous spermatids, at various stages of differentiation, are embedded in the apical part of the cytoplasm (Fig. 20.3 and Plate 20.2).
- Near the basement membrane, spermatocytes and spermatogonia indent the sustentacular cell cytoplasm.
- The lateral surface of the adjoining sustentacular cells is connected by tight junctions that divide the wall of the seminiferous tubule into deep **basal** and superficial **adluminal** compartments. The basal occluded junctions form the **blood–testis barrier** that isolates the adluminal compartment from connective tissue. This protects the developing spermatozoa from immune system. Otherwise the newly formed germ cells would be considered foreign cells (as they have different chromosome number and surface membrane receptor), and antispermic antibody will produce and lead to the suppression of spermatogenesis.
- The basal compartment contains spermatogonia cells, and the adluminal compartment contains primary and secondary spermatocytes and spermatids. The spermatids are drawn within the upper part of cells for spermiogenesis until mature spermatozoa is released into the lumen.
- Sustentacular cells contain abundant mitochondria, endoplasmic reticulum, and other organelles. It also contains an abundant microfilaments and microtubules for providing structural support to the developing spermatozoa.
- In the adult testis, sustentacular cells are less prominent than germ cells but more prominent than germ cells before puberty and in old age.

Functions

- They provide physical and nutritional support to the developing germ cells.
- The phagocytosis of the residual cytoplasm that remains after conversion of spermatids to spermatozoa.
- They establish blood–testis barrier and protect the developing spermatozoa from immune system.
- They secrete fructose-rich fluid that helps to transport the spermatozoa along the seminiferous tubules. This fluid is rich in testosterone that may stimulate activity of cells lining the epididymis.
- Sertoli cells secrete a **Müllerian inhibitory substance** or **anti-Müllerian** hormone that suppresses the development of the Müllerian ducts in male fetuses. They are also believed to produce a substance that inhibits spermatogenesis before puberty.
- Follicle-stimulating hormone (FSH) from anterior pituitary activates Sertoli cells to secrete **androgen-binding protein (ABP)**, and luteinizing hormone stimulates interstitial cells to secrete testosterone. ABP

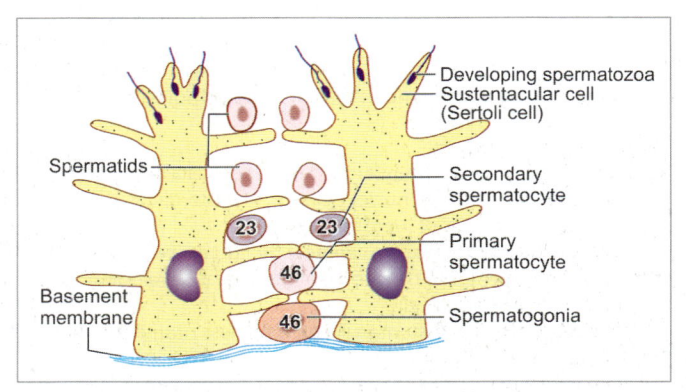

Fig. 20.3: A sustentacular cell and some related germ cells (schematic representation).

Plate 20.2: Testis (High magnification)

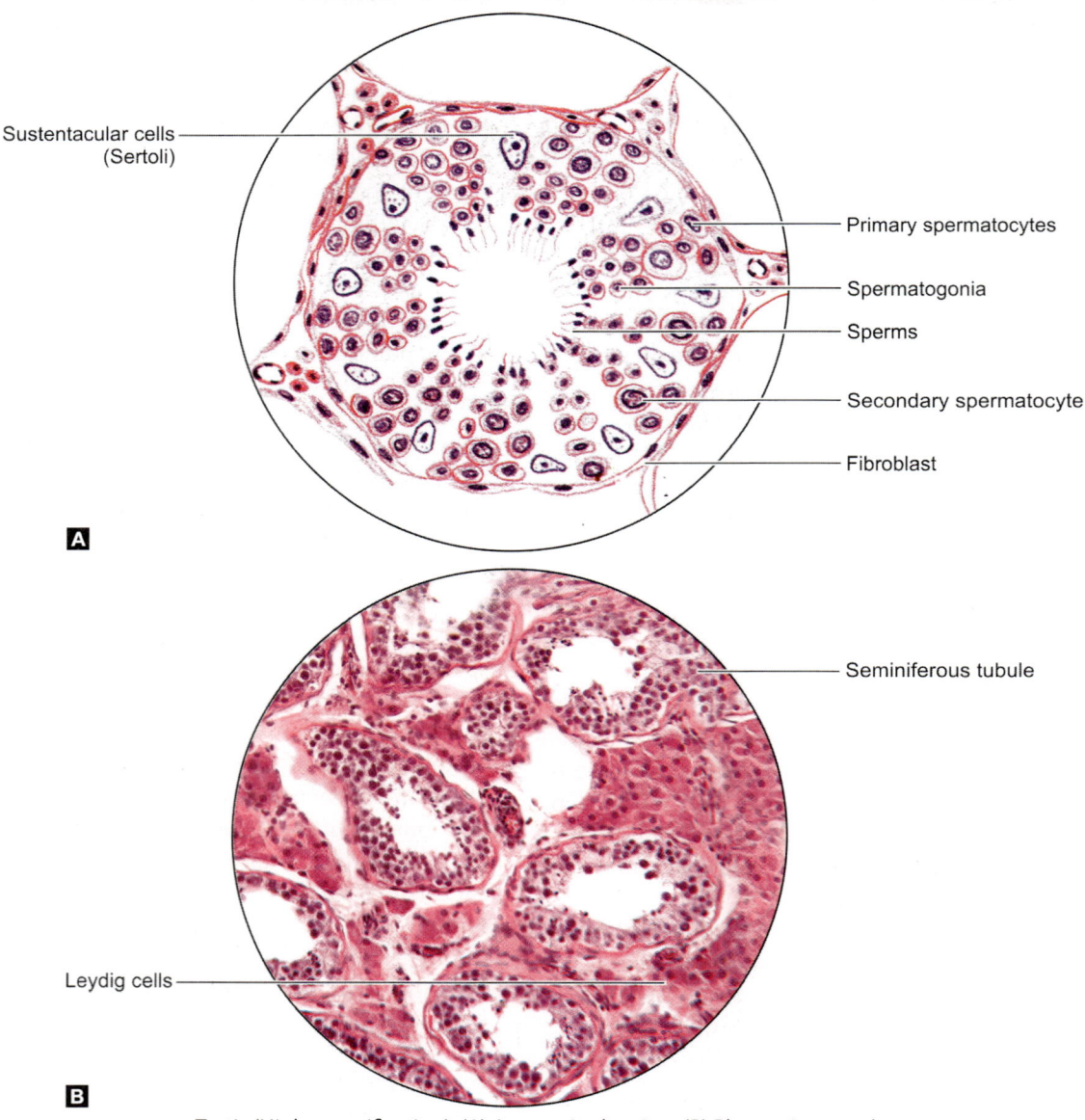

Testis (High magnification): (A) As seen in drawing; (B) Photomicrograph.
Courtesy (B): Ivan Damjanov. Atlas of Histopathology, 1st edition. New Delhi: Jaypee Brothers Medical Publishers (P) Ltd; 2012. p. 203.

Points of identification
Details of cells lining a seminiferous tubule seen at a high magnification. Note that the cell boundaries are indistinct, and nuclei are prominent.
- The outermost row of nuclei belongs to sustentacular cells (Sertoli) and to spermatogonia, some of which are undergoing mitosis (note very dense nucleus of irregular shape)
- Passing inwards toward the center of the tubule we have large darkly staining nuclei of spermatocytes, and many smaller nuclei of spermatids
- Toward the center of the tubule a number of developing spermatozoa are seen. The sperms are often found in clusters embedded in the cytoplasm of Sertoli cells
- In the adult testis, sustentacular cells are less prominent than germ cells. They are more prominent than germ cells before puberty and in old age
- In the drawing, groups of interstitial cells can be seen in the connective tissue between the seminiferous tubules (not seen in photomicrograh).

Note: In the practical class you may not be able to recognize these cells. Observe that the presence of many cells located at different levels gives the appearance of a stratified epithelium which are actually the spermatogonia at different stages of maturation.

CHAPTER 20: Male Reproductive System

binds to testosterone and increases its concentration within seminiferous tubules. It also secretes an ***inhibin hormone*** which inhibits the secretion of FSH. Testosterone, FSH, and ABP along with low scrotal temperature is necessary for proper spermatogenesis (Flowchart 20.1).

Interstitial Cells of Leydig

- The interstitial cells of Leydig are the large, round, or polyhedral cells lying in the connective tissue that intervenes between the coils of seminiferous tubules within the lobule (Plate 20.1A). They have single eccentrically placed nucleus and the cytoplasm stains lightly and often has a foamy appearance.
- They are typically steroid-secreting cells which have mitochondria with tubular cristae, numerous smooth endoplasmic reticulum, and well-developed Golgi complex. Rod-shaped Reinke's crystalloids are also present in the cytoplasm. Yellow-brown pigment (lipofuscin) is seen in some cells.
- The Leydig cells are abundant if fetal testis disappear after birth and reappear at puberty and persist throughout the reproductive life. The growth of the cells in fetal life is regulated by placental gonadotropin hormone and in puberty by interstitial stimulating hormone.
- Interstitial cells secrete male sex hormone testosterone. Secretion is stimulated by the interstitial cell stimulating hormone from hypophysis cerebri. Interstitial cells help in the descent of testis in fetal life, and in puberty, they stimulate the growth of secondary sex characters, initiate heterosexual drive, and play a role in growth of epithelial cells of prostate and seminal vesicles.
- Some interstitial cells may be present in the mediastinum testis, in the epididymis, or even in the spermatic cord. Apart from interstitial cells, the interstitial tissue contains collagen fibers, fibroblasts, macrophages, mast cells, blood vessels, and lymphatics.

Structure of Rete Testis and Efferent Ductules

- The rete testis consists of anastomosing tubules that are lined by flattened or cuboidal cells. They bear microvilli. The epithelium is surrounded by connective tissue of the mediastinum testis.
- The efferent ductules are lined by ciliated columnar epithelium, and some nonciliated cells bearing microvilli are also present. The tubules are surrounded by circularly placed smooth muscle. Movement of spermatozoa through the tubules is facilitated by ciliary action, and by peristaltic contraction of smooth muscle.

SPERMATOGENESIS

The process of the formation of spermatozoa from type A spermatogonia is called ***spermatogenesis*** (Flowchart 20.2). This process occurs in waves along the length of seminiferous tubules, and it takes about 64 days to complete. It consists of several stages as described in Figure 20.4.

Stages of Spermatogenesis (Flowchart 20.3)

- The stem cells from which all stages in the development of spermatozoa are derived are called ***spermatogonia*** which are derived from primitive male sex cells. Spermatogonia lie near the basal lamina and contain diploid chromosomes (46, XY). Spermatogonia undergo several mitotic divisions and give rise to more spermatogonia, and to primary spermatocytes.
- Spermatogonia consists of ***dark type-A, paletype-A, and type-B*** types. Each germ cell divides into two dark type-A spermatocytes, which acts as stem cells. Each dark A divides into one dark A cell as a reserve and one pale A cell. Pale A undergo mitosis into two pale A cells, one as a reserve and another one divides into type B cell. Each type B cell undergoes mitosis, and four generations of type B spermatogonia are formed. B cells undergo

Flowchart 20.1: Scheme to show control of male genital system.

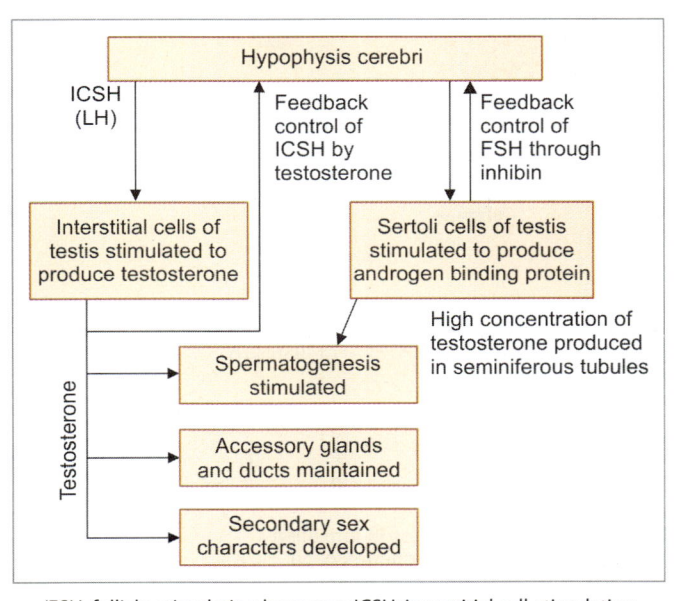

(FSH: follicle-stimulating hormone; ICSH: interstitial cell-stimulating hormone; LH: luteinizing hormone)

Flowchart 20.2: Spermatogenesis.

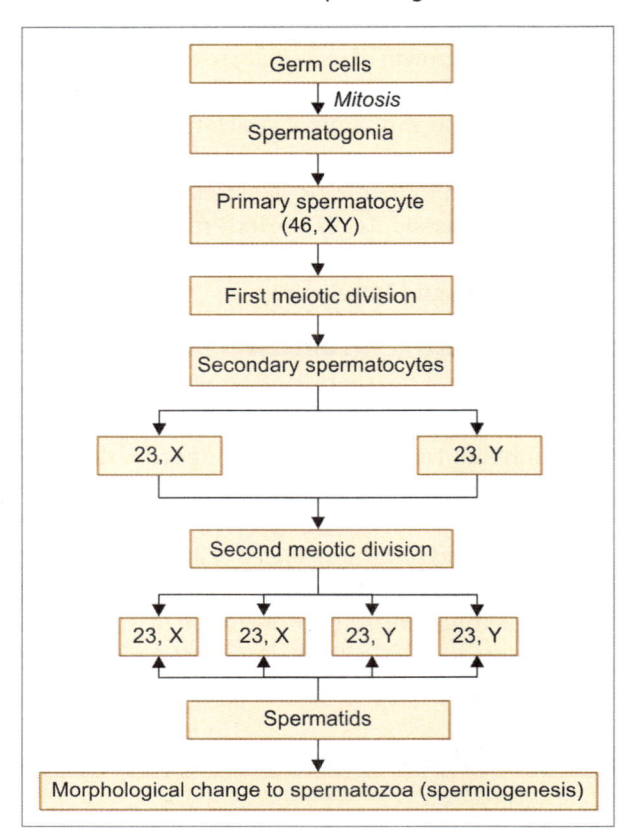

```
Germ cells
    │ Mitosis
    ▼
Spermatogonia
    │
    ▼
Primary spermatocyte
(46, XY)
    │
    ▼
First meiotic division
    │
    ▼
Secondary spermatocytes
    │
  ┌─┴─┐
  ▼   ▼
23, X  23, Y
  │   │
  ▼   ▼
Second meiotic division
  │   │
┌─┴─┐ ┌─┴─┐
▼   ▼ ▼   ▼
23,X 23,X 23,Y 23,Y
    │
    ▼
Spermatids
    │
    ▼
Morphological change to spermatozoa (spermiogenesis)
```

mitotic division to form primary spermatocytes with diploid chromosomes.

- **Primary spermatocytes** are the largest cells with large spherical nuclei occupying the middle region of the seminiferous epithelium. Primary spermatocytes undergo **first meiotic division (reduction division)** to form two secondary spermatocytes with haploid chromosomes (23 X/23 Y) and **2n** deoxyribonucleic acid (DNA). Primary spermatocytes enter into prolonged prophase of first meiotic division.
- **Secondary spermatocytes** are smaller than primary spermatocytes and undergo **second meiotic division** to form two spermatids with haploid chromosomes with **1n** DNA and some residual bodies between them. There is no further reduction in chromosome number. They are scarcely seen in sections as they undergo second meiotic division as soon as they are formed.
- Each **spermatid** is a rounded cell with a spherical nucleus and present near the inner zone of seminiferous tubule epithelium. Older spermatids are plunge into the cytoplasm of Sertoli cells until the mature spermatozoa is released into the lumen of seminiferous tubules. The spermatid undergoes changes in shape and in the orientation of its organelles to form a spermatozoon. This process is called **spermiogenesis**.

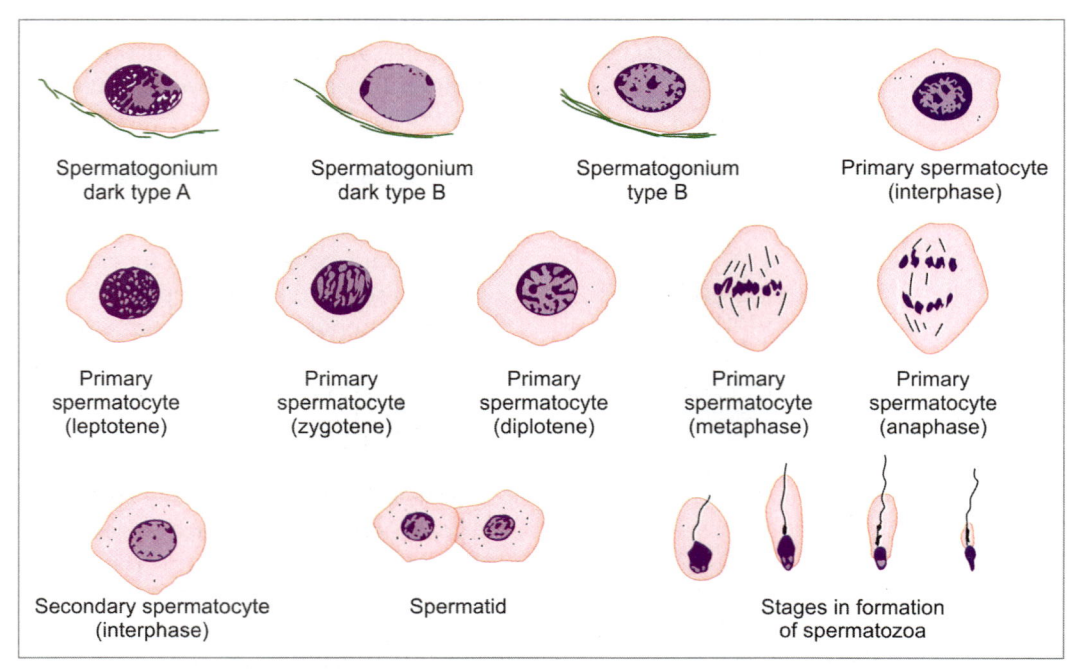

Spermatogonium dark type A | Spermatogonium dark type B | Spermatogonium type B | Primary spermatocyte (interphase)

Primary spermatocyte (leptotene) | Primary spermatocyte (zygotene) | Primary spermatocyte (diplotene) | Primary spermatocyte (metaphase) | Primary spermatocyte (anaphase)

Secondary spermatocyte (interphase) | Spermatid | Stages in formation of spermatozoa

Fig. 20.4: Some stages in spermatogenesis as seen in the walls of seminiferous tubules (schematic representation).

CHAPTER 20: Male Reproductive System

Flowchart 20.3: Stages of spermatogenesis.

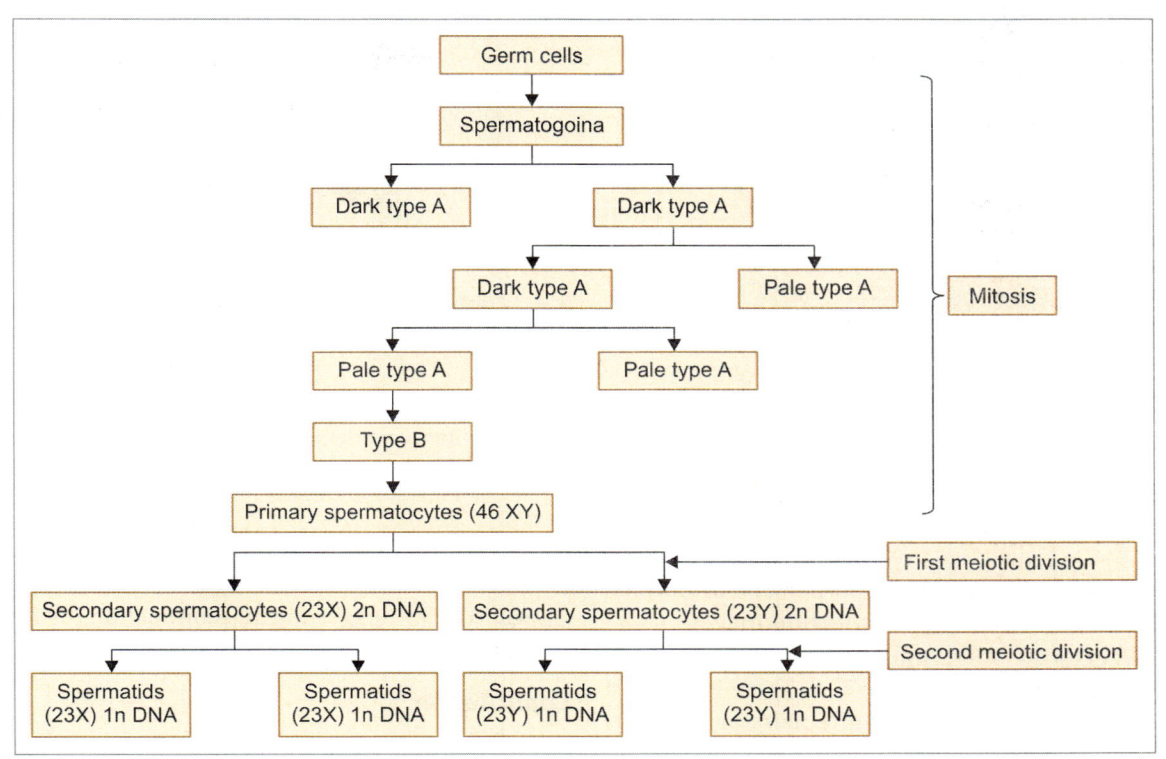

```
                    Germ cells
                        ↓
                   Spermatogoina
                     ↓      ↓
           Dark type A    Dark type A  ⎫
                           ↓      ↓    ⎪
                     Dark type A   Pale type A  ⎬ Mitosis
                       ↓      ↓                  ⎪
                  Pale type A   Pale type A     ⎭
                       ↓
                    Type B
                       ↓
           Primary spermatocytes (46 XY)
                  ↓           ↓           ← First meiotic division
   Secondary spermatocytes (23X) 2n DNA   Secondary spermatocytes (23Y) 2n DNA
          ↓         ↓              ↓         ↓   ← Second meiotic division
    Spermatids  Spermatids    Spermatids  Spermatids
    (23X) 1n DNA (23X) 1n DNA (23Y) 1n DNA (23Y) 1n DNA
```

Spermiogenesis

- The process by which a spermatid becomes a spermatozoon is called *spermiogenesis* (or *spermateleosis*). The spermatid is a more or less circular cell containing a nucleus, Golgi complex, centriole, and mitochondria. All these components take part in forming the spermatozoon.
- The nucleus undergoes condensation and changes shape to form the head. The Golgi complex is transformed into the acrosomic cap that comes to lie over one side of the nucleus. The acrosome marks the future anterior pole of the spermatozoon.
- The centriole divides into two parts and migrates away from acrosome to the pole of the cell. The axial filament grows out of the distal centriole. The region occupied by the two centrioles later becomes the neck of the spermatozoon. The proximal centriole probably forms the basal body.
- The part of the axial filament between the head and the annulus becomes surrounded by mitochondria and together with them forms the middle piece.
- Most of the cytoplasm of the spermatid is shed and is phagocytozed by Sertoli cells. The cell membrane persists as a covering for the spermatozoon.

Structure of a Mature Spermatozoon

- The spermatozoon has a *head*, neck, and *tail*. The *tail* is made of three pieces, i.e. middle piece, principal piece, and endpiece.
- The *head* is covered by a cap called the *acrosomic cap*, *anterior nuclear cap*, or *galea capitis* (Fig. 20.5). It is flattened from before backward so that it is oval when seen from the front but appears to be pointed or in section. It is occupied by nucleus with extremely condensed chromatin. This condensation makes it highly resistant to various physical stresses.
- The *neck* of the spermatozoon is narrow. It contains a funnel-shaped *basal body* and a spherical *centriole*.
- The *basal body* also called the *connecting piece* helps to establish an intimate union between the head and the remainder of the spermatozoon. It is composed of cylindrical arrangement of the nine columns of the connecting piece that encircles the centriole. Each of the columns is continuous distally with one coarse fiber of the axial filament.
- An *axial filament* begins just behind the centriole. It passes through the middle piece and extends into the tail. At the point where the middle piece joins the tail, this axial filament passes through a ring-like *annulus*. The

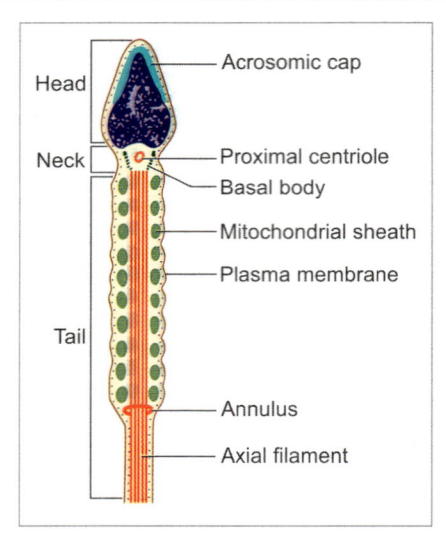

Fig. 20.5: Structure of spermatozoon as seen by electron microscope (schematic representation).

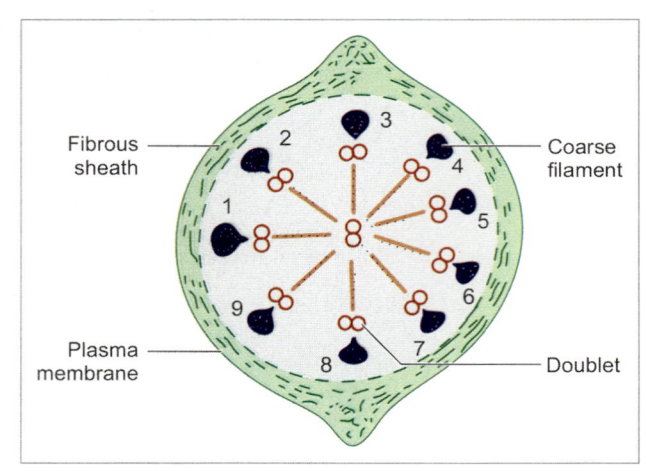

Fig. 20.6: Transverse section across the tail of a spermatozoon to show the arrangement of fibrils (schematic representation).

axial filament that lies in the middle piece is surrounded by a *spiral sheath* made up of mitochondria.

- The **axial filament** is composed of several fibrils arranged as illustrated in Figure 20.6. There is a pair of central fibrils, surrounded by nine pairs or **doublets** arranged in a circle around the central pair. In addition to these doublets, there are nine coarser petal-shaped fibrils present outside each doublet. These coarse fibrils are present in the middle piece and most of the tail, but do not extend into the terminal part of the tail. These fibrils are surrounded by fibrous sheath, and the fibrous sheath is surrounded by spirally arranged mitochondria. The entire sperm is enclosed in a plasma membrane.
- The part of tail connected to neck is middle piece. The middle piece contains the mitochondrial sheath and provides energy for sperm maturation. Principal piece contains the 9 + 2 pattern of microtubules in the central core surrounded by nine coarse fibers enclosed in a fibrous sheath (Fig. 20.6). End piece contains 9 + 2 axonema enclosed by plasma membrane.

Maturation and Capacitation of Spermatozoa

Maturation

- As fully formed spermatozoa pass through the male genital passages, they undergo a process of **maturation**. Spermatozoa acquire some motility only after passing through the epididymis. The secretions of the epididymis, seminal vesicles, and the prostate have a stimulating effect on sperm motility, but spermatozoa become fully motile only after ejaculation.
- When introduced into the vagina, spermatozoa reach the uterine tubes much sooner than their own motility would allow, suggesting that contractions of uterine and tubal musculature exert a sucking effect.

Capacitation

- Spermatozoa acquire the ability to fertilize the ovum only after they have been in the female genital tract for sometime. This final step in their maturation is called **capacitation**. During capacitation, some proteins and glycoproteins are removed from the plasma membrane overlying the acrosome.
- When the sperm reaches near the ovum, changes take place in membranes over the acrosome and enable release of lysosomal enzymes present within the acrosome. This is called the **acrosome reaction**. The substances released include hyaluronidase that helps in separating corona radiata cells present over the ovum. *Trypsin-like substances* and a substance called *acrosin* help in digesting the zona pellucida and penetration of the sperm through it. Changes in the properties of the zona pellucida constitute the **zona reaction**.

EPIDIDYMIS

- The epididymis is a highly convoluted tubule and a comma-shaped structure present on the posterolateral aspect of testis.
- It consists of head, body, and tail. The **head** is formed by the union of the 10–20 efferent ductules, becomes highly coiled and continuous body. These are lined by ciliated columnar epithelium (Plate 20.3). At the lower end of

CHAPTER 20: Male Reproductive System

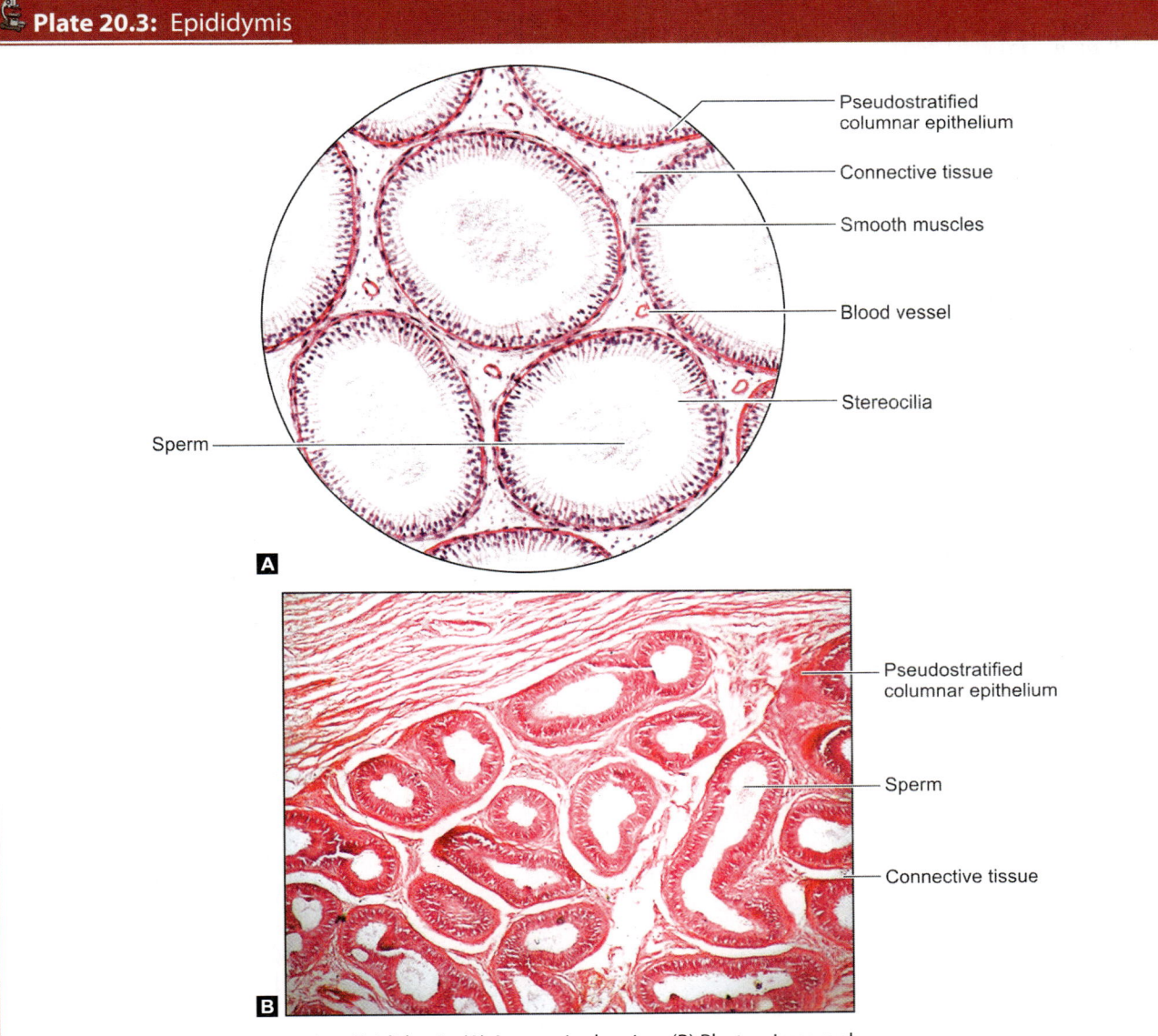

Plate 20.3: Epididymis

Epididymis: (A) As seen in drawing; (B) Photomicrograph.

Points of identification
- The body of the epididymis is a long convoluted duct
- A section shows number of tubules lined by pseudostratified columnar epithelium in which there are tall columnar cells and shorter basal cells that do not reach the lumen. The columnar cells bear stereocilia
- Smooth muscles are present in the wall of the duct
- Clumps of spermatozoa are present in the lumen of the duct.

the head of the epididymis, these tubules join to form a single tube called the **duct of the epididymis**.
- The **body** and **tail** of the epididymis are made up of the duct of the epididymis that is greatly coiled on itself. The terminal part of the tail which stores spermatozoa loses its convolutions and continuous with ductus deferens.
- The duct is lined by pseudostratified columnar epithelium which is composed of two types of cells called tall columnar *principal cells* and shorter *basal cell*.
- The **basal cells** are short, and they do not reach the lumen. Basal cells are pyramidal or polyhedral with rounded nuclei with large accumulation of heterochromatin, and

it stains dark. The basal cells function as stem cells to replace the principal and basal cells.

- The tall **principal cells** have irregular, oval nuclei with one or two nucleoli. The nuclei stains light compared to basal cells and are located at the base of the cell. The cytoplasm has abundant rough endoplasmic reticulum, lysosomes, and a prominent Golgi complex. The luminal surfaces of each columnar cell bear long, branched, irregular microvilli, and nonmotile projections stereocilia, absorbs 90% of fluid and creates fluid current that moves the immobile sperm from the seminiferous tubles.
- These cells are supported on a basal lamina by circularly arranged smooth muscle fibers and loose connective tissue rich in blood capillaries. This muscle layer increases in thickness gradually from head to tail and may be organized into the inner circular and outer longitudinal layers in the tail region. This muscle layer helps to move the sperm along the duct.

Functions

- Phagocytosis of defective spermatozoa and residual bodies that are eliminated during spermatogenesis
- Absorption of excess fluid
- Secretion of substances (sialic acid, glycerylphosphorylcholine) that play a role in maturation of spermatozoa.

DUCTUS DEFERENS

The ductus deferens (deferent duct or vas deferens) is a thick cord-like muscular tube, about 45 cm in length extending from the lower end of epididymis to the prostatic urethra. The wall of the ductus deferens consists of three layers from inside outward:
1. Mucous membrane
2. Muscular layer
3. Connective tissue

Mucous Membrane

The mucous membrane shows a number of longitudinal folds so that the lumen appears to be stellate in section, and it is lined by simple columnar throughout and pseudostratified at the distal end of the vas deferens. Epithelium is similar to epididymis but principal cells are shorter. The cells are ciliated in the extra abdominal part of the duct. The epithelium is supported by a lamina propria in which there are many elastic fibers.

Muscle

The muscle coat is very thick and consists of three layers of smooth muscle. It is arranged in the form of an inner circular layer and an outer longitudinal layer. An inner and outer longitudinal layer and middle circular layer are present.

Connective Tissue

The fibroelastic connective tissue forms the adventitial layer containing blood vessels and nerves.

The terminal dilated part of the ductus deferens is called the **ampulla**, which joints the duct of seminal vesicles to form ejaculatory duct. It has the same structure as that of the seminal vesicle (Plate 20.4).

SEMINAL VESICLE

- The seminal vesicle (Plate 20.5) is a sac-like mass, located adjacent to the posterior wall of the prostate gland, and secretes a viscous fluid that constitutes about 70% of the ejaculate.
- The wall of the seminal vesicle consists of three layers from inside outwardwhich are as follows:
  1. Mucous membrane
  2. Muscular layer
  3. Connective tissue

Mucous Membrane

- The mucous membrane is highly convoluted, forming labyrinth-like cul-de-sac with lumen. The lumen is lined by pseudostratified columnar epithelium consists of short basal cells and low columnar cells. Goblet cells are also present in the epithelium.
- Columnar cells have numerous short microvilli, and cytoplasm contains rough endoplasmic reticulum, Golgi apparatus, numerous mitochondria, and abundant secretory granules. The height of the cell varies directly with the blood testosterone level.

Muscle

The seminal vesicles consist of a thin intermediate layer of smooth muscles. The muscle layer contains outer longitudinal and inner circular fibers.

Connective Tissue

The outer covering of loose connective tissue forms the adventitial layer containing blood vessels and nerves.

Functions

- The seminal vesicles produce a thick secretion that forms about 70% of the semen. The secretion contains fructose which provides nutrition to spermatozoa.
- It also contains amino acids, proteins, prostaglandins, fibrinogen, ascorbic acid, and citric acid. This secretion

CHAPTER 20: Male Reproductive System

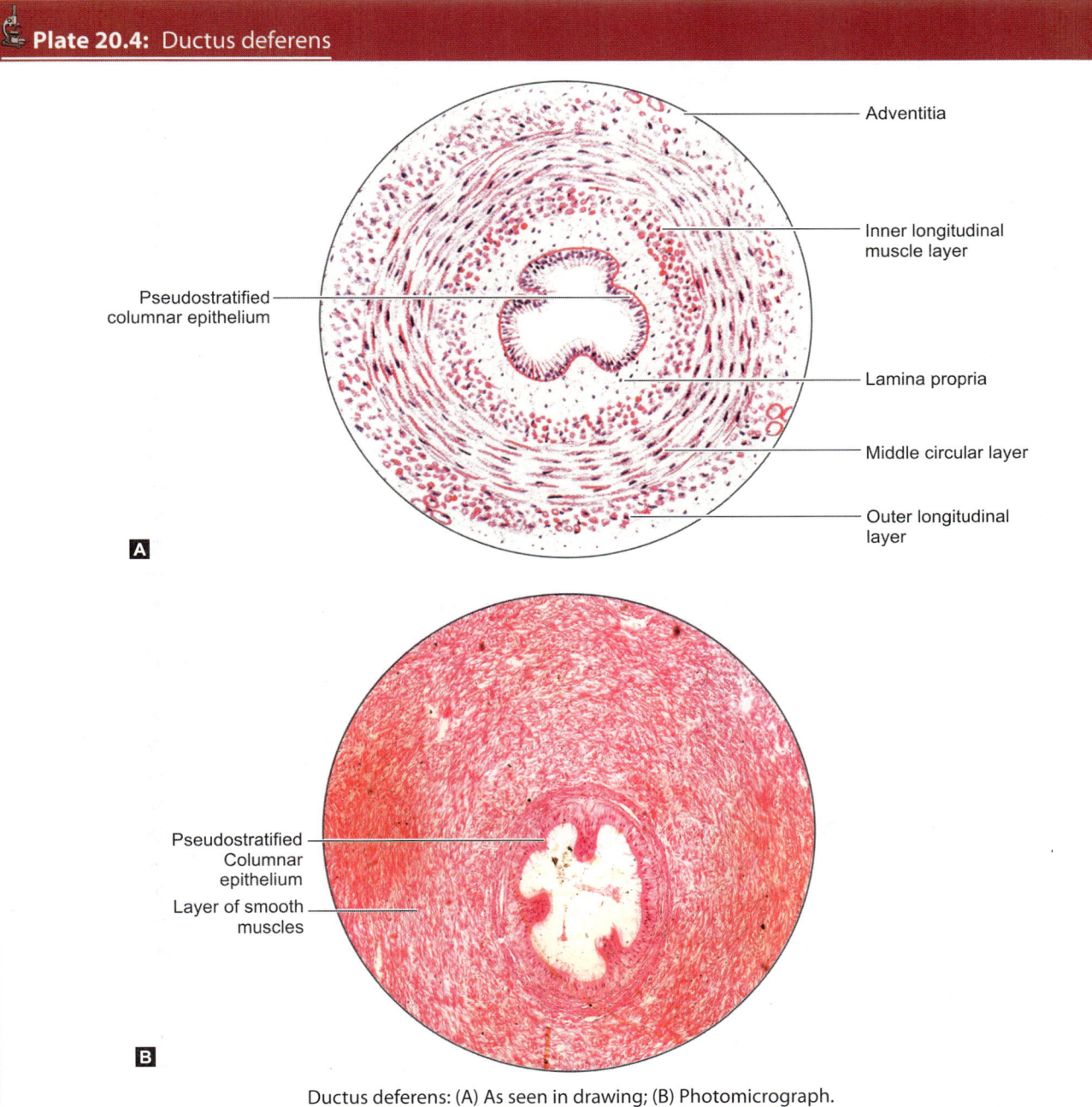

Plate 20.4: Ductus deferens

Ductus deferens: (A) As seen in drawing; (B) Photomicrograph.
Courtesy (B): Balakrishna Shetty, Sweekritha H Poonja. HISTOLOGY Practical Manual, 4th edition. New Delhi: Jaypee Brothers Medical Publishers (P) Ltd; 2019. p. 120.

Points of identification
This tubular structure displays:
- A small irregular lumen
- Mucous membrane lined by pseudostratified columnar epithelium with underlying lamina propria
- The muscle coat is very thick. Three layers, inner longitudinal, middle circular, and outer longitudinal are seen
- Outer most layer is adventitia composed of collagen fibers and containing blood vessels.

Plate 20.5: Seminal vesicle (Low magnification)

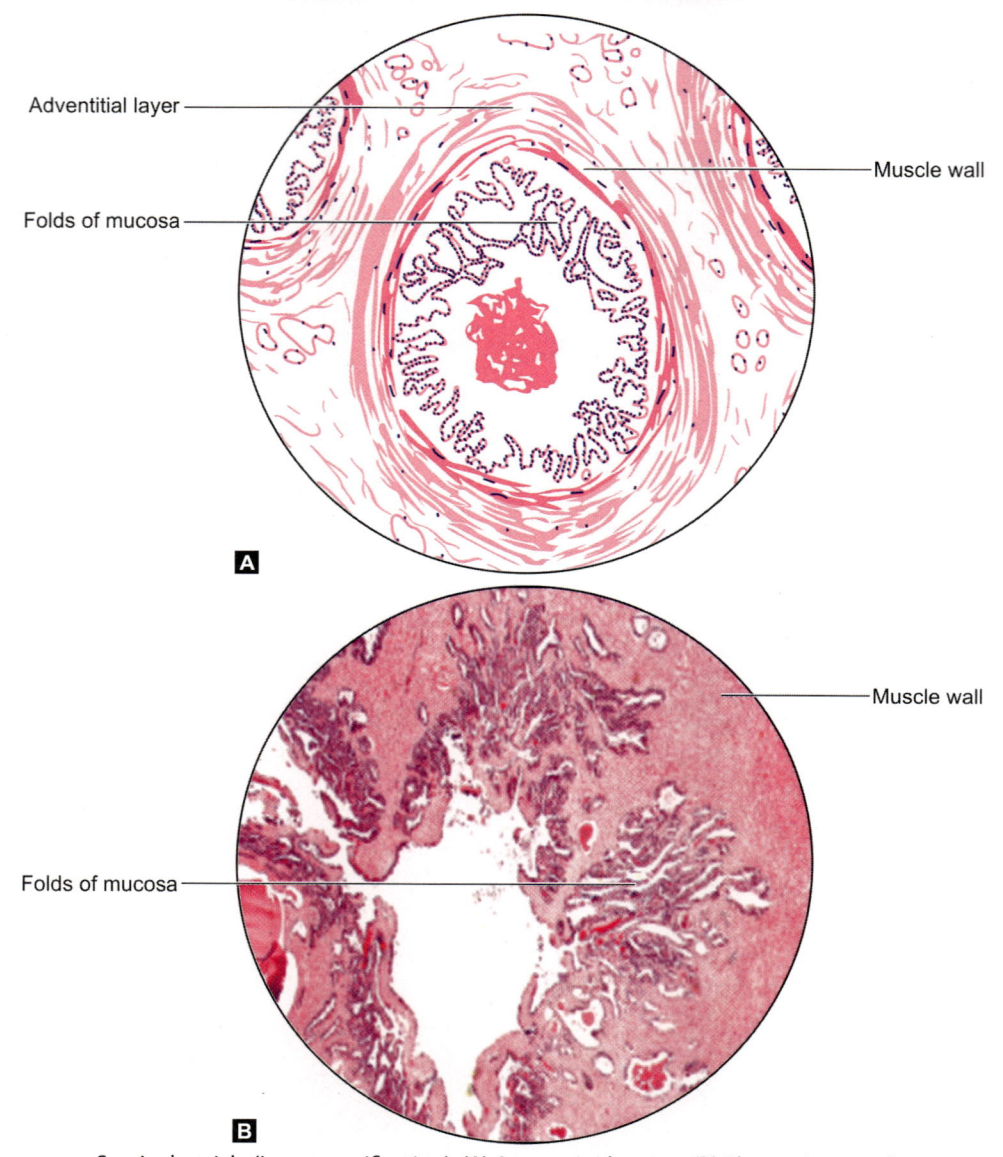

Seminal vesicle (Low magnification): (A) As seen in drawing; (B) Photomicrograph.

Points of identification
- The seminal vesicle is made up of a convoluted tubule
- The tube has an outer covering of connective tissue, a thin layer of smooth muscle and an inner mucosa
- The mucosal lining is thrown into numerous folds that branch and anastomose to form a network
- The lining epithelium is usually simple columnar or pseudostratified.

is expelled during ejaculation by the contraction of the smooth muscle of the vesicle wall.
- Prostaglandins stimulate activity in the female genital tract. Fibrinogen allows semen to coagulate after ejaculation.

PROSTATE

- The prostate is the largest accessory sex gland. It is a dense conical organ extending from the neck of the urinary bladder and surrounds the beginning of urethra.
- It is made up of 30–50 compound tubuloalveolar glands that are embedded in the fibromuscular stroma. The glandular part of the prostate is poorly developed at birth. It undergoes considerable proliferation at puberty and degenerates in old age.
- The prostate is covered by inner true and outer false capsules. True capsule is formed by condensation of the fibrous stroma of the gland, and false capsule is derived from visceral layer of pelvic fascia. The space between the two capsules is occupied by prostatic venous plexus.
- The prostate consists of one-fourth of fibrous, one-fourth of muscular, and half of glandular tissue.
- In sections, the glandular tissue is seen in the form of numerous follicles that are lined by simple to pseudostratified columnar epithelium (Plate 20.6). The epithelium is thrown into numerous folds along with some underlying connective tissue. The foldings are formed after puberty, and in old age, infoldings of follicles disappear. The follicles drain into 12–20 excretory ducts that open into the prostatic urethra. The ducts are lined by a double layered epithelium. The superficial luminal layer is columnar, and the deeper layer is cuboidal.
- Gland consists of four zones: The **transition zone** surrounds the proximal part of urethra and comprises of 5% of the glandular tissue. The **central zone** comprises of 20% and surrounds ejaculatory duct behind the transition zone. The **peripheral zone** comprises of 70%, and it is cup-shaped which surrounds the central and transition zones as well as prostatic urethra except in front. The *fibromuscular stroma* with no glandular tissue is present in front of prostatic urethra between the peripheral zones.
- The glands of prostate are arranged in three concentric layers around the urethra and from within outward (Figs. 20.7 and 20.8):
    1. **Inner mucous glands**: They are simple tubular surrounds the preprostatic urethra open into the prostatic sinuses above the colliculus.
    2. **Intermediate submucous glands** with less follicle and smaller ducts open into the sinuses at the level of colliculus.
    3. **Outer main glands** are long branched glands with numerous follicles, and longer ducts open in the prostatic sinuses below the colliculus. Ducts join with the urethra.
- Small rounded masses of uniform or lamellated structure are found within the lumen of the follicles called **amyloid bodies** or **corpora amylacea**. These are more abundant in older individuals. They are rich in condensed glycoprotein and keratin sulfate without any clinical significance. They are often calcified.
- The fibromuscular tissue forms a conspicuous feature of sections of the prostate. It contains collagen fibers and smooth muscle. Within the gland the fibromuscular tissue forms septa that separate the glandular elements. These septa are continuous with a fibrous capsule that surrounds the prostate. The capsule contains numerous veins and parasympathetic ganglion cells.
- The prostate gland is traversed by the prostatic urethra and the ejaculatory ducts.

Functions

- The prostate produces a secretion that forms a considerable part of semen. The secretion is serous white fluid and rich in enzymes (acid phosphatase, amylase, and protease) and in citric acid.
- The prostate also produces **prostaglandins** that have numerous actions.

PENIS

- The penis is the erectile copulatory organ in males and consists of two parts, *root* and *a body/corpus*. The *root* is fixed to the perineum, and the **body/corpse** is free part.
- The penis is covered all round by thin skin that is attached loosely to underlying tissue (Fig. 20.9).
- The substance of the penis is made up of three columns of erectile tissue, two dorsal and one ventral, and each enclosed by its own dense fibrous connective tissue capsule, the tunica albuginea. The dorsal columns are the right and left *corpora cavernosa*, while the ventral column is the *corpus spongiosum*.
- The corpus spongiosum ends distally in an enlarged, bulbous portion, the *glans penis*.
- Erectile tissue of the penis contains numerous variably shaped, endothelially lined spaces, and they are separated from each other by connective tissue trabeculae and smooth muscle cells. The vascular spaces of the corpora

Plate 20.6: Prostate (Low magnification)

A

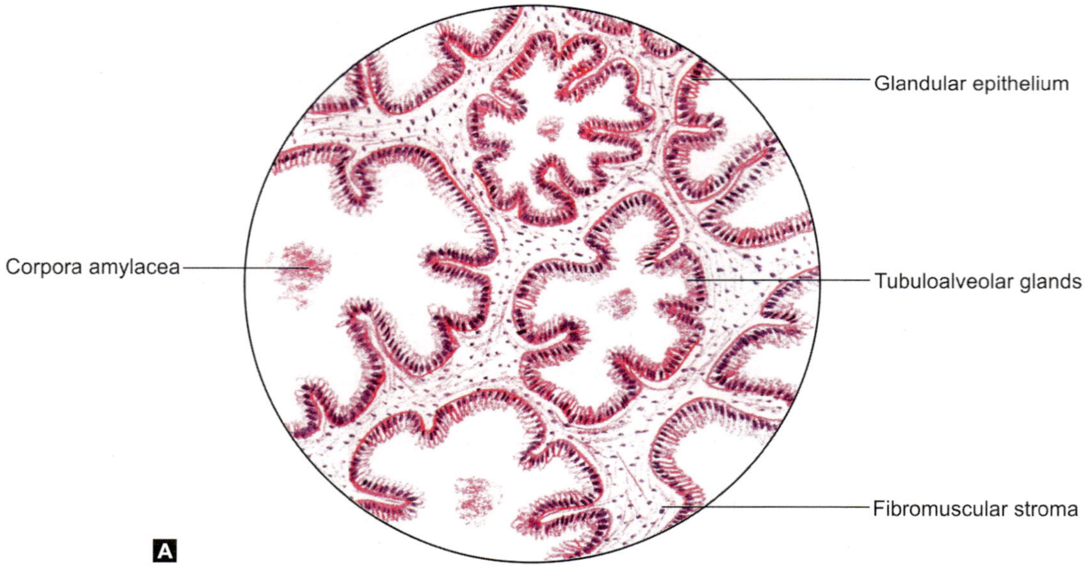

- Glandular epithelium
- Corpora amylacea
- Tubuloalveolar glands
- Fibromuscular stroma

B

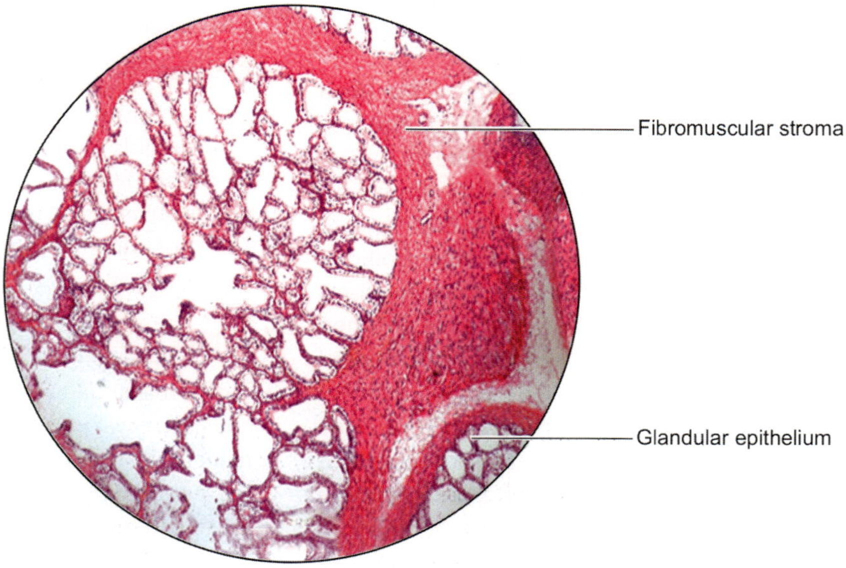

- Fibromuscular stroma
- Glandular epithelium

Prostate (low magnification): (A) As seen in drawing (Low magnification); (B) Photomicrograph (low magnification).

Points of identification
- The prostate consists of glandular tissue embedded in prominent fibromuscular stroma
- The glandular tissue is in the form of follicles with serrated edges. They are lined by columnar epithelium. The lumen may contain amyloid bodies
- The follicles are separated by broad bands of fibromuscular tissue.

cavernosa are larger centrally and smaller peripherally, whereas spaces of the spongiosum are similar in size throughout. The trabeculae of corpus spongiosum contain more elastic fibers and fewer muscle fibers than corpora cavernosa.

- The spaces are in communication with arteries and veins but normally they are empty. They are filled with blood under pressure during erection of the penis.
- Each corpus cavernosum is surrounded by a dense sheath containing collagen fibers, elastic fibers, and

CHAPTER 20: Male Reproductive System

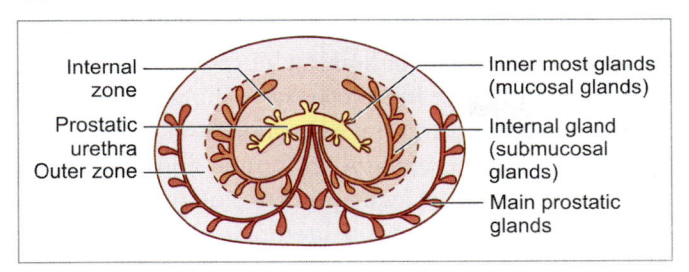

Fig. 20.7: Arrangement of glandular tissue in prostate (schematic representation).

some smooth muscle. In the midline the sheaths of the right and left corpora cavernosa fuse to form a median septum. The corpora cavernosa lie side by side and are separated only by a median fibrous septum.

- The corpus spongiosum is placed in the midline ventral to the corpora cavernosa. The corpus spongiosum is also surrounded by a sheath, but this sheath is much thinner than that around the corpora cavernosa. The corpus spongiosum is traversed by the penile urethra throughout its length.
- The tip of urethra at glans penis is lined by stratified squamous nonkeratinized epithelium. Many small mucous glands of Littre are scattered along the length of urethra, which secrete mucus and have lubricating functions.
- Many sensory nerve endings are present in the penis, particularly on the glans.

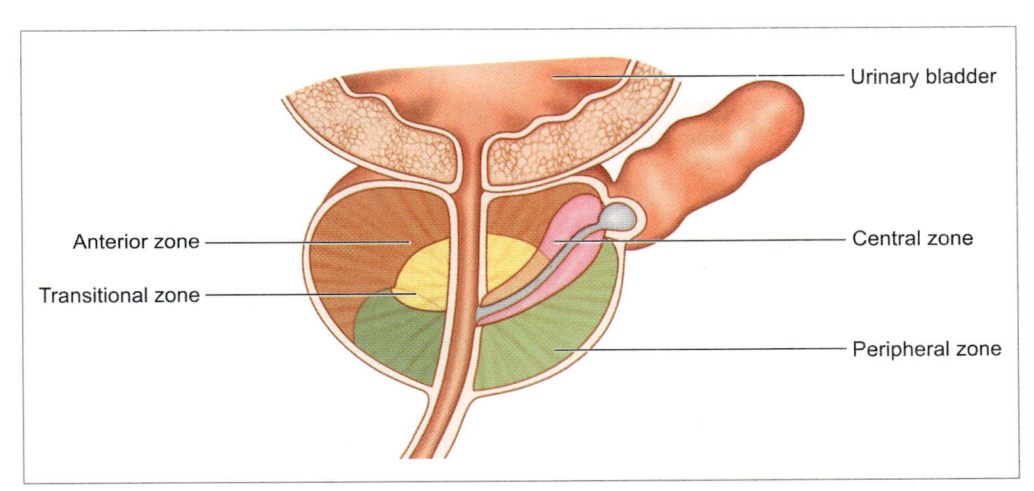

Fig. 20.8: Lobes of prostate gland.

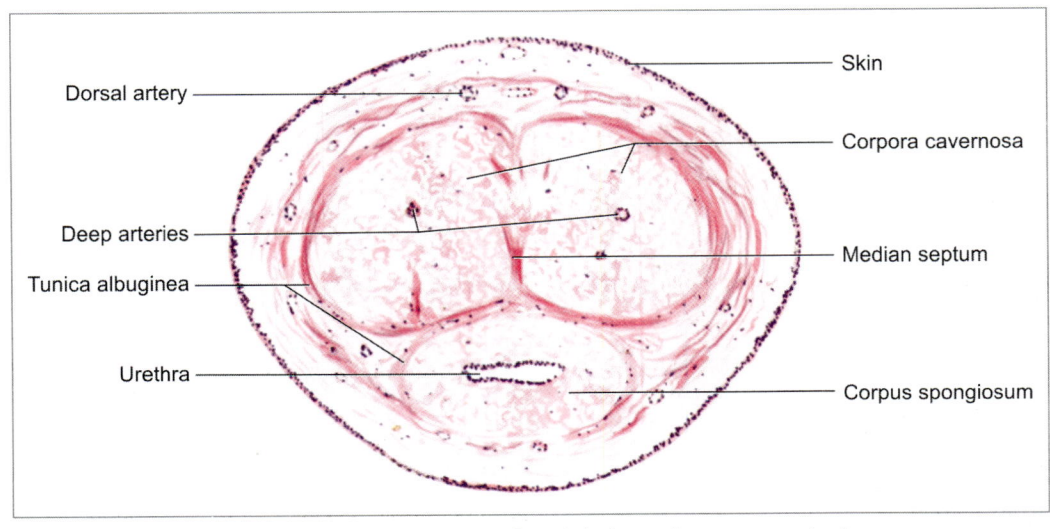

Fig. 20.9: Transverse section of penis (schematic representation).

APPLIED HISTOLOGY

- Testicular tumors can arise from germ cells (germ cell tumors), stroma (sex cord stromal tumors), or both (combined germ cell-sex cord-stromal tumors). Examples of germ cell tumors are seminoma, embryonal carcinoma, teratoma, and choriocarcinoma; sex cord stromal tumors are Leydig cell tumor, Sertoli cell tumor, and granulosa cell tumor. Gonadoblastoma is an example of combined germ cell-sex cord-stromal tumors.
- Germ cell tumors comprise approximately 95% of all testicular tumors and are more frequent before the age of 45 years. Testicular germ cell tumors are almost always malignant.
- Fructose content in seminal fluid: in the cases of male infertility, on semen analysis, the absence of fructose suggests congenital absence of seminal vesicle or portion of the ductal system or both.
- **Benign prostatic hypertrophy**: It mainly affects the transition zone, and the enlargement of the prostate is a very common condition in men and considered by some as normal aging process. Enlargement of the prostate can compress the urethra leading to difficulty in micturition.
- **Carcinoma of prostate**: It mostly arises from the peripheral zone, and many a times, carcinoma of the prostate is small and detected as microscopic foci in a prostate removed for benign enlargement of prostate or found incidentally at autopsy.
- Central zone is rarely involved in any disease.

MULTIPLE CHOICE QUESTIONS

1. Which of the following structure is incorrectly matched with their lining epithelium?
    a. Rete testis—simple cuboidal epithelium
    b. Ductuli efferentes—pseudostratified epithelium
    c. Ductus epididymidis—pseudostratified columnar with stereocilia
    d. Ductus deferens—simple columnar ciliated epithelium
2. Testosterone is secreted by which cell?
    a. Sertoli   b. Leydig
    c. Spermatogonia   d. Spermatocytes
3. All of the following are the functions of Sertoli cells *except*:
    a. Physical and nutritional support to the developing germ cells
    b. Phagocytosis of the residual cytoplasm
    c. Establish blood–testis barrier
    d. They secrete fructose less fluid
4. Which of the following is true?
    a. There is one corpus cavernosa and one corpus spongiosum
    b. There is one corpus cavernosa and two corpora spongiosum
    c. There are two corpora cavernosa and one corpus spongiosum
    d. There are two corpora cavernosa and two corpora spongiosum
5. What is the most commonly seen type of epithelium in the prostate?
    a. Transitional   b. Pseudostratified squamous
    c. Simple squamous   d. Simple cuboidal
6. What are the spherical structures seen in some prostatic alveoli called?
    a. Corpora arenacea   b. Hassall's corpuscles
    c. Prostatic concretions d. Pacinian corpuscles
7. What type of gland composes the prostate?
    a. Simple tubular gland
    b. Simple alveolar gland
    c. Compound tubular gland
    d. Compound tubuloalveolar gland
8. What constitutes the stroma of the prostate?
    a. Loose irregular connective tissue
    b. Smooth muscle
    c. Fibromuscular
    d. Adipose tissue
9. How many seminiferous tubules are found in each testis of an average man?
    a. 4–6   b. 40–60
    c. 400–600   d. 4,000–6,000
10. Anti-Müllerian hormone is secreted by which cells?
    a. Sertoli   b. Androgen-binding protein
    c. Testosterone   d. All of the above
11. What is the surface modification seen on the cells of the epididymis?
    a. Flagella and microvilli
    b. Stereocilia and cilia
    c. Cilia and microvilli
    d. Microvilli and stereocilia

Answers
1. b   2. b   3. d   4. c   5. b   6. a   7. d   8. c   9. c
10. a 11. d

CHAPTER 21

Female Reproductive System

Learning objectives

To study the:
- Structure of ovary
- Steps in oogenesis
- Formation of ovarian follicles and ovulation
- Structure of uterine tube
- Structure of uterus
- Structure of cervix, vagina and external genitalia
- Structure of mammary gland
- Applied histology

IDENTIFICATION POINTS

Ovary	Uterus		Uterine tube	Mammary gland	
	Proliferative phase	*Secretory phase*		*Resting phase*	*Lactating phase*
☐ Covered by single layer of cuboidal cells as germinal epithelium ☐ Presence of cortex and medulla ☐ The *medulla* consists of loose connective tissue, smooth muscles, blood vessels, lymphatics, and nerves ☐ Cortex contains ovarian follicle at different stages of development: Primary, primordial, secondary, and mature Graafian follicles ☐ Presence of corpus luteum and atretic follicle in the cortex.	☐ Presence of endometrium, myometrium, and epimetrium ☐ Highly cellular and nonedematous ☐ Uterine glands are elongated, straight, and tubular without secretion ☐ Glands are lined by columnar epithelium ☐ Spiral arteries are less coiled, do not reach the superficial part of endometrium.	☐ Presence of endometrium, myometrium, and epimetrium ☐ Highly vascular and edematous ☐ Uterine glands are dilated, tortuous with watery secretion ☐ Glands are lined by columnar epithelium ☐ Spiral arteries are more coiled, reach superficial part of endometrium.	☐ Uterine tube is made up of three layers: Inner mucous, middle muscular, and outer serosa layers ☐ Presence of numerous branching mucosal folds ☐ The mucosa is lined by ciliated columnar epithelium ☐ Muscular layer consists of inner, circular, and outer longitudinal muscle layer.	☐ Presence of tubuloalveolar glands separated by connective and fatty tissues ☐ Contain more connective tissue and less glandular tissue ☐ Presence of few poorly developed alveoli ☐ Alveoli is lined by cuboidal epithelium and wider lumen ☐ Presence of narrow empty ducts.	☐ Presence of compound tubuloalveolar glands separated by connective and fatty tissues ☐ Contain more glandular and less connective tissue ☐ Presence of numerous well-developed alveoli ☐ Alveoli is lined by columnar epithelium and narrow lumen ☐ Presence of wider ducts and filled with secretions.

INTRODUCTION

The female reproductive system includes (Fig. 21.1):
- A pair of ovaries
- A pair of uterine tubes
- Uterus
- Vagina
- External genitalia
- Mammary glands.

OVARY

- The ovaries are the female gonads, responsible for the formation of ova.
- Each ovary is an oval structure about 3 cm long in diameter and situated on each side of the uterus and attached to the posterior layer of the broad ligament below and behind the uterine tubes.

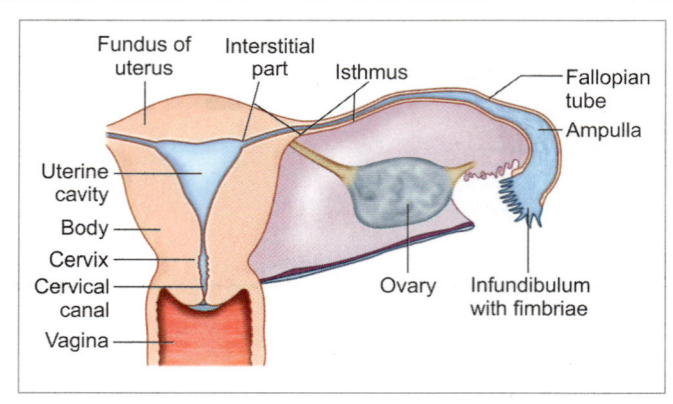

Fig. 21.1: Parts of female reproductive system (schematic representation).

- Before puberty, its surface is smooth; thereafter due to repeated ovulations and cicatrization, the surface becomes irregular.
- They also produce hormones estrogen and progesterone that are responsible for the development of the female secondary sex characters, and produce marked cyclical changes in the uterine endometrium.

General Structure

- The ovary is covered by a single layer of cubical cells known as germinal epithelium. This epithelium is continuous with the mesothelium lining the peritoneum, and represents a modification of the latter.
- The germinal epithelium rests on a connective tissue layer called the **tunica albuginea** which is thinner and less dense than that of the testis. Tunica albuginea is a dense, irregular collagenous connective tissue capsule and collagen fibers run parallel to ovarian surface.
- The substance of the gland consists of inner medulla and outer cortex (Fig. 21.2 and Plate 21.1):

Cortex: Cortex composed of connective tissue stroma made up of reticular fibers and numerous fusiform cells that resemble mesenchymal cells called stromal/interstitial cells. Stroma also contains **ovarian follicles** at various stages of development.

- **At birth**: Cortex contains a numerous *primordial follicles*. Each primordial follicle consists of a centrally placed sex cell known as *primary oocyte* and surrounded by a single layer of *follicular cells* derived from the somatic tissue.
- **In childbearing period**: During this period, the primordial follicles are divided into primary, secondary, and tertiary follicular stages. During reproductive life, the cortex contains the ovarian follicles and corpora lutea at different stages of development, atretic follicles, and corpora albicantia.
- **After menopause**: The cortex becomes fibrotic and contains interstitial cells and corpora albicantia.

Medulla: It **consists** of loose connective tissue, smooth muscles, blood vessels, lymphatics, and nerves. The hilum of the ovary is the site for entry of blood vessels and lymphatics and it is continuous with the medulla. The hilum also contains some remnants of the mesonephric

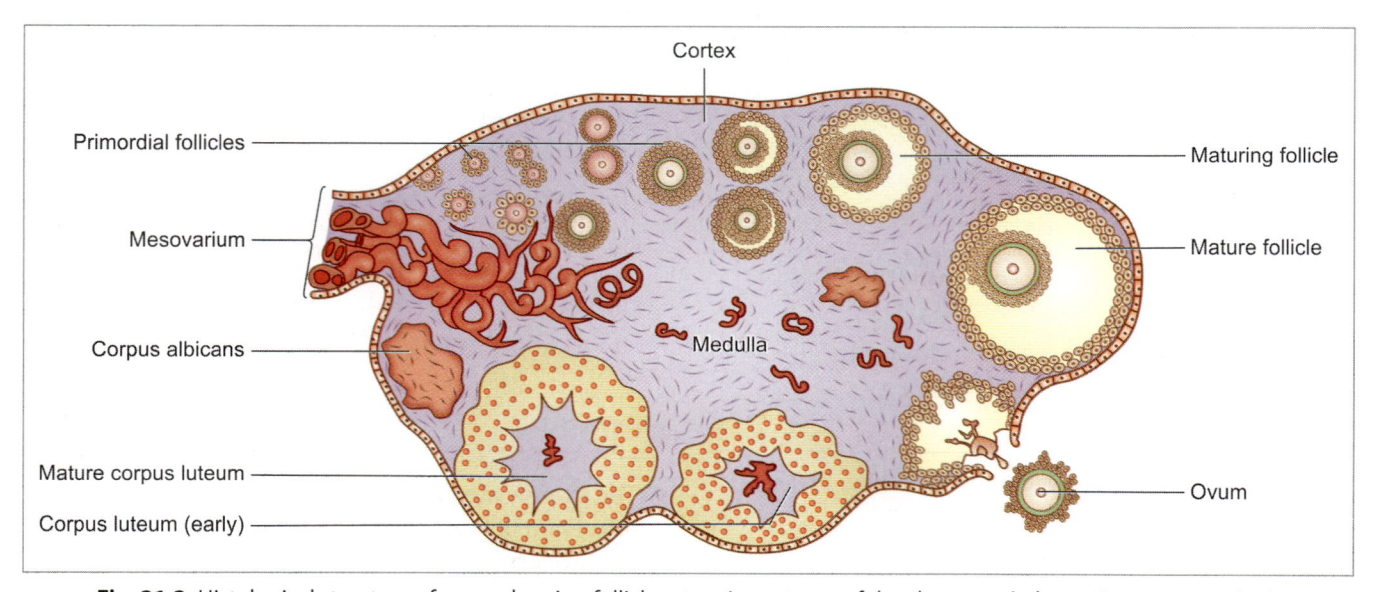

Fig. 21.2: Histological structure of ovary showing follicles at various stages of development (schematic representation).

CHAPTER 21: Female Reproductive System

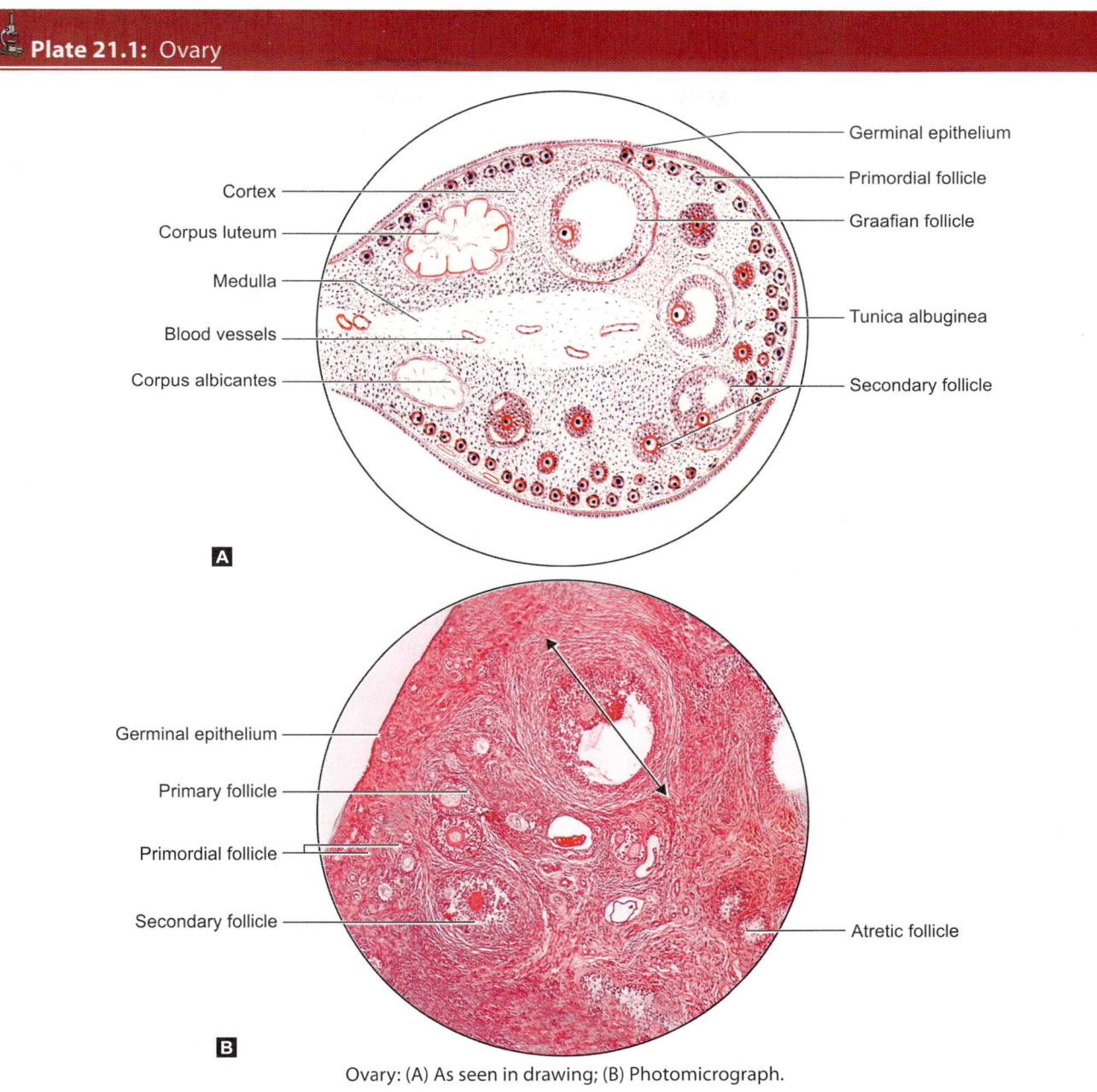

Plate 21.1: Ovary

Ovary: (A) As seen in drawing; (B) Photomicrograph.

Courtesy (B): Balakrishna Shetty, Sweekritha H Poonja. HISTOLOGY Practical Manual, 4th edition. New Delhi: Jaypee Brothers Medical Publishers (P) Ltd; 2019. p. 126.

Points of identification
- The surface is covered by a cuboidal epithelium. Deep to the epithelium, there is a layer of connective tissue that constitutes the tunica albuginea
- The substance of the ovary has an outer cortex in which follicles of various sizes are present, and an inner medulla consisting of connective tissue containing numerous blood vessels
- Just deep to the tunica albuginea, many primordial follicles each of which contains a developing ovum surrounded by flattened follicular cells are present
- Large follicles have a follicular cavity surrounded by several layers of follicular cells
- The cells surrounding the ovum constitute the cumulus oophorus
- The follicle is surrounded by a condensation of connective tissue which forms a capsule for it
- The capsule consists of an inner cellular part (the theca interna), and an outer fibrous part (the theca externa) collectively called as theca folliculi. The follicle is surrounded by a stroma made up of reticular fibers and fusiform cells.

ducts, and **hilus cells** that are similar to interstitial cells of the testis and secrete androgens.

Note: The term germinal epithelium is a misnomer. The epithelium does not produce germ cells. The cells of this epithelium bear microvilli, and contain numerous mitochondria. They become larger in pregnancy.

Oogenesis

The process of formation of ovum from the stem cells is called oogenesis (Flowchart 21.1).

- ❖ **Oogonia** are large round stem cells from which ova are derived and they are present in the cortex of the ovary. Oogonia develop in the yolk sac endoderm from primordial stem cells and undergo mitotic division and during 6th week of gestation migrate to the cortex of developing ovary.
- ❖ Oogonia undergo mitotic division till 5th month of gestation and about 5 to 7 million oogonia are formed. Only about 1 million of oogonia is surrounded by follicular cells and survive till the birth and remaining oogonia undergo atresia, degenerate, and die.
- ❖ All oogonia to be used throughout the life of a woman are produced before birth and do not multiply thereafter.

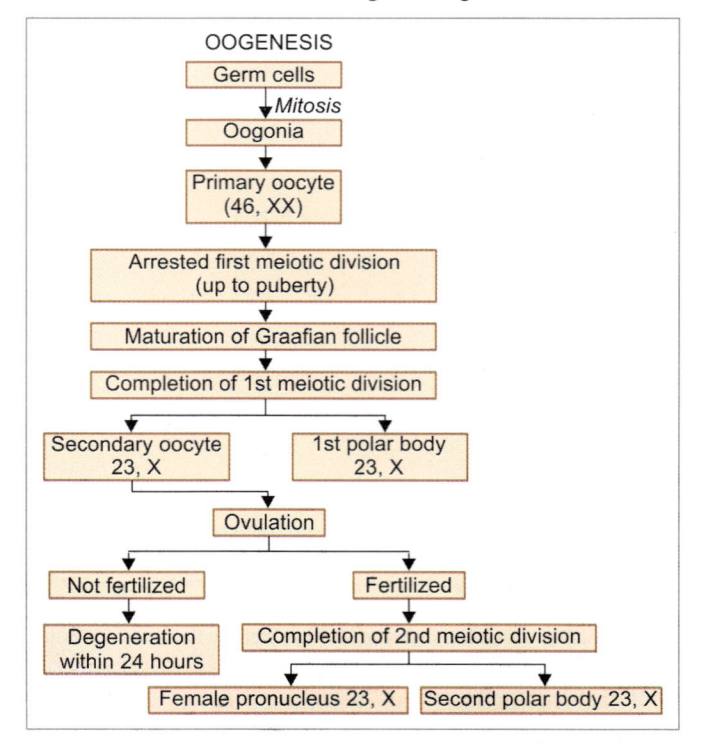

Flowchart 21.1: Stages of oogenesis.

```
                OOGENESIS
                Germ cells
                    ↓ Mitosis
                 Oogonia
                    ↓
              Primary oocyte
                (46, XX)
                    ↓
         Arrested first meiotic division
              (up to puberty)
                    ↓
         Maturation of Graafian follicle
                    ↓
         Completion of 1st meiotic division
                 ↙       ↘
       Secondary oocyte   1st polar body
          23, X              23, X
              ↓
           Ovulation
          ↙      ↘
  Not fertilized  Fertilized
       ↓             ↓
  Degeneration   Completion of 2nd meiotic division
  within 24 hours       ↙         ↘
              Female pronucleus 23, X  Second polar body 23, X
```

- ❖ An oogonium enlarges to form a **primary oocyte**. The primary oocyte contains the diploid number of chromosomes, i.e. 46. It is spherical with acentric nucleus containing single nucleolus.
- ❖ Primary oocyte is arrested in the prophase stage of 1st meiosis. It completes the 1st meiotic division just before ovulation to form two daughter cells each of which has 23 chromosomes. The primary oocytes remain in prophase and do not complete their first meiotic division until they begin to mature and are ready to ovulate.
- ❖ With each menstrual cycle, about 5 to 30 primary oocytes begin to mature and complete the first meiotic division just before ovulation.
- ❖ The cytoplasm of the primary oocyte is not equally divided. Most of it goes to one daughter cell that is large and is called the **secondary oocyte**. The second daughter cell has hardly any cytoplasm, and forms the **first polar body**.
- ❖ The secondary oocyte immediately enters the second meiotic division. Ovulation takes place while the oocyte is in metaphase. The secondary oocyte remains arrested in metaphase till fertilization occurs.
- ❖ The second meiotic division is completed only if fertilization occurs. The secondary oocyte undergoes the second meiotic division and the daughter cells being again unequal in size. The larger daughter is the **mature ovum** and the smaller daughter cell which has hardly any cytoplasm is the **second polar body**. Thus, one primary oocyte ultimately gives rise to only one ovum.

Formation of Ovarian Follicles

- ❖ **Ovarian follicles** consist of a developing ova surrounded by follicular cells. The development and maturation of an ovarian follicle passes through four stages (primordial, primary, secondary, and Graafian) and the process is called folliculogenesis (Figs. 21.2 and 21.3).
- ❖ **Primordial follicle** (Fig. 21.3A) is the most primitive follicles. It is composed of primary oocyte surrounded by a single layer of flattened cells called *follicular cells/ granulosa cells*. Primordial follicles are the smallest and simplest in structure located at the periphery of the cortex. Numerous primordial follicles are present in the ovary at birth. They undergo further development only at puberty.
- ❖ A primordial follicle develops into **primary follicle**. The flattened follicular cells become cuboidal. Oocyte surrounded by a single layer of cuboidal follicular cells is called as **unilaminar primary follicle**. The follicular

CHAPTER 21: Female Reproductive System

cells proliferate and stratify to form several layers of cells and now the primary follicle with many layers of follicular cells is called as **multilaminar primary follicle** (Fig. 21.3B).

- A homogeneous membrane, the *zona pellucida*, appears between the follicular cells and the oocyte. Cytoplasmic extensions from follicular cells invade the zona pellucida, come in contact with the oocyte plasmalemma and form gap junctions through which they communicate with oocyte.
- Stromal cells organize around multilaminar primary follicle forming an inner cellular layer called ***theca interna*** and outer fibrous layer called ***theca externa***. Granulosa cells are separated from the theca interna by thick basal lamina. Theca interna cells express receptors for luteinizing hormone (LH) to produce *androstenedione* which gets converted to estrogen by granulosa cells.
- **Secondary follicle**: Multilaminar primary follicle develops and increases in size and the follicular cells proliferate to form several layers of cells that constitute the ***membrana granulosa***. The oocyte enlarges and reaches its maximum size (125 μm) (Figs. 21.3A and B).
- Intercellular spaces develop within the masses of granulosa cells and filled with the fluid called ***liquor folliculi*** and the follicle is called as ***secondary follicle***. Under the influence of FSH, number of layers of granulosa cells increase as well as the fluid-filled cavity. As more fluid is produced, individual cavity coalesces to form single cavity called ***antrum***.
- ***Graafian follicle***: The granulosa cells are rearranged and now the primary oocyte lies eccentrically and surrounded by small group of granulosa cells that projects into the cavity called as ***cumulus oophorus***. The granulosa cells that attach the oocyte to the wall of the follicle constitute the ***discus proligerus*** (Fig. 21.4). The innermost layer of cumulus oophorus that lies directly adjacent to the zona pellucida is called ***corona radiata***.

Ovulation

- By 14th day of menstrual cycle, blood estrogen level increases causes surge of LH. The ovarian follicle is at first very small compared to the thickness of the ovarian cortex. As the follicle enlarges, it becomes so big that it not only reaches the surface of the ovary, but forms a bulging in this situation. As a result, the stroma and the theca on this side of the follicle are stretched and become very thin (Fig. 21.5).
- An avascular area *(stigma)* appears over the most convex point of the follicle. At the same time, the cells of the cumulus oophorus become loosened by accumulation of fluid between them. The follicle ultimately ruptures and the ovum is shed from the ovary.
- The shedding of the ovum is called ***ovulation***. The "ovum" that is shed from the ovary is not fully mature.

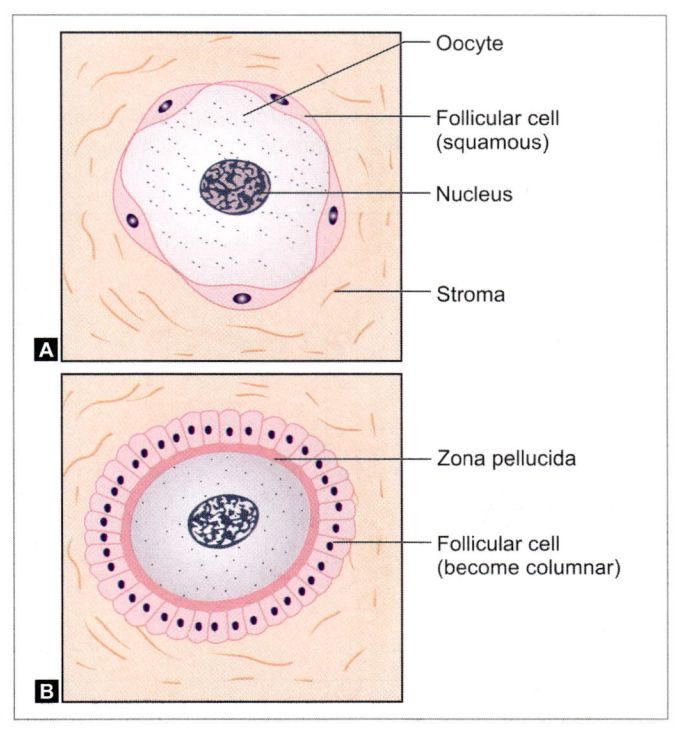

Figs. 21.3A and B: (A) Primordial follicle; (B) Primary follicle (schematic representation).

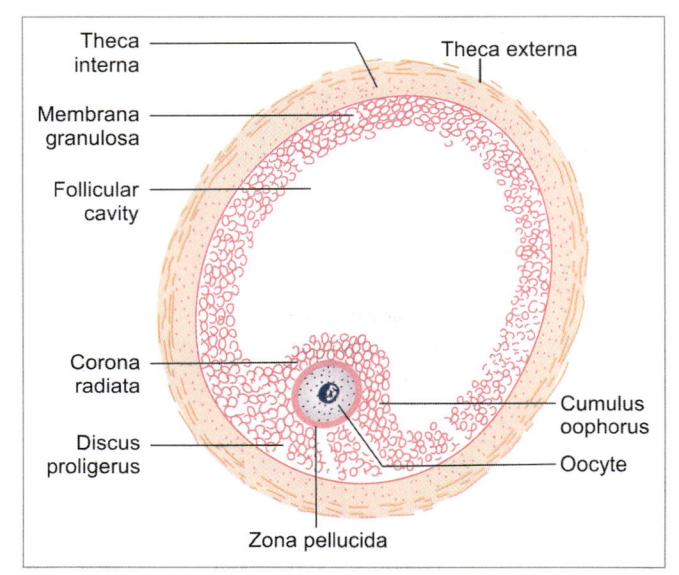

Fig. 21.4: Mature ovarian follicle (schematic representation).

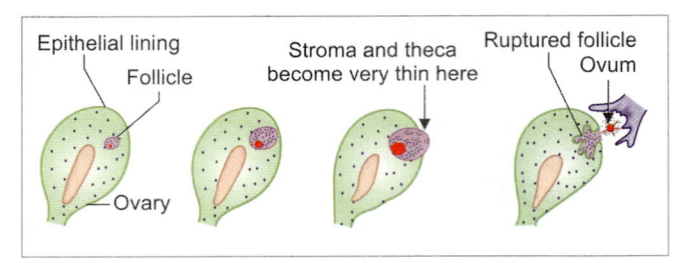

Fig. 21.5: Relationship of a growing ovarian follicle to the ovary (schematic representation).

It is really a secondary oocyte surrounded by zona pellucida and corona radiata (Fig. 21.6).

Fate of the Ovum

- The ovum is carried into the fallopian tube partly by the follicular fluid discharged from the follicle and partly by the activity of ciliated cells lining the tube.
- The ovum slowly travels through the tube toward the uterus, taking three to four days to do so.
- If fertilization takes place, then the ovum begins to develop into an embryo. It travels to the uterus and gets implanted in its wall. If the ovum is not fertilized, it dies in 12 to 24 hours and it passes through the uterus into the vagina and is discharged.

Corpus Luteum

- After ovulation, the follicle ruptures and its wall collapses and becomes folded. Sudden reduction in pressure caused by rupture of the follicle results in bleeding into the follicle. The follicle filled with blood is called the ***corpus hemorrhagicum***. At this stage, the follicular cells are small and rounded.
- The cells now enlarge rapidly and as they increase in size, their walls press against those of neighboring cells so that the cells acquire a polyhedral shape (Figs. 21.7 and 21.8). Their cytoplasm becomes filled with a yellow pigment called ***lutein***. The presence of this yellow pigment gives the structure a yellow color, and that is why it is called the corpus luteum (= yellow body) which functions as endocrine gland.
- The granulosa cells are modified into large pale staining cells called ***granulosa-lutein cells***, which constitutes about 80% of cell population and present in the center of the follicle. They produce progesterone and convert androgens produced by theca cells to estrogen.
- The theca interna cells modified into dark staining cells called theca lutein cells, which constitutes about 20%

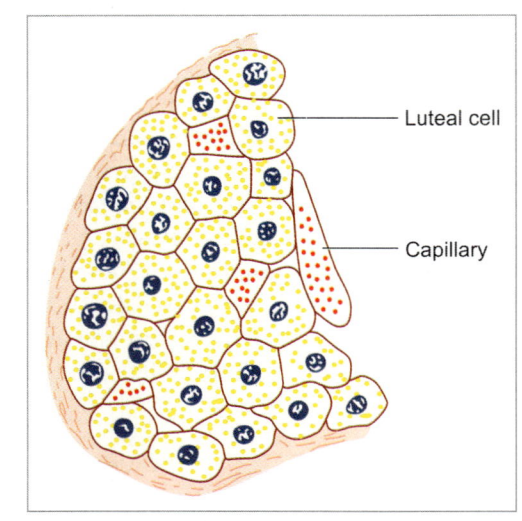

Fig. 21.7: Corpus luteum. Note the large hexagonal cells filled with yellow granules (schematic representation).

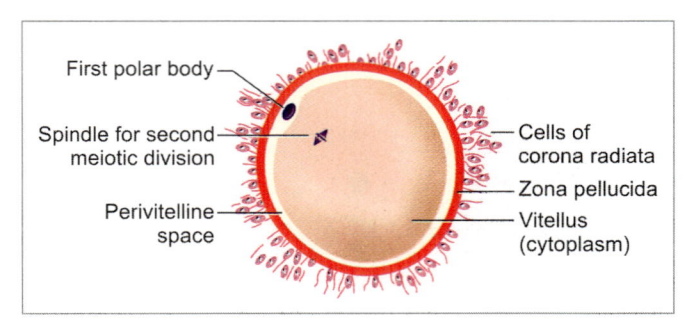

Fig. 21.6: Structure of ovum at the time of ovulation (schematic representation).

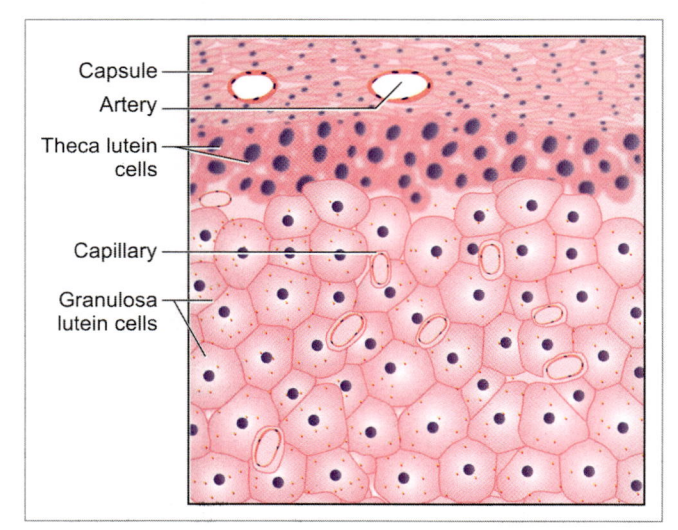

Fig. 21.8: Corpus luteum (high magnification) (schematic representation).

of cell population and present near the periphery. They produce progesterone, some estrogen, and androgens.

- The subsequent fate of the corpus luteum depends on whether the ovum is fertilized or not. If the ovum is not fertilized, the corpus luteum persists for about 14 days. During this period, it secretes progesterone. It remains relatively small and is called the **corpus luteum of menstruation**.
- If the ovum is fertilized and pregnancy results, the corpus luteum persists for three to four months. It is larger than the corpus luteum of menstruation, and is called the **corpus luteum of pregnancy**. The progesterone secreted by it is essential for the maintenance of pregnancy in the first few months. After the fourth month, the corpus luteum is no longer needed, as the placenta begins to secrete progesterone.
- The corpus luteum is invaded by fibroblasts, becomes fibrotic and ceases to function and the mass of fibrous tissue is called as the **corpus albicans** (= white body) (Fig. 21.9). The remnants of the corpus albicans persist as a scar on the surface of the ovary.

Fate of Ovarian Follicles

- The series of changes that begin with the formation of an ovarian follicle and end with the degeneration of the corpus luteum constitute what is called an **ovarian cycle**.
- In each ovarian cycle, one follicle reaches maturity, sheds an ovum, and becomes a corpus luteum. At the same time, several other follicles also begin to develop but do not reach maturity. These follicles do not persist into the next ovarian cycle but undergo degeneration and eventually phagocytosed by macrophages. Follicles that undergo degeneration are known as **atretic follicles**.
- The ovum and granulosa cells of each follicle disappear. The cells of the theca interna, however, proliferate to form the **interstitial glands**, also called the **corpora atretica**. These glands are believed to secrete estrogens. After a period of activity, each gland becomes a mass of scar tissue indistinguishable from the corpus albicans formed from the corpus luteum.
- The cortex of an ovary of woman in the reproductive period can show ovarian follicles at various stages

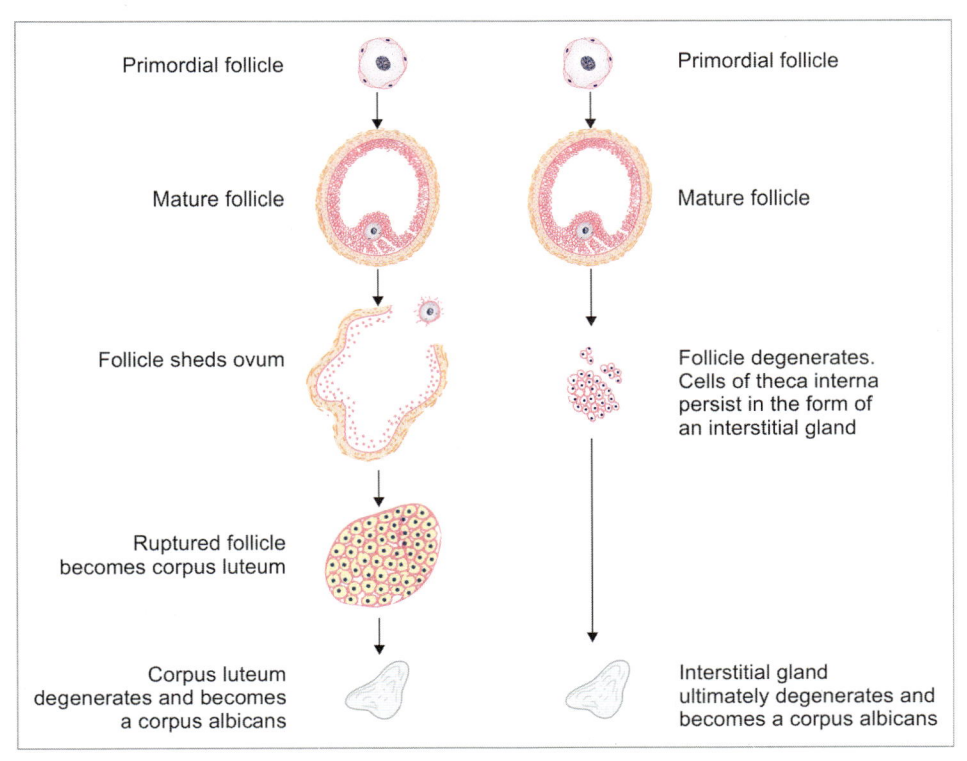

Fig. 21.9: Comparison of fate of ovarian follicles that shed an ovum and of those that do not (schematic representation).

of maturation (corpora lutea, corpora albicantia, and corpora atretica).

UTERINE TUBES

General Features

- Uterine tubes are paired muscular tubes which convey the ova from ovary to uterine cavity and they are called *fallopian tubes/oviducts*.
- Each uterine tube has a medial or uterine end attached to the uterus, and a lateral end that opens into the peritoneal cavity near the ovary.
- From medial to lateral side, the tube has:
  - A *uterine/intramural part* that passes through the thick uterine wall
  - A relatively narrow, thick-walled part called the *isthmus*
  - A thin-walled dilated part called the *ampulla*
  - Funnel-shaped *infundibulum*. It is prolonged into a number of finger-like processes or *fimbriae*.

Microscopic Features

The wall of the uterine tube consists of mucous, muscular, and serous layers from within outward.

- **Mucous membrane** shows three to six longitudinal folds, which give rise to a number of secondary and tertiary folds that almost fill the lumen of the tube (Plate 21.2). These folds are most conspicuous in the ampulla. It is lined by columnar epithelium that rests on a basement membrane. The epithelium consists of *ciliated, secretory, and intercalary* cells.
  - **Ciliated cells** help to move the ova.
  - **Secretory cells** are also called as *peg cells*, they contain secretory granules and are not ciliated and their surface shows microvilli. Secretion from the cells provides nutrition to the fertilized ovum and the spermatozoa.
  - **Intercalary cells** are sandwiched between the basement membrane and the epithelium. They act as precursors of the ciliated and secretory cells.
- **Muscular layer** consists of outer longitudinal and inner circular layers of smooth muscles. The intramural part may have innermost longitudinal layer. The circular muscle is abundant at the isthmus where the lumen is narrow and suggesting of existence of anatomical sphincter.
- **Serosa layer** is derived from the peritoneum and covers the entire tube except the lower border and the intramural part.

Functions

- The uterine tube conveys ova, shed by the ovary, to the uterus. Ova enter the tube at its fimbriated end. Spermatozoa enter the uterine tube through the vagina and uterus.
- Fertilization normally takes place in the ampulla. When fertilization occurs, the fertilized ovum travels toward the uterus through the tube.
- Secretions present in the tubes provide nutrition, oxygen, and other requirements for ova and spermatozoa passing through the tube.

UTERUS

General Features

- Uterus is an inverted pear-/pyriform-shaped muscular organ located in the pelvic cavity between urinary bladder below urinary bladder in front and sigmoid colon, rectum behind.
- On each side, it receives the opening of the uterine tube at the superolateral angle/cornu and communicates below with vagina through external os.
- The uterus consists of three parts from above downward: *Fundus*, *body*, and *cervix*. The fundus is the upper dome-shaped part which is above the attachment of the fallopian tube. The body extends from the fundus to the isthmus; the isthmus is a narrow constricted part separating the body of the uterus from the cervix. Below the isthmus, the uterus becomes cylindrical in shape; this part is known as cervix.
- The uterus has a very thick wall consists of endometrium, myometrium, and perimetrium from within outward.

Microscopic Features

Endometrium

- The mucous membrane of the uterus is called the *endometrium*.
- The endometrium consists of a lining epithelium and lamina propria/stroma. Numerous uterine glands are present in the stroma.
  - **Lining epithelium** is columnar. Before menarche, the cells are ciliated, during reproductive life, it is lined by simple columnar epithelium because cilia cannot grow due to repeated destruction of superficial part of endometrium.
  - **Lamina propria/stroma** contains embryonic stromal cells, numerous blood vessels, lymphatics, nerves, and tubular uterine glands.

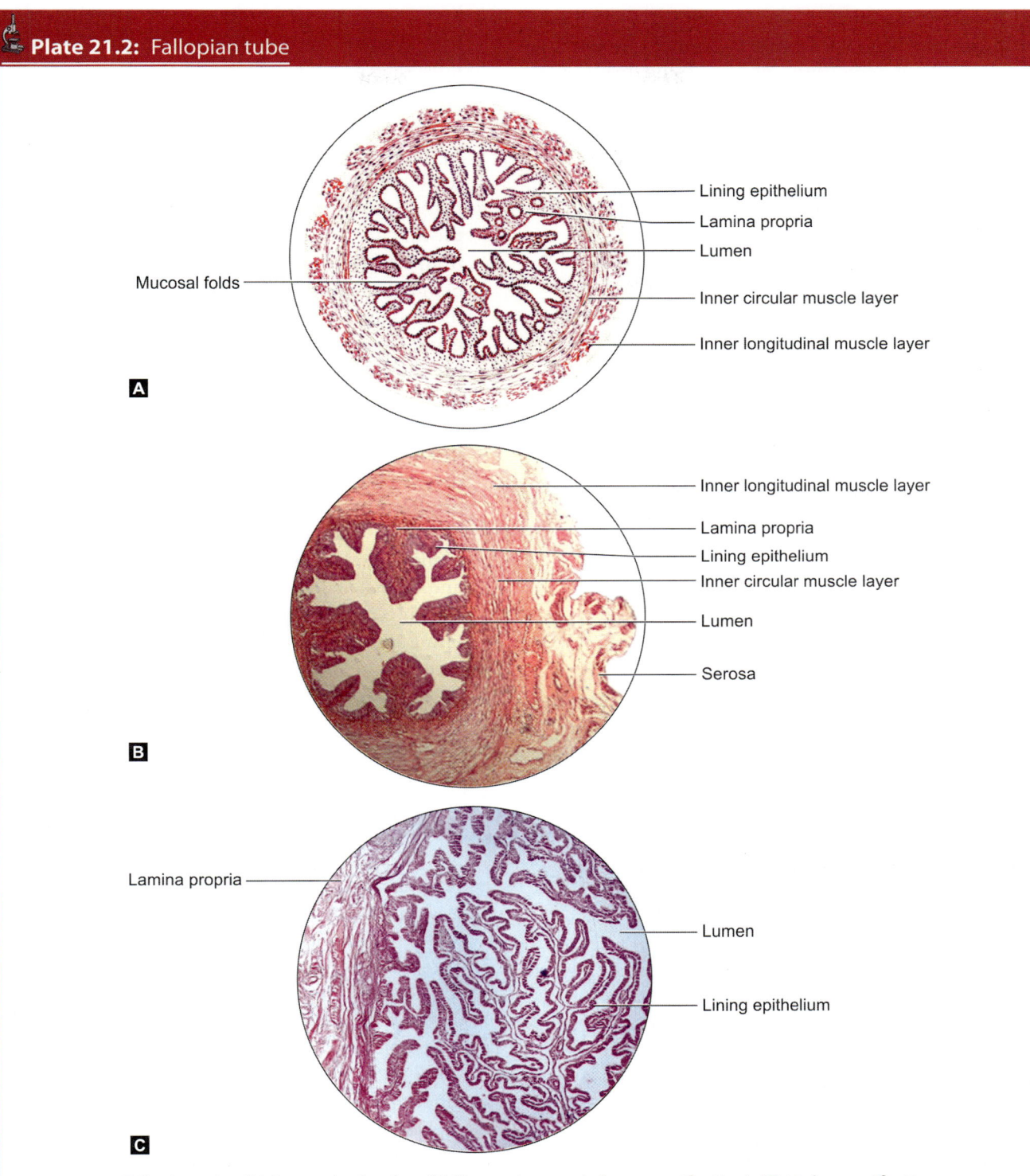

CHAPTER 21: Female Reproductive System

Plate 21.2: Fallopian tube

A — Labels: Mucosal folds; Lining epithelium; Lamina propria; Lumen; Inner circular muscle layer; Inner longitudinal muscle layer

B — Labels: Inner longitudinal muscle layer; Lamina propria; Lining epithelium; Inner circular muscle layer; Lumen; Serosa

C — Labels: Lamina propria; Lumen; Lining epithelium

Fallopian tube: (A) As seen in drawing; (B) Photomicrograph (low magnification); (C) High magnification.

Points of identification
- The uterine tube is characterized by the presence of numerous branching mucosal folds that almost fill the lumen of the tube
- The mucosa is lined by ciliated columnar epithelium
- The uterine tube has a muscular wall with an inner circular and outer longitudinal muscle layer.

- **The glands** are lined by simple columnar epithelium and extend up to the inner surface of myometrium.
❖ Functionally, endometrium consists of outer basal layer and inner functional layer.
  - Functional layer undergoes changes during the menstrual cycle and it cast off in each month during menstruation. Basal layer remains practically unaltered and helps in regeneration of the epithelial lining after menstruation.
  - The basal layer is supplied by straight basal arteries from myometrium and functional layer is supplied by spiral arteries which allow diminished blood flow and undergo vasoconstriction before menstruation.

Endometrial changes in menstrual cycle

❖ The endometrium undergoes marked cyclical changes that constitute the **menstrual cycle**. The cycle is calculated from the beginning of one menstrual bleeding to the beginning of the next bleeding and an average of 28 days duration. Ovulation takes place at the middle of the cycle. Preovulatory cycle is regulated by estrogen of ovarian follicle and postovulatory cycle is regulated by progesterone of corpus luteum.
❖ The endometrial changes are divided into **menstrual**, **postmenstrual/regenerative**, **proliferative**, and **secretory** (Table 21.1).
  - The **menstrual phase** is manifested by uterine bleeding which persists for 3 to 4 days. There is exfoliation of functional layer of endometrium due to sudden withdrawal of progesterone after the regression of corpus luteum.

- In the **postmenstrual phase**, the endometrium is thin. It progressively increases in thickness being thickest at the end of the secretory phase.
- The **regenerative phase** takes 1 to 3 days to complete. The epithelial cells from the uterine glands proliferate by mitosis and cover the denuded surface of mucous membrane. Estrogen helps in regeneration.
- During **proliferative/follicular/estrogenic phase**, the functional layer gradually increases in thickness from 1 mm to 3 mm before the ovulation. The proliferation is stimulated by estrogen. There is increase in the population of stroma cells, elongation of uterine glands, and spiral arteries of the endometrium. The uterine glands are straight in the proliferative phase. Proliferative phase may extend 1–2 days after ovulation till the formation of corpus luteum (Plate 21.3).
- In **secretory/luteal phase**, the functional layer is increased in thickness 2 to 3 times more than the proliferative phase. Enlargements of the stroma cells due to appearance of cytoplasmic glycogen, accumulation of tissue fluid around the stroma cells, and by distension of uterine glands with secretion showing raggedy appearance of the epithelial cells lining the glandular lumen. As the endometrium increases in thickness, the glands elongate, increase in diameter, and become twisted on themselves and they have a saw-toothed appearance in sections. Glycogen-filled stroma cells are known as decidual cells which provide nutrition to the embedded ovum. Secretory phase is under the control of estrogen and progesterone. Implantation of fertilized ovum takes place in secretory phase (Plate 21.4).
- **Premenstrual phase** is 1 to 2 days prior to the onset of next menstrual cycle. In this phase, there is a reduction in thickness of the functional layer due to regression of corpus luteum. The spiral arteries shorten and become more coiled. Blood appear in the uterine lumen with shedding of flakes of endometrium (Fig. 21.10).

❖ At the time of menstruation, the greater parts of the uterine glands are lost along with the entire lining epithelium leaving behind only their most basal parts.
❖ The lining epithelium is reformed after the cessation of menstruation by proliferation of epithelial cells in the basal parts of the glands.

Myometrium

❖ The muscle layer of the uterus is called the **myometrium** and it consists of bundles of smooth muscle. Along with,

Table 21.1: Differences between proliferative and secretory phase.

	Proliferative phase	Secretory phase
Duration	6th to 13th day in a 28-day cycle	15th to 28th day in a 28-day cycle
Thickness of endometrium	It is about 2–3 mm thick	It is about 5 mm thick
Lining epithelium	Simple columnar	Simple columnar
Stroma	Highly cellular and nonedematous	Highly vascular and edematous
Uterine glands	Uterine glands are elongated, straight, and tubular without secretion	Uterine glands are dilated, tortuous, and giving a saw-toothed appearance with watery secretion
Spiral artery	Less coiled, do not reach the superficial part of endometrium	More coiled, reach superficial part of endometrium
Hormones	Estrogen is secreted	Progesterone is secreted

CHAPTER 21: Female Reproductive System

Plate 21.3: Uterus (Proliferative phase)

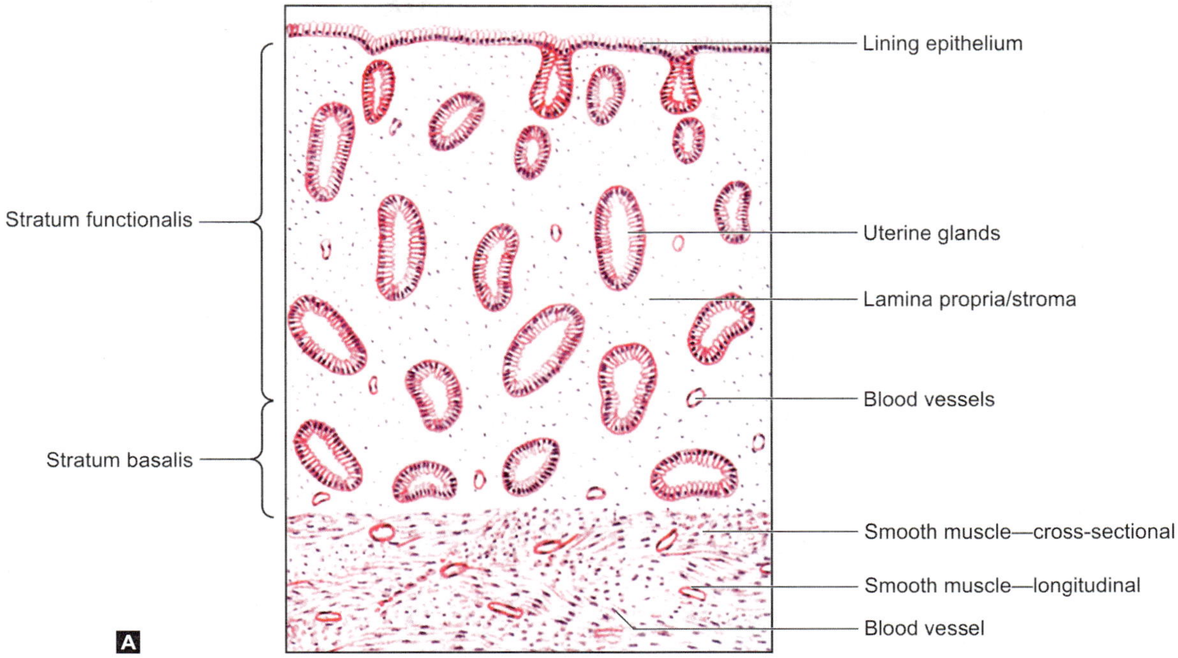

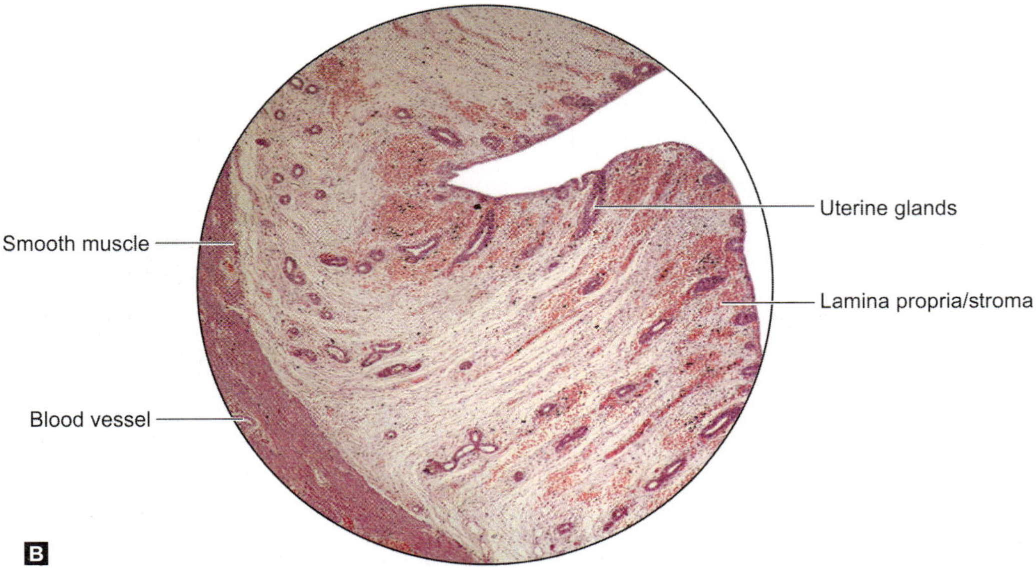

A — labels: Stratum functionalis, Stratum basalis, Lining epithelium, Uterine glands, Lamina propria/stroma, Blood vessels, Smooth muscle—cross-sectional, Smooth muscle—longitudinal, Blood vessel

B — labels: Smooth muscle, Blood vessel, Uterine glands, Lamina propria/stroma

Uterus (Proliferative phase): (A) As seen in drawing; (B) Photomicrograph.

Points of identification
- The wall of the uterus consists of a mucous membrane (called the endometrium) and a very thick layer of muscle (the myometrium). The thickness of the muscle layer helps to identify the uterus easily
- The endometrium has a lining of columnar epithelium that rests on a stroma of connective tissue
- Numerous tubular uterine glands dip into the stroma
- The appearance of the endometrium varies considerably depending upon the phase of the menstrual cycle. The endometrium is thin and progressively increases in thickness. The uterine glands are straight and tubular in this phase.

Plate 21.4: Uterus (Secretory phase)

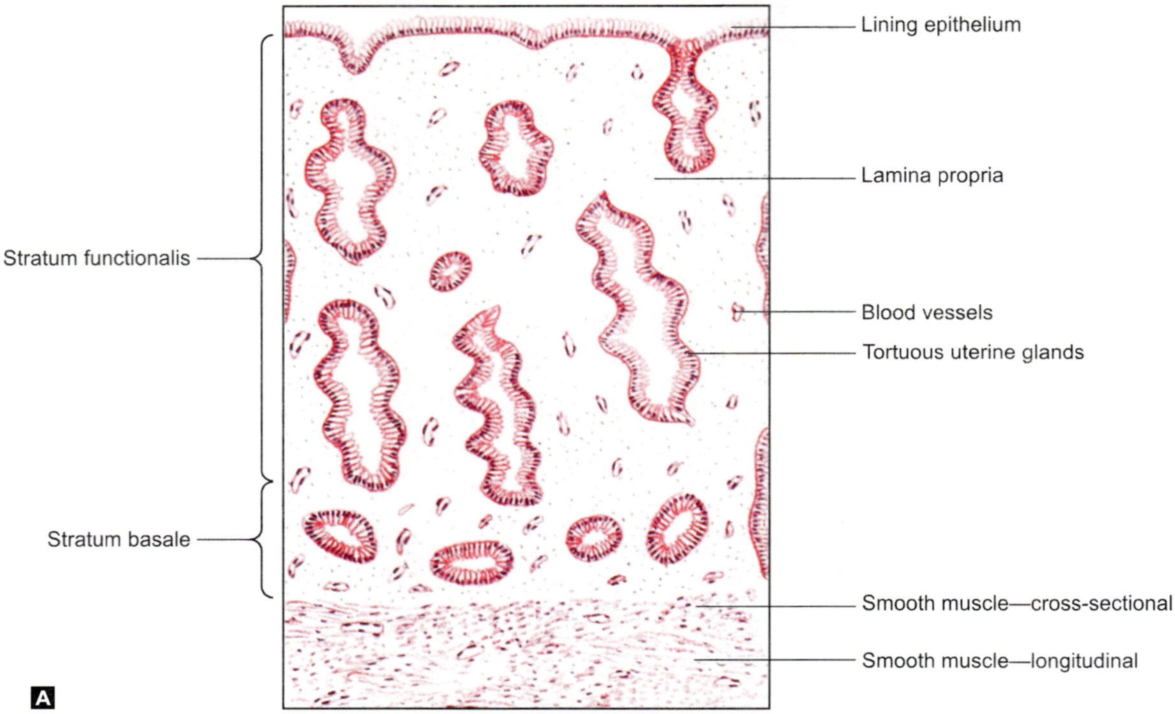

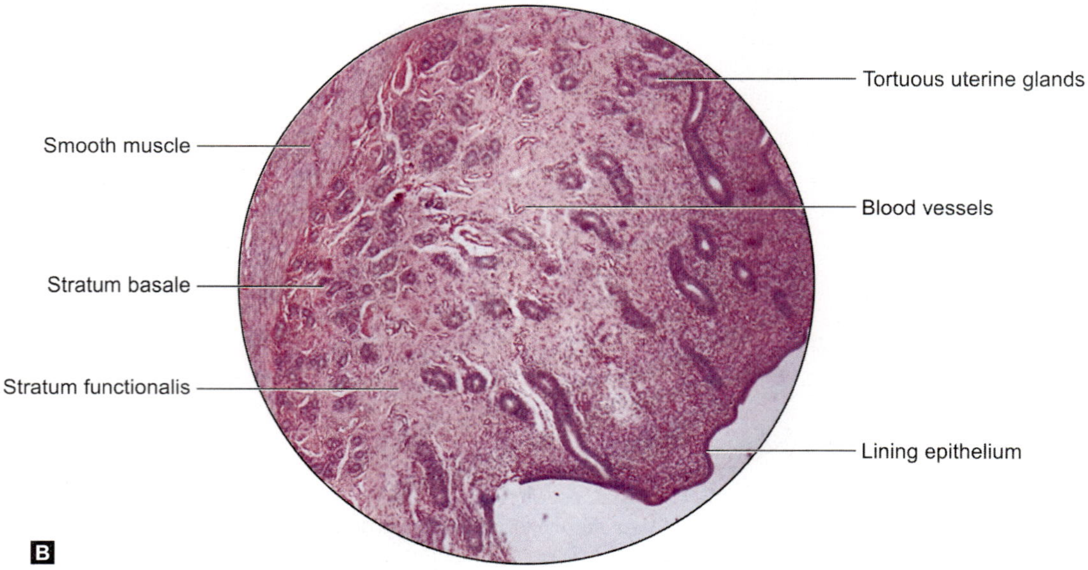

Uterus (Secretory phase): (A) As seen in drawing; (B) Photomicrograph.

Points of identification
In the secretory phase:
- The thickness of the endometrium is much increased
- The uterine glands elongate, become dilated, and tortuous as a result of which they have saw-toothed margins in sections
- Blood vessels extend in the upper portion of endometrium.

CHAPTER 21: Female Reproductive System

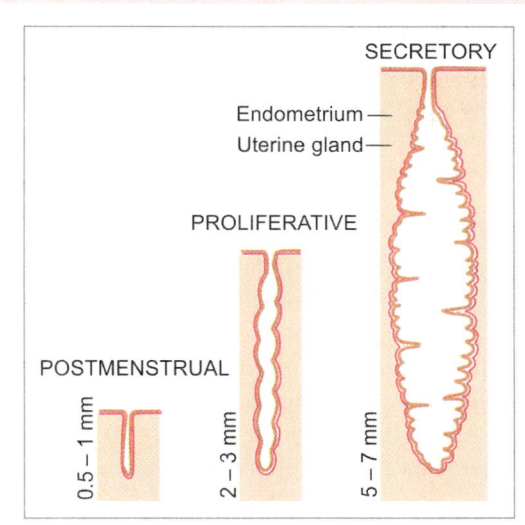

Fig. 21.10: Uterine glands at various stages of menstrual cycle. The thickness of endometrium is also indicated (schematic representation).

there is connective tissue, blood vessels, nerves, and lymphatics.
- The muscle fibers run in various directions and distinct layers are difficult to define. The myometrium consists of three ill-defined layers as **outer longitudinal**, **middle circular**, **and inner reticular**. In the middle layer, there is a mixture of bundles running in various directions.
    - The longitudinal muscles are continuous with the corresponding muscles of the uterine tubes. Longitudinal muscle helps in the anchorage of uterus and expels the uterine contents to the exterior.
    - Middle layer contains vascular bed, the stratum vasculare. Circular muscle of this layer forms a sphincter to retain the uterine contents (product of conception).
    - Endometrial vessels pass through the interstices of inner reticular arrangement of smooth muscle layer. On contraction, the muscle stops the bleeding in menstruation or during placental separation. Inner layer acts as *living ligature of the uterus*.
    - Growth of myometrium is stimulated by estrogen. The muscle cells increase in number (**hyperplasia**) and in size (**hypertrophy**) during pregnancy. Contractions of the myometrium are responsible for expulsion of the fetus at the time of childbirth.

Perimetrium
- The perimetrium/serous coat is derived from the peritoneum and covers the entire organ except two lateral borders, anterior surface of the supravaginal part of the cervix and the vaginal part of the cervix.
- Posterior surface of the uterus is adherent to the underlying muscle but in the anterior surface, it is adherent in the upper part but separated from the muscle by loose areolar tissue in the lower part.

> **Added Information**
>
> **Hormones influencing ovulation and menstruation**
> The changes taking place in the uterine endometrium during the menstrual cycle occur under the influence of:
> - **Estrogens** produced by the thecal gland (theca interna) and by the interstitial gland cells, and possibly by granulosa cells.
> - **Progesterone** produced by the corpus luteum.
> The development of the ovarian follicle and of the corpus luteum is in turn dependent on hormones produced by the anterior lobe of the hypophysis cerebri. These are:
> - The **follicle-stimulating hormone** (FSH), which stimulates the formation of follicles and the secretion of estrogens by them, and the **luteinizing hormone** (LH), which helps to convert the ovarian follicle into the corpus luteum, and stimulates the secretion of progesterone.
> - Secretion of FSH and LH is controlled by a **gonadotropin-releasing hormone** (GnRH) produced by the hypothalamus. Production of LH is also stimulated by feedback of estrogens secreted by follicular cells of the ovary. A sudden increase (surge) in the level of LH takes place near the middle of the menstrual cycle, and stimulates ovulation that takes place about 36 hours after the surge.
>
> Apart from hormones, nervous and emotional influences may affect the ovarian and menstrual cycles. An emotional disturbance may delay or even prevent menstruation.

CERVIX

General Features
The cervix is the lower, narrow cylindrical part of the uterus. The cervical canal is narrow and communicates with the uterine cavity at its upper end and with vagina at its lower end. The upper and lower openings are referred to as internal and external os, respectively. The lower portion of cervix, which projects into vagina, is called as ***portio vaginalis***.

Microscopic Features
- The structure of the cervix of the uterus is somewhat different from that of the body. Here, the mucous membrane (or ***endocervix***) has a number of obliquely placed ***palmate folds***. It contains deep branching glands that secrete mucous.
- The mucosa also shows small cysts that probably represent glandular elements that are distended with secretion. These cysts are called the ***Ovula Nabothi***.

- The mucous membrane of the upper two-thirds of the cervical canal is lined by ciliated columnar epithelium, but over its lower one-third the epithelium is nonciliated columnar. Near the external os, the canal is lined by stratified squamous epithelium.
- The part of the cervix that projects into vagina has an external surface that is covered by stratified squamous epithelium.
- The cervix has few smooth muscle fibers and mainly (85%) consists of dense connective tissue.
- The mucosa does not undergo remarkable changes during the menstrual cycle and does not desquamate during menstruation.
- During pregnancy, the cervical mucous glands proliferate and secrete a more viscous and abundant mucus.
- The lumen of the cervix is normally a narrow canal. It has tremendous capacity for dilation and, at the time of childbirth, it becomes large enough for the fetal head to pass through.

VAGINA

General Features

- The vagina is the female organ of copulation and forms the lower part of the birth canal.
- The vagina is a fibromuscular elastic tube that extends from lower part of the cervix to the external genitalia. It is about 8 cm long. It is capable of considerable elongation and distension, this being helped by the rich network of elastic fibers in its wall.

Microscopic Features

From within outward, the wall of the vagina consists of mucous, muscular, and serous layers (Plate 21.5).

Mucous Membrane

- The mucous membrane shows numerous longitudinal folds, and is firmly fixed to the underlying muscle layer. It consists of lamina propria and epithelium.
- It is lined by stratified squamous nonkeratinized epithelium and devoid of mucous glands. The vaginal surface being kept moist by secretions of glands in the cervix of the uterus. The vaginal fluid is derived from the transudate present in the lamina propria and secretions from cervix.
- The epithelial cells are rich in glycogen. Naturally occurring vaginal bacterial flora metabolize the glycogen forming lactic acid and protects the vagina from invasion of pathogenic bacteria. Bacterial infection of the vagina is common during childhood and after menopause as the acidity is low.
- The lamina propria is composed of loose connective tissue and contains plexus of blood vessels, lymphatics, and nerves. The tissue is rich in elastic fibers.

Muscle Coat

- The muscle coat is made up of an outer longitudinal and a much thinner inner circular layers of smooth muscles layers.
- Many elastic fibers are present among the muscle fibers.
- The lower end of the vagina is surrounded by striated muscle fibers (bulbospongiosus muscle) that form the sphincter at its external opening.

Adventitia/Serous

The muscle wall is surrounded by an adventitia made up of fibrous tissue containing many elastic fibers. It is derived from peritoneum and covers only the posterior fornix of vagina.

FEMALE EXTERNAL GENITALIA

The external genitalia consist of labia majora, labia minora, vestibule, and clitoris.

- **Labia majora** are two folds of skin with adipose tissue and a thin layer of smooth muscle. It is covered by coarse hair on their external surface and is devoid of hair on the inner surface. Numerous sebaceous and sweat glands are present. The homolog of this is scrotum in the male.
- **Labia minora** are present medial to and slightly deep to the labia majora. They are two smaller folds of skin without hair follicles and adipose tissue. The mucous membrane is made up of a core of connective tissue that is covered by stratified squamous epithelium. Modified sebaceous glands are present. It is the homolog of urethral surface of penis in male.
- The cleft between the two labia minora is the **vestibule**. It receives the secretions of the glands of Bartholin, which are paired mucous glands. Orifices of vagina and urethra are located here.
- **Clitoris** is regarded as a miniature penis, with the important difference that the urethra does not pass through it. Two erectile bodies called *corpora cavernosa* and a *glans* are present. The surface of the clitoris is covered by mucous membrane and not skin that is lined by stratified squamous epithelium. The mucosa is richly supplied with nerves.

CHAPTER 21: Female Reproductive System

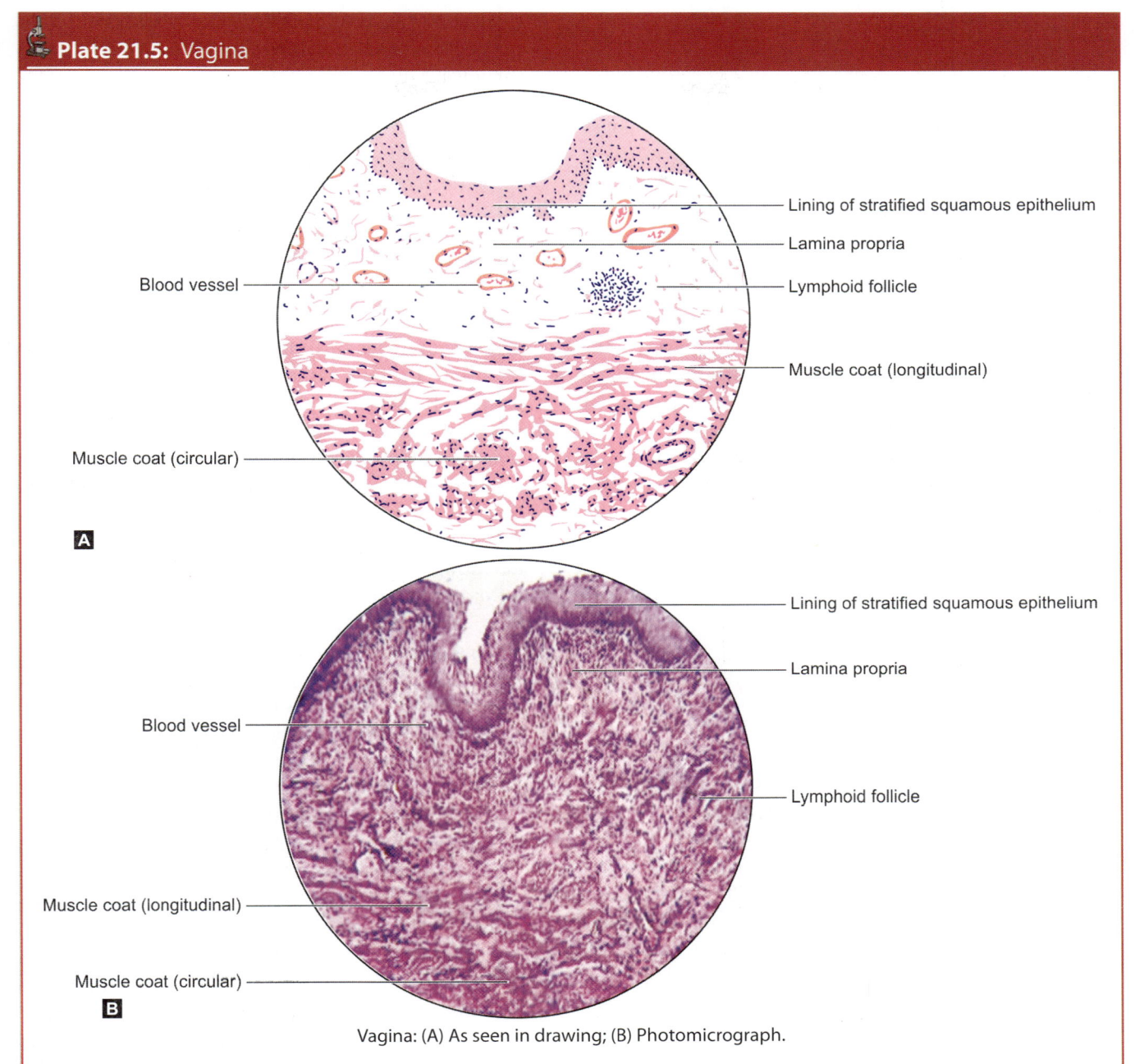

Plate 21.5: Vagina

Vagina: (A) As seen in drawing; (B) Photomicrograph.

Points of identification
- The vagina is a fibromuscular structure consisting of an inner mucosa, a middle muscular layer, and an outer adventitia
- The mucosa consists of stratified squamous nonkeratinized epithelium and loose fibroelastic connective tissue lamina propria with many blood vessels and no glands
- The mucosa of vagina is rich in glycogen and hence, the cells are pale stained which distinguishes it from esophagus
- Muscular layer consists of smooth muscle fibers.

MAMMARY GLAND

General Features

- The mammary glands are present in both sexes but they remain rudimentary in the male and are well-developed in females after puberty.
- Mammary glands secrete milk which contains protein, lipids, lactose, lymphocytes and monocytes, antibodies, minerals, and fat-soluble vitamins to provide nourishment for the newborn.
- Mammary gland is a modified sweat gland. Each gland is a soft rounded elevation present over the pectoral region. The skin over the center of the elevation shows a darkly pigmented circular area called the *areola* and overlying the central part of the areola there is a projection called the *nipple*.
- Each mammary gland is covered by skin and deep to which it is made up of glandular, fibrous, and interlobar fatty tissue. The glandular masses are separated by connective tissue and of adipose tissue (Plate 21.6). The fascia covering the gland is connected to overlying skin by fibrous processes called the **suspensory ligaments** of Cooper.

Microscopic Features

The gland is made up of stroma and parenchyma. Parenchyma is mainly constituted by lactiferous glands with their ducts.

- The **glandular tissue** are of compound tubule alveolar type and arranged as 15 to 20 pyramidal lobes, each being drained by a separate **lactiferous duct**. The lobes are arranged in radiating manner and converge toward the areola. Near the areola, each duct dilates to form the **lactiferous sinus** and act as a reservoir of milk and finally the ducts open on to the nipple. Each duct drains a smaller segmental ducts and lobules. Each segmental duct divides into number of terminal ducts and from the latter numerous secretory glands pouch out to form **alveoli**.
- The area of parenchyma drained by one terminal duct is known as the **lobule**. The lobules are separated by fibro-fatty dense connective tissue and the alveoli are embedded in this intralobular connective tissue.
- The cells lining the alveoli vary in appearance in accordance with functional activity. In the "resting" phase, they are cuboidal and in actively producing alveoli, the cells become columnar. Myoepithelial cells are present between the cells and the basement membrane. Once the secretions are poured into lumen, reduction in the size lining cells to cuboid is observed but never to initial size. The cells are filled with secretory vacuoles.

Structure of Glandular Elements

The structure of the glandular elements of the mammary gland varies considerably at different periods of life as follows:

- **Before the onset of puberty**, the glandular tissue consists entirely of ducts.
- **Between puberty and the first pregnancy**, the duct system proliferates. At the end of each duct, solid masses of polyhedral cells are formed, but proper alveoli are few or absent. The bulk of the breast consists of connective tissue and fat that widely separate the glandular elements.
- **Resting/nonsecreting** mammary glands have same structure as the lactating gland except that they are smaller and they contain more connective tissue and less glandular tissue. The alveoli are lined by cuboidal epithelium and have a large lumen (Plate 21.6).
- **Lactating/active mammary glands (Plate 21.7):**
    - Mammary glands are activated by elevated level of estrogen and progesterone during pregnancy to become lactating glands.
    - During pregnancy, there is a proliferation and epithelial growth of terminal ducts and lobules with increase in the number of alveoli per lobule. The terminal portions of the ducts branch and grow and the alveoli develop and mature. Each lobe is filled with compound tubuloalveolar gland.
    - The development of breast tissue during pregnancy takes place under the influence of hormones produced by the hypophysis cerebri. Cells lining glandular tissue bear receptors for these hormones.
    - As the pregnancy progress, there is a hypertrophy of the glandular parenchyma and engorgement with **colostrum**, a protein-rich fluid. True milk secretion starts after a few days of delivery with the suckling of the newborn.
    - The alveoli are lined by columnar epithelium and surrounded by myoepithelial cells. The secretory cells possess abundant rough endoplasmic reticulum, mitochondria, several Golgi apparatus, lipid droplets, and numerous vesicles. Different alveoli display varying degrees of preparation for synthesis of milk substance.
    - Alveolar cells secrete lipid and proteins. Lipids are stored as droplets in the cytoplasm and released from the cells by **apocrine** mode of exocytosis. Proteins

CHAPTER 21: Female Reproductive System

Plate 21.6: Mammary gland (Resting)

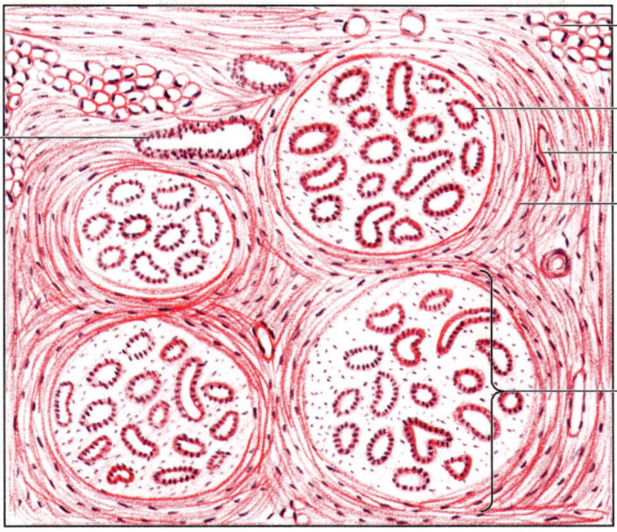

A — Labels: Interlobular duct, Adipose tissue, Alveoli, Blood vessel, Interlobular connective tissue, Lobule

B — Labels: Alveoli, Interlobular connective tissue, Interlobular duct, Lobule

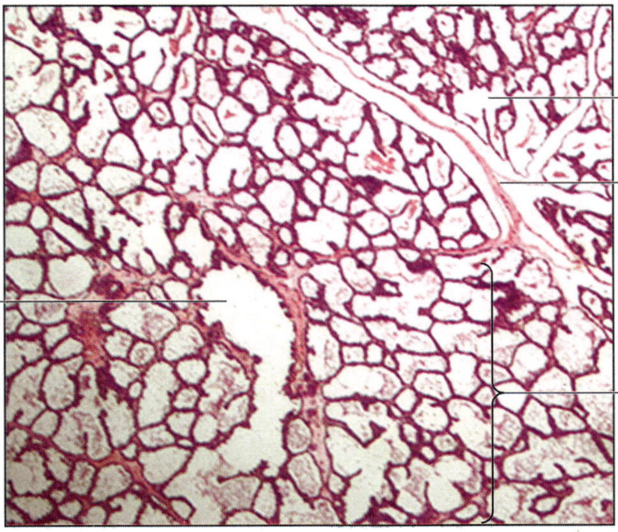

Mammary gland (Resting): (A) As seen in drawing; (B) Photomicrograph.

Points of identification
- Mammary gland consists of lobules of glandular tissue separated by considerable quantity of connective tissue and fat
- Nonlactating mammary glands contain more connective tissue and less glandular tissue
- The glandular elements or alveoli are distinctly tubular. They are lined by cuboidal epithelium and have a large lumen so that they look like ducts. Some of them may be in form of solid cords of cells
- Extensive branching of duct system seen.

are secreted from the cells by **merocrine** mode of exocytosis.

■ After lactation stops, the alveoli shrink, remaining milk is absorbed, and the glandular tissue returns to the resting condition. It undergoes atrophy after menopause.

Ducts System

❖ Each lobe drains into a ***lactiferous duct*** that opens at the summit of the nipple (Fig. 21.11). Beneath the nipple, the lactiferous duct dilates into ***lactiferous sinus***, which functions as a reservoir of milk.

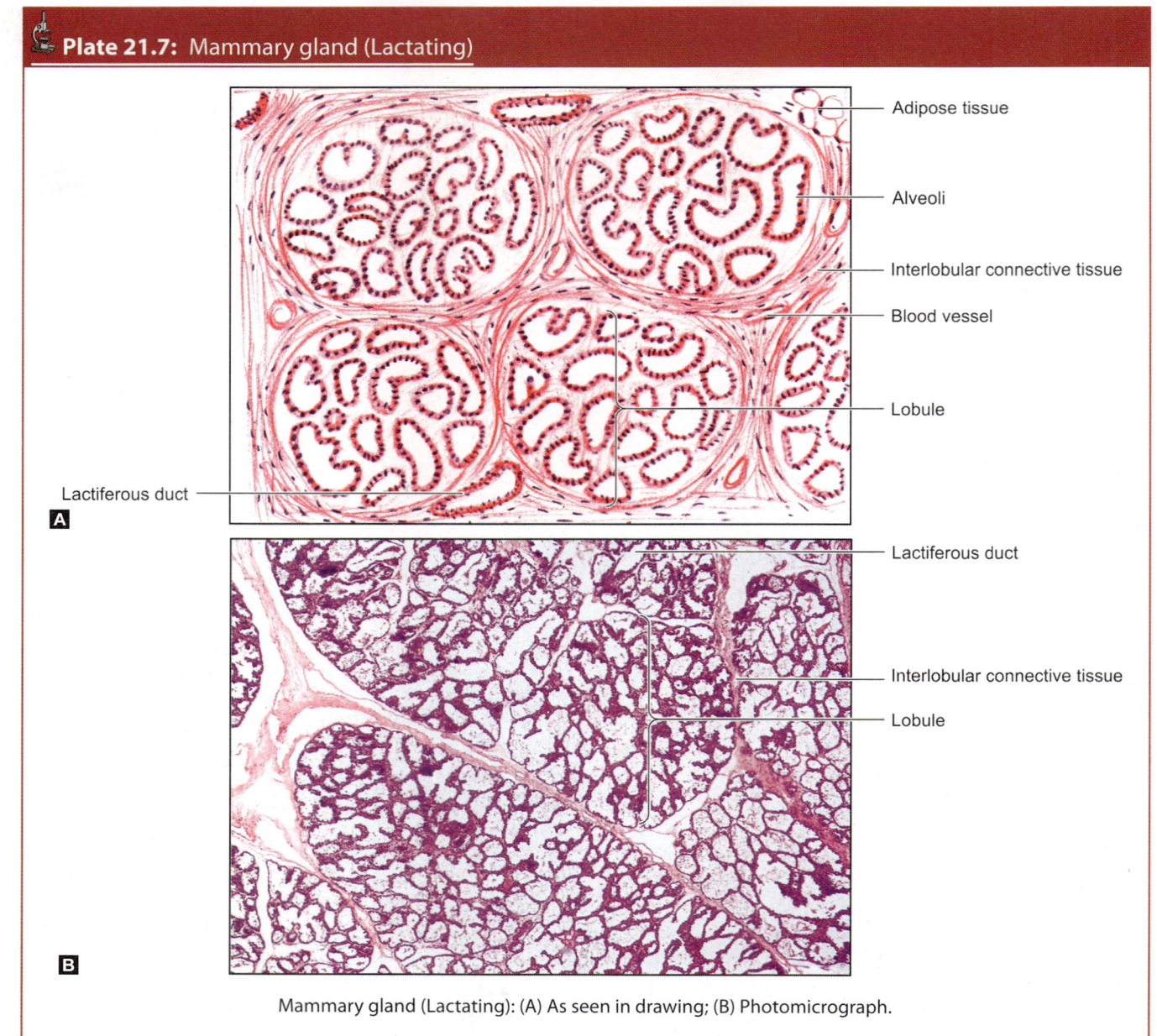

Plate 21.7: Mammary gland (Lactating)

Mammary gland (Lactating): (A) As seen in drawing; (B) Photomicrograph.

Points of identification
- In lactating mammary gland, the glandular elements proliferate so that they become relatively more prominent than the connective tissue
- The interlobular connective tissue septum is very thin
- The lobules are formed by compactly arranged alveoli
- The alveoli are lined by simple cuboidal secretory epithelium and associated myoepithelial cells. Their lumen contains eosinophilic secretory material which appears vacuolated due to the presence of fat droplets.

- The smaller ducts are lined by columnar epithelium but the larger ducts are lined by two or more layers of columnar epithelium and near their openings on the nipple, the lining becomes stratified squamous keratinized epithelium. Between the epithelium and the basement membrane of the ducts, the myoepithelial cells are present.
- Difference between structure of resting and lactating mammary gland is provided in Table 21.2.

CHAPTER 21: Female Reproductive System

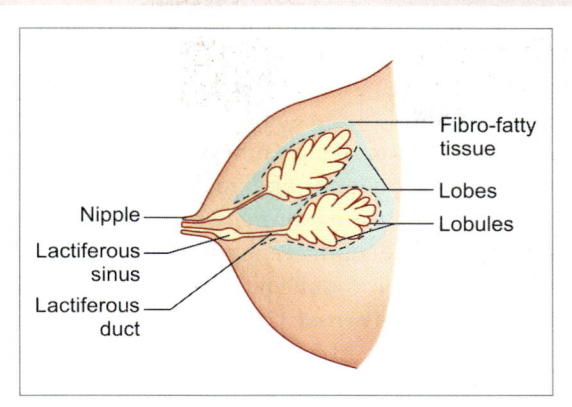

Fig. 21.11: Human female breast (schematic representation).

Table 21.2: Differences between resting and lactating mammary gland.

	Resting mammary gland	Lactating mammary gland
Stroma	Contains more connective tissue and less glandular tissue	Contains more glandular tissue and less connective tissue
Secretory units	Secretory units are few and poorly developed	Secretory units are numerous and are more developed
Alveoli	Lined by cuboidal epithelium and wider lumen	Lined by columnar epithelium and narrow lumen
Excretory ducts	Narrow and empty	Wider and filled with milk

Nipple and Areola

- The nipple is the conical projection below the center of the breast and is pierced by 15–20 lactiferous ducts.
- The nipple is covered by keratinized stratified squamous epithelium. It consists of dense connective tissue and smooth muscles arranged circularly and longitudinally. A circular muscle erects the nipple for suckling and longitudinal muscle retracts the nipple.
- Nipple has rich nerve supply and provided with sensory receptors for suckling.
- The pigmented skin around the nipple is called *areola*. The pigmentation is irreversibly darkened after pregnancy.
- The skin of the areola lacks hair follicles. Outer margin of the areola contains a number of modified sebaceous glands, which are enlarged during pregnancy and lactation and are known as **tubercles of Montgomery**. Oily secretion of these glands provides lubrication during lactation.
- Areola also contains sweat and accessory mammary glands. Skin of areola is devoid of hair and subcutaneous fat.

> **Added Information**
> - In the resting mammary gland, glandular epithelium is surrounded by an avascular zone containing fibroblasts. It has been claimed that this zone constitutes an *epitheliostromal junction* that controls passage of materials to glandular cells.
> - In the male, the mammary gland is rudimentary and consists of ducts that may be represented by solid cords of cells. The ducts do not extend beyond the areola.
> - During menstrual cycle, at the time of ovulation, there is increase in the estrogen level which leads to proliferation of the cells of the ducts.
> - Premenstrual phase breast engorgement is due to greater hydration of connective tissue.

APPLIED HISTOLOGY

Ovary

- **Ovarian tumors**: 70% of ovarian tumors arise from the epithelial surface.
- **Polycystic ovarian disease**: Ovaries are filled with numerous fluid-filled follicular cysts. This is associated with anovulation, irregular, or scanty menstruation. Also called as Stein–Leventhal syndrome.
- **Ovulation pain**: During ovulation, about 45% of women experience mid-cycle pain ("mittelschmerz") which is sharp, lower abdominal that lasts from a few minutes to as long as 24 hours.
- **Pregnancy test**: Human chorionic gonadotropin (hCG) produced by corpus luteum of pregnancy can be detected in urine as early as 10 to 14 days of pregnancy. It forms the basis of urine pregnancy test kits.

Fallopian Tube

Ectopic tubal pregnancy: The implantation of a fertilized ovum in the uterine tube is called as ectopic pregnancy. The most frequent site of tubal pregnancy is the ampullary portion and the least common is interstitial pregnancy.

Uterus

- **Dysfunctional uterine bleeding**: Dysfunctional uterine bleeding (DUB) is defined as excessive bleeding occurring during or between menstrual periods without a causative uterine lesion such as tumor, polyp, infection, hyperplasia, trauma, blood dyscrasia, or pregnancy.
- **Endometriosis**: Endometriosis refers to the presence of endometrial glands and stroma in abnormal locations

outside the uterus. Most common site being ovary followed by pouch of Douglas.

- **Adenomyosis**: Adenomyosis is defined as abnormal distribution of histologically benign endometrial tissue within the myometrium along with myometrial hypertrophy, due to either a metaplasia or estrogenic stimulation due to endocrine dysfunction of the ovary.

Vagina

Vaginitis: The most common causes of vaginitis are *Candida* (moniliasis) and *Trichomonas* (trichomoniasis). These infections are particularly common in pregnant and diabetic women and may involve both vulva and vagina. However, the adult vaginal mucosa is relatively resistant to gonococcal infection because of its structure.

Mammary Gland

- **Fibroadenoma**: Fibroadenoma or adenofibroma is a benign tumor of fibrous and epithelial elements. It is the most common benign tumor of the female breast. Though it can occur at any age during reproductive life, most patients are between 15 and 30 years of age. Clinically, fibroadenoma generally appears as a solitary, discrete, and freely mobile nodule within the breast.
- **Carcinoma of the breast**: Cancer of the breast is among the most common of human cancers throughout the world. The incidence of breast cancer is highest in the perimenopausal age group and is uncommon before the age of 25 years. Clinically, the breast cancer usually presents as a solitary, painless, and palpable lump which is detected quite often by self-examination.

MULTIPLE CHOICE QUESTIONS

1. What are developing gametes called?
   a. Oogenesis
   b. Ovary
   c. Oocyte
   d. Ova
2. Which stage of the follicle is arrested in prophase?
   a. Primordial follicle
   b. Primary follicle
   c. Secondary follicle
   d. Mature follicle
3. What is the cavity within a secondary follicle?
   a. Graafian follicle
   b. Theca folliculi
   c. Zona pellucida
   d. Antrum
4. Which of these correctly describe the sequence of the follicular phase?
   a. Graafian follicle stage, secondary (antral follicle) stage, growing follicle stage, and primary follicle stage
   b. Graafian follicle stage, growing follicle stage, primary follicle stage, and secondary (antral follicle) stage
   c. Growing follicle stage, primary follicle stage, secondary (antral follicle) stage, and Graafian follicle stage
   d. Primary follicle stage, growing follicle stage, secondary (antral follicle) stage, and Graafian follicle stage
5. Which of these secrete androgens in corpus luteum?
   a. Connective septa
   b. Granulosa-lutein cells
   c. Theca lutein cells
   d. Corpus albicans
6. Which of these secrete progesterone in corpus luteum?
   a. Connective septa
   b. Granulosa-lutein cells
   c. Theca lutein cells
   d. Corpus albicans
7. What is the name given to the type of cells surrounding oocyte which are cuboidal?
   a. Granulosa
   b. Leydig
   c. Sertoli
   d. Theca
8. What is the layer which is thick glycoprotein and acid proteoglycan between oocyte and granulosa cells?
   a. Antrum
   b. Mature follicle
   c. Theca
   d. Zona pellucida
9. Which of the following cells have a haploid chromosome number?
   a. Spermatogonia
   b. Oogonia
   c. Primary oocyte
   d. Secondary spermatocyte
10. Intralobular ducts drain into interlobular ducts which join to form a single excretory duct—the lactiferous duct.
    a. True
    b. False
11. What types of glands are found in the areola that alter pH and discourages bacterial growth?
    a. Sweat
    b. Montgomery
    c. Eccrine
    d. Ebner's
12. Uterine tube is lined by -------------- epithelium.
    a. Simple columnar
    b. Ciliated columnar
    c. Stratified columnar
    d. Pseudostratified columnar
13. Palmate folds are present in which part of uterus?
    a. Fundus
    b. Body
    c. Cervix
    d. Vagina
14. Alveoli of lactating mammary gland is lined by ---------- epithelium.
    a. Squamous
    b. Cuboidal
    c. Columnar
    d. Stratified

Answers

1. d 2. a 3. d 4. c 5. c 6. b 7. a 8. d 9. d
10. a 11. b 12. b 13. c 14. c

CHAPTER 22

Endocrine System

Learning objectives

To study the:
- Chemical structure of hormones
- Distribution of endocrine cells
- Hypophysis cerebri—parts, cells, secretion, and function
- Blood supply of pituitary gland
- Thyroid gland—cells, synthesis of hormone, and function
- Parathyroid gland—cells, secretion, and function
- Suprarenal gland (cortex and medulla)—layers, cells, secretion, and function
- Pineal gland
- Paraganglia, aortic bodies, and carotid body
- Applied histology

IDENTIFICATION POINTS

Pituitary gland	Thyroid gland	Adrenal gland
☐ Pars anterior, pars intermedia, and pars posterior ☐ Presence of chromophils and chromophobes in the anterior lobe ☐ Presence of unmyelinated nerve fibers with pituicytes and Herring bodies in the posterior lobe ☐ Follicles in pars intermedia.	☐ Colloid-filled follicles are seen ☐ Follicles are lined by cuboidal/columnar epithelium ☐ Parafollicular cells between follicular cells and basement membrane/ in between follicles are seen.	☐ Outer cortex and inner medulla ☐ Cortex is divided into zona glomerulosa, zona fasciculata, and zona reticularis ☐ Chromaffin cells are seen in medulla.

INTRODUCTION

- Endocrine glands are ductless glands whose secretions are carried to specific destinations through vascular system.
- The secretions of endocrine cells are called **hormones** (*Gr—hormaein* = to excite). They interact with specific hormone receptors to alter biologic activity of the target cells.
- Along with the autonomic nervous system, the endocrine organs coordinate and control the metabolic activities and the internal environment of the body.
- Feedback mechanisms (positive or negative) regulate hormonal function.
- Endocrine tissues are highly vascular. The secretory pole of an endocrine cell is toward the wall of a capillary (or sinusoid).
- Endocrine gland includes pituitary, suprarenal, thyroid, and parathyroid glands, etc.

HORMONES

- Hormones are chemical messengers that are produced by endocrine glands and delivered by bloodstream to target cells or organs.
- A hormone acts on cells that bear specific receptors for it. Some hormones act only on one organ or on one type of cell, while other hormones may have widespread effects.
- On the basis of their chemical structure, hormones belong to four main types:
  1. **Amino acid derivatives**, for example, adrenalin, noradrenalin, and thyroxine.
  2. **Small peptides**, for example, encephalin, vasopressin, and thyroid-releasing hormone.
  3. **Proteins**, for example, insulin, parathormone, and thyroid-stimulating hormone.
  4. **Steroids**, for examples, progesterone, estrogens, testosterone, and cortisol.

DISTRIBUTION OF ENDOCRINE CELLS

Endocrine cells are distributed in three different ways:
1. Some **organs** are entirely endocrine in function. They are referred to as **endocrine glands** (or **ductless glands**). Example are the hypophysis cerebri/pituitary, the pineal gland, the thyroid gland, the parathyroid glands, and the suprarenal/adrenal glands.
2. **Groups of endocrine cells** may be present in organs that have other functions. They include the islets of the pancreas, the interstitial cells of the testes, and the follicles and corpora lutea of the ovaries. Hormones are also produced by some cells in the kidneys, the thymus, and the placenta. Some authors describe the liver as being partly an endocrine gland.
3. **Isolated endocrine cells** may be distributed in the epithelial lining of an organ like gastrointestinal tract (GIT) and respiratory tract. Cells in many locations in the body produce amines that have endocrine functions. Many of these amines also act as neurotransmitters or as neuromodulators. These widely distributed cells are grouped together as the **neuroendocrine system** or the amine precursor uptake and decarboxylation **(APUD) cell system**.

HYPOPHYSIS CEREBRI

- ❖ The hypophysis cerebri is also called the **pituitary gland** and is approximately the size of a pea.
- ❖ It is suspended from the floor of the third ventricle (of the brain) by a narrow funnel-shaped stalk called the **infundibulum**, and lies in a depression on the upper surface of the sphenoid bone, called **sella turcica**.
- ❖ It produces several hormones some of which profoundly influence the activities of other endocrine tissues and is sometimes referred as "**master endocrine gland**". Its own activity is influenced by the hypothalamus, and by the pineal body.
- ❖ The hypophysis cerebri is divided into **adenohypophysis and neurohypophysis** (Fig. 22.1).
    - ■ **Adenohypophysis/anterior lobe**: The pars anterior also called the **pars distalis** and the **pars**

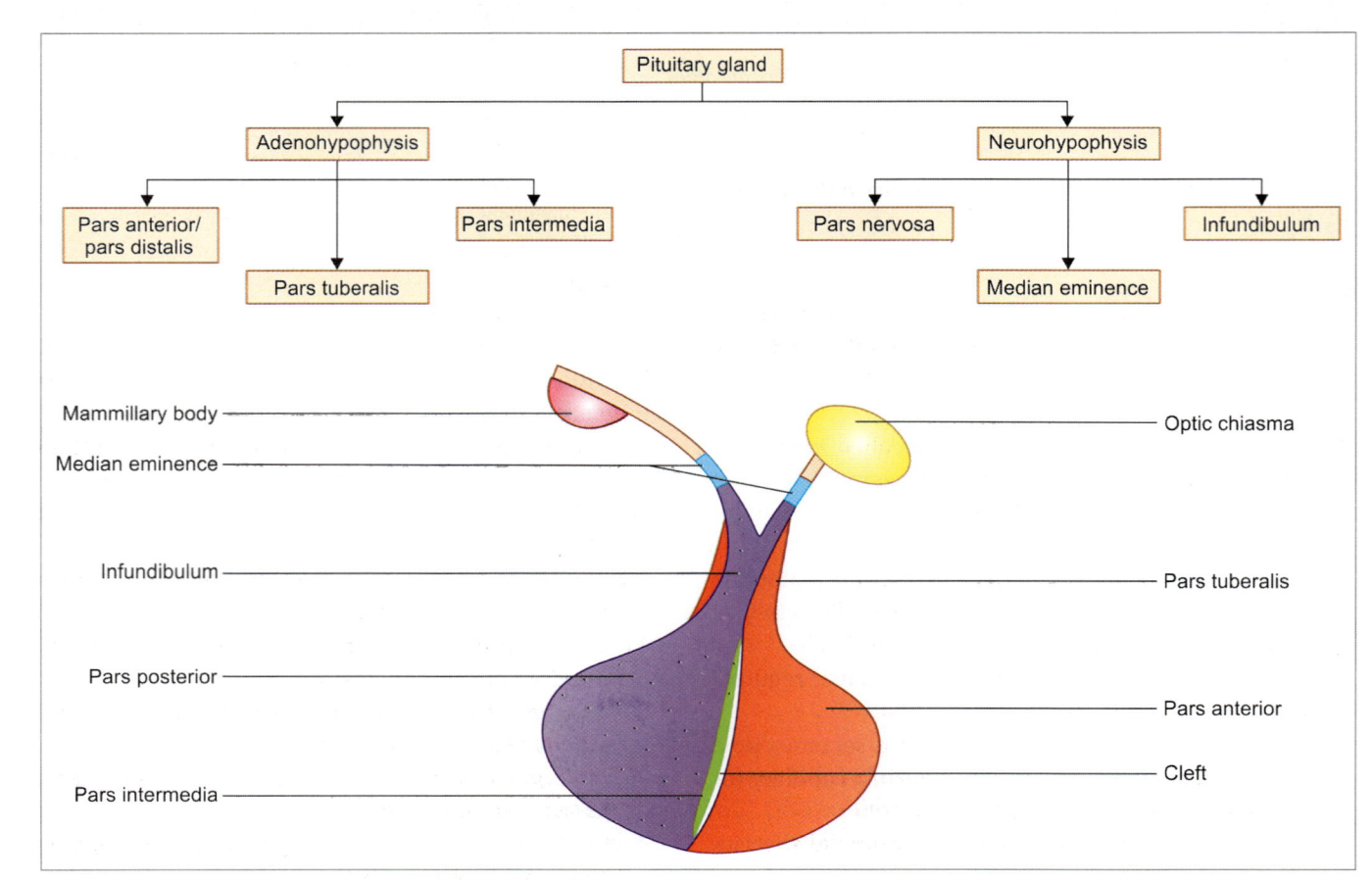

Fig. 22.1: Subdivisions of the hypophysis cerebri (schematic diagram).

CHAPTER 22: Endocrine System

intermedia, are both made up of cells having a direct secretory function. They are collectively referred to as the **adenohypophysis**. An extension of the pars anterior surrounds the central nervous core of the infundibulum. Because of its tubular shape, this extension is called the **pars tuberalis**. The pars tuberalis is part of the adenohypophysis.

- **Neurohypophysis/posterior lobe**: The pars posterior contains numerous nerve fibers. It is directly continuous with the central core of the infundibular stalk which is made up of nervous tissue. The pars posterior and infundibular stalks are together referred to as the **neurohypophysis**. The area in the floor of the third ventricle (tuber cinereum) immediately adjoining the attachment to it of the infundibulum is called the **median eminence**. Some authorities include the median eminence in the neurohypophysis.

Adenohypophysis (Plate 22.1)

Pars Anterior/Pars Distalis/Anterior Lobe

- Anterior lobe is covered by fibrous capsule and consists of cords of cells separated by fenestrated sinusoids.
- The parenchymal cells of the pars anterior consist of chromophils (cells have affinity for dyes) and chromophobes (cells have no affinity for dyes). (a) *Chromophil cells* that have brightly staining granules in their cytoplasm and (b) *Chromophobe cells* in which granules are not prominent.

Chromophil cells

- Chromophil cells have affinity for histological dyes and are further classified as *acidophil* when their granules stain with acid dyes (like eosin or orange G), or *basophil* when the granules stain with basic dyes (like hematoxylin). Basophil granules are also periodic acid-Schiff (PAS) stain positive. The acidophil cells are often called *alpha cells*, and the basophils are called *beta cells* (Plate 22.2).
- Electron microscope (EM) examination shows that both acidophil and basophil cells contain abundant dense cored vesicles in the cytoplasm.
- **Acidophils**: Acidophils are most abundant cells in pars anterior. Acidophils can be divided into subtypes on the basis of the size and shape of the granules in them.
  Types of acidophil cells:
  - *Somatotrophs* produce the **somatotropic hormone/ somatotropin (STH)**, or **growth hormone (GH)**. This hormone controls body growth, especially before puberty.

- *Mammotrophs/lactotrophs* produce the **mammotropic hormone** [also called **mammotropin, prolactin (PRL), lactogenic hormone**, or LTH] which stimulates the growth and activity of the female mammary gland during pregnancy and lactation.

- **Basophil cells**: Basophils stain blue with basic dyes and it is usually located at the periphery of pars distalis.
  Types of basophilic cells:
  - *Corticotrophs* (or *corticotropes*) produce the **corticotropic hormone/adrenocorticotropin** or ACTH. This hormone stimulates the secretion of some hormones of the adrenal cortex. The staining characters of these cells are intermediate between those of acidophils and basophils. Other corticotropic hormones that have been identified are β-lipotropin (β-LPH), α-melanocyte-stimulating hormone (α-MSH), and β-endorphin.
  - *Thyrotrophs* (or *thyrotropes*) produce the **thyrotropic hormone** (**thyrotropin** or TSH) which stimulates the activity of the thyroid gland.
  - *Gonadotrophs* (*gonadotropes*, or *delta basophils*) produce two types of hormones, each type having a different action in the male and female.
    - In the female, the first of these hormones stimulates the growth of ovarian follicles. It is, therefore, called the **follicle-stimulating hormone** (FSH). It also stimulates the secretion of estrogens by the ovaries. In the male, the same hormone stimulates spermatogenesis.
    - In the female, the second hormone stimulates the maturation of the corpus luteum, and secretion of progesterone by it. It is called the **luteinizing hormone** (LH). In the male, the same hormone stimulates the production of androgens by the interstitial cells of the testes, and is called the **interstitial cell-stimulating hormone** (ICSH).

Chromophobe cells

- These cells do not stain darkly as they contain very few granules in their cytoplasm. Immunocytochemistry shows that they represent cells similar to the various types of chromophils mentioned earlier (including mammotrophs, somatotrophs, thyrotrophs, gonadotrophs, or corticotrophs).
- They are probably degranulated chromophils.
  i. Somatotrophs constitute about 50%, mammotrophs about 25%, corticotrophs 15–20%, and gonadotrophs about 10% of the cell population of the pars anterior.

Plate 22.1: Hypophysis cerebri

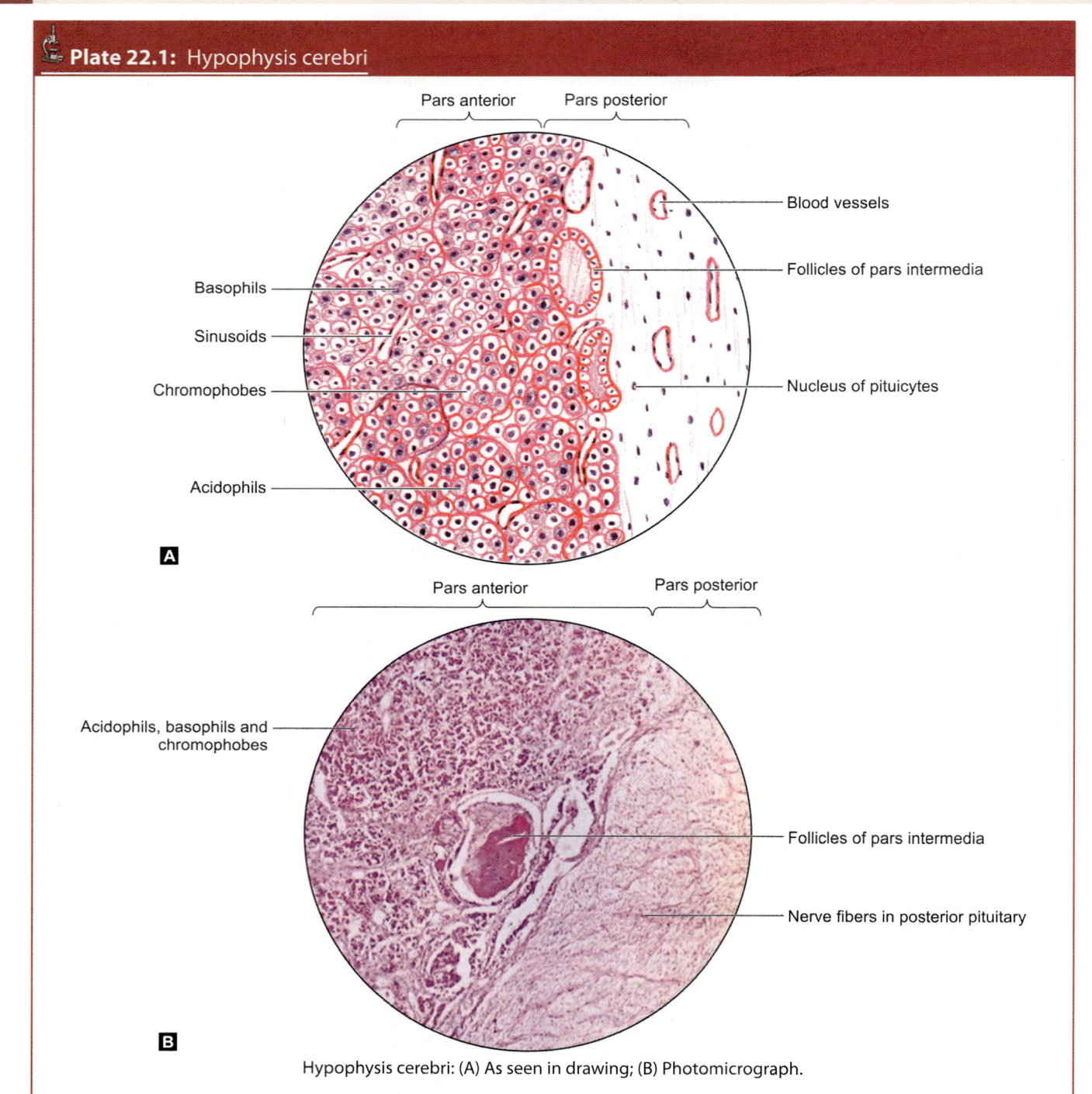

Hypophysis cerebri: (A) As seen in drawing; (B) Photomicrograph.

Points of identification
The hypophysis cerebri consists of three main parts:
- Pars anterior is cellular
- Pars intermedia is variable in structure
- Pars posterior consists of fibers, and is lightly stained.

CHAPTER 22: Endocrine System

Plate 22.2: Pars anterior

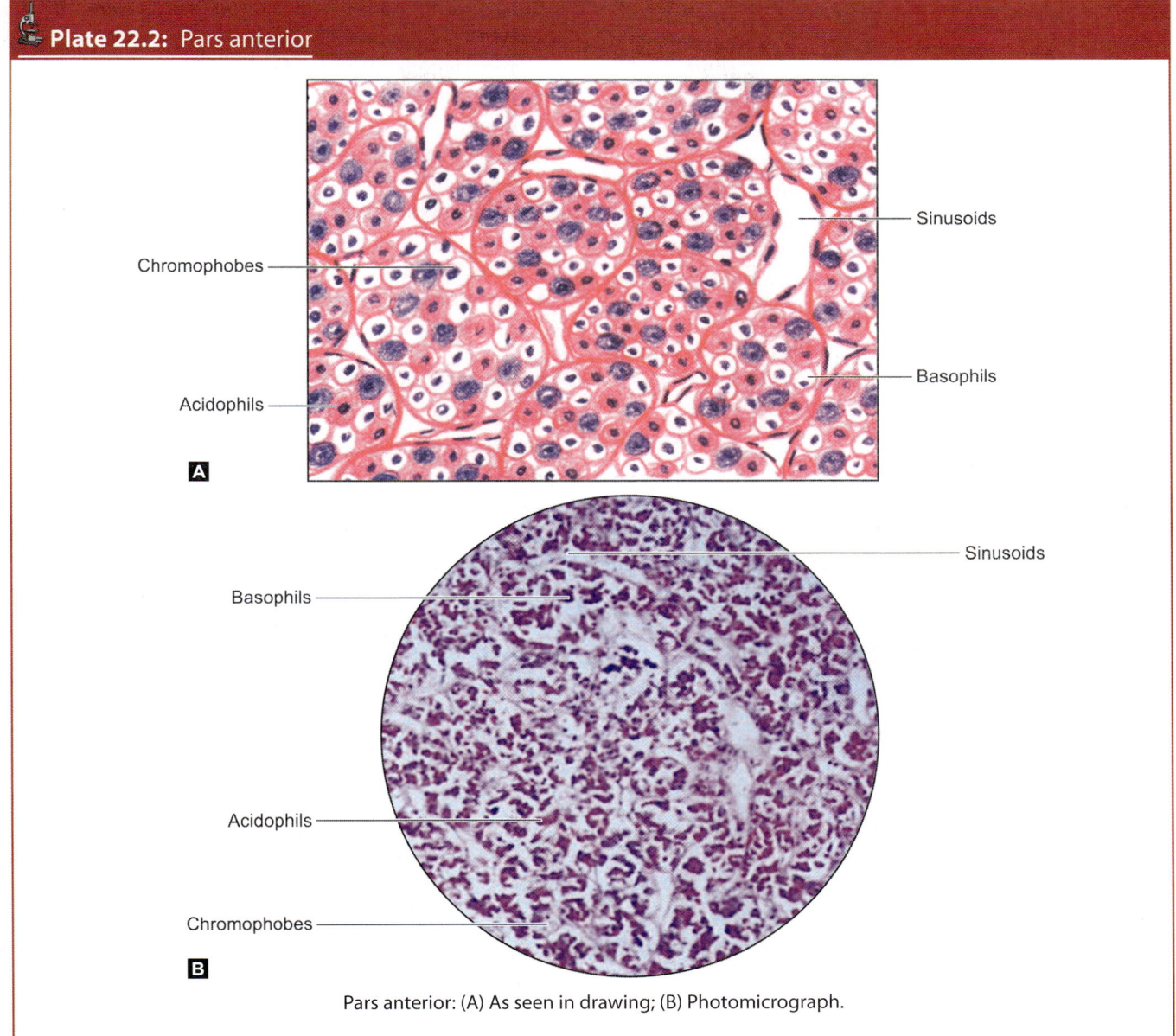

Pars anterior: (A) As seen in drawing; (B) Photomicrograph.

Points of identification
- It consists of groups or cords of cells.
- The cells are of three types:
  1. The pink staining cells are alpha cells or acidophils
  2. The cells with bluish cytoplasm are beta cells or basophils
  3. Cells in which the cytoplasm is not conspicuous, and the nuclei are closely packed, are chromophobe cells
- Numerous sinusoids are present between the groups of cells.

ii. Somatotrophs are located mainly in the lateral parts of the anterior lobe. Thyrotrophs are concentrated in the anterior, median part; and corticotrophs in the posterior, median part. Gonadotrophs and mammotrophs are scattered throughout the anterior lobe.

Pars Tuberalis

The pars tuberalis surrounds the infundibulum of neurohypophysis and consists mainly of undifferentiated cells. Some acidophil and basophil cells are also present.

Pars Intermedia

- This is poorly developed in the human hypophysis. In ordinary preparations, the most conspicuous feature is the presence of colloid-filled vesicles/follicles (Fig. 22.2). The vesicles are remnants of the pouch of Rathke.
- Beta cells, other secretory cells, and chromophobe cells are present. Some cells of the pars intermedia produce the *melanocyte-stimulating hormone* (MSH) which causes increased pigmentation of the skin. Other cells produce ACTH. *Endorphins* are present in the cytoplasm of secretory cells.

Note: The secretion of hormones from the adenohypophysis is under control of the hypothalamus as described later.

Neurohypophysis

Pars Posterior/Pars Nervosa

- The pars posterior consists of numerous unmyelinated nerve fibers which are the axons of secretory neurons located in supraoptic and paraventricular nuclei of the hypothalamus (Fig. 22.2).
- Situated between these axons, there are supporting cells of a special type called **pituicytes**. These cells have long dendritic processes many of which lie parallel to the nerve fibers.
- The pars posterior of the hypophysis is associated with the release of vasopressin and oxytocin. The axons descending into the pars posterior from the hypothalamus end in terminals closely related to capillaries.
- The neurosecretions/hormones secreted by supraoptic and paraventricular nuclei travel through these neurons and stored along the axons as well as at dilated nerve terminals. Collection of secretory granules at nerve terminal is called **Herring bodies** (Fig. 22.3).
- Hormones released at pars nervosa are vasopressin from supraoptic and oxytocin from paraventricular nuclei. Here, they are released into the capillaries of the region and enter the general circulation.
  - *Vasopressin* (also called the *antidiuretic hormone* or ADH): This hormone controls reabsorption of water by kidney tubules.
  - *Oxytocin*: It controls the contraction of smooth muscle of the uterus and also of the mammary gland.

Blood Supply of Hypophysis Cerebri

- The hypophysis cerebri is supplied by superior and inferior branches arising from the internal carotid arteries. Some branches also arise from the anterior and posterior cerebral arteries.
- The inferior hypophyseal arteries are distributed mainly to the pars posterior.
- Branches from the superior set of arteries supply the median eminence and infundibulum.
- Superior hypophyseal arteries divide into a plexus of fenestrated capillaries. These plexus join to form portal vessels. These portal vessels descend through the infundibular stalk and end in the pars anterior as secondary capillary plexus called sinusoids. The sinusoids are drained by veins that end in neighboring venous sinuses.
- The earlier arrangement is unusual in that two sets of capillaries intervene between the arteries and veins.

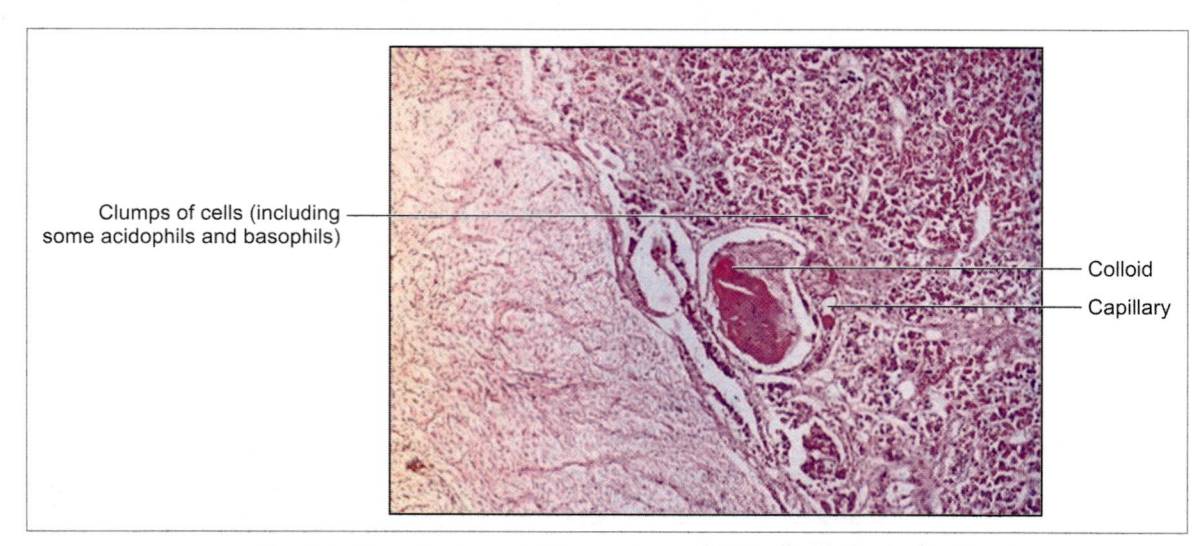

Fig. 22.2: Hypophysis cerebri. Pars posterior (left) and pars intermedia (right).

CHAPTER 22: Endocrine System

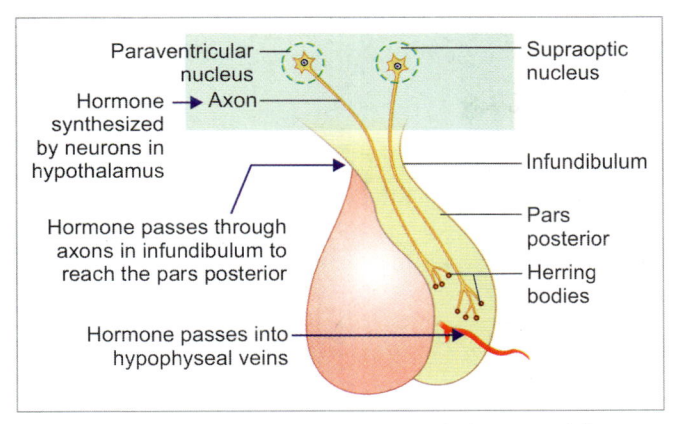

Fig. 22.3: The relationship between hypothalamus and the pars posterior of the hypophysis cerebri (schematic representation).

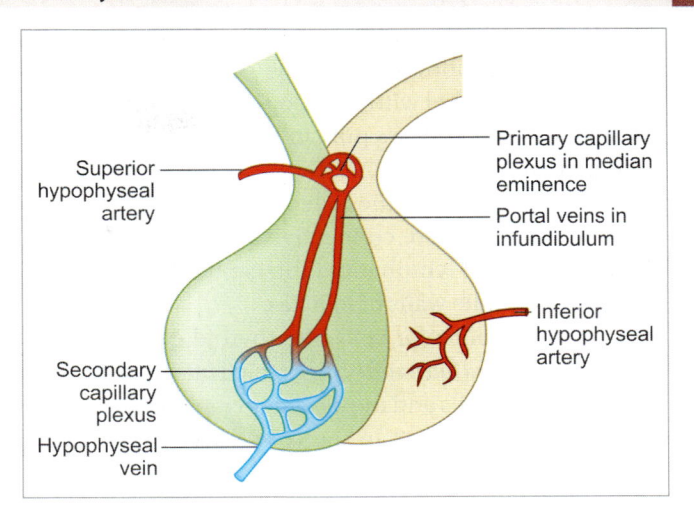

Fig. 22.4: Hypothalamo-hypophyseal portal system (schematic representation).

One of these is in the median eminence and the upper part of the infundibulum. The second set of capillaries is represented by the sinusoids of the pars anterior. This arrangement is referred to as the **hypothalamo-hypophyseal portal system** (Fig. 22.4).

Control of Secretion of Hormones

- The secretion of hormones by the adenohypophysis takes place under higher control of neurons in the hypothalamus, notably those in the median eminence and in the infundibular nucleus. The axons of these neurons end in relation to capillaries in the median eminence and in the upper part of the infundibulum.
- Different neurons produce specific *releasing factors* (or releasing hormones) for each hormone of the adenohypophysis. These factors are released into the capillaries.
- Portal vessels arising from the capillaries carry these factors to the pars anterior of the hypophysis. Here, they stimulate the release of appropriate hormones.
- Some factors inhibit the release of hormones. The synthesis and discharge of releasing factors by the neurons are under nervous control.
- As these neurons serve as intermediaries between nerve impulse and hormone secretion, they have been referred to as **neuroendocrine transducers**. Some cells called *tanycytes*, present in ependyma, may transport releasing factors from neurons into the cerebrospinal fluid (CSF), or from CSF to blood capillaries. They may, thus, play a role in control of the adenohypophysis.
- The entire neurohypophysis (from the median eminence to the pars posterior) is permeated by a continuous network of capillaries in which blood may flow **in either direction**. The capillaries provide a route through which hormones released in the pars posterior can travel back to the hypothalamus, and into CSF. Some veins draining the pars posterior pass into the adenohypophysis. Secretions by the adenohypophysis may, thus, be controlled not only from the median eminence, but by the entire neurohypophysis. Blood flow in veins connecting the pars anterior and pars posterior may be reversible providing a feedback from adenohypophysis to the neurohypophysis.

THYROID GLAND

General Features

- Thyroid is a bilobed gland. Each lobe is situated on either side of trachea, below larynx, and in lower neck.
- The two lobes are connected to each other by **isthmus** in front of trachea.
- Peculiarities: (a) stores hormone in the form of colloid, (b) superficially located, and (c) depends on environment for secretion (iodine).

Microscopic Features

- The thyroid gland is covered by a dense irregular connective tissue capsule derived from deep cervical fascia. Parathyroid glands are embedded within the capsule on posterior aspect of the thyroid gland. Septa extending into the gland from the capsule divide it into lobules.
- On microscopic examination, each lobule is seen to be made up of an aggregation of *follicles*.

- Each follicle is lined by **follicular cells** that rest on a basement membrane.
- The follicle is filled with a homogeneous material called **colloid** which appears pink in hematoxylin and eosin-stained sections (Plate 22.3).
- The spaces between the follicles are filled by a stroma made up of delicate connective tissue with numerous capillaries and lymphatics. The capillaries lie in close contact with the walls of follicles.
- Apart from follicular cells, the thyroid gland contains C-cells (or **parafollicular cells**) which intervene between the follicular cells and the basement membrane and also between the follicles in the connective tissue stroma (Plate 22.3).

Follicular Cells

- The follicular cells vary in shape from squamous, cuboidal, and to columnar depending on the level of their activity (Fig. 22.5).
- Highly active follicle is lined by columnar cells with scanty colloid, moderate active follicle is lined by cuboidal cells with moderate colloid, and inactive follicle is lined by squamous cells with abundant colloid. Different follicles may show different levels of activity (Fig. 22.5).
- Follicular cells have a round to ovoid nucleus with two nucleoli and basophilic cytoplasm.
- With the EM, a follicular cell shows the presence of apical microvilli, abundant granular endoplasmic reticulum, and a prominent supranuclear Golgi complex. Lysosomes, microtubules, and microfilaments are also present. The apical part of the cell contains many secretory vacuoles (Fig. 22.6).
- The activity of follicular cells is influenced by the thyroid-stimulating hormone (TSH or thyrotropin) produced by the hypophysis cerebri.
- The follicular cells secrete triiodothyronine (T3) with three atoms of iodine and tetraiodothyronine (T4) or thyroxine with four atoms of iodine in each molecule. These hormones influence the rate of metabolism.

C-cells (Parafollicular Cells)

- They are also called **clear cells**, or **light cells**. C-cells share features of the APUD cell system and derived from neural crest cells.
- The cells are polyhedral with oval eccentric nuclei.
- Typically, they lie between the follicular cells and their basement membrane. They may, however, lie between adjoining follicular cells, but they do not reach the lumen and may also lie in the connective tissue between the follicles in groups.

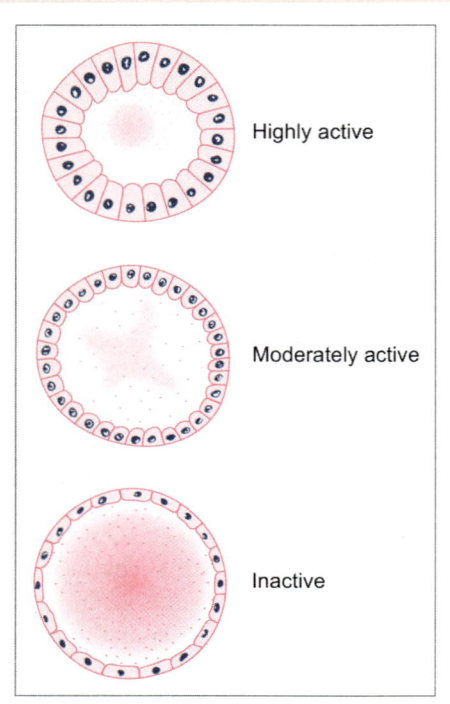

Fig. 22.5: Variations in appearance of thyroid follicles at different levels of activity (schematic representation).

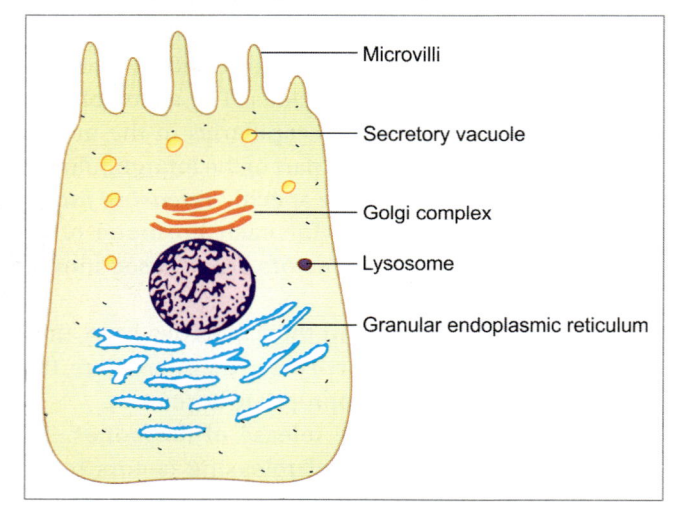

Fig. 22.6: Ultrastructure of a follicular cell of the thyroid gland (schematic representation).

- With the EM, the cells show well-developed granular endoplasmic reticulum, Golgi complexes, numerous mitochondria, and membrane-bound secretory granules.
- C-cells secrete the hormone **calcitonin**.
- This hormone has an action opposite to that of the parathyroid hormone on calcium metabolism.

CHAPTER 22: Endocrine System

Plate 22.3: Thyroid gland

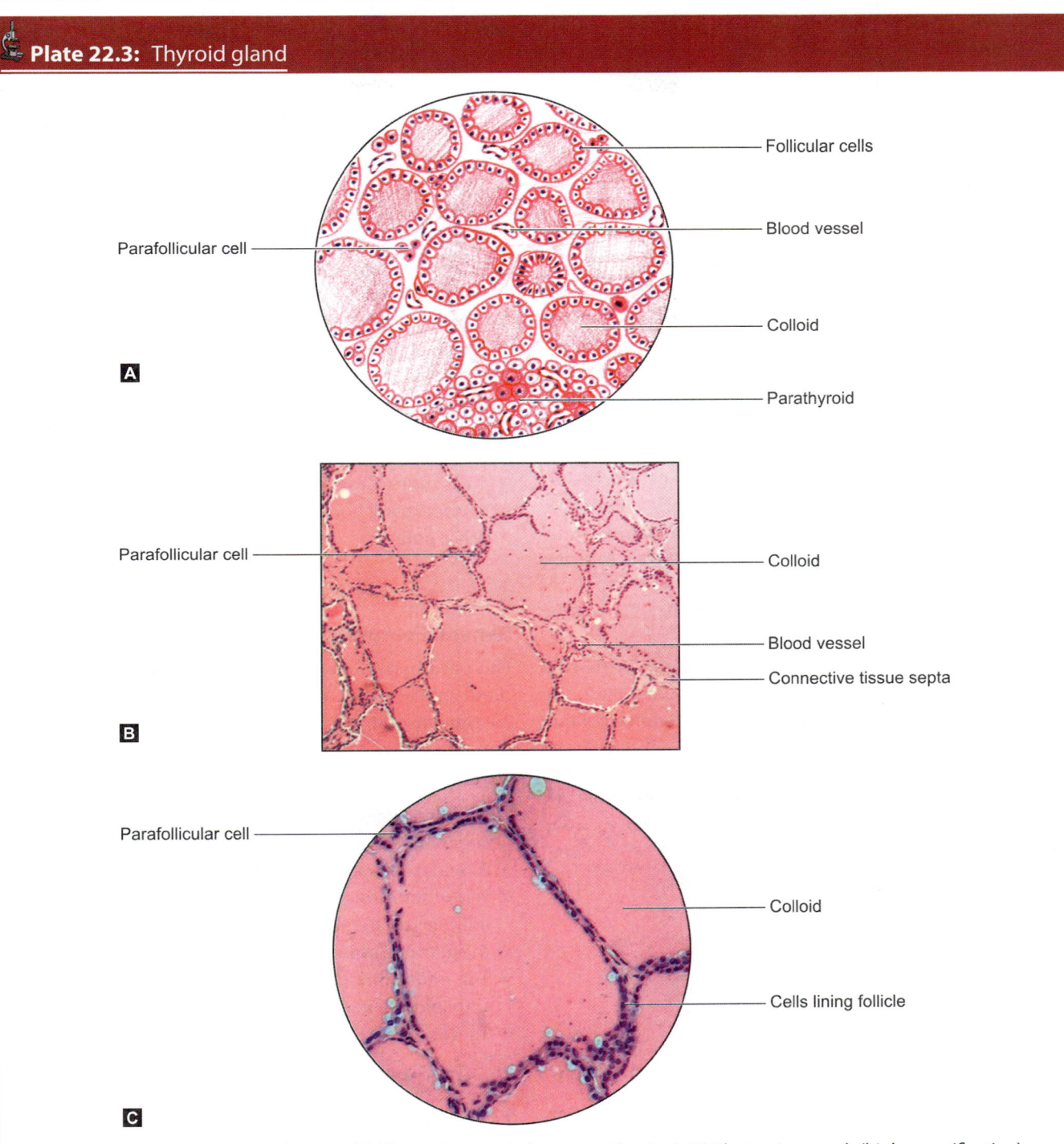

A — Labels: Parafollicular cell, Follicular cells, Blood vessel, Colloid, Parathyroid

B — Labels: Parafollicular cell, Colloid, Blood vessel, Connective tissue septa

C — Labels: Parafollicular cell, Colloid, Cells lining follicle

Thyroid gland: (A) As seen in drawing; (B) Photomicrograph (low magnification); (C) Photomicrograph (high magnification).

Points of identification
- The thyroid gland is made up of follicles lined by cuboidal epithelium
- In photomicrograph, in low magnification, it can be seen that follicles vary in shape and size
- Each follicle is filled with a homogenous pink colloid proteinaceous material composed primarily of thyroglobulin that has been produced by the follicular epithelial cells
- Parafollicular cells are present in relation to the follicles and also as groups in the connective tissue
- In the intervals between the follicles, there is some connective tissue and blood vessels between follicles.

- It mainly lowers the blood calcium level when serum calcium level is high by suppressing release of calcium ions from bone. This is achieved by suppressing bone resorption by osteoclasts.
- Secretion of calcitonin is stimulated by increase in blood calcium level.

Synthesis of Thyroid Hormone

- The synthesis of thyroid hormones is regulated by iodine levels and TSH binding to TSH receptors of follicular cells.
- The synthesis and accumulation of thyroid hormone takes place in four stages: Synthesis of thyroglobulin, uptake of iodine from the blood, activation of iodine, and iodination of the tyrosine residues of thyroglobulin (Flowchart 22.1).
  - **Synthesis of thyroglobulin**: Thyroglobulin (a glycoprotein) is synthesized by granular endoplasmic reticulum and is packed into secretory vacuoles in the Golgi complex. The vacuoles travel to the luminal surface where they release thyroglobulin into the follicular cavity by exocytosis.
  - The **uptake of circulating iodine** by follicular cells by a membrane transport protein.
  - **Activation of iodine**: Iodine is **oxidized** by thyroid peroxidase and transported into the follicle. Here, the thyroglobulin combines with iodine to form colloid. Colloid is iodinated thyroglobulin.
  - **Iodination**: Within the colloid, the **iodination of the tyrosine residues of thyroglobulin** resulting in the formation of monoiodothyronine and diiodothyronine. The coupling of these molecules produces T3 and T4 hormones.
- Release of thyroid hormones: When stimulated by TSH, follicular cells take up the colloid into the cell by endocytosis. Within the cell, the iodinated thyroglobulin is acted upon by enzymes present in lysosomes-releasing hormones T3 and T4 which pass basally through the cell and are released into blood capillaries.
- Hormone produced in the thyroid gland is mainly T4. In the liver, the kidneys, and some other tissues, T4 is converted to T3 by removal of one iodine molecule. T3 and T4 circulating in blood are bound to a protein called thyroxine-binding globulin, TBG and the bound form of hormone is not active.
- T4 is more abundant than T3, constitutes almost 90% of circulating hormones but T3 acts more rapidly and is more potent.

PARATHYROID GLANDS

General Features

The parathyroid glands are located behind the thyroid gland, one at each end of upper and lower pole and within the capsule of thyroid gland.

Microscopic Features

- Gland is covered by connective tissue capsule from which septa extend into the gland substance and merge with reticular fibers which supports the secretory cells.
- With increasing age, secretory cells are replaced with adipocytes and almost it constitutes more than 50% of the gland in older age (Plate 22.4).
- The endocrine cells are arranged in cords. Numerous sinusoids lie in close relationship to the cells.
- There are two types of cells: Chief cells and oxyphil cells.

Chief Cells/Principal Cells

- The chief cells are more numerous than the oxyphil cells.
- With the light microscope, the chief cells are seen to be small polygonal cells with vesicular nucleus and light staining and slightly eosinophil/acidophilic cytoplasm.
- Sometimes, the cell accumulates glycogen and lipids and looks "clear".
- Three types of chief cells: light, dark, and clear have been described.

Flowchart 22.1: Some steps in the formation of hormones by the thyroid gland.

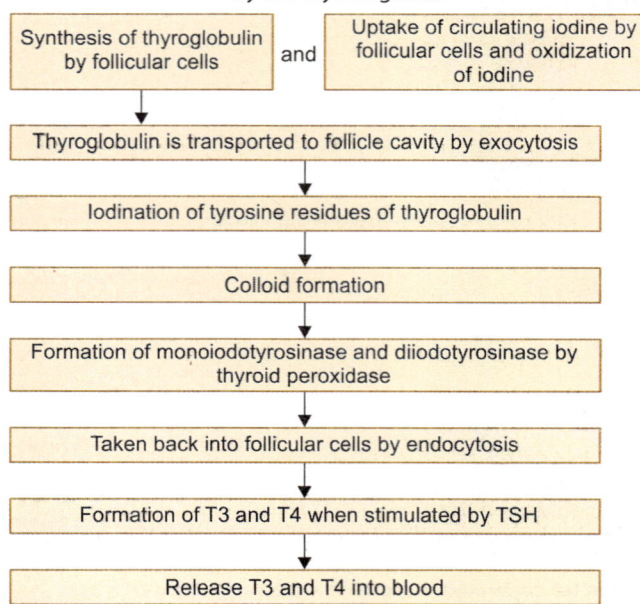

```
Synthesis of thyroglobulin     and     Uptake of circulating iodine by
by follicular cells                    follicular cells and oxidization
                                       of iodine
                        ↓
Thyroglobulin is transported to follicle cavity by exocytosis
                        ↓
Iodination of tyrosine residues of thyroglobulin
                        ↓
Colloid formation
                        ↓
Formation of monoiodotyrosinase and diiodotyrosinase by
thyroid peroxidase
                        ↓
Taken back into follicular cells by endocytosis
                        ↓
Formation of T3 and T4 when stimulated by TSH
                        ↓
Release T3 and T4 into blood
```

CHAPTER 22: Endocrine System

Plate 22.4: Parathyroid gland

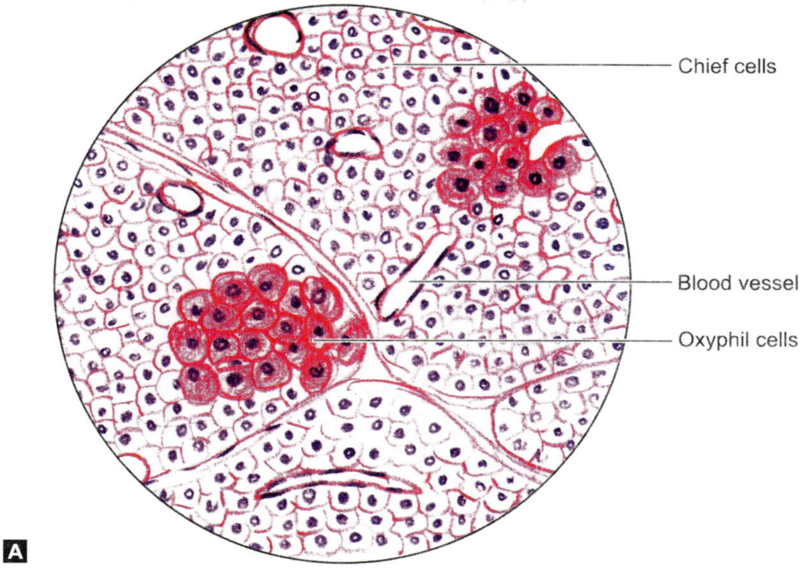

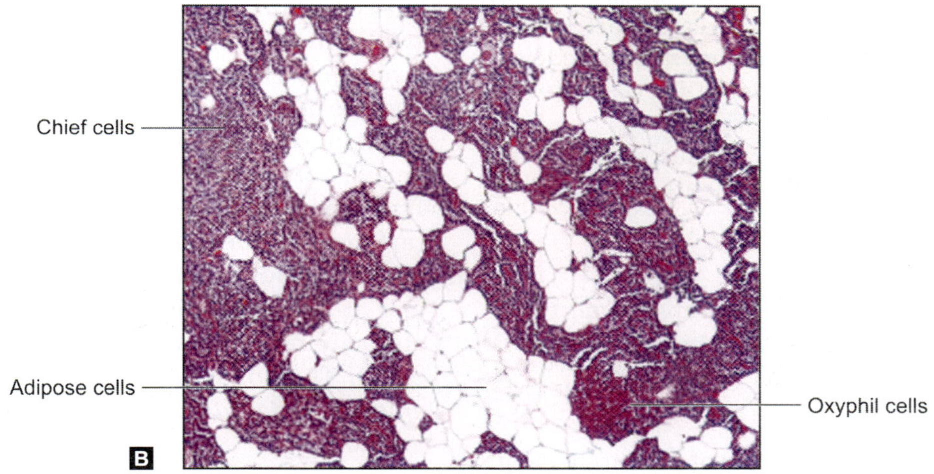

Parathyroid gland: (A) As seen in drawing; (B) Photomicrograph.
Courtesy: Damjanov I. Atlas of Histopathology, 1st edition. New Delhi: Jaypee Brothers Medical Publishers (P) Ltd; 2012. p. 290.

Points of identification
- These glands are made up of masses of cells with numerous capillaries in between
- Most of the cells (of which only nuclei are seen) are the chief cells which appear as small basophilic cells
- Oxyphil cells appear as large as eosinophilic (pink) cells
- Oxyphil cells are few in number
- Adipose cells are also seen.

❖ With the EM, active chief cells are seen to have abundant granular endoplasmic reticulum and well-developed Golgi complexes. Small secretory granules are seen, especially in parts of the cytoplasm near adjacent blood sinusoids.
❖ The chief cells produce the **parathyroid hormone or parathormone**.
❖ Parathormone tends to increase the serum calcium level by: Increasing the bone resorption through stimulation of osteoclastic activity, calcium resorption from renal tubules, and calcium absorption from the gut.

Oxyphil Cells

- The oxyphil cells are much larger than the chief cells and contain granules that stain strongly with acid dyes.
- Their nuclei are smaller and stain more intensely than those of chief cells.
- They are less numerous than the chief cells.
- The oxyphil cells are absent in the young and appear a little before the age of puberty.
- With the EM, it is seen that the granules of oxyphil cells are really mitochondria, large numbers of which are present in the cytoplasm.
- True secretory granules are not present. The functions of oxyphil cells are unknown.

SUPRARENAL GLANDS/ADRENAL GLANDS

General Features

- Suprarenal glands are paired organs and lie near the superior poles of the kidney in the abdomen. In many animals, they do not occupy a "supra" renal position, but lie near the kidneys therefore, called as *adrenal glands*.
- The gland is made up of two functionally distinct parts—a yellow superficial part called the *cortex*, and a reddish-brown deep part called the *medulla*. The volume of the cortex is about ten times that of the medulla.
- Cortex and medulla have distinct origins, functions, and morphological characteristics that are united during development.

Microscopic Features

Gland is covered by a connective tissue capsule from which septa extend into the gland substance. Stroma has network of reticular fibers that supports the secretory cells.

Suprarenal Cortex

- The suprarenal cortex is made up of cells arranged in cords. Sinusoids intervene between the cords.
- On the basis of the arrangement of the cells, the cortex can be divided into three layers: (a) Outermost zona glomerulosa, (b) Middle zona fasciculata, and (c) Inner zona reticularis (Plate 22.5).
- The cells of adrenal cortex have the typical structure of steroid-secreting cells. They do not store the secretory products but they secrete when needed.

Zona glomerulosa

- It is the outermost layer and constitutes the outer one-fifth of the cortex.
- Here, the cells are arranged in closely packed inverted U-shaped cords or rounded like acinus groups and surrounded by capillaries.
- With the light microscope, the cells of the zona glomerulosa are seen to be small polyhedral or columnar with basophilic cytoplasm and deeply staining nuclei.
- Produce the mineralocorticoid hormones **aldosterone** and **deoxycorticosterone**. These hormones influence the electrolyte and water balance of the body. The secretion of aldosterone is influenced by renin secreted by juxtaglomerular cells of the kidney. The secretion of hormones by the zona glomerulosa appears to be largely **independent** of the hypophysis cerebri.

Zona fasciculata

- It is the middle layer and forms the middle three-fifths of the cortex.
- The cells are arranged in straight columns with two cells thick at right angles to the surface. Sinusoids intervene between the columns.
- With the light microscope, the cells of the zona fasciculata are seen to be large, polyhedral with basophilic cytoplasm, and vesicular nuclei.
- The cells of the zona fasciculata are very rich in lipids. With routine staining methods, the lipids are dissolved giving the cells an "empty" or vacuolated appearance. Because of their vacuolization, the cells are also called **spongiocytes**. These cells also contain considerable amounts of vitamin C.
- Produce the glucocorticoids **cortisone** and **cortisol** (**dihydrocortisone**). These hormones have widespread effects, including those on carbohydrate metabolism and protein metabolism. They appear to decrease antibody response and have an anti-inflammatory effect. The zona fasciculata also produces small amounts of **dehydroepiandrosterone** (DHA) which is an androgen.

Zona reticularis

- The inner one-fifth layer of the cortex is called the **zona reticularis**.
- It is called as reticularis because it is made up of cords that branch and anastomose with each other to form a kind of reticulum.
- The cells in this layer are smaller and more acidophilic.
- With the light microscope, the cells of the zona reticularis are seen to be similar to those of the zona fasciculata but the lipid content is less. Their cytoplasm is often eosinophilic. The cells often contain brown lipofuscin pigment granules.
- With the EM, the cells in all layers of the cortex are characterized by the presence of abundant smooth

CHAPTER 22: Endocrine System

Plate 22.5: Suprarenal gland

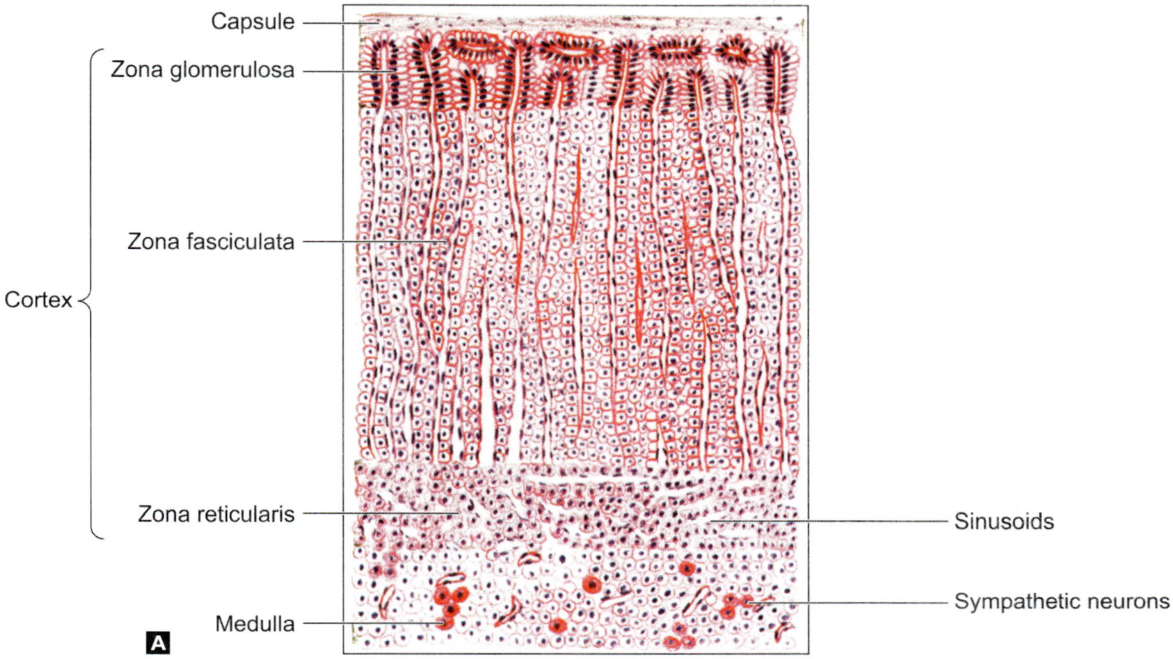

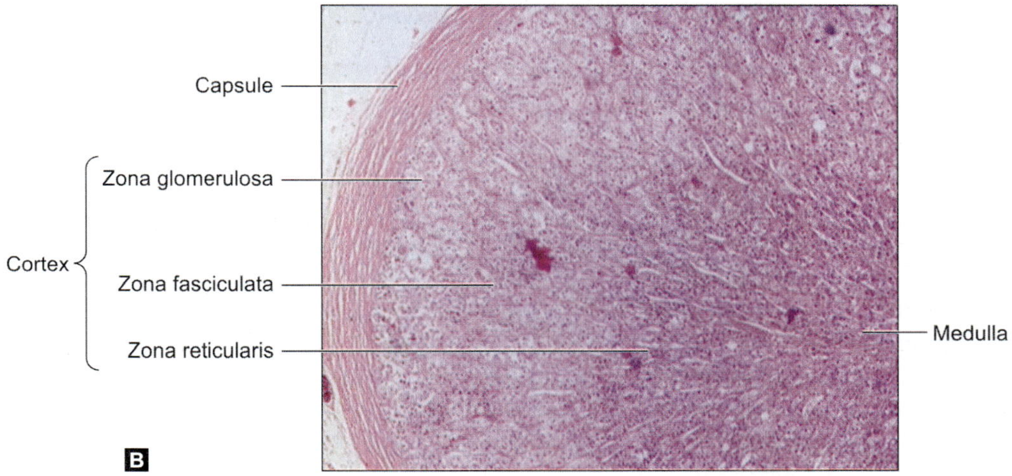

Suprarenal gland: (A) As seen in drawing; (B) Photomicrograph.

Points of identification
- The suprarenal gland is made up of a large number of cells arranged in layers. It consists of an outer cortex and an inner medulla
- The cortex is divisible into three zones
- The zona glomerulosa is most superficial. Here, the cells are arranged in the form of inverted U-shaped structures or acinus-like groups
- In the zona fasciculata, the cells are arranged in straight columns (typically two-cell thick). Sinusoids intervene between the columns
- The zona reticularis is made up of cords of cells that branch and form a network
- The medulla is made up of groups of cells separated by wide sinusoids. Some sympathetic neurons are also present.

endoplasmic reticulum. The Golgi complex is best developed in cells of the zona fasciculata. Mitochondria are elongated in the glomerulosa, spherical in the fasciculata, and unusual with tubular cisternae (instead of the usual plates) in the reticularis (Fig. 22.7).

❖ Produce some glucocorticoids, and sex hormones, both estrogens and androgens.

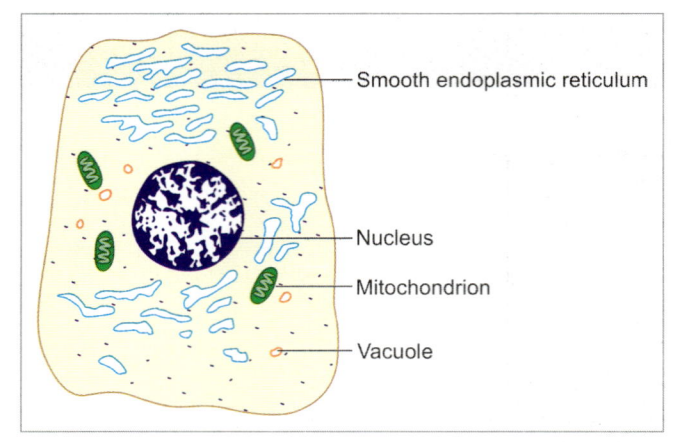

Fig. 22.7: Some features of ultrastructure of a cell from the adrenal cortex (schematic representation).

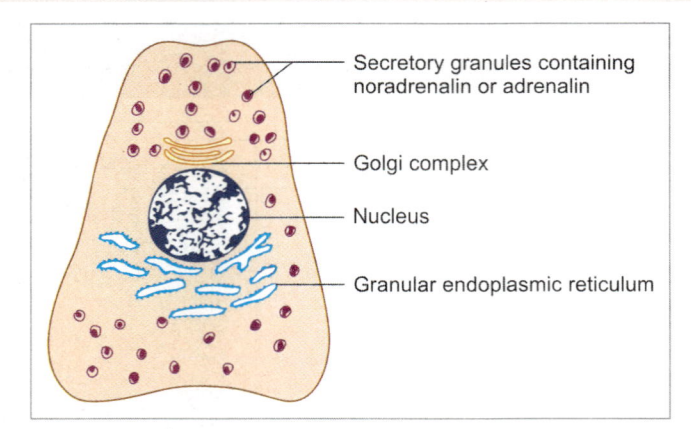

Fig. 22.8: Some features of ultrastructure of a cell from the adrenal medulla (schematic representation).

Suprarenal Medulla

- Both functionally and embryologically, the medulla of the suprarenal gland is distinct from the cortex.
- Functions as a modified sympathetic ganglion with postganglionic sympathetic cells without axons and dendrites.
- It has chromaffin cells and sympathetic ganglion cells which are scattered throughout.
- They are derived from neural crest cells. Cells are nothing but modified postganglionic neurons that have a secretory function.
- Chromaffin cells are columnar or polyhedral and have a basophilic cytoplasm arranged in cords or clumps. The cell groups or columns are separated by wide sinusoids.
- With the EM, the cells of the adrenal medulla are seen to contain abundant granular endoplasmic reticulum and a prominent Golgi complex (Fig. 22.8). The cells also contain membrane-bound secretory vesicles. In some cells, these vesicles are small and electron dense while in others, they are large and not so dense. The former contains noradrenalin and the latter adrenalin.
- In contrast to the suprarenal cortex, the medulla is not essential for life as its functions can be performed by other chromaffin tissues.
- Chromaffin cells secrete noradrenalin (norepinephrine) and adrenalin (epinephrine) into the blood. This secretion takes place mainly at times of stress (fear and anger) and results in widespread effects similar to those of stimulation of the sympathetic nervous system (e.g. increase in heart rate and blood pressure).
- A secretion of suprarenal medulla is controlled by splanchnic nerves.

PINEAL GLAND

General Features

- The pineal gland (or pineal body) is a small piriform structure present in relation to the posterior wall of the third ventricle of the brain. It is also called the *epiphysis cerebri*.
- The secretions of the gland are influenced by the light and dark periods of the day and it is most active during night.

Microscopic Features

- The gland is covered by pia mater forming a capsule from which septa extends into the gland and divides it into incomplete lobules.
- Sections of the pineal gland stained with hematoxylin and eosin shows a mass of cells among which there are blood capillaries and nerve fibers.
- A distinctive feature of the pineal in sections is the presence of irregular masses made up mainly of calcium salts. These masses constitute the *corpora arenacea* or *brain sand* (Fig. 22.9).
- The gland composed of pinealocytes and interstitial cells.

Pinealocytes

- Pinealocytes cell have a polyhedral body containing a spherical, oval, or irregular nucleus.
- The cell body gives off long processes with expanded *terminal buds* that end in relation to the walls of capillaries, or in relation to the ependyma of the third ventricle.
- The cell bodies of pinealocytes contain both granular and agranular endoplasmic reticulum, a well-developed Golgi complex, and many mitochondria. An organelle of unusual structure made up of groups of microfibrils and perforated lamellae may be present *(canaliculate lamellar bodies)*.

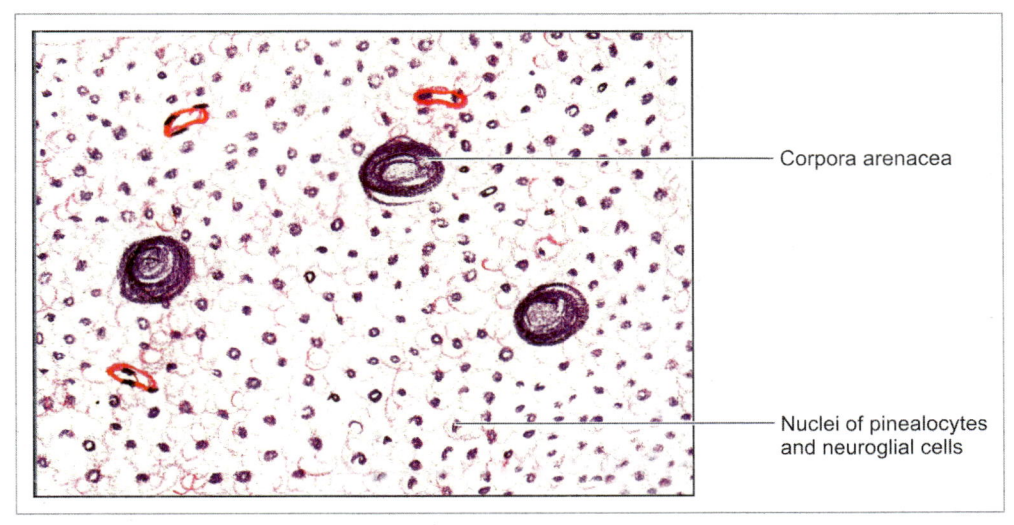

Fig. 22.9: Pineal body as seen with a light microscope (schematic representation).

- Hormone produced by pinealocytes: The pinealocytes produce a number of hormones which are chemically indolamines or polypeptides. The best known hormone of the pineal gland is the amino acid **melatonin** (so called because it causes changes in skin color in amphibia). Large concentrations of melatonin are present in the pineal gland. It is released at night and inhibits the release of growth hormone and gonadotropin hormones. It also induces the feeling of sleepiness and can be used as a supplement to combat sleep disorders.

Interstitial Cells

- The pinealocytes are separated from one another by neuroglial cells that resemble astrocytes in structure.
- They lie in proximity to blood vessel and pinealocytes.
- Cells are dark staining elongated nucleus with well-developed rough endoplasmic reticulum.

> **Added Information**
>
> **Cyclic activity of pineal gland**
> - Because of the light-mediated response, the pineal gland may act as a kind of biological clock which may produce circadian rhythms (variations following a 24-hour cycle) in various parameters.
> - The suprachiasmatic nucleus of the hypothalamus plays an important role in the cyclic activity of the pineal gland.
> - This nucleus receives fibers from the retina. In turn, it projects to the tegmental reticular nuclei located in the brainstem. Reticulospinal fibers arising in these nuclei influence the sympathetic preganglionic neurons located in the first thoracic segment of the spinal cord. Axons of these neurons reach the superior cervical ganglion from where the **nervus conarii** arises and supplies the pineal gland.

SOME OTHER ORGANS HAVING ENDOCRINE FUNCTIONS

Paraganglia

- Aggregations of cells similar to those of the adrenal medulla are to be found at various sites. They are collectively referred to as paraganglia because most of them are present in close relation to autonomic ganglia.
- The cells of paraganglia give a positive chromaffin reaction, receive a preganglionic sympathetic innervation, and have secretory granules containing catecholamines in their cytoplasm.
- Like the cells of the adrenal medulla, paraganglia are believed to develop from cells of the neural crest.
- Paraganglia are richly vascularized. They are regarded as endocrine glands that serve as alternative sites for the production of catecholamines in the fetus, and in early postnatal life, when the adrenal medulla is not yet fully differentiated.
- Most of the paraganglia retrogress with age, but some persist into adult life.

Note: Some workers include the para-aortic bodies and carotid bodies among paraganglia.

Para-aortic Bodies

- These are two elongated bodies that lie, one on each side of the aorta, near the origin of the inferior mesenteric artery.
- The two masses may be united to each other by a band passing across the aorta.

* These bodies have a structure similar to that of the adrenal medulla. The cells secrete noradrenalin. The aortic bodies retrogress with age.

Carotid Bodies

* These are small oval structures, present one on each side of the neck, at the bifurcation of the common carotid artery (i.e. near the carotid sinus).
* The carotid bodies contain a network of capillaries in the intervals between which there are several types of cells.

Cells of Carotid Bodies

* The most conspicuous cells of the carotid body are called *glomus cells* (or type I cells) (Fig. 22.10). These are large cells that have several similarities to neurons as follows:
  ▪ They give off dendritic processes.
  ▪ Their cytoplasm contains membrane-bound granules which contain a number of neuropeptides. In the human carotid body, the most prominent peptide present is encephalin. Others present include dopamine, serotonin, catecholamines, vasoactive intestinal peptide (VIP), and substance P.
  ▪ The cells are in synaptic contact with afferent nerve terminals of the glossopharyngeal nerve. Chemoreceptor impulses pass through these fibers to the brain. Some glomus cells also show synaptic connections with the endings of preganglionic sympathetic fibers, and with other glomus cells.
  ▪ The organization of endoplasmic reticulum in them shows similarities to that of Nissl substance.
  ▪ They are surrounded by sheath cells that resemble neuroglial elements.
* Because of these similarities to neurons, and because of the possibility that the cells release dopamine (and possibly other substances), they are sometimes described as neuroendocrine cells (and are included in the APUD cell category).
* The exact significance of the glomus cells, and of their nervous connections, is not understood at present. They could possibly be sensory receptors sensitive to oxygen and carbon dioxide tension. Dopamine released by them may influence the sensitivity of chemoreceptor nerve endings. They may also serve as interneurons.
* Apart from the glomus cells, other cells present in the carotid bodies are as follows:
  ▪ Sheath cells (or type II cells) that surround the glomus cells.

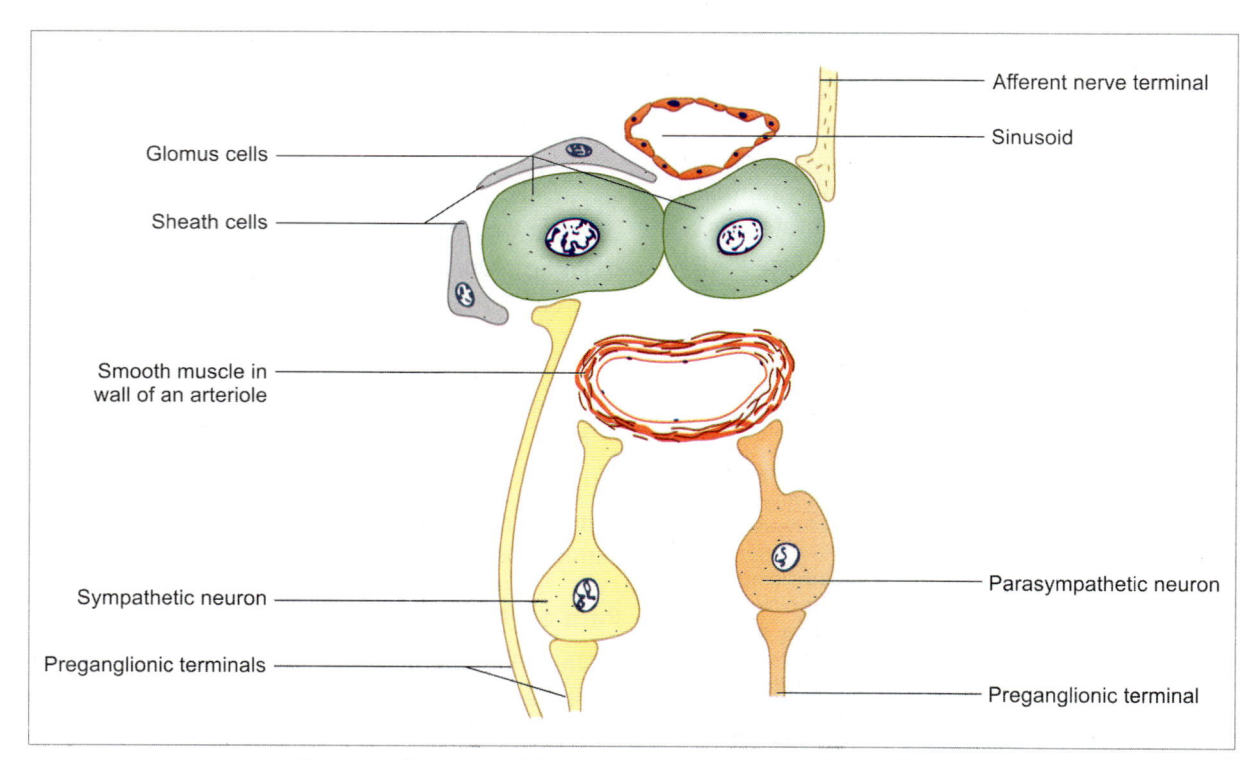

Fig. 22.10: Structure of the carotid body (schematic representation).

CHAPTER 22: Endocrine System

- A few sympathetic and parasympathetic postganglionic neurons.
- Endothelial cells of blood vessels, and muscle cells in the walls of arterioles.
- Some connective tissue cells.

Nerve Supply of Carotid Bodies

The carotid body is richly innervated as follows:
- Afferent nerve terminals from the glossopharyngeal nerve form synapses with glomus cells.
- Preganglionic sympathetic and parasympathetic fibers end on the corresponding ganglion cells. Some preganglionic sympathetic fibers end by synapsing with glomus cells.
- Postganglionic fibers arising from the sympathetic and parasympathetic nerve cells within the carotid body innervate muscle in the walls of arterioles.

Functions of Carotid Bodies

- The main function of the carotid bodies is that they act as chemoreceptors that monitor the oxygen and carbon dioxide levels in blood.
- They reflexly control the rate and depth of respiration through respiratory centers located in the brainstem.
- In addition to this function, the carotid bodies are also believed to have an endocrine function.

Note: The precise mechanism by which the carotid bodies respond to changes in oxygen and carbon dioxide tension is not understood. It is not certain as to which cells, or nerve terminals are responsible for this function.

> **Added Information**
>
> **Diffuse neuroendocrine or APUD cell system**
> - Apart from the discrete endocrine organs considered in this chapter, there are groups of endocrine cells scattered in various parts of the body. These cells share some common characteristics with each other, and also with the cells of some discrete endocrine organs.
> - All these cells take up precursor substances from the circulation and process them (by decarboxylation) to form amines or peptides. They are, therefore, included in what is called the **APUD cell system**. These peptides or amines serve as hormones.
> - Many of them also function as neurotransmitters. Hence, the APUD cell system is also called the **diffuse neuroendocrine system**. The cells of this system contain spherical or oval membrane-bound granules with a dense core. There is an electron-lucent halo around the dense core.
> - The diffuse neuroendocrine system is regarded as representing a link between the autonomic nervous system on the one hand, and the organs classically recognized as endocrine on the other, as it shares some features of both.
>
> *Contd...*

> *Contd...*
>
> - The effects of the amines or peptides produced by the cells of the system are sometimes "local" (like those of neurotransmitters) and sometimes widespread (like those of better known hormones).
>
> The cell types included in the APUD cell system are as follows:
> - Various cells of the adenohypophysis.
> - Neurons in the hypothalamus that synthesize the hormones of the neurohypophysis (oxytocin, vasopressin), and the cells that synthesize releasing factors controlling the secretion of hormones by the adenohypophysis.
> - The chief cells of the parathyroid glands producing parathyroid hormone.
> - The C-cells (parafollicular cells) of the thyroid, producing calcitonin.
> - Cells of the adrenal medulla (along with some outlying chromaffin tissues) that secrete adrenalin and noradrenalin. These include the SIF cells of sympathetic ganglia.
> - Cells of the gastroenteropancreatic endocrine system which includes cells of pancreatic islets producing insulin, glucagon, and some other amines. It also includes endocrine cells scattered in the epithelium of the stomach and intestines producing one or more of the following: 5-hydroxytryptamine, glucagon, dopamine, somatostatin, substance P, motilin, gastrin, cholecystokinin, secretin, vasoactive intestinal polypeptide (VIP), and some other peptides.
> - Glomus cells of the carotid bodies producing dopamine and noradrenalin.
> - Melanocytes of the skin producing promelanin.
> - Some cells in the pineal gland, the placenta, and modified myocytes of the heart called **myoendocrine cells**.
> - Renin-producing cells of the kidneys.

APPLIED HISTOLOGY

Pituitary Gland

- **Gigantism**: When growth hormone (GH) excess occurs prior to epiphyseal closure, gigantism is produced. The main clinical feature in gigantism is the excessive and proportionate growth of the child. There is enlargement as well as thickening of the bones resulting in considerable increase in height and enlarged thoracic cage.
- **Acromegaly**: Acromegaly results when there is overproduction of GH in adults following cessation of bone growth and is more common than gigantism. The term "acromegaly" means increased growth of extremities (*acro* = extremity). There is enlargement of hands and feet, coarseness of facial features with increase in soft tissues, prominent supraorbital ridges, and a more prominent lower jaw which when clenched results in protrusion of the lower teeth in front of upper teeth (**prognathism**).

- **Diabetes insipidus**: Deficient secretion of ADH due to inflammatory and neoplastic lesions of the hypothalamo-hypophyseal axis, destruction of neurohypophysis due to surgery, radiation, head injury, etc., causes diabetes insipidus. The main features of diabetes insipidus are excretion of a very large volume of dilute urine of low specific gravity (below 1.010), polyuria, and polydipsia.
- The vessels descending through the infundibular stalk are easily damaged in severe head injuries. This leads to loss of function in the anterior lobe of the hypophysis cerebri.

Thyroid Gland

- **Hyperthyroidism**: Hyperthyroidism, also called thyrotoxicosis, is a hypermetabolic clinical and biochemical state caused by excess production of thyroid hormones. The condition is more frequent in females.
- **Hypothyroidism**: Hypothyroidism is a hypometabolic clinical state resulting from inadequate production of thyroid hormones for prolonged periods, or rarely, from resistance of the peripheral tissues to the effects of thyroid hormones. Depending upon the age at onset of disorder, it is divided into two forms:
  1. **Cretinism** or congenital hypothyroidism is the development of severe hypothyroidism during infancy and childhood.
  2. **Myxedema** is the adulthood hypothyroidism.
- **Graves' disease**: Graves' disease, also known as Basedow's disease, primary hyperplasia, exophthalmic goiter, and diffuse toxic goiter, is characterized by a triad of features:
  - Hyperthyroidism (thyrotoxicosis)
  - Diffuse thyroid enlargement
  - Ophthalmopathy.

The disease is more frequent between the age of 30 years and 40 years and has five-fold increased prevalence among females.

Parathyroid Gland

- **Hyperparathyroidism**: Hyperfunction of the parathyroid glands occurs due to excessive production of parathyroid hormone. It is classified into three types—primary, secondary, and tertiary.
  1. **Primary hyperparathyroidism** occurs from oversecretion of parathyroid hormone due to disease of the parathyroid glands.
  2. **Secondary hyperparathyroidism** is caused by diseases in other parts of the body.
  3. **Tertiary hyperparathyroidism** develops from secondary hyperplasia after removal of the cause of secondary hyperplasia.
- **Hypoparathyroidism**: Deficiency or absence of parathyroid hormone secretion causes hypoparathyroidism.

Suprarenal Gland

- **Addison's disease**: Condition with decreased secretion of the adrenocortical hormones due to destruction of suprarenal cortex.
- **Cushing's disease**: A small tumors in the basophils of the anterior pituitary lead to increase in ACTH output leading to enlargement of suprarenal cortex resulting in overproduction of cortisol.

MULTIPLE CHOICE QUESTIONS

1. Which of the following is not a characteristic of the endocrine system?
    a. Products secreted into blood
    b. Glands with ducts
    c. Secretes hormones
    d. Nonlocalized response
2. Calcitonin is a hormone of which of following?
    a. Adrenal cortex
    b. Thyroid gland
    c. Pituitary gland
    d. Thymus gland
3. Calcium level in the blood is regulated by the:
    a. Thyroid
    b. Parathyroid
    c. Posterior pituitary
    d. Adrenal medulla
    e. a and b
4. Which gland is called the "master gland"?
    a. Adrenal medulla
    b. Adrenal cortex
    c. Thyroid
    d. Pituitary
5. Which cell type secretes ACTH?
    a. Lactotropic
    b. Thyrotropic
    c. Corticotropic
    d. Gonadotropic
6. Which cell type is involved in the secretion of thyroglobulin?
    a. Principal cells
    b. Oxyphil cells
    c. Parafollicular cells
    d. Follicular cells
7. Which part of the adrenal gland secretes glucocorticoids?
    a. Chromaffin cells
    b. Zona reticularis
    c. Zona glomerulosa
    d. Zona fasciculata
8. Which part of pituitary gland contains Herring bodies?
    a. Pars nervosa
    b. Pars intermedia
    c. Pars anterior
    d. Pars distalis

Answers

1. b   2. b   3. a   4. d   5. c   6. c   7. d   8. a

CHAPTER 23

Special Senses: Eye

Learning objectives

To study the:
- Structure of eyeball
- Outer fibrous coat—sclera, cornea
- Middle vascular coat or uvea
- Retina
- Lens
- Accessory visual organs—eyelid, conjunctiva
- Lacrimal gland
- Applied histology

IDENTIFICATION POINTS

Cornea
- The cornea is made up of five layers: Corneal epithelium, anterior limiting membrane, or Bowman's membrane, corneal stroma, posterior limiting lamina, and endothelium
- The corneal epithelium is nonkeratinized stratified squamous epithelium
- The substantia propria is made up of collagen fibers embedded in a ground substance
- Endothelium is lined by a single layer of flattened or cuboidal cells.

Retina
- Made up of ten layers: Pigment epithelium, layer of rods and cones, external limiting membrane, outer nuclear layer, outer plexiform layer, inner nuclear layer, inner plexiform layer, ganglionic cell layer, nerve fiber layer, and internal limiting membrane
- Outer pigment epithelium is made up of simple cuboidal epithelium
- The outer nuclear layer is thicker with densely packed nuclei than in the inner nuclear layer
- Ganglion cell layer is made up of a single row of cells of varying size.

INTRODUCTION

- The eyes are peripheral organs for vision and are located in the bony orbit.
- Each eyeball is like a camera. It has a ***lens*** that produces images of objects that we look at. The images fall on a light sensitive membrane called the ***retina***. Cells in the retina convert light images into nerve impulses that pass through the optic nerve, and other parts of the visual pathway to reach visual areas in the cerebral cortex. It is in the cortex that vision is actually perceived.

STRUCTURE OF EYEBALL

The wall of an eyeball consists of three layers:
1. *Outer fibrous coat*: That includes **sclera and cornea**
2. *Middle vascular coat*: That includes **choroid, ciliary body, and iris**
3. *Inner nervous coat*: Called **retina**.

- The space between the iris and the cornea is called the ***anterior chamber***, while the space between the iris and the front of the lens is called the ***posterior chamber***. These chambers are filled with a fluid called the ***aqueous humor***. The part of the eyeball behind the lens is filled by a jelly-like substance called the ***vitreous body***.
- The main parts of eyeball (as seen in section) are shown in Figure 23.1.

OUTER FIBROUS COAT

Sclera

- The outer wall of the eyeball is formed (in its posterior five-sixths) by a thick white opaque membrane called the ***sclera***. The sclera consists of white fibrous tissue (collagen). Some elastic fibers and connective tissue cells (mainly fibroblasts) are also present. Some of the cells are pigmented.

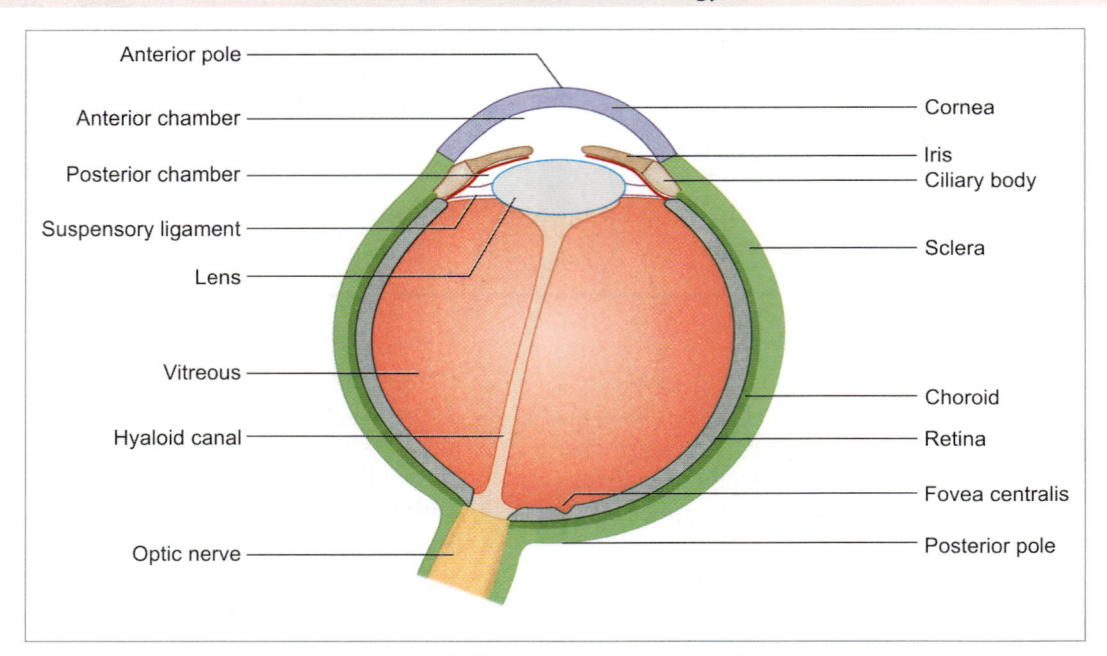

Fig. 23.1: Section across the eyeball to show its main parts (schematic representation).

- Externally, the sclera is covered in its anterior part by the ocular conjunctiva, and posteriorly by a fascial sheath (or *episclera*). The deep surface of the sclera is separated from the choroid by the *perichoroidal space*. Delicate connective tissue present in this space constitutes the *suprachoroid lamina* (or *lamina fusca*).
- Anteriorly, the sclera becomes continuous with the cornea at the *corneoscleral junction* (also called *sclerocorneal junction* or *limbus*). A circular channel called the *sinus venosus sclerae* (or *canal of Schlemm*) is located in the sclera just behind the corneoscleral junction (Fig. 23.2). A triangular mass of scleral tissue projects toward the cornea just medial to this sinus. This projection is called the *scleral spur*.
- The optic nerve is attached to the back of the eyeball, a short distance medial to the posterior pole. Here, the sclera is perforated like a sieve, and the area is, therefore, called the *lamina cribrosa*. Bundles of optic nerve fibers pass through the perforations of the lamina cribrosa.

Functions

- The sclera (along with the cornea) collectively forms the *fibrous tunic* of the eyeball and provides protection to delicate structures within the eye.
- It resists intraocular pressure and maintains the shape of the eyeball.
- Its smooth external surface allows eye movements to take place with ease.

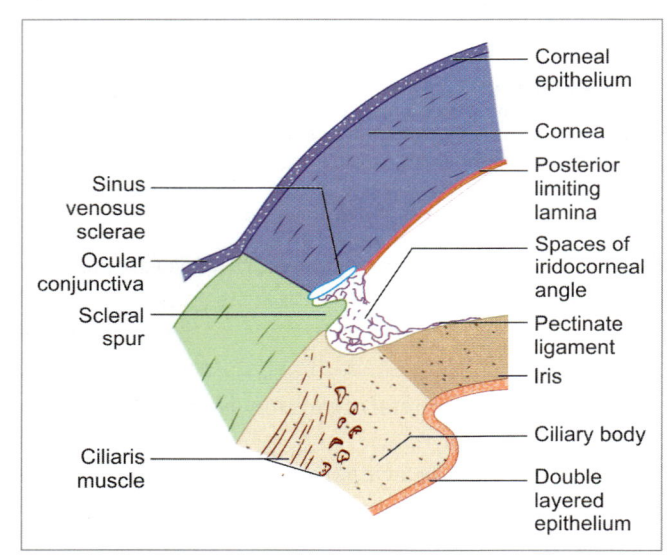

Fig. 23.2: Some features of the eyeball to be seen at the junction of the cornea with the sclera (schematic representation).

- The sclera also provides attachment to muscles that move the eyeball.

Cornea

In the anterior one-sixth of the eyeball, the sclera is replaced by a transparent disc called the *cornea*. The cornea is convex forward. It is colorless and avascular but has a very rich nerve supply.

Microscopic features

The cornea is made up of five layers:

1. **Anterior corneal epithelium**:
   - The outermost layer is of nonkeratinized stratified squamous epithelium (corneal epithelium).
   - The cells in the deepest layer of the epithelium are columnar; in the middle layers, they are polygonal; and in the superficial layers, they are flattened. The cells are arranged with great regularity.
   - With the electron microscope (EM), the cells on the superficial surface of the epithelium show projections either in the form of microvilli or folds of plasma membrane. These folds are believed to play an important role in retaining a film of fluid over the surface of the cornea.
   - The corneal epithelium regenerates rapidly after damage.

2. **Bowman's membrane**:
   - The corneal epithelium rests on the anterior limiting lamina (also called Bowman's membrane).
   - With the light microscope, this lamina appears to be structureless, but with the EM, it is dense homogeneous, made up of fine collagen fibrils embedded in matrix.
   - It gives great stability and strength to the cornea. It also acts as barrier to spread of infections.
   - Once damaged, it cannot regenerate, leading to scar formation and permanent impairment of vision.

3. **Corneal stroma**:
   - Most of the thickness of the cornea is formed by the substantia propria (or corneal stroma).
   - The substantia propria is made up of type 1 collagen fibers embedded in a ground substance containing sulfated glycosaminoglycans. They are arranged with great regularity and form lamellae (around 200–250 layers).
   - The fibers within one lamellus are parallel to one another, but the fibers in adjoining lamellae run in different directions forming obtuse angles with each other.
   - The transparency of the cornea is due to the regular arrangement of fibers, and because of the fact that the fibers and the ground substance have the same refractive index.
   - Fibroblasts are present in the substantia propria. They appear to be flattened in vertical sections through the cornea, but are seen to be star-shaped on surface view. They are also called keratocytes or corneal corpuscles.

4. **Descemet's membrane**:
   - Deep to the substantia propria, there is a thin homogeneous acellular layer called the posterior limiting lamina (or Descemet's membrane). It is a true basement membrane.
   - They can regenerate after injury.
   - At the margin of the cornea, the posterior limiting membrane becomes continuous with fibers that form a network in the angle between the cornea and the iris (iridocorneal angle).
   - The spaces between the fibers of the network are called the spaces of the iridocorneal angle. Some of the fibers of the network pass onto the iris as the pectinate ligament (Fig. 23.2).

5. **Endothelium**:
   - The posterior surface of the cornea is lined by a single layer of flattened cells that constitute the endothelium of the anterior chamber. This layer is in contact with the aqueous humor of the anterior chamber.
   - The endothelial cells are adapted for transport of ions. They possess numerous mitochondria.
   - They are united to neighboring cells by desmosomes and by occluding junctions. The cells pump out excessive fluid from cornea, and thus, ensure its transparency (Plate 23.1).

Causes for transparency of cornea

- Avascularity
- The regular arrangement of fibers in substantia propria
- The collagen fibers and the ground substance have the same refractive index
- Uniform and regular arrangement of anterior epithelium
- Relative state of corneal dehydration.

Nutrition of cornea

- Lacrimal fluid forming thin capillary layer on the surface of cornea
- Aqueous humor in anterior chamber
- Blood vessels at sclerocorneal junction.

Vascular Coat or Uvea

Deep to the sclera, there is a vascular coat (uvea) that consists of:
- Choroid
- Ciliary body
- Iris.

Plate 23.1: Cornea

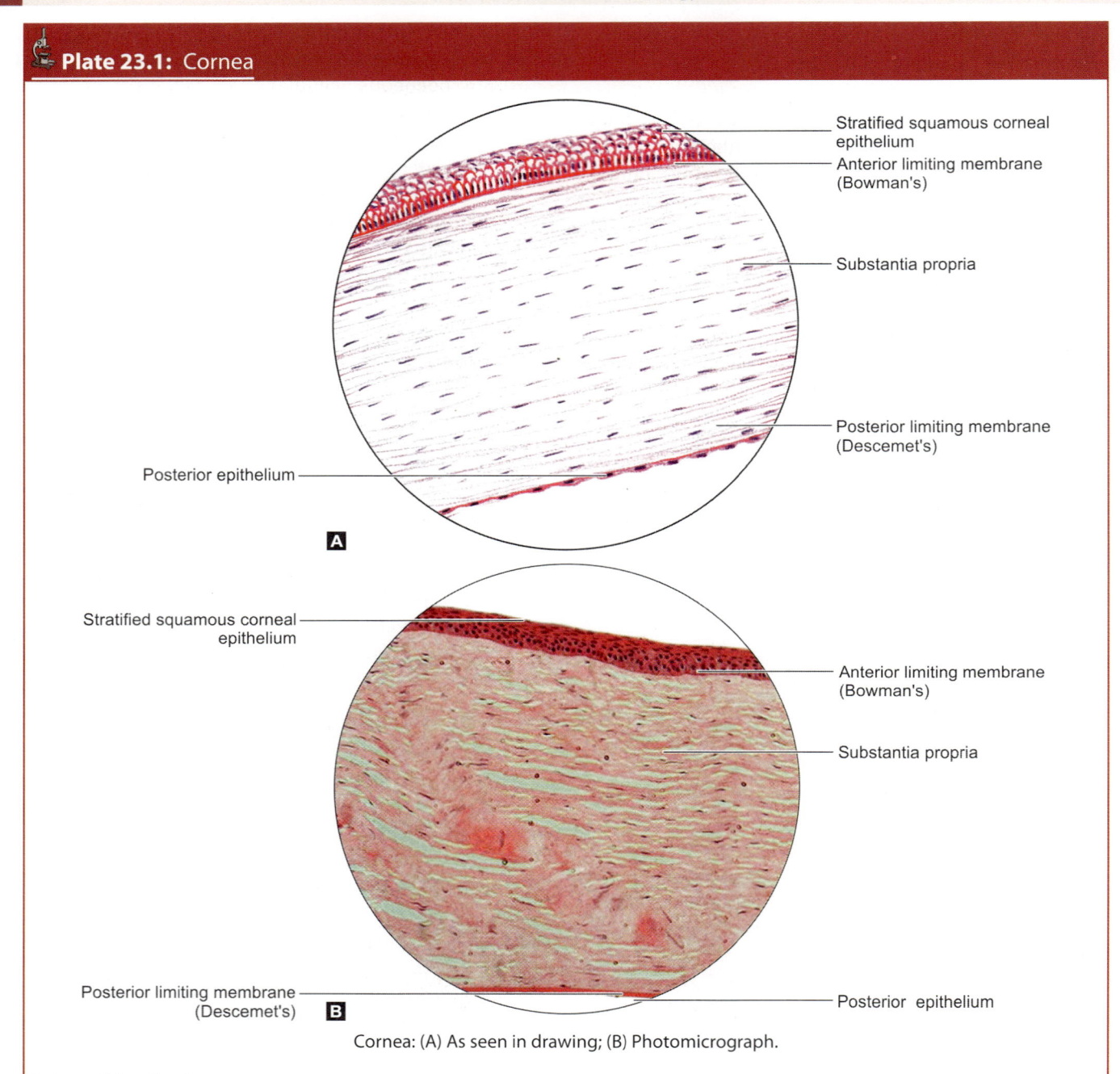

Cornea: (A) As seen in drawing; (B) Photomicrograph.

Points of identification
- The cornea is made up of five layers: Corneal epithelium, anterior limiting membrane, or Bowman's membrane, corneal stroma, posterior limiting lamina, and endothelium
- The corneal epithelium is nonkeratinized stratified squamous epithelium
- The substantia propria is made up of collagen fibers embedded in a ground substance
- Endothelium is lined by a single layer of flattened or cuboidal cells.

Choroid

The choroid consists of:
- **Choroid proper**
- **Suprachoroid lamina** that separates the choroid proper from the sclera
- **Basal lamina (membrane of Bruch)**, which intervenes between the choroid proper and the retina (Fig. 23.3).

Choroid proper

- The choroid proper consists of a network of blood vessels supported by connective tissue in which many pigmented cells are present, giving the choroid a dark color. This color darkens the interior of the eyeball. The pigment also prevents reflection of light within the eyeball. Both these factors help in formation of sharp images on the retina.
- The choroid proper is made up of an outer *vascular lamina* containing small arteries and veins, and lymphatics, and an inner *capillary lamina* (or *choroidocapillaris*). The connective tissue supporting the vessels of the vascular lamina is the *choroidal stroma*. Apart from collagen fibers, it contains melanocytes, lymphocytes, and mast cells. The capillary lamina is not pigmented. Nutrients diffusing out of the capillaries pass through the basal lamina to provide nutrition to the outer layers of the retina.

Suprachoroid lamina

The suprachoroid lamina is also called the *lamina fusca*. It is nonvascular. It is made up of delicate connective tissue containing collagen, elastic fibers, and branching cells containing pigment. A plexus of nerve fibers is present. Some neurons may be seen in the plexus.

Basal lamina

With the light microscope, the basal lamina (or *membrane of Bruch*) appears to be a homogeneous layer. However, with the EM, the membrane is seen to have a middle layer of elastic fibers, on either side of which there is a layer of delicate collagen fibers. The basal lamina is said to provide a smooth surface on which pigment cells and receptors of the retina can be arranged in precise orientation.

Ciliary Body

- The ciliary body represents an anterior continuation of the choroid. It is a ring-like structure continuous with the periphery of the iris.
- It is connected to the lens by the suspensory ligament.
- The ciliary body is made up of vascular tissue, connective tissue, and muscle.
- The muscle component constitutes the *ciliaris muscle*. The ciliaris muscle is responsible for producing alterations in the convexity of the lens (through the suspensory ligament) enabling the eye to see objects at varying distances from it. In other words, the ciliaris is responsible for accommodation.
- The inner surface of the ciliary body is lined by a double-layered epithelium. The outer cell layer is pigmented,

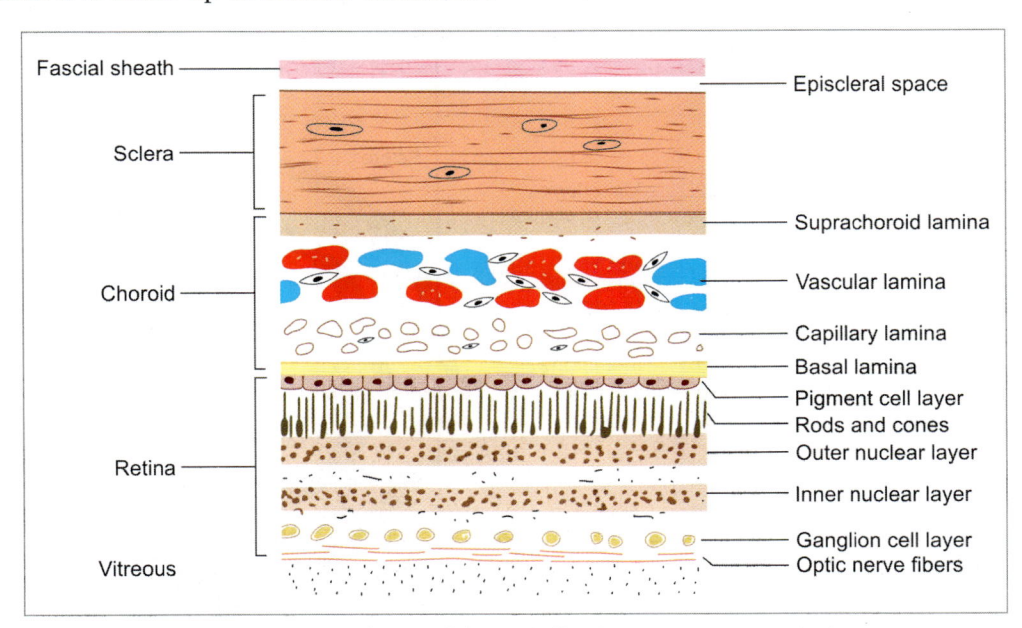

Fig. 23.3: Various layers of the eyeball (schematic representation).

whereas the inner cell layer (facing the posterior chamber) is nonpigmented. The cells of the inner layer secrete aqueous humor.
* The anterior part of the inner surface of the ciliary body has short processes toward the lens, known as **ciliary processes**.

Iris

* The iris is the most anterior part of the vascular coat of the eyeball.
* It forms a diaphragm placed immediately in front of the lens. At its periphery, it is continuous with the ciliary body. In its center, there is an aperture the **pupil**. The pupil regulates the amount of light passing into the eye.
* The iris is composed of a stroma of connective tissue containing numerous pigment cells, and in which are embedded blood vessels and smooth muscle.
* Some smooth muscle fibers are arranged circularly around the pupil and constrict it. They form the **sphincter pupillae**. Other fibers run radially and form the **dilator pupillae**.
* The posterior surface of the iris is lined by a double layer of epithelium continuous with that over the ciliary body. This epithelium represents a forward continuation of the retina. The cells of this epithelium are deeply pigmented.

Retina

This is the inner coat of eyeball and lines its posterior three-fourths of surface. The retina contains photoreceptors (rods and cones) which are essential for vision.

Embryological Considerations

To understand the structure of the retina, brief reference to its development is necessary (Figs. 23.4A and B).

* The retina develops as an outgrowth from the brain (diencephalon). The proximal part of the diverticulum remains narrow and is called the **optic stalk**. It later becomes the optic nerve. The distal part of the diverticulum forms a rounded hollow structure called the **optic vesicle**.
* This vesicle is invaginated by the developing lens (and other surrounding tissues) so that it gets converted into a two-layered **optic cup**.
* At first, each layer of the cup is made up of a single layer of cells. The outer layer persists as a single-layered epithelium that becomes pigmented. It forms the **pigment cell layer** of the retina. Over the greater part of the optic cup, the cells of the inner layer multiply to form several layers of cells that become the **nervous layer of the retina**.
* In the anterior part, both layers of the optic cup remain single layered. These two layers line: (1) the inner surface of the ciliary body forming the **ciliary part of the retina**, and (2) the posterior surface of the iris forming the **iridial part of the retina**.
* Retina has a specialized area where vision is most acute, called as fovea centralis or macula (Fig. 23.5). This area contains only cones which are essentially bare (the overlying layers are pushed to the side).
* The retina also has a "blind spot", the optic disc, where the optic nerve leaves the eye and there are no photoreceptor cells.

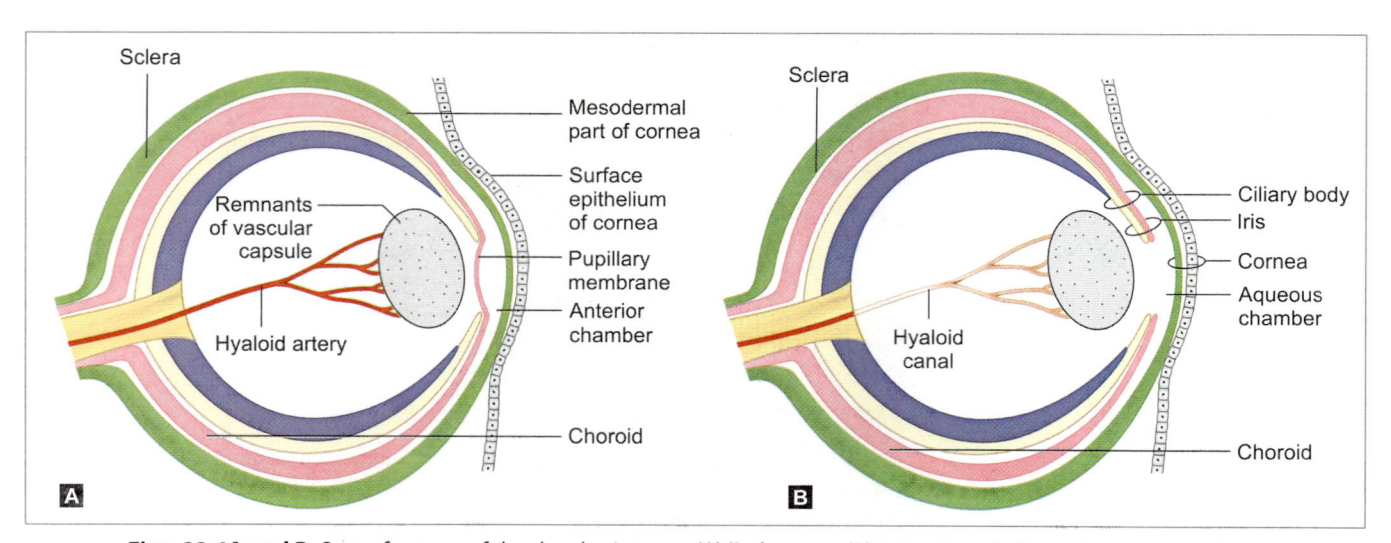

Figs. 23.4A and B: Some features of the developing eye: (A) Early stage; (B) Later stage (schematic representation).

CHAPTER 23: Special Senses: Eye

- Opposite the posterior pole of the eyeball, the retina shows a central region about 6 mm in diameter. This region is responsible for sharp vision. In the center of this region, an area about 2 mm in diameter has a yellow color and is called the macula lutea (Fig. 23.5). In the center of the macula lutea, there is a small depression that is called the fovea centralis. The floor of the fovea centralis is often called the foveola. This is the area of clearest vision.

- The optic nerve is attached to the eyeball a short distance medial to the posterior pole. The nerve fibers arising from the retina converge to this region, where they pass through the lamina cribrosa. When viewed from the inside of the eyeball, this area of the retina is seen as a circular area called the optic disc.

Basic Structure of the Retina

When we examine sections through the retina (stained by hematoxylin and eosin, Fig. 23.2), a number of layers can be distinguished. The significance of the layers becomes apparent, however, only if we study the retina using special methods. A highly schematic presentation of the layers of the retina, and of the cells present in them is shown in Figure 23.6. The retina can be said to have an external surface that is in contact with the choroid, and an internal surface that is in contact with the vitreous.

From outside to inside, retina consists of following **ten** layers:

1. ***Pigment cell layer***: It is the outermost layer of retina which is separated from choroid by Bruch's membrane. This consists of a single layer of low cuboidal cells containing melanin pigment. Processes from pigment cells extend into the next layer.

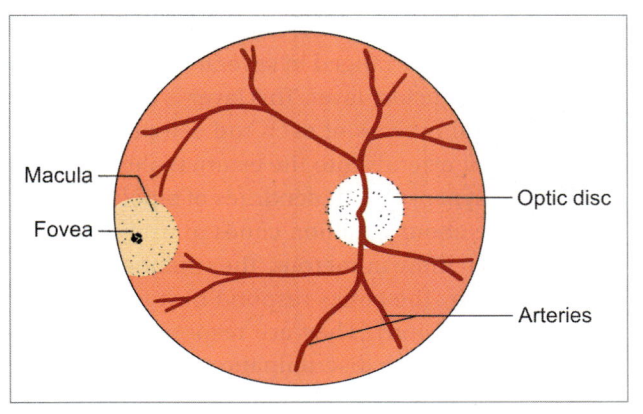

Fig. 23.5: Some features of the retina as seen through an ophthalmoscope (schematic representation). Note the arteries emerging through the optic disc.

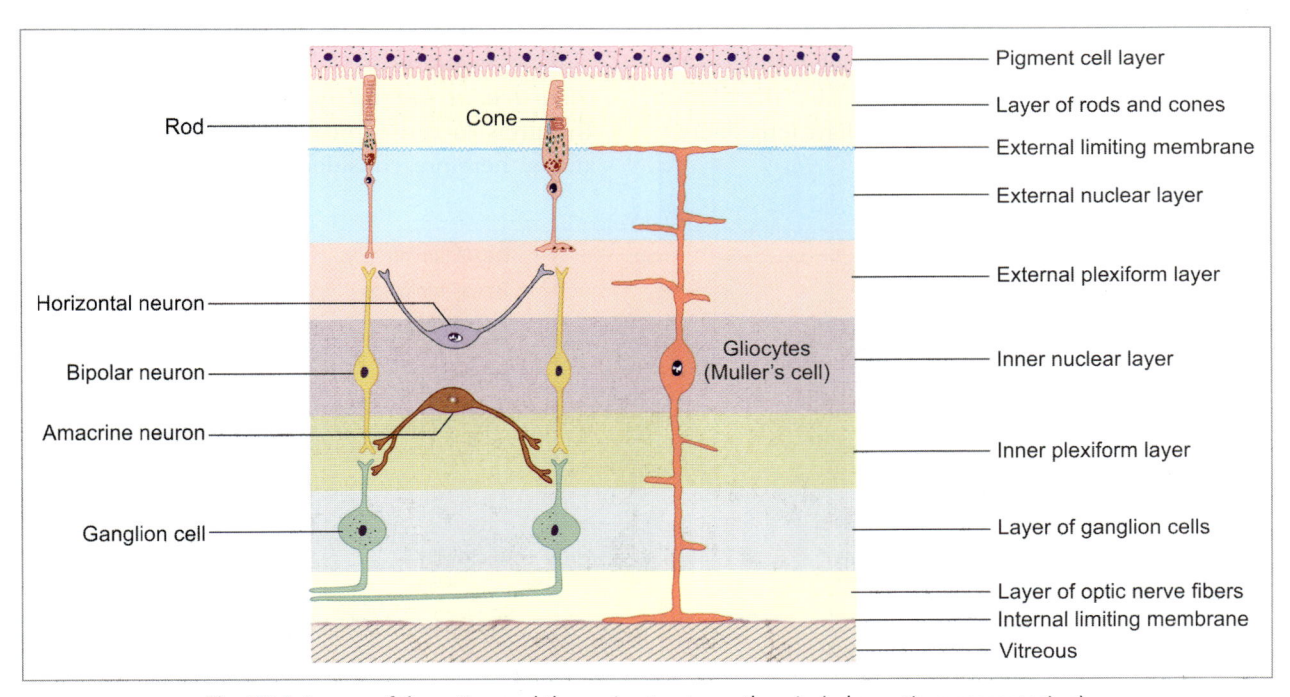

Fig. 23.6: Layers of the retina and the main structures therein (schematic representation).

This layer performs the following functions:
- It absorbs and prevents back reflection of light that has passed through the neural layers of the retina.
- The pigment cells phagocytose the shed membranous discs of the outer segment of rods and cones.
- These cells also produce melanin.
- They may play a role in regular spacing of rods and cones and may provide mechanical support to them.
- They have a phagocytic role. They "eat up" the ends of rods and cones which are constantly.

Pigment cells appear to be rectangular in vertical section, their width being greater than their height (Fig. 23.7). In surface view, they are hexagonal. The nucleus is basal in position. The pigment in the cytoplasm is melanin. With the EM, it can be seen that the surface of the cell shows large microvilli that contain pigment. These microvilli project into the intervals between the processes of rods and cones. Each pigment cell is related to about a dozen rods and cones. The plasma membrane at the base of the cell shows numerous infoldings.

2. **Layer of rods and cones**: The rods are processes of rod cells, and cones are processes of cone cells. The peripheral process is rod-shaped in the case of rod cells, and cone-shaped in the case of cone cells.

3. **Outer limiting membrane or lamina**: Between second and third layer, there is presence of a pink linear marking called as outer limiting membrane or lamina. This results because of zonula adherens of the glial cells (Müller cells) with the cell bodies of photoreceptor cells. The Müller cells are supporting cells of retina. They have long slender body that is radially oriented in retina.

4. **External nuclear layer**: The external nuclear layer contains the cell bodies and nuclei of rod cells and of cone cells.

Rods and cones:
- These cells are photoreceptors that convert the stimulus of light into nerve impulses.
- Each rod cell or cone cell can be regarded as a modified neuron. It consists of a cell body, a peripheral (or external) process, and a central (or internal) process. The peripheral processes lie in the layer of rods and cones described above. The nuclei of these cells are arranged in several layers in the form of external nuclear layer. This layer is darkly stained. The central process of each rod cell or cone cell is an axon. It extends into the external plexiform layer where it synapses with dendrites of bipolar neurons.
- There are about 7 million cones in each retina. The rods are far more numerous. They number more than 100 million. The cones respond best to bright light (photopic vision). They are responsible for sharp vision and for the discrimination of color. Rods can respond to poor light (scotopic vision) and especially to movement across the field of vision.
- Each rod is about 50 µm in length and about 2 µm thick. Cones are about 40 µm in length and 3–5 µm thick (Fig. 23.8).
- The pigment in the rods is **rhodopsin**, and that in the cones is **iodopsin**.

Ultrastructure of rod and cone cells:
The ultrastructure of rod cells and of cone cells is similar and is, therefore, considered together.

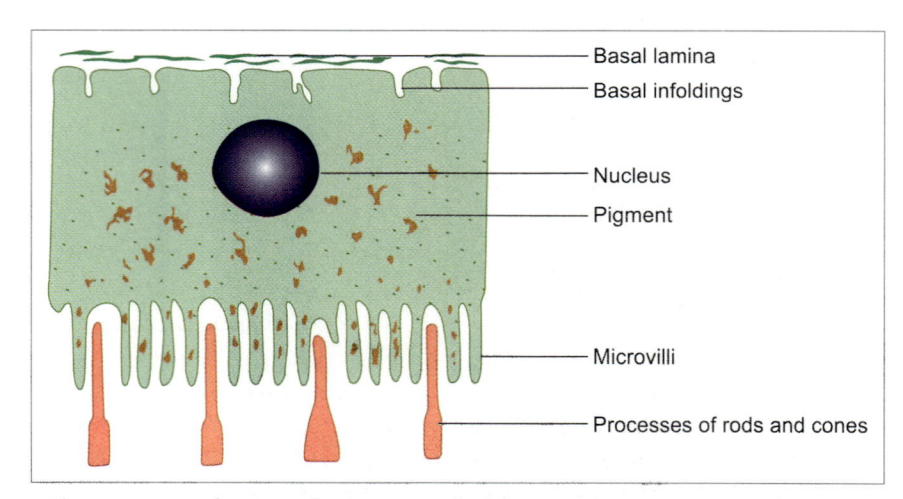

Fig. 23.7: Some features of a pigment cell of the retina (schematic representation).

CHAPTER 23: Special Senses: Eye

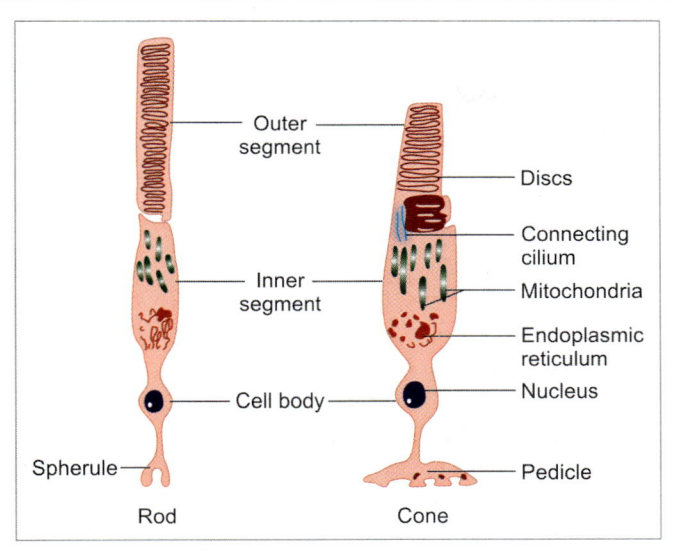

Fig. 23.8: The main parts of rods and cones (schematic representation).

- Each rod or cone cell consists of a cell body containing the nucleus, and of external and internal processes, an inner fiber and spherule (Fig. 23.9). The parts of cone cells are almost same except the terminal part which is called pedicle instead of spherule.
- The cell body (lying in the external nuclear layer) gives off two "fibers", inner and outer. The **outer fiber** passes outward up to the external limiting membrane and becomes continuous with the rod process, or the cone process.
- The process itself can be divided into an ***inner segment***, and an ***outer segment***. The outer segment is the real photoreceptor element. It contains a large number of membranous discs stacked on one another. It is believed that the discs are produced by the cilium (see below) and gradually move toward the tip of the outer segment. Here, old discs are phagocytosed by pigment cells.
- The outer segments of rods and cones contain photosensitive pigments that are concerned with the conversion of light into nerve impulses. The pigments are believed to be bound to the membranes of the sacs of the outer segments.
- Cones are believed to be of three types, red sensitive, green sensitive, and blue sensitive. Iodopsin has, therefore, to exist in three forms, one for each of these colors. However, the three types of cones cannot be distinguished from one another on the basis of their ultrastructure.

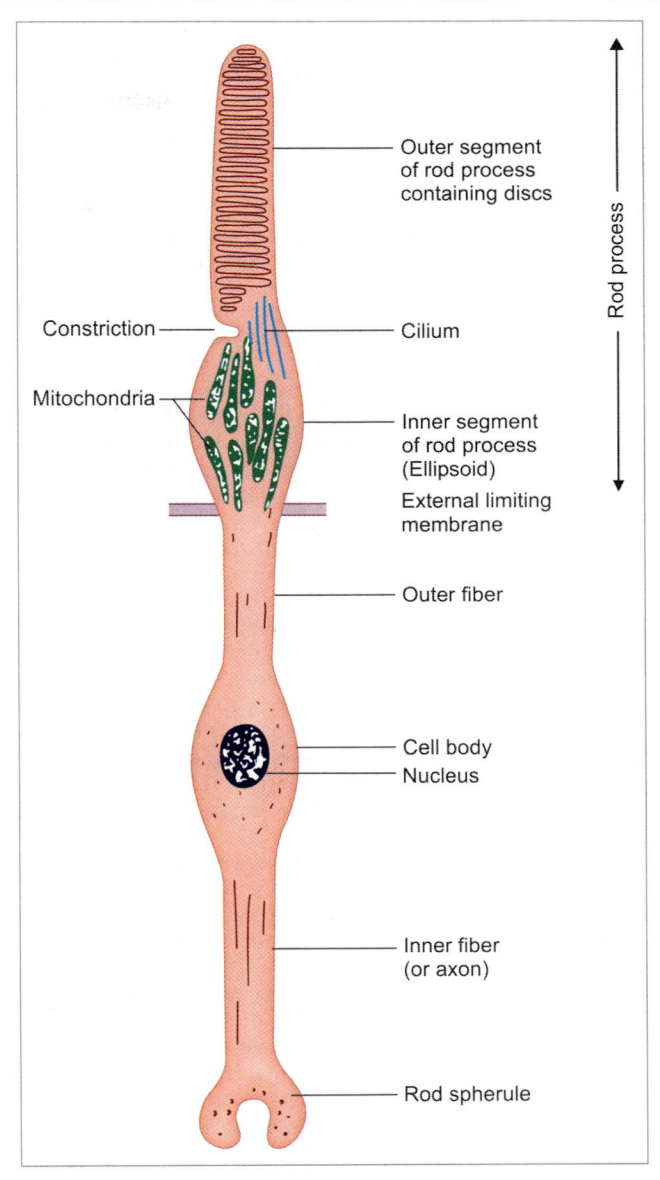

Fig. 23.9: Structure of a rod cell as seen by electron microscope (schematic representation).

5. ***External plexiform layer***: The external plexiform layer (or outer synaptic zone) consists only of nerve fibers that form a plexus. The axons of rods and cones synapse here with dendrites of bipolar neurons and horizontal cells. This layer stains lightly.
6. ***Internal nuclear layer***: The internal nuclear layer contains the cell bodies and nuclei of three types of neurons:
   i. **Bipolar cells**: They give off dendrites that enter the external plexiform layer to synapse with the axons of

Added Information

- The inner segment of the rod or cone process is wider than the outer segment. It contains a large number of mitochondria that are concentrated in a region that is called the **ellipsoid**.
- At the junction of the inner and outer segments of the rod or cone process, there is an indentation of the plasma membrane on one side, so that the connection becomes very narrow. This narrow part contains a fibrillar **cilium** in which the microfibrils are orientated as in cilia elsewhere. This cilium is believed to give rise to the flattened discs of the outer segment.
- The part of the rod cell between the cell body and the external limiting membrane is the outer fiber. The length of the outer fiber varies from rod to rod, being greatest in those rods that have cell bodies placed "lower down" in the external nuclear layer. The outer fiber is absent in cones, the inner segment of the cone process being separated from the cone cell body only by a slight constriction.
- The **cell bodies** of rod cells and of cone cells show no particular peculiarities of ultrastructure.
- The **inner fibers** of rod and cone cells resemble axons. At its termination, each rod axon expands into a spherical structure called the **rod spherule**, while cone axons end in expanded terminals called **cone pedicles** (Figs. 23.10 and 23.11). The rod spherules and cone pedicles form complex synaptic junctions with the dendrites of bipolar neurons, and with processes of horizontal cells. Each rod spherule synapses with processes of two bipolar neurons, and with processes of horizontal neurons.
- Each cone pedicle has numerous synapses with processes from one or more bipolar cells, and with processes of horizontal cells. In many situations, the cone pedicle bears several invaginations that are areas of synaptic contacts. Each such area receives one process from a bipolar dendrite, and two processes, one each from two horizontal neurons. Such groups are referred to as **triads**. Each cone pedicle has 24 such triads. Apart from triads, the cone pedicle bears numerous other synaptic contacts in areas intervening between the triads. These areas synapse with dendrites of diffuse bipolar cells. Some pedicles also establish synaptic contacts with other cone pedicles.

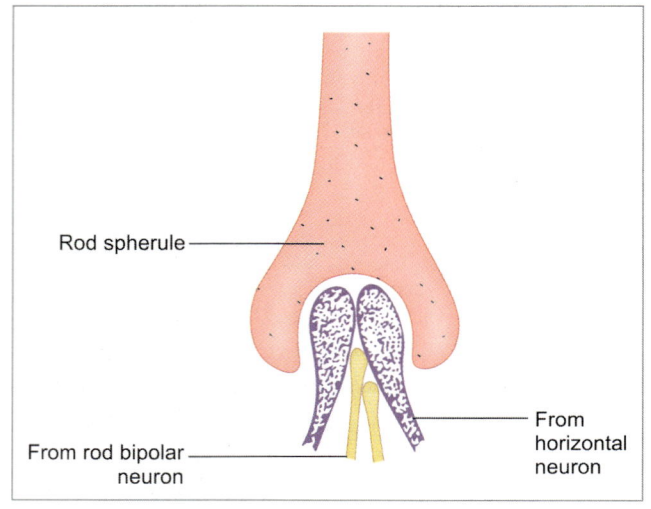

Fig. 23.10: Rod spherule synapsing with terminals of rod bipolar cells and horizontal cells (schematic representation).

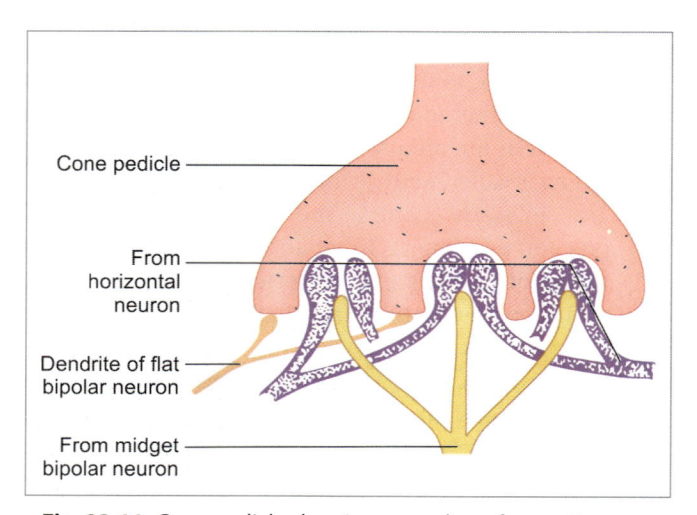

Fig. 23.11: Cone pedicle showing a number of synaptic areas, each area receiving three terminals (schematic representation).

rod and cone cells, and axons that enter the internal plexiform layer where they synapse with dendrites of ganglion cells. The bipolar cells are oriented perpendicular to the layers of retina.

ii. **Horizontal cells**: They give off processes that run parallel to the retinal surface. These processes enter the outer plexiform layer and synapse with rods, cones, and dendrites of bipolar cells. The horizontal cells are oriented parallel to the layers of retina.

Horizontal neurons are of two types, **rod horizontals** and **cone horizontals**, depending on whether they synapse predominantly with rods or cones. Each horizontal cell gives off one long process, and a number of short processes (7 in case of rod horizontal cells, and 10 in case of cone horizontal cells). The short processes are specific for the type of cell: those of rod horizontals synapse with a number of rod spherules, and those of cone horizontals synapse with cone pedicles. The long processes synapse with both rods and cones (which are situated some distance away from the cell body of the horizontal neuron). The long and short processes of horizontal cells cannot be distinguished as dendrites or axons, and each process probably conducts in both directions.

iii. **Amacrine cells** also lie horizontally in the retina. Their processes enter the inner plexiform layer where they synapse with axons of bipolar cells, and with dendrite of ganglion cells.

The term amacrine is applied to neurons that have no true axon. Like the processes of horizontal cells, those of amacrine neurons also conduct impulses in both directions. Each cell gives off one or two thick processes that divide further into a number of branches. The amacrine cells are believed to play a very important role in the interaction between adjacent areas of the retina resulting in production of sharp images. They are also involved in the analysis of motion in the field of vision.

Müller cells: Apart from bipolar, horizontal, and amacrine neurons, the internal nuclear layer also contains the nuclei of retinal gliocytes or **cells of Müller** (Fig. 23.6). These cells give off numerous protoplasmic processes that extend through almost the whole thickness of the retina. Externally, they extend to the junction of the layer of rods and cones with the external nuclear layer. Here, the processes of adjoining gliocytes meet to form a thin *external limiting membrane*. Internally, the gliocytes extend to the internal surface of the retina where they form an *internal limiting membrane*. The retinal gliocytes are neuroglial in nature. They support the neurons of the retina and may ensheath them. They probably have a nutritive function as well.

7. *Internal plexiform layer*: The *internal plexiform layer* (or *inner synaptic zone*) consists of synapsing nerve fibers. The axons of bipolar cells synapse with dendrites of ganglion cells, and both these processes synapse with processes of amacrine cells. The internal plexiform layer also contains some horizontally placed *internal plexiform cells*, and also a few ganglion cells.
8. *Layer of ganglion cells*: The layer of ganglion cells contains the cell bodies of ganglion cells. The dendrites of these cells enter the internal plexiform layer to synapse with processes of bipolar cells and of amacrine cells. Each ganglion cell gives off an axon that forms a fiber of the optic nerve.
9. *Layer of optic nerve fibers*: The layer of optic nerve fibers is made up of axons of ganglion cells. The fibers converge on the optic disc where they pass through foramina of the lamina cribrosa to enter the optic nerve.
10. *Internal limiting membrane*: The processes of adjoining Müller cells extend to the internal surface of the retina to form an *internal limiting membrane*. This membrane separates the retina from the vitreous.

Appearance of the Retina in Sections stained by H&E (Plate 23.2)

- ❖ The inner and outer nuclear layers can be made out even at low magnification.
- ❖ The outer nuclear layer is thicker, and the nuclei in it are more densely packed than in the inner nuclear layer. This (outer nuclear) layer contains the nuclei of rods and cones. The cone nuclei are oval and lie in a single row adjoining the layer of rods and cones. The remaining nuclei are those of rods.
- ❖ The nuclei in the inner nuclear layer belong to bipolar cells, horizontal cells, amacrine cells, and gliocytes.
- ❖ The layer of ganglion cells is (at most places) made up of a single row of cells of varying size. The cell outlines are indistinct, but the nuclei can be made out. They are of various sizes. On the whole, they are larger and stain more lightly than nuclei in the inner and outer nuclear layers.
- ❖ The layer of pigment cells resembles a low cuboidal epithelium. All the nuclei in this layer are of similar size, and lie in a row.
- ❖ The remaining layers (layers of rods and cones, inner and outer plexiform layers, and the layer of optic nerve fibers) are seen as light staining areas in which no detail can be made out. The layer of rods and cones may show vertical striations.

Blood–Retinal Barrier

The blood vessels that ramify in the retina do not supply the rods and cones. These are supplied by diffusion from choroidal vessels. The endothelial cells of capillaries in the retina are united by tight junctions to prevent diffusion of substances into the rods and cones. This is referred to as the blood–retinal barrier.

LENS

The lens of the eye is a transparent biconvex avascular structure. It is suspended between the iris and the vitreous by the zonules, which connect the lens with the ciliary body. It is surrounded by an elastic capsule which is a semipermeable membrane. The posterior surface of the lens is more curved than the anterior surface.

The lens consists of three parts:

1. Lens capsule
2. Lens epithelium
3. Lens substance (Fig. 23.12).

Plate 23.2: Retina

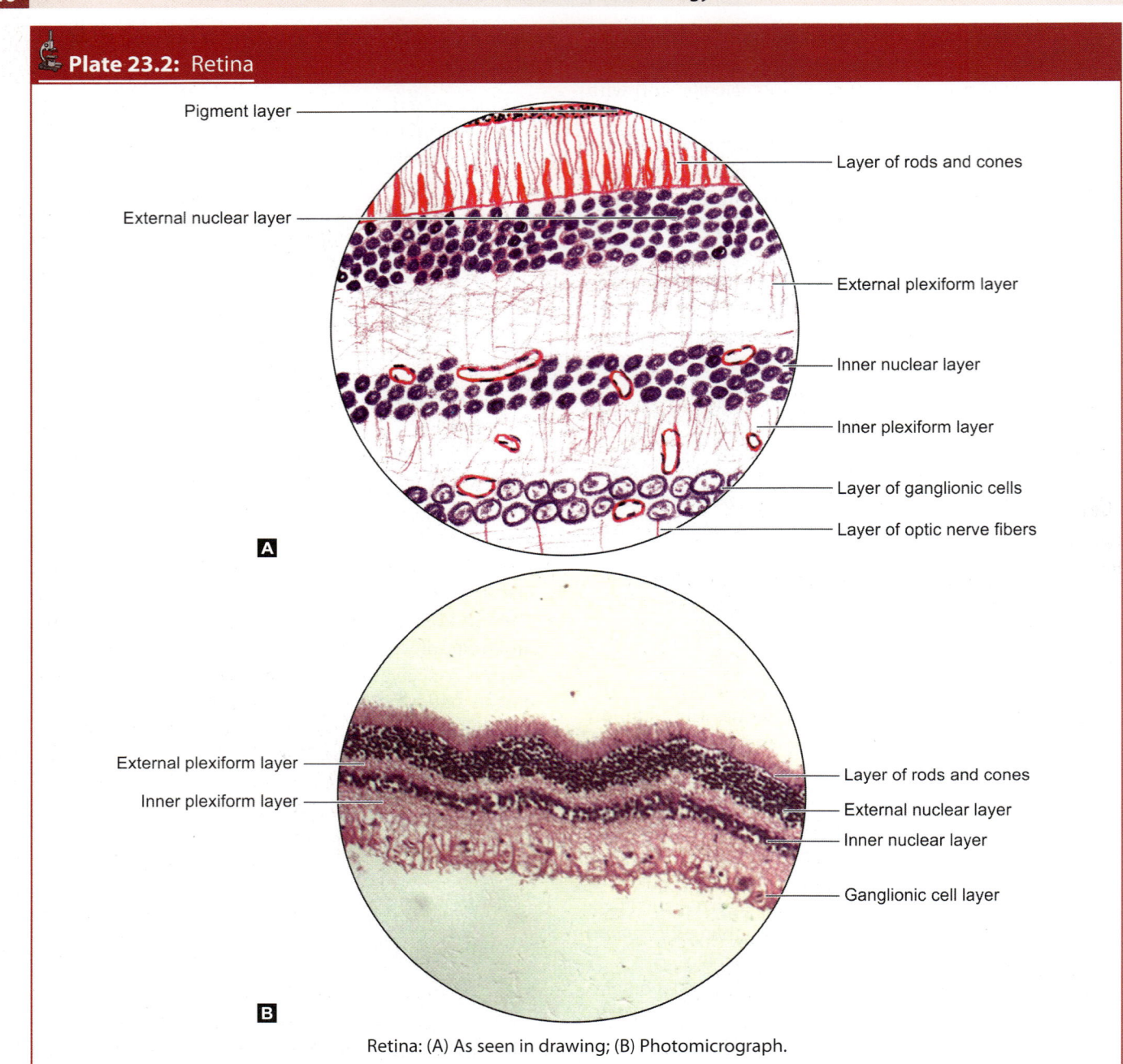

Labels on A (drawing):
- Pigment layer
- Layer of rods and cones
- External nuclear layer
- External plexiform layer
- Inner nuclear layer
- Inner plexiform layer
- Layer of ganglionic cells
- Layer of optic nerve fibers

Labels on B (photomicrograph):
- External plexiform layer
- Inner plexiform layer
- Layer of rods and cones
- External nuclear layer
- Inner nuclear layer
- Ganglionic cell layer

Retina: (A) As seen in drawing; (B) Photomicrograph.

Points of identification
- Made up of ten layers: Pigment epithelium, layer of rods and cones, external limiting membrane, outer nuclear layer, outer plexiform layer, inner nuclear layer, inner plexiform layer, ganglionic cell layer, nerve fiber layer, and internal limiting membrane
- Outer pigment epithelium is made up of simple cuboidal epithelium
- The outer nuclear layer is thicker with densely packed nuclei than in the inner nuclear layer
- Ganglion cell layer is made up of a single row of cells of varying size.

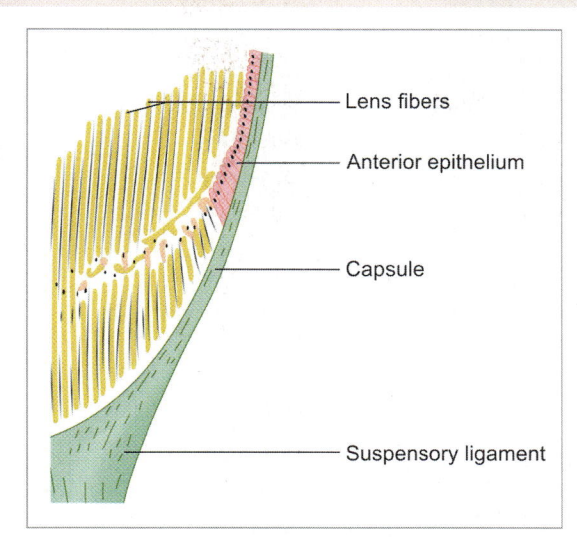

Fig. 23.12: Section through part of the lens near its margin (schematic representation).

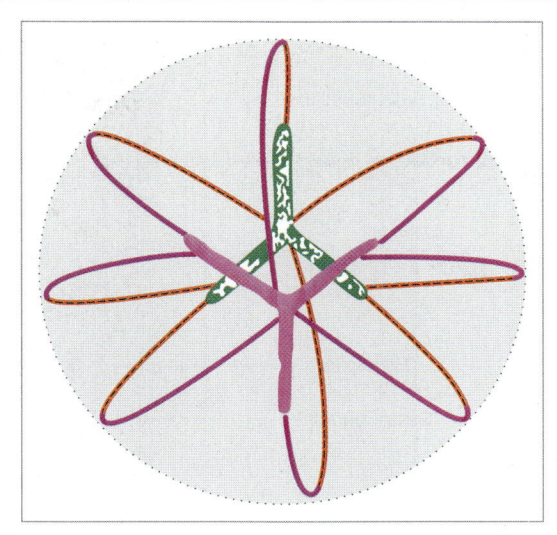

Fig. 23.13: Arrangement of fibers within the lens. Note the Y-shaped lines on the front and back of the lens (schematic representation).

Lens Capsule

- It is a transparent, homogeneous, and highly elastic collagenous basement membrane. It is made up mainly of type IV collagen and glycoproteins.
- The capsule is thicker in front than behind.
- It is secreted by the lens epithelium.

Lens Epithelium

- Deep to the capsule, the lens is covered on its anterior surface by a lens epithelium.
- The cells of the epithelium are cuboidal. However, toward the periphery of the lens, the cells become progressively longer. Ultimately, they are converted into long fibers that form the substance of the lens.
- The cells of epithelium are metabolically active, contain Na^+-K^+-ATPase, and generate adenosine triphosphate (ATP) to meet the energy demand of the lens.
- The cells show high mitotic activity and form new cells which migrate toward the equator. The lens epithelial cells continue to divide and develop into the lens fibers.

Lens Fibers

- The *lens fibers* develop from the lens epithelial cells that continue to divide and get elongated and transformed into lens fibers.
- They are mainly composed of soluble proteins called *crystallins*.
- The fibers formed earlier lie in the deeper plane (nucleus of the lens), the newer ones occupy a more superficial plane.

- When the lens is examined from the front, or from behind, three faint lines are seen radiating from the center to the periphery. In the fetus, these lines form a "Y" that is upright on the front of the lens, and inverted at the back (Fig. 23.13). The lines become more complex in the adult. These lines are called **sutural lines**. They are made up of amorphous material. The ends of lens fibers are attached at these lines. Each lens fiber starts on one surface at such a line, and follows a curved course to reach the opposite surface where it ends by joining another such line.

ACCESSORY VISUAL ORGANS

The accessory visual organs include the extraocular muscles and related fascia, the eyebrows, the eyelids, the conjunctiva, and the lacrimal gland.

Eyelids

Eyelids are two movable skin folds that protect the eye from injury and keep the cornea clean and moist.

The basic structure of an eyelid is shown in Figure 23.14.

- Anteriorly, there is a layer of true skin with which a few small hair and sweat glands are associated. The skin is thin.
- Deep to the skin, there is a layer of delicate connective tissue that normally does not contain fat.
- Considerable thickness of the lid is formed by fasciculi of the palpebral part of the orbicularis oculi muscle (skeletal muscle).

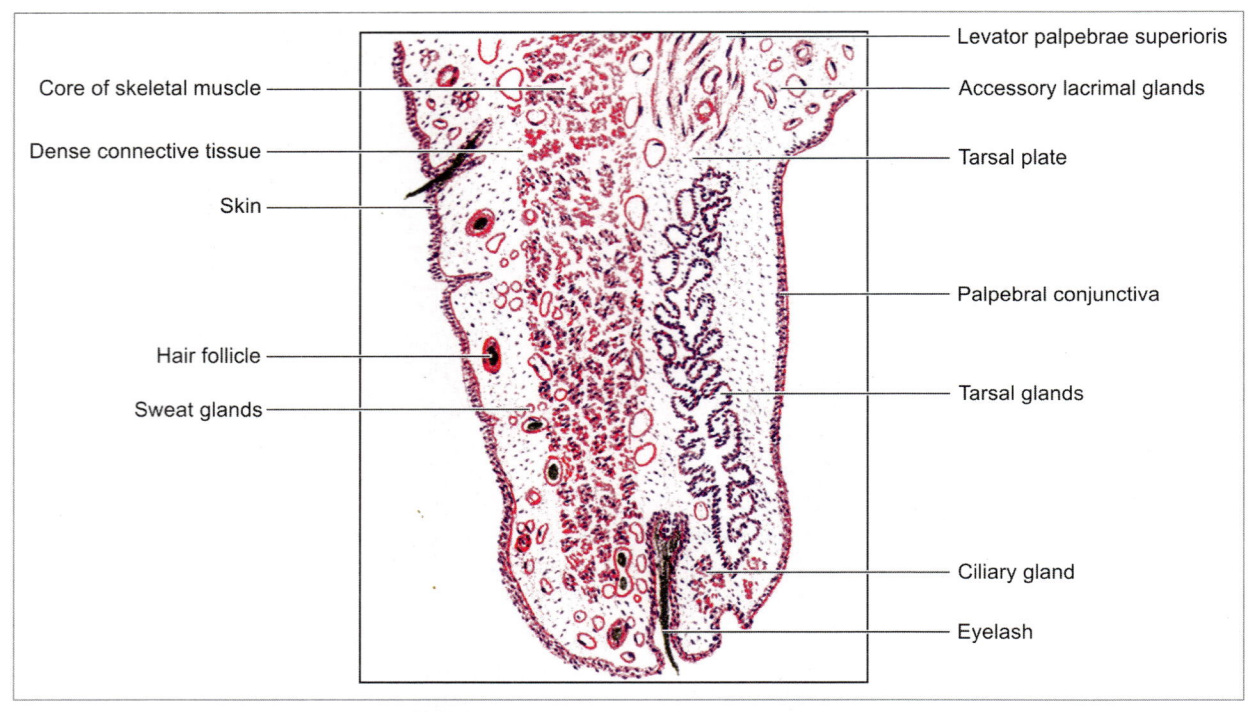

Fig. 23.14: Eyelid (schematic representation).

- The "skeleton" of each eyelid is formed by a mass of fibrous tissue called the *tarsus*, or *tarsal plate*.
- On the deep surface of the tarsal plate, there are a series of vertical grooves in which *tarsal glands* (or *meibomian glands*) are lodged. Occasionally, these glands may be embedded within the tarsal plate. Each gland has a duct that opens at the free margin of the lid. The tarsal glands are modified sebaceous glands. They produce an oily secretion, a thin film of which spreads over the lacrimal fluid (in the conjunctival sac) and delays its evaporation.
- Modified sweat glands, called *ciliary glands* (or *glands of Moll*), are present in the lid near its free edge. Sebaceous glands present in relation to eyelashes constitute the *glands of Zeis*. They open into hair follicles. Accessory lacrimal glands are often present just above the tarsal plate (*glands of Wolfring*).
- The inner surface of the eyelid is lined by the palpebral conjunctiva.

Conjunctiva

- The conjunctiva is a thin transparent membrane that covers the inner surface of each eyelid (*palpebral conjunctiva*) and the anterior part of the sclera (*ocular conjunctiva*).
- At the free margin of the eyelid, the palpebral conjunctiva becomes continuous with skin, and at the margin of the cornea, the ocular conjunctiva becomes continuous with the anterior epithelium of the cornea.
- When the eyelids are closed, the conjunctiva forms a closed *conjunctival sac*. The line along which palpebral conjunctiva is reflected onto the eyeball is called the *conjunctival fornix*: superior, or inferior.
- Conjunctiva consists of an epithelial lining that rests on connective tissue. Over the eyelids, this connective tissue is highly vascular and contains much lymphoid tissue. It is much less vascular over the sclera.
- The epithelium lining the palpebral conjunctiva is typically two layered. There is a superficial layer of columnar cells, and a deeper layer of flattened cells. At the fornix, and over the sclera, the epithelium is three layered; there being an additional layer of polygonal cells between the two layers mentioned above. The three-layered epithelium changes to stratified squamous at the sclerocorneal junction.

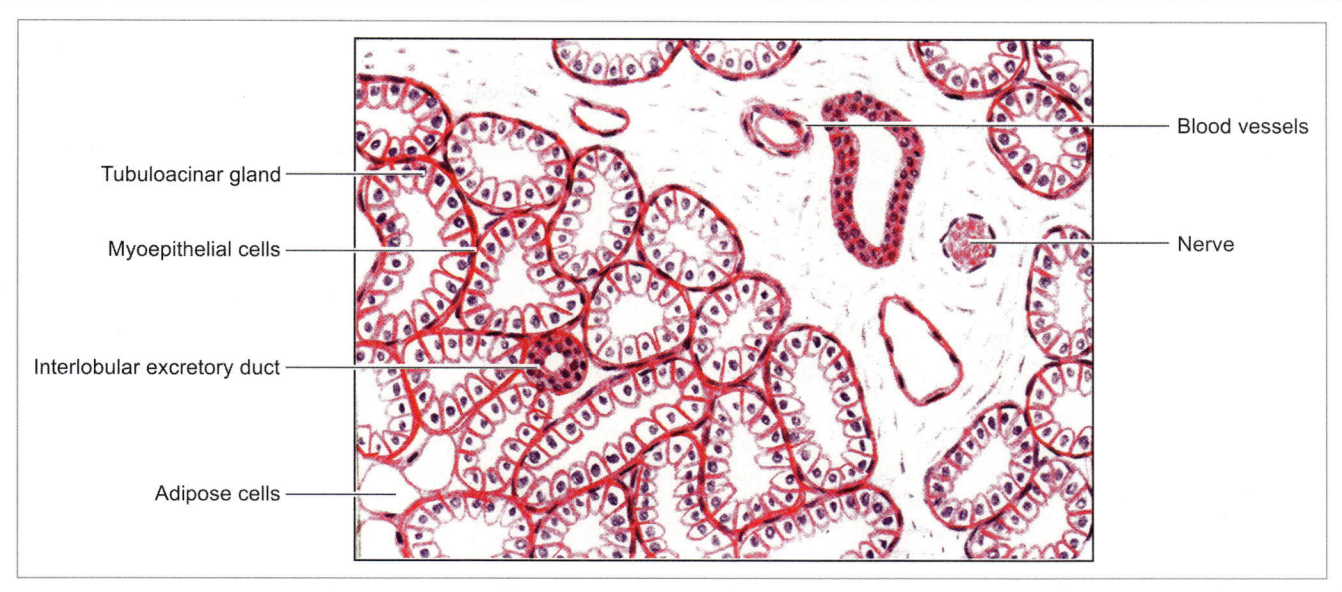

Fig. 23.15: Lacrimal gland (schematic representation).

Lacrimal Gland

- The lacrimal gland is a compound tubuloalveolar gland and consists of a number of lobes that drain through about 20 ducts. It is a tear-secreting gland.
- The structure of the lacrimal gland is similar to that of a serous salivary gland (Fig. 23.15). But it can be distinguished from those of serous salivary glands because of the following features:
  - The acini are larger, and have wider lumina.
  - All cells appear to be of the same type. They are low columnar in shape and stain pink with hematoxylin and eosin.
  - The profiles of the acini are often irregular or elongated.
  - The walls of adjacent acini within a lobule may be pressed together, there being very little connective tissue between them. However, the acini of different lobules are widely separated by connective tissue. Myoepithelial cells are present as in salivary glands.
- Small ducts of the lacrimal gland are lined by cuboidal or columnar epithelium. Larger ducts have a two-layered columnar epithelium or a pseudostratified columnar epithelium.
- Electron microscope studies on the human lacrimal gland reveal that the secretory cells may be of several types, including both mucous and serous cells.
- The ducts of the lacrimal gland open into the lateral part of the superior conjunctival fornix. Lacrimal fluid keeps the conjunctiva moist.
- Accessory lacrimal glands are present near the superior conjunctival fornix (*glands of Krause*).

Added Information

Density of rods and cones in retina

The density of rods and cones in different parts of the retina is shown schematically in Figure 23.16. Note the following points:

- The density of cones is greatest in the fovea (about 1.5 million/mm^2). Their density decreases sharply in proceeding to the margin of the central area, but thereafter the density is uniform up to the ora serrata (about 5,000/mm^2).
- The density of rods is greatest at the margin of the central area (about 1.5 million/mm^2). It decreases sharply on proceeding toward the margin of the central area. There are no rods in the foveola. The density of rods also decreases in passing toward the ora serrata (where it is about 30,000/mm^2).

Bipolar neurons

Bipolar cells of the retina are of various types. The terminology used for them is confusing as it is based on multiple criteria. The main points to note are as follows:

- The primary division is into bipolars that synapse with rods (rod bipolars), and those that synapse with cones (cone bipolars).
- As there are three types of cones, responding to the colors red, green, and blue, we can distinguish three corresponding types of cone bipolars (red cone bipolar, green cone bipolar, and blue cone bipolar).
- When a photoreceptor (rod or cone) is exposed to light, it releases neurotransmitter at its synapse with the bipolar cell. Some bipolars respond to neurotransmitter by depolarization (and secretion of neurotransmitter at their synapses with ganglion cells). These are called ON bipolars as they are "switched on" by light. Other bipolars respond to release of neurotransmitter by hyperpolarization. In other words, they are "switched off" by light and are called OFF bipolars.

Contd...

Contd...

- On the basis of structural characteristics, and the synapses established by them, cone bipolars are divided into three types: *midget*, *blue cone*, and *diffuse*.
  - A midget bipolar establishes synapses with a single cone (which may be red or green sensitive). Some midget bipolars synapse with indented areas on cone pedicles forming triads (Fig. 23.11). These are ON bipolars. Other midget bipolars establish "flat" synapses with the cone pedicle (and are also referred to as flat bipolars). These are OFF bipolars.
  - A blue cone bipolar connects to one blue cone, and establishes triads. It may be of the ON or OFF variety.
  - Diffuse cone bipolars establish synapses with several cone pedicles. They are not color specific.

Axons of rod bipolar neurons synapse with up to four ganglion cells, but those of one midget bipolar neuron synapse with only one (midget) ganglion cell, and with amacrine neurons.

Ganglion cells

- The dendrites of ganglion cells synapse with axons of bipolar cells, and also with processes of amacrine cells. The axons arising from ganglion cells constitute the fibers of the optic nerve.
- Ganglion cells are of two main types. Those that synapse with only one bipolar neuron are **monosynaptic**, while those that synapse with many bipolar neurons are **polysynaptic**. Monosynaptic ganglion cells are also called *midget ganglion cells*. Each of them synapses with one midget bipolar neuron. We have seen that midget bipolars in turn receive impulses from a single cone. This arrangement is usual in the central region of the retina, and allows high resolution of vision to be attained.
- Polysynaptic ganglion cells are of various types. Some of them synapse only with rod bipolars (*rod ganglion cells*). Others have very wide dendritic ramifications that may synapse with several 100 bipolar neurons (*diffuse ganglion cells*). This arrangement allows for summation of stimuli received through very large numbers of photoreceptors facilitating vision in poor light. On physiological grounds, ganglion cells are also classified as "ON" or "OFF" cells.

Horizontal neurons

Horizontal neurons establish numerous connections between photoreceptors (Fig. 23.17). Some of them are excitatory, while others are inhibitory. In this way, these neurons play a role in integrating the activity of photoreceptors located in adjacent parts of the retina. As they participate in synapses between photoreceptors and bipolar neurons, horizontal neurons may regulate synaptic transmission between these cells.

Amacrine neurons

Different types of amacrine neurons are recognized depending upon the pattern of branching. We have seen that the processes of amacrine neurons enter the internal plexiform layer where they may synapse with axons of several bipolar cells, and with the dendrites of several ganglion cells (Fig. 23.18). They also synapse with other amacrine cells. At many places, an amacrine process synapsing with a ganglion cell is accompanied by a bipolar cell axon. The two are referred to as a *dyad*.

Contd...

Internal plexiform cells (present in the internal plexiform layer) represent a third variety of horizontally oriented neurons in the retina.

- Apart from integration of impulses from rods and cones, horizontal, amacrine, and internal plexiform cells act as "gates" that can modulate passage of inputs from rods and cones to ganglion cells. In this connection, it is to be noted that processes of amacrine neurons are interposed between processes of bipolar cells and ganglion cells, while processes of horizontal cells are interposed between photoreceptors and bipolar cells.
- While there are well over a 100 million photoreceptors in each retina, there are only about 1 million ganglion cells, each giving origin to one fiber of the optic nerve (the bipolar cells are intermediate in number between photoreceptors and ganglion cells). In passing from the photoreceptors to the ganglion cells, there has, therefore, to be considerable convergence of impulses (Fig. 23.19). Each ganglion cell would be influenced by impulses originating in several photoreceptors. On functional considerations, it would be expected that such convergence would be most marked near the periphery of the retina, and that it would involve the rods much more than the cones. It has been estimated that in the peripheral parts of the retina, one ganglion cell may be connected to as many as 300 rods or to 10 cones. Convergence leads to summation of impulses arising in many photoreceptors and allows vision even in very dim light. It would also be expected that convergence would be minimal in the macula, and absent in the foveola to allow maximal resolution.
- The second highly important fact about intraretinal connections is the presence of numerous arrangements for interaction of adjacent regions of the retina as follows:
  - Firstly, cone pedicles establish numerous contacts with other cone pedicles and with adjacent rod spherules.
  - Except in the fovea, most photoreceptors are connected to more than one bipolar cell. In turn, each bipolar cell is usually connected to more than one ganglion cell.
  - The vertically arranged elements of the retina (photoreceptors, bipolar cells, and ganglion cells) are intimately interconnected to adjacent elements through horizontal neurons and amacrine neurons.

Mechanism of firing of bipolar neurons

- When no light falls on the retina, photoreceptors are depolarized. Exposure to light causes hyperpolarization.
- When a photoreceptor is depolarized, it releases inhibitor at its junction with a bipolar neuron. This prevents the bipolar neuron from firing. Release of inhibitor is controlled by voltage-gated calcium channels.
- Hyperpolarization of photoreceptor, caused by exposure to light, leads to closure of Ca^{++} gates and release of inhibitor is stopped. This causes the bipolar neuron to fire. As explained earlier, this description applies to ON bipolars.
- Rhodopsin, present in photoreceptors, is a complex of a protein *opsin* and *cis-retinal* that is sensitive to light. When exposed to light, cis-retinal is transformed to trans-retinal. This leads to decrease in concentration of cyclic GMP that in turn leads to closure of sodium channels. Closure of sodium channels results in hyperpolarization of photoreceptor (Flowchart 23.1).

Contd...

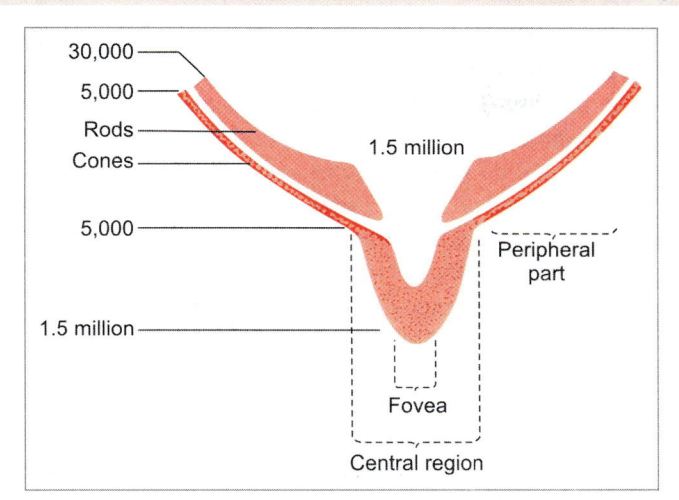

CHAPTER 23: Special Senses: Eye

Fig. 23.16: Scheme to show the relative number of rods and cones in different parts of the retina. The figures represent number of receptors per mm². The diagram is not drawn to scale.

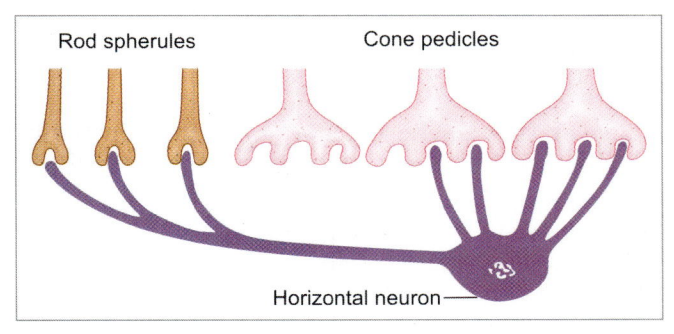

Fig. 23.17: Connections of a cone horizontal neuron (schematic representation).

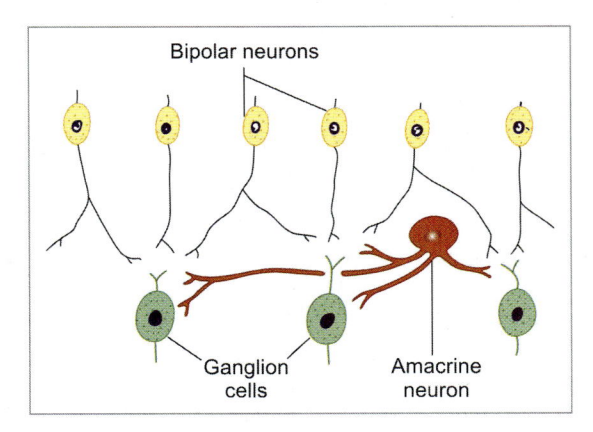

Fig. 23.18: Connections of an amacrine neuron (schematic representation).

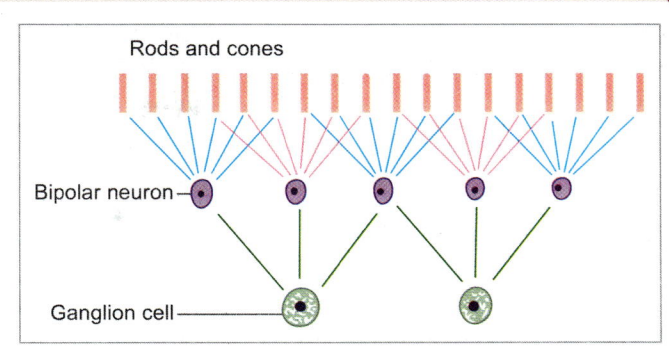

Fig. 23.19: How impulses arising in several photoreceptors concentrate on one ganglion cell (schematic representation)?

Flowchart 23.1: Mechanism of firing of bipolar neurons.

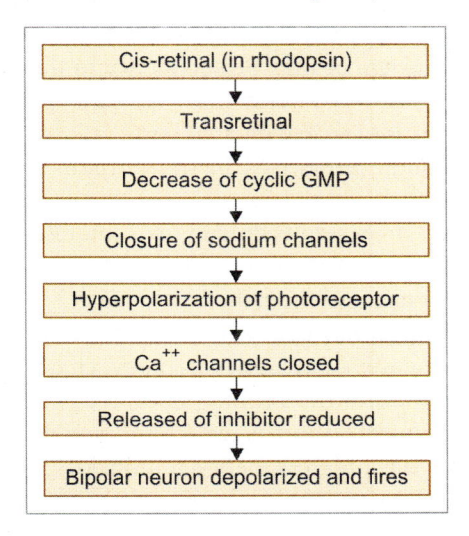

Cis-retinal (in rhodopsin) → Transretinal → Decrease of cyclic GMP → Closure of sodium channels → Hyperpolarization of photoreceptor → Ca^{++} channels closed → Released of inhibitor reduced → Bipolar neuron depolarized and fires

APPLIED HISTOLOGY

Cornea

Corneal ulcer: It is an inflammatory or infective condition of the cornea involving disruption of epithelial layer and corneal stroma.

Keratitis: It is an inflammation of cornea, may be or may not be associated with infection. Noninfectious keratitis may be due to minor injuries or contact lens, long wear, or foreign body.

Corneal opacity: It occurs when the cornea becomes scarred. This stops light from passing through the cornea to the retina and may cause the cornea to appear white or clouded over.

Corneal abrasion: The loss of the surface epithelial layer of the eye's cornea as a result of trauma to the surface of the eye.

Corneal neovascularization: Excessive ingrowth of blood vessels from the limbal vascular plexus into the cornea, caused by deprivation of oxygen from the air.

Keratoconus: A degenerative disease, the cornea thins and changes shape to be more like a cone.

Wilson's disease: Copper pigment deposited in the Descemet's membrane.

Retina

- **Retinal detachment**: It is the separation of the neurosensory retina from the retinal pigment epithelium. It may occur spontaneously in older individuals past 50 years of age or may be secondary to trauma in the region of head and neck. There are three pathogenetic mechanisms of retinal detachment:
  1. Pathologic processes in the vitreous or anterior segment
  2. Collection of serous fluid in the subretinal space
  3. Accumulation of vitreous under the retina through a hole or a tear in the retina.
- **Retinitis pigmentosa**: It is a group of systemic and ocular diseases of unknown etiology, characterized by degeneration of the retinal pigment epithelium. The earliest clinical finding is night blindness due to loss of rods and may progress to total blindness.
- **Retinoblastoma**: This is the most common malignant ocular tumor in children. It may be present at birth or recognized in early childhood before the age of 4 years. About 60% cases of retinoblastoma are sporadic and the remaining 40% are familial. Familial tumors are often multiple and multifocal and transmitted as an autosomal dominant trait by retinoblastoma gene (Rb gene) located on chromosome 13. Such individuals have a higher incidence of bilateral tumors and have increased risk of developing second primary tumor, particularly osteogenic sarcoma. Clinically, the child presents with leukokoria, i.e. white pupillary reflex.

Lens

Cataract: It is the opacification of the normally crystalline lens which leads to gradual painless blurring of vision. The various causes of cataract are: Senility, congenital (e.g. Down syndrome, rubella, galactosemia), traumatic (e.g. penetrating injury, electrical injury), metabolic (e.g. diabetes, hypoparathyroidism), drug-associated (e.g. long-term corticosteroid therapy), smoking, and heavy alcohol consumption.

Eyelid

- **Stye or "external hordeolum"** is an acute suppurative inflammation of the sebaceous glands of Zeis, the apocrine glands of Moll, and the eyelash follicles.
- **Chalazion** is a very common lesion and is the chronic inflammatory process involving the meibomian glands. It occurs as a result of obstruction to the drainage of secretions. The inflammatory process begins with destruction of meibomian glands and duct and subsequently involves tarsal plate.

MULTIPLE CHOICE QUESTIONS

1. Which structure is transparent?
   a. Choroid
   b. Ciliary body
   c. Iris
   d. Cornea
2. What type of neurons is present in the retina?
   a. Unipolar
   b. Pseudounipolar
   c. Bipolar
   d. Multipolar
3. Which layer of the cornea is acellular?
   a. Epithelium
   b. Endothelium
   c. Descemet's membrane
   d. Substantia propria
4. Which of the following is the receptor for color?
   a. Rods
   b. Cones
   c. Bipolar cells
   d. Ganglion cells
5. Nutrition of cornea are all, *except*:
   a. Lacrimal fluid on the surface of cornea
   b. Aqueous humor in anterior chamber
   c. Blood vessels at sclerocorneal junction
   d. Central artery of retina
6. All of the following are the functions of pigment layer, *except*:
   a. It absorbs and prevents back reflection of light
   b. Convert light to electrical energy
   c. Provide mechanical support to them
   d. They have a phagocytic role
7. Cell that form the internal limiting membrane is:
   a. Ganglion
   b. Müller
   c. Bipolar
   d. Amacrine
8. Keratitis is a inflammation of:
   a. Sclera
   b. Retina
   c. Cornea
   d. Choroid

Answers
1. d   2. c   3. c   4. d   5. d   6. b   7. b   8. c

CHAPTER 24

Special Senses: Ear

Learning objectives

To study the:
- Parts of ear
- Components and structure of external ear
- Components of middle ear
- Bony labyrinth and its parts
- Membranous labyrinth and its parts
- Specialized end organs in membranous labyrinth
- Mechanism of hearing
- Applied histology

IDENTIFICATION POINTS

Pinna
- The pinna has a core of elastic cartilage covered on both sides by true skin in which hair follicles and sweat glands are seen.

Cochlea
- The cochlea is embedded in the petrous temporal bone
- It is in the form of a spiral canal and is, therefore, cut up six times
- The cone-shaped mass of bone surrounded by these turns of the cochlea is called the modiolus which contains a canal through which fibers of the cochlear nerve pass
- A mass of neurons belonging to the spiral ganglion lies to the inner side of each turn of the cochlea
- The parts to be identified in each turn of the cochlea are the scala vestibuli, scala media, the scala tympani, the vestibular membrane, the basilar membrane, the membrana tectoria, and the organ of Corti, and the spiral lamina
- Outer wall of the cochlear turn is the spiral ligament and it is lined by avascularized epithelium (stria vascularis).

INTRODUCTION

- Ear is the peripheral sense organ concerned with hearing and equilibrium.
- Anatomically speaking, the ear is made up of three main parts called the ***external ear***, the ***middle ear***, and the ***internal ear***.
- The external and middle ears are concerned exclusively with hearing. The internal ear has a ***cochlear part*** concerned with hearing, and a ***vestibular part*** which provides information to the brain regarding the position and movements of the head.

The main parts of the ear are shown in Figure 24.1.

EXTERNAL EAR

- The external ear consists of ***auricle*** or ***pinna*** and ***external acoustic meatus (external auditory canal)***.
- The part of the ear that is seen on the surface of the body (i.e. the part that the lay person calls the ear) is anatomically speaking, the auricle or pinna. Leading inward from the auricle, there is a tube called the external acoustic meatus.
- The inner end of the external acoustic meatus is closed by a thin membranous diaphragm called the ***tympanic membrane***. This membrane separates the external acoustic meatus from the middle ear.

Auricle (Pinna)

- The auricle consists of a thin plate of elastic cartilage covered on both sides by true skin (Plate 24.1).
- The skin is closely adherent to the cartilage on its lateral surface while it is comparatively loose on medial surface. Epithelium is squamous keratinizing. Hair follicles, sebaceous glands, and sweat glands are present in the skin; adipose tissue is present only in lobule.

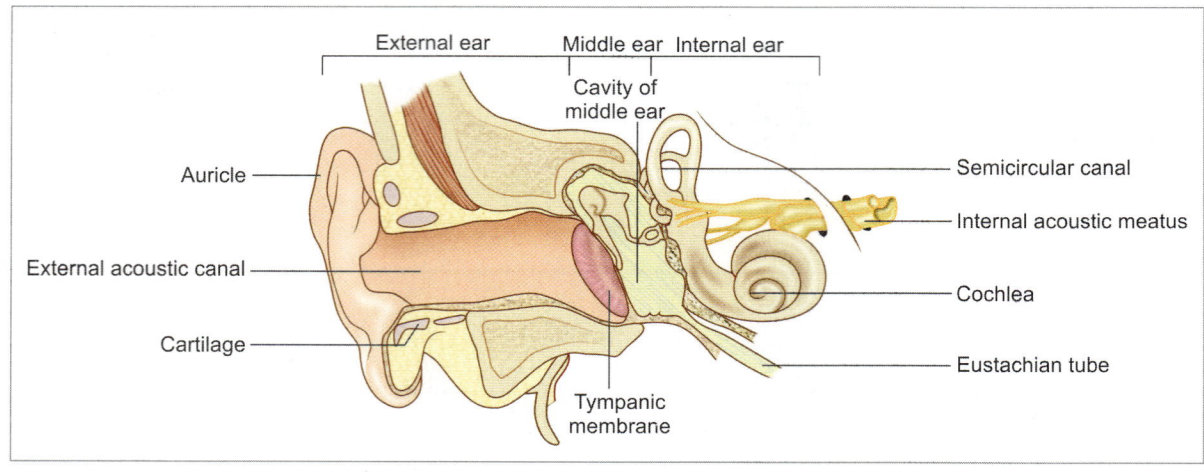

Fig. 24.1: The main parts of the ear (schematic representation).

Plate 24.1: Pinna

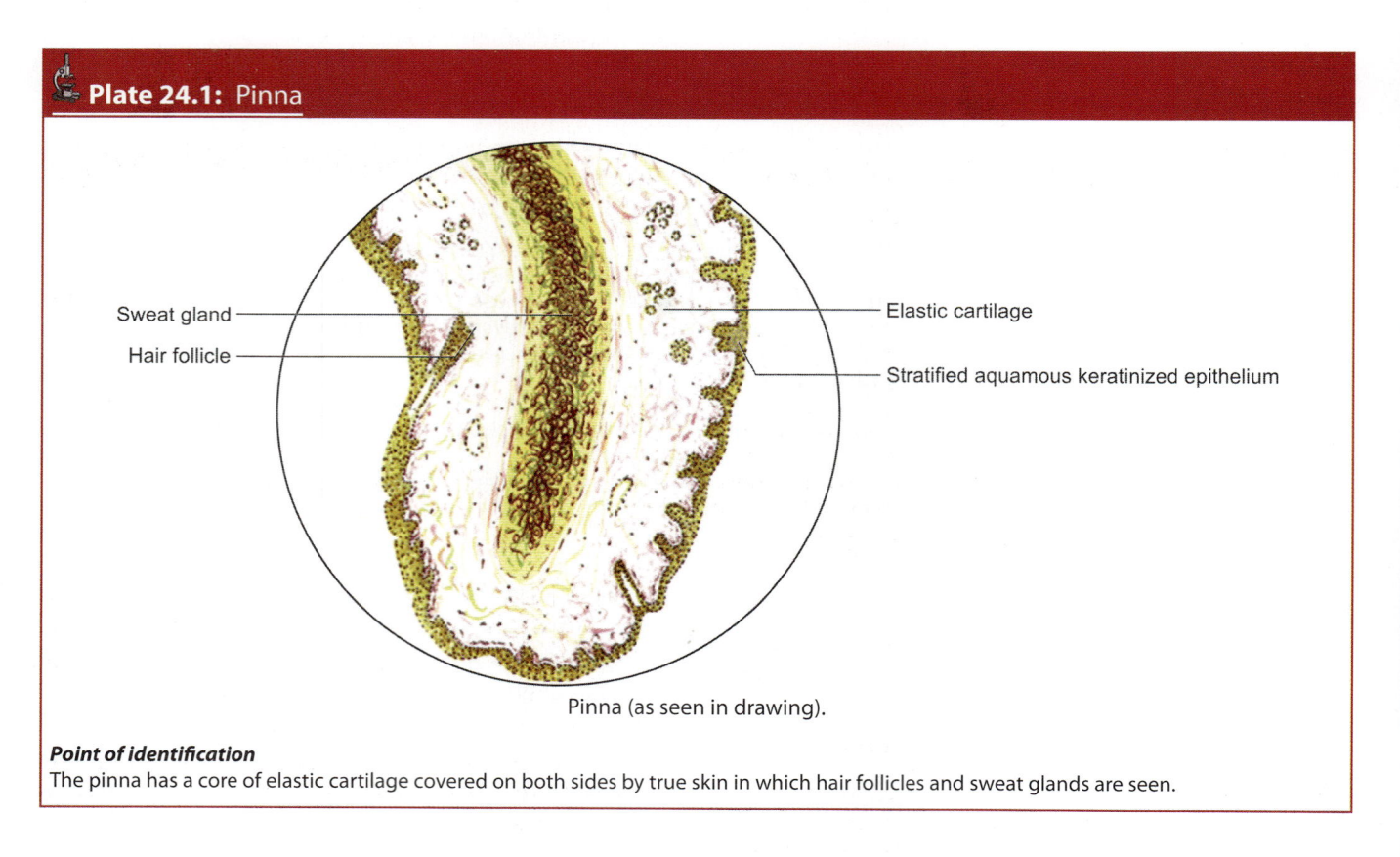

Pinna (as seen in drawing).

Point of identification
The pinna has a core of elastic cartilage covered on both sides by true skin in which hair follicles and sweat glands are seen.

External Acoustic Meatus

- External auditory canal (EAC) measures about 24 mm and extends from the concha to the tympanic membrane.
- EAC is usually divided into two parts: (1) cartilaginous and (2) bony. Its outer one-third (8 mm) is cartilaginous and its inner two-thirds (16 mm) is bony.

- **Cartilaginous EAC:** It is a continuation of the cartilage that forms the framework of the pinna. The skin of the cartilaginous canal is thick and contains hair follicles, ceruminous and pilosebaceous glands that secrete wax. The ceruminous glands secrete the wax of the ear. They are modified sweat glands lined by a columnar, cuboidal, or squamous epithelium.

- **Bony EAC**: It is mainly formed by the tympanic portion of temporal bone but roof is formed by the squamous part of the temporal bone. Skin of the bony EAC is thin and continuous over the tympanic membrane. Skin is devoid of subcutaneous layer, hair follicles, and ceruminous glands.
- **Isthmus**: Approximately 6 mm lateral to tympanic membrane, bony EAC has a narrowing called the isthmus.

Tympanic Membrane

- Its dimensions are: 9–10 mm height and 8–9 mm width. It is 0.1 mm thick.
- Tympanic membrane (TM) is a partition wall between the EAC and the middle ear. It is positioned obliquely. It forms angle of 55° with deep EAC.
- **Structure**: Tympanic membrane consists of the following three layers:
  - **Outer epithelial layer**: It is continuous with the EAC skin.
  - **Middle fibrous layer**: The middle layer is made up of fibrous tissue, which is lined on the outside by skin (continuous with that of the external acoustic meatus), and on the inside by mucous membrane of the tympanic cavity.
  - The fibrous layer contains collagen fibers and some elastic fibers. The fibers are arranged in two layers. In the outer layer, they are placed radially, while in the inner layer, they run circularly.
  - **Inner mucosal layer**: The mucous membrane is lined by an epithelium which may be cuboidal or squamous. It is said that the mucosa over the upper part of the tympanic membrane may have patches of ciliated columnar epithelium, but this is not borne out by EM studies.
- **Otoscopy**: Normal tympanic membrane is shiny and pearly gray in color. Its transparency varies from person to person.

MIDDLE EAR

- The *middle ear* is a small space placed deep within the petrous part of the temporal bone. It is also called the *tympanum*.
- Medially, the middle ear is closely related to parts of the internal ear. It is lined with mucous membrane.
- The cavity of the middle ear is continuous with that of the nasopharynx through a passage called the *auditory tube*. Within the cavity of the middle ear, there are three small bones or *ossicles*: the *malleus*, the *incus*, and the *stapes*. They form a chain that is attached on one side to the tympanic membrane, and at the other end to a part of the internal ear.

Tympanic Cavity

- The walls of the tympanic cavity are formed by bone which is lined by mucous membrane.
- The mucous membrane also covers the ossicles.
- The lining epithelium varies from region to region. Typically, it is cuboidal or squamous. At places, it may be ciliated columnar. The ossicles of the middle ear consist of compact bone, but do not have marrow cavities.

Auditory Tube (Eustachian Tube)

- It is a channel connecting the tympanic cavity with the nasopharynx. The length of Eustachian tube (ET) is 36 mm. Its lateral third is bony and medial two-thirds (i.e. 24 mm) is fibrocartilaginous.
- The bone or cartilage is covered by mucous membrane which is lined by ciliated columnar epithelium. Near the pharyngeal end of the tube, the epithelium becomes pseudostratified columnar.
- Goblet cells and tubuloalveolar mucous glands are also present. A substantial collection of lymphoid tissue, present at the pharyngeal end, forms the **tubal tonsil**.

INTERNAL EAR

- The *internal ear* is in the form of a complex system of cavities lying within the petrous temporal bone. It has sense organs for both hearing and balance.
- It has a central part called the *vestibule*. Continuous with the front of the vestibule, there is a spiral-shaped cavity called the *cochlea*. Posteriorly, the vestibule is continuous with three *semicircular canals*.
- Because of the complex shape of these intercommunicating cavities, the internal ear is also called the *labyrinth*. It consists of a bony labyrinth contained within the petrous part of temporal bone (Fig. 24.2). The space bounded by bone is *bony labyrinth*. Its wall is made up of bone that is denser than the surrounding bone. Its inner surface is lined by periosteum. Lying within the bony labyrinth, there is a system of ducts which constitute the *membranous labyrinth*.
- The space within the membranous labyrinth is filled by a fluid called the endolymph. The space between the membranous labyrinth and the bony labyrinth is filled by another fluid called the perilymph.

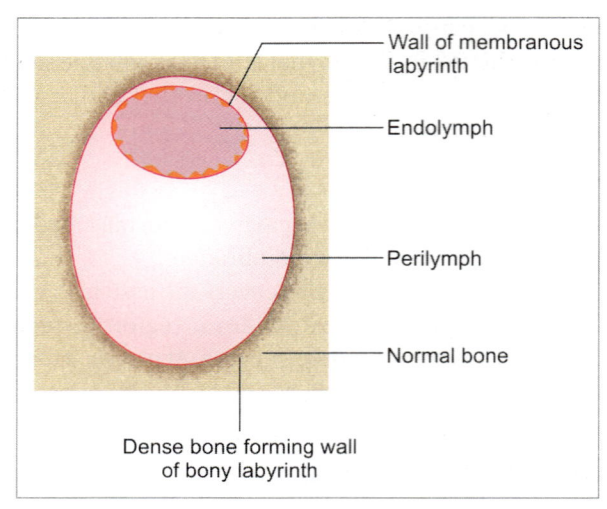

Fig. 24.2: Basic structure of internal ear as seen in a section through a semicircular canal (schematic representation).

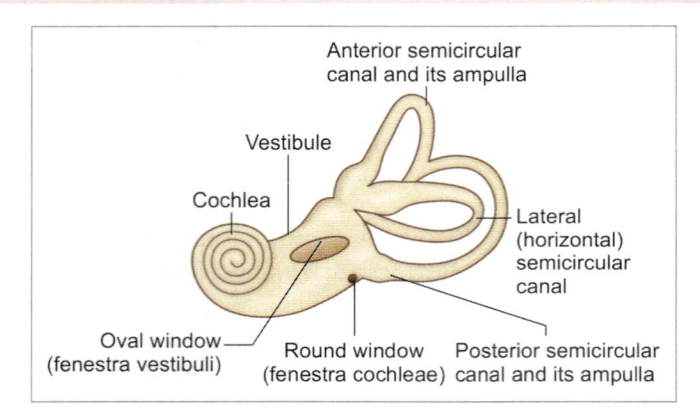

Fig. 24.3: Bony labyrinth as seen from the lateral side (schematic representation).

Bony Labyrinth

The bony labyrinth consists of three parts:
1. Vestibule
2. Semicircular canals
3. The bony cochlea.

Vestibule

Vestibule is the central part (Fig. 24.3). It is continuous anteriorly with the **cochlea**, and posteriorly with three **semicircular canals**.

Semicircular Canals

- There are three semicircular canals (SCCs): Lateral (horizontal), posterior, and superior (anterior).
- Each canal occupies two-thirds of a circle and has a diameter of 0.8 mm. They lie in planes at right angles to one another.
- Each canal has two ends: Ampullated and nonampullated. All the three ampullated ends and nonampullated end of lateral SCC open independently and directly into the vestibule. The nonampullated ends of posterior and superior canals join and form a crus commune (4 mm length), which then opens into the medial part of vestibule. So, the three SCCs open into the vestibule by five openings.

Bony Cochlea

- The cochlea has a striking resemblance to a snail shell. It is basically a tube that is coiled on itself for two and three-fourth turns. The "turns" rest on a solid core of bone called the **modiolus**.

Note: Because of the spiral nature of the cochlea, the mutual relationships of the structures within it differ in different parts of the cochlea. A structure that is "inferior" in the upper part of the canal becomes "superior" in the lower part. For descriptive convenience, the structures lying next to the modiolus are described as "inner" and those away from it as "outer". These terms as used here are not equivalents of "medial" and "lateral" as normally used. The words "superior" and "inferior" indicate relationships as they exist in the lowest (or basal) turn of the cochlea. In sections, through the middle of the cochlea, the cochlear canal is cut up six times as shown in Plate 24.2.

- The cochlear canal is partially divided into two parts by a bony lamina that projects outward from the modiolus. This bony projection is called the **spiral lamina**.
- Passing from the tip of the spiral lamina to the opposite wall of the canal, there is the **basilar membrane**.
- The spiral lamina and the basilar membrane together divide the cochlear canal into three parts—scala vestibuli, scala tympani, and scala media (membranous cochlea). The lower most channel is the **scala tympani**. When traced proximally, the scala tympani opens in the medial wall of the middle ear through an aperture **fenestra cochleae (round window)**, which is closed by the **secondary tympanic membrane**.
- The part of the cochlear canal above the basilar membrane is further divided into two parts by an obliquely placed **vestibular membrane (of Reissner)**. The part above the vestibular membrane is the **scala vestibuli**. When traced proximally, it becomes continuous with the vestibule (Fig. 24.4).
- At the apex of the cochlea, the scala vestibuli becomes continuous with the scala tympani called helicotrema.

CHAPTER 24: Special Senses: Ear

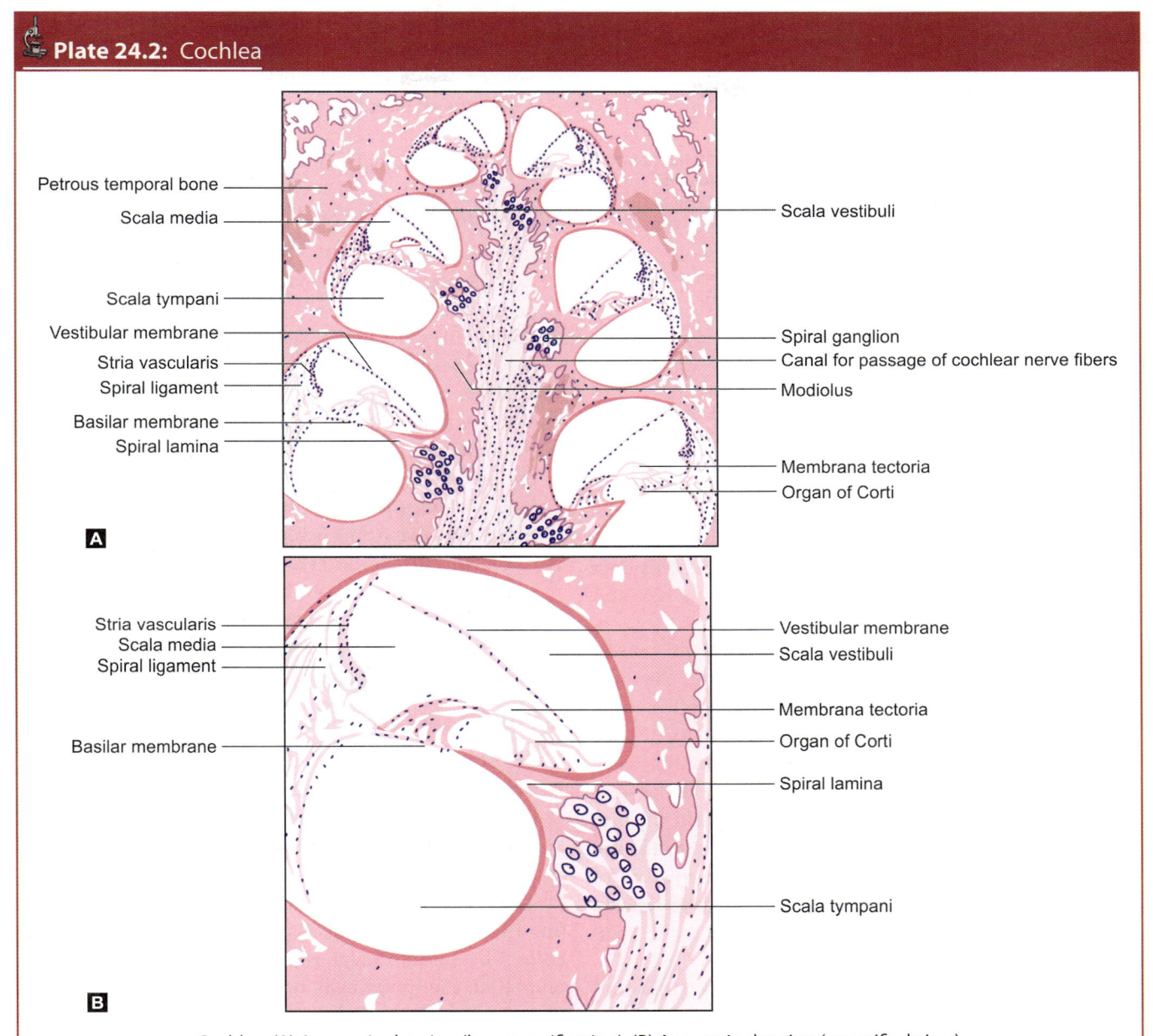

Plate 24.2: Cochlea

Cochlea: (A) As seen in drawing (low magnification); (B) As seen in drawing (magnified view).

Points of identification
- The cochlea is embedded in the petrous temporal bone
- It is in the form of a spiral canal and is, therefore, cut up six times
- The cone-shaped mass of bone surrounded by these turns of the cochlea is called the modiolus which contains a canal through which fibers of the cochlear nerve pass
- A mass of neurons belonging to the spiral ganglion lies to the inner side of each turn of the cochlea
- The parts to be identified in each turn of the cochlea are the scala vestibuli, scala media, the scala tympani, the vestibular membrane, the basilar membrane, the membrana tectoria, and the organ of Corti, and the spiral lamina
- Outer wall of the cochlear turn is the spiral ligament and it is lined by avascularized epithelium (stria vascularis).

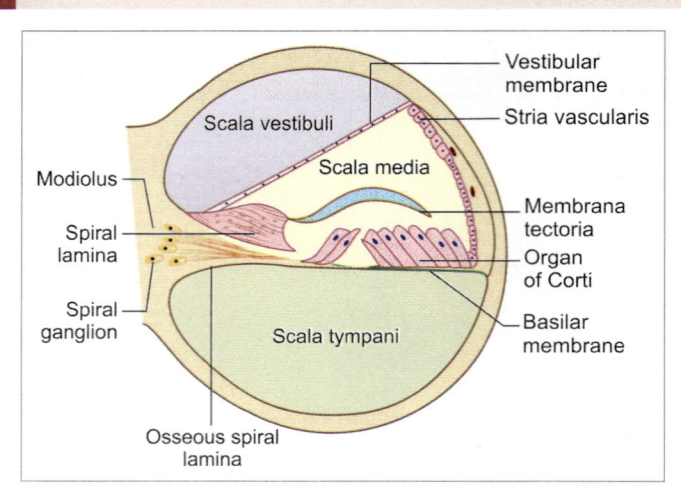

Fig. 24.4: Structure of cochlear canal to show scala vestibuli and tympani (schematic representation).

Both scala vestibuli and scala tympani are filled with perilymph.
- The triangular space between the basilar and vestibular membranes is called the **duct of the cochlea**. This duct represents the membranous labyrinth of the cochlea and contains endolymph.
- The vestibular membrane consists of a basal lamina lined on either side by squamous cells. Some of the cells show an ultrastructure indicative of a fluid transport function. The cells of the membrane form a barrier to the flow of ions between endolymph and perilymph so that these two fluids have different concentrations of electrolytes.
- The basilar membrane is divisible into two parts. The part supporting the organ of Corti is the **zona arcuata**. The part lateral to the zona arcuata is the **zona pectinata**. The zona arcuata is made up of a single layer of delicate filaments of collagen. The zona pectinata is made up of three layers of fibers.
- *Aqueduct of cochlea*: The scala tympani is connected with the subarachnoid space through the aqueduct of cochlea. It is thought to regulate perilymph and pressure in bony labyrinth.

Inner Ear Fluids

Perilymph fills the space between bony and membranous labyrinth while endolymph fills the entire membranous labyrinth.

Perilymph
- It resembles extracellular fluid and is rich in sodium ions. The aqueduct of cochlea provides communication between scala tympani and subarachnoid space. Perilymph percolates through the arachnoid type connective tissue present in the aqueduct of cochlea.
- *Source*: There are two theories:
  1. Filtrate of blood serum from the capillaries of spiral ligament.
  2. CSF reaching labyrinth via aqueduct of cochlea.

Endolymph
- It resembles intracellular fluid and is rich in potassium ions. Protein and glucose contents are less than in perilymph.
- *Source*: They are believed to be following:
  - Stria vascularis
  - Dark cells of utricle and ampullated ends of semicircular ducts.
- *Absorption*: There are following two opinions regarding the absorption of endolymph:
  1. **Endolymphatic sac**: The longitudinal flow theory believes that from cochlear duct, endolymph reaches saccule, utricle, and endolymphatic duct and is then absorbed by endolymphatic sac.
  2. **Stria vascularis**: The radial flow theory believes that endolymph is secreted as well as absorbed by the stria vascularis.

Membranous Labyrinth (Fig. 24.5)

It consists of:
- Utricle and saccule within vestibule
- Cochlear duct in the cochlea
- Three semicircular ducts within each semicircular canal
- Endolymphatic duct and sac.

The wall of the membranous labyrinth is trilaminar. The outer layer is fibrous and is covered with **perilymphatic cells**. The middle layer is vascular. The inner layer is epithelial, the lining cells being squamous or cuboidal. Some of the cells (called **dark cells**) have an ultrastructure indicative of active ionic transport. They probably control the ionic composition of endolymph.

Utricle
- The utricle, which is oblong and irregular, has anteriorly upward slope at an approximate angle of 30°.
- It lies in the posterior part of bony vestibule and receives the five openings of the three semicircular ducts. The utricle (4.33 mm^2) is bigger than saccule (2.4 mm^2) and lies superior to saccule.
- The utricle is connected with the saccule through utriculosaccular duct.

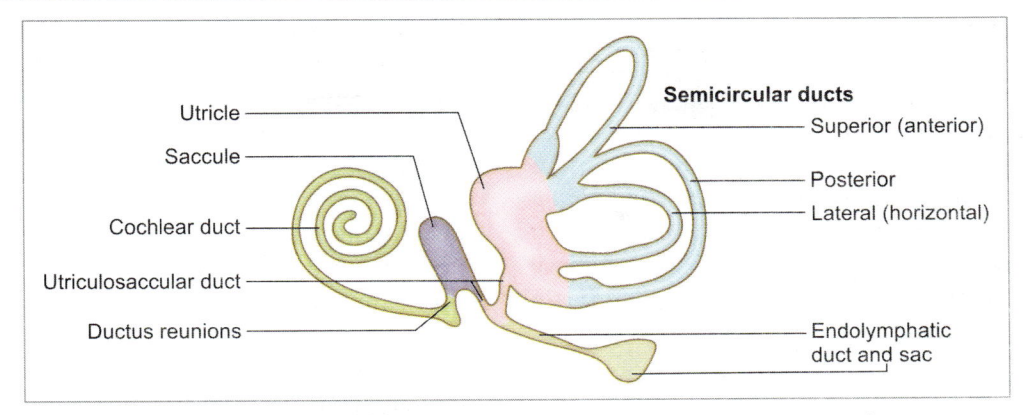

Fig. 24.5: Parts of the membranous labyrinth (schematic representation).

- Its sensory epithelium, which is called macula, is concerned with linear acceleration and deceleration.

Saccule

- The saccule lies anterior to the utricle opposite the stapes footplate in the bony vestibule.
- Its sensory epithelium, macula, responds to linear acceleration and deceleration. The saccule is connected to the cochlea through the thin reunion duct.

Cochlear Duct

The cochlear duct is a triangular canal lying between the basilar membrane and the vestibular membrane (Figs. 24.4 to 24.6).

- The endosteum on the outer wall of the cochlear canal is thickened. This thickened endosteum forms the outer wall of the duct of the cochlea. The basilar and vestibular membranes are attached to this endosteum.

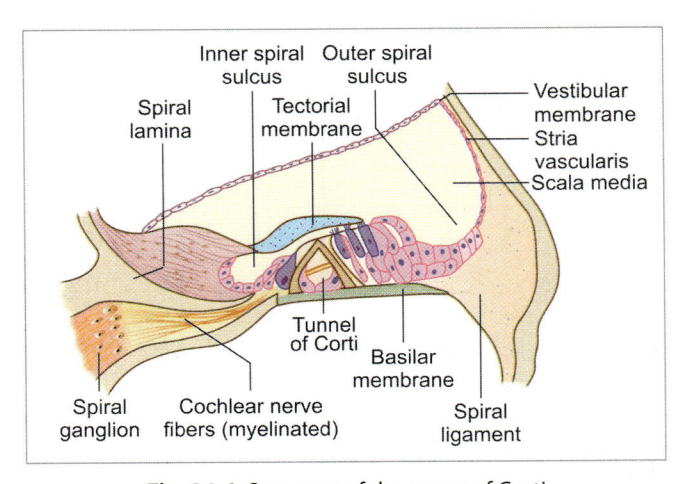

Fig. 24.6: Structure of the organ of Corti (schematic representation).

- The thickened endosteum shows a projection in the region of attachment of the basilar membrane: This projection is called the *spiral ligament*.
- A little above the spiral ligament the thickened endosteum shows a much larger rounded projection into the cochlear duct: This is the *spiral prominence*. The spiral prominence forms the upper border of a concavity called the *outer spiral sulcus*.
- Between the spiral prominence and the attachment of the vestibular membrane, the thickened endosteum is covered by a specialized epithelium that is called the *stria vascularis*. The region is so called because there are capillaries within the thickness of the epithelium (this is the only such epithelium in the whole body). The epithelium of the stria vascularis is made up of three layers of cells: Marginal, intermediate, and basal.
- The cells of the marginal layer are called *dark cells*. They are in contact with the endolymph filling the duct of the cochlea. These cells have a structure and function similar to that of the dark cells already described in the planum semilunatum. These dark cells may be responsible for the formation of endolymph. The basal parts of the dark cells give off processes that come into intimate contact with the intraepithelial capillaries. The capillaries are also in contact with processes arising from cells in the intermediate and basal layers of the stria vascularis.
- Spiral lamina is a bony projection into the cochlear canal. Near the attachment of the spiral lamina to the modiolus, there is a spiral cavity in which the *spiral ganglion* is lodged. This ganglion is made up of bipolar cells. Central processes arising from these cells form the fibers of the cochlear nerve. Peripheral processes of the ganglion cells pass through canals in the spiral lamina to reach the spiral organ of Corti.

- The periosteum on the upper surface of the spiral lamina is greatly thickened to form a mass called the ***limbus lamina spiralis*** (or ***spiral limbus***). The limbus is roughly triangular in shape. It has a flat "lower" surface attached to the spiral lamina, a convex "upper" surface to which the vestibular membrane is attached, and a deeply concave "outer" surface. The concavity is called the ***internal spiral sulcus***. This sulcus is bounded above by a sharp ***vestibular lip*** and below by a ***tympanic lip*** which is fused to the spiral lamina.

Specialized End Organs in Membranous Labyrinth

The internal ear is a highly specialized end organ that performs the dual functions of hearing and of providing information about the position and movements of the head. The impulses in question are converted into nerve impulses by a number of structures that act as transducers.

- These are ***spiral organ*** (***of Corti***) for hearing and maculae (singular = ***macula***) present in the utricle and saccule for changes in position of the head (Fig. 24.7).
- Information about angular movements of the head is provided by end organs called the ***ampullary crests*** (or ***cristae ampullae***). One such crest is present in each semicircular duct. One end of each semicircular duct is dilated to form an ***ampulla***, and the end organ lies within this dilatation. These end organs are described here.

Macula

- They lie in otolith organs (utricle and saccule). Macula of the utricle is situated in its floor in a horizontal plane in the dilated superior portion of the utricle. Macula of saccule is situated in its medial wall in a vertical plane. The macula utriculi (approximately 33,000 hair cells) are larger than saccular macula (approximately 18,000 hair cells).
- The striola, which is a narrow curved line in center, divides the macula into two areas. They appreciate position of head in response to gravity and linear acceleration. A macula consists mainly of two parts: A sensory neuroepithelium and an otolith membrane.
    1. ***Sensory neuroepithelium***: It is made up of type 1 and type 2 cells, which are similar to the hair cells of the ampullary cristae. Type I cells are in higher concentration in the area of striola and change orientation (mirror-shaped) along the line of striola with opposite polarity. The kinocilia face striola in the utricular macula, whereas in saccule, they face away from the striola. The polarity and curvilinear shape of striola offer CNS wide range of neural information of angles in all the three dimensions for optimal perception and compensatory correction. During tilt, translational head movements and positioning, visual stimuli combined with receptors of neck muscles, joint, and ligaments play an important part.
    2. ***Otolithic membrane***: The otolithic membrane consists of a gelatinous mass, a subgelatinous space, and the crystals of calcium carbonate called otoliths (otoconia or statoconia) (Fig. 24.8). The otoconia, which are multitude of small cylindrical

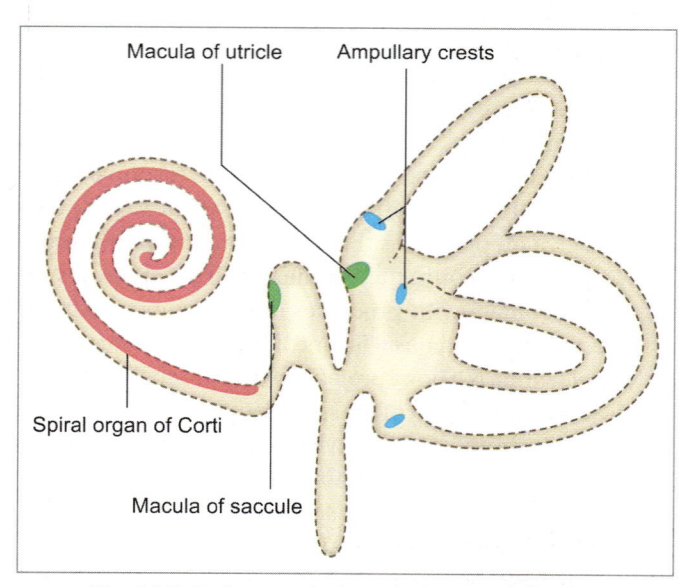

Fig. 24.7: End organs in the membranous labyrinth (schematic representation).

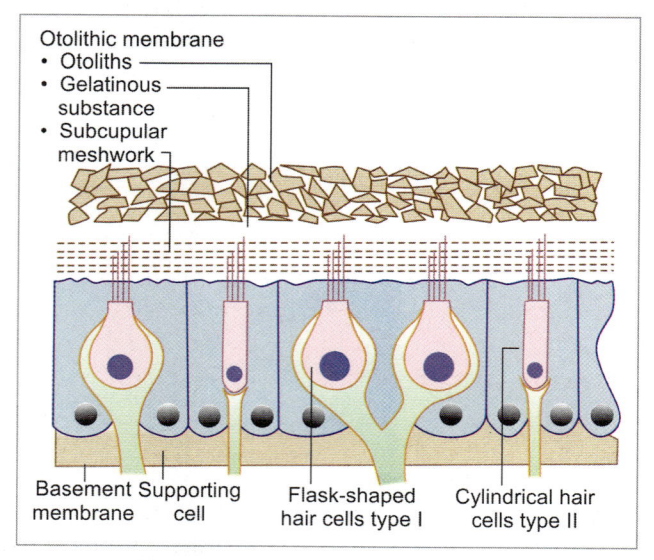

Fig. 24.8: Macula of otolith organs utricle and saccule (schematic representation).

and hexagonally-shaped bodies with pointed ends, consists of an organic protein matrix together with crystallized calcium carbonate. The otoconia (3–19 μm long) lie on the top of the gelatinous mass. The cilia of hair cells project into the gelatinous layer. The linear, gravitational, and head tilt movements result into the displacement of otolithic membrane, which stimulate the hair cells lying in different planes.
- The maculae give information about the position of the head and are organs of *static balance*. In contrast, the ampullary crests are organs of *kinetic balance*.
- The macula of the saccule may be concerned with the reception of low frequencies of sound. Impulses arising from the ampullary crests and the maculae influence the position of the eyes. They also have an influence on body posture (through the vestibular nuclei).

Spiral Organ of Corti

- This sensory organ of the hearing is situated on the basilar membrane. It is spread like a ribbon along the entire length of basilar membrane (Figs. 24.4 and 24.6).
- The spiral organ of Corti is so called because (like other structures in the cochlea) it extends in a spiral manner through the turns of the cochlea. It is made up of epithelial cells that are arranged in a complicated manner.
- The cells are divisible into the true receptor cells or *hair cells*, and supporting elements which are given different names depending on their location.
- The cells of the spiral organ are covered from above by a gelatinous mass called the *membrana tectoria*. It consists of delicate fibers embedded in a gelatinous matrix. This material is probably secreted by cells lining the vestibular lip of the limbus lamina spiralis.
- The tunnel of Corti, which is situated between the inner and outer rod cells and contains a fluid called cortilymph (Fig. 24.9). The base of the tunnel lies over the basilar membrane.
- To the internal side of the inner rod cells, there is a single row of *inner hair cells*. The inner hair cell is supported by tall cells lining the tympanic lip of the internal spiral sulcus.
- On the outer side of each external rod cell, there are three or four *outer hair cells*. The outer hair cells do not lie directly on the basilar membrane, but are supported by the *phalangeal cells* (*of Deiters*) which rest on the basilar membrane.
- To the outer side of the outer hair cells and the phalangeal cells, there are tall supporting cells (*cells of Hensen*). Still more externally, the outer spiral sulcus is lined by cubical cells (*cells of Claudius*).
- A narrow space the *cuniculum externum* intervenes between the outermost hair cells and the cells of Hensen. A third space, the *cuniculum medium* (or *space of Nuel*) lies between the outer rod cell and the outer hair cells. The spaces are filled with perilymph (or *cortilymph*).

Rod cells (Fig. 24.9)

- Each rod cell (or *pillar cell*) has a broad *base* (or *footplate*, or *crus*) that rests on the basilar membrane, an elongated middle part (*rod* or *scapus*), and an expanded upper end called the *head* or *caput*.
- The bases of the rod cells are greatly expanded and contain their nuclei. The bases of the inner and outer rod cells meet each other forming the base of the tunnel of Corti.
- The heads of these cells also meet at the apex of the tunnel. Here, a convex prominence on the head of the outer rod cell fits into a concavity on the head of the inner rod cell. The uppermost parts of the heads are expanded into horizontal plates called the *phalangeal processes*. These processes join similar processes of neighboring cells to form a continuous membrane called the *reticular lamina*.

Hair cells

- These important receptor cells of hearing transduce sound energy into electrical energy.
- The hair cells are so called because their free "upper" or apical ends bear a number of "hairs". The hairs are really stereocilia.
- Each cell is columnar or piriform. The hair cells are distinctly shorter than the rod cells.

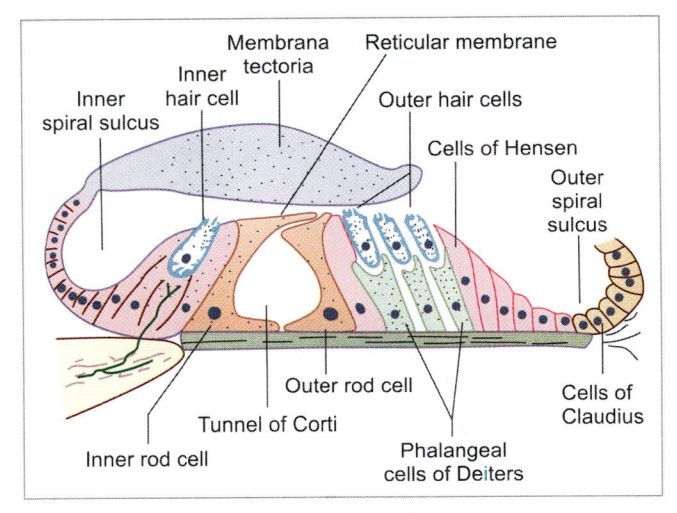

Fig. 24.9: The cells in the organ of Corti (schematic representation).

- ❖ Their apices are at the level of the reticular lamina. Their lower ends (or bases) do not reach the basilar membrane. They rest on phalangeal cells. The plasma membrane at the base of each hair cell forms numerous synaptic contacts with the terminations of the peripheral processes of neurons in the spiral ganglion. Some efferent terminals are also present. The apical surface of each hair cell is thickened to form a *cuticular plate* the edges of which are attached to neighboring cells.
- ❖ There are two types of hair cells—*inner and outer* (Table 24.1).
  1. **Inner hair cells**: Inner hair cells (IHCs) form a single row and are richly supplied by afferent cochlear fibers. These are flask-shaped cells and relatively short (Fig. 24.10). They are very important in the transmission of auditory impulses. Their nerve fibers are mainly afferent.
  2. **Outer hair cells**: Outer hair cells (OHCs) are arranged in three or four rows and mainly receive efferent innervation from the olivary complex. These are long cylindrical cells which modulate the function of inner hair cells (Fig. 24.11). Their nerve fibers are mainly efferent. The lower end of each outer hair cell fits into a depression on the upper end of a phalangeal cell, but the inner hair cells do not have such a relationship. The "hairs" of the outer hair cells are somewhat longer and more slender than those on inner hair cells. They are arranged as a shallow "U" rather than a "V". Occasionally, the outer hair cells may have more than three rows of hair, and the rows may assume the shape of a "W" (instead of a "V").

Outer phalangeal cells and reticular lamina

- ❖ These are the cells that support the outer hair cells.
- ❖ They lie lateral to the outer rod cells. Their bases rest on the basilar membrane. Their apical parts have a complicated configuration. The greater part of the apex forms a cup-like depression into which the base of an outer hair cell fits.
- ❖ Arising from one side (of the apical part) of the cell, there is a thin rod-like *phalangeal process*. This process passes "upward", in the interval between hair cells, to reach the

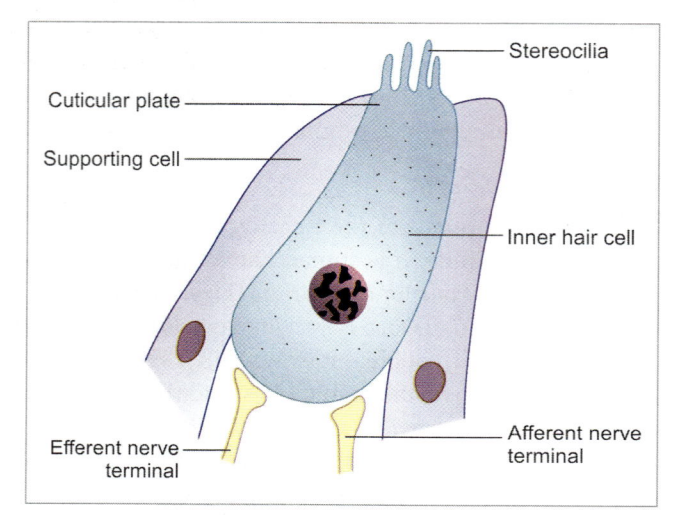

Fig. 24.10: Structure of the inner hair cell (schematic representation).

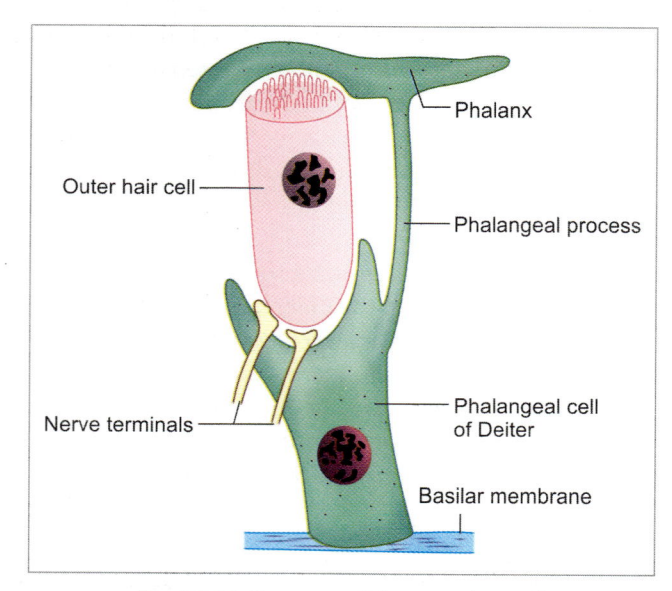

Fig. 24.11: Structure of the outer hair cell (schematic representation).

Table 24.1: Differences between inner hair cells (IHCs) and outer hair cells (OHCs).

	Inner hair cells	Outer hair cells
Cells numbers	3,500	12,000
Rows	One	Three or four
Shape	Flask	Cylindrical
Nerve supply	Mainly afferent fibers	Mainly efferent fibers
Development	Early	Late
Function	Transmit auditory stimuli	Modulate function of inner hair cells
Ototoxicity	More resistant	More sensitive and easily damaged
High intensity noise	More resistant	More sensitive and easily damaged
Generation of otoacoustic emissions	No	Yes

level of the apices of hair cells. Here, the phalangeal process expands to form a transverse plate called the ***phalanx***.

❖ The edges of the phalanges of adjoining phalangeal cells unite with each other to form a membrane called the ***reticular lamina*** (the reticular lamina also receives contributions from the heads of hair cells). The apices of hair cells protrude through apertures in this lamina. The cell edges forming the reticular lamina contain bundles of microtubules embedded in dense cytoplasm. Adjacent cell margins are united by desmosomes, occluding junctions, and gap junctions. The reticular lamina forms a barrier impermeable to ions except through the cell membranes. It also forms a rigid support between the apical parts of hair cells thus, ensuring that the hair cells rub against the membrana tectoria when the basilar membrane vibrates.

Ampullary Crests (Fig. 24.12)

❖ One ampullary crest is present in the ampullated end of each of the three semicircular ducts. Each crest is an elongated ridge projecting into the ampulla, and reaching almost up to the opposite wall of the ampulla. The long axis of the crest lies at right angles to that of the semicircular duct.

❖ The crest is lined by a columnar epithelium in which two kinds of cells are present. These are ***hair cells*** which are specialized mechanoreceptors, and ***supporting*** (or ***sustentacular***) ***cells***.

❖ **Hair cells**: The hair cells occupy only the upper half of the epithelium. The luminal surface of each hair cell bears "hairs". When examined by EM, the "hairs" are seen to be of two types as follows:

1. There is one large kinocilium which is probably nonmotile.
2. There are a number of stereocilia (large microvilli).

❖ These "hair" extend into a gelatinous (protein polysaccharide) material which covers the crest and is called the ***cupula***. The hair processes of the hair cells are arranged in a definite pattern, the orientation being specific for each semicircular duct. This orientation is of functional importance.

❖ Each hair cell is innervated by terminals of afferent fibers of the vestibular nerve. Efferent fibers that can alter the threshold of the receptors are also present.

❖ Hair cells can be divided into two types depending on their shape and on the pattern of nerve endings around them. Type I hair cells (inner hair cell) are flask shaped. They have a rounded base and a short neck. The nucleus lies in the expanded basal part (outer hair cell). The basal part is surrounded by a goblet-shaped nerve terminal (or ***calix***). Type II hair cells are columnar. Both types of hair cells receive nerve terminals which are afferent (nongranular) as well as efferent (granular).

❖ Both in the ampullae of semicircular ducts, and in the maculae of the utricle and saccule, each hair cell is polarized with regard to the position of the kinocilium relative to the stereocilia. Each hair cell (in an ampulla) can be said to have a side that is toward the utricle, and a side that faces in the opposite direction. In the lateral semicircular duct, the kinocilia lie on the side of the cells which are toward the utricle, while in the anterior and posterior semicircular ducts, the kinocilia lie on the opposite side. When stereocilia are bent toward the kinocilium, the cell is hyperpolarized. It is depolarized when bending is away from the kinocilium. Depolarization depends on the opening up of Ca^{++} channels.

❖ The **supporting (or sustentacular) cells** are elongated and may be shaped-like hourglasses (narrow in the middle and wide at each end). They support the hair cells and provide them with nutrition. They may also modify the composition of endolymph.

❖ **Functioning of ampullary crests**: The ampullary crests are stimulated by movements of the head (especially by acceleration). When the head moves, a current is produced in the endolymph of the semicircular ducts (by inertia). This movement causes deflection of the cupula to one side distorting the hair cells. It appears likely that distortion of the crest in one direction causes stimulation of nerve impulses, while distortion in the

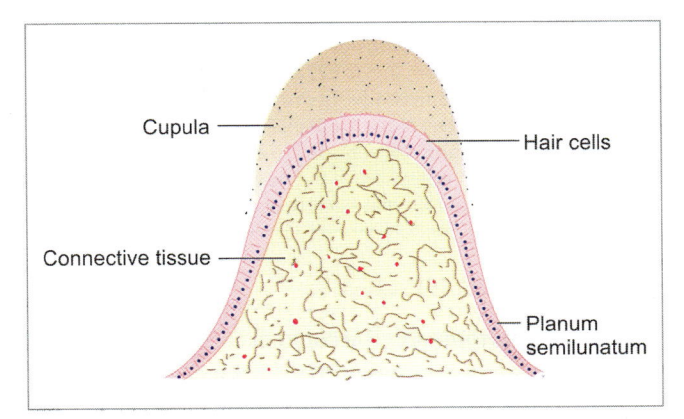

Fig. 24.12: Structure of an ampullary crest (schematic representation).

opposite direction produces inhibition. In any given movement, the cristae of some semicircular ducts are stimulated while those of others are inhibited. Perception of the exact direction of movement of the head depends on the precise pattern formed by responses from the various cristae.

SOME ELEMENTARY FACTS ABOUT THE MECHANISM OF HEARING

- Sound waves traveling through air pass into the external acoustic meatus and produce vibrations in the tympanic membrane. These vibrations are transmitted through the chain of ossicles to perilymph in the vestibule.
- In this process, the force of vibration undergoes considerable amplification because: (a) the chain of ossicles acts as a lever, and (b) the area of the tympanic membrane is much greater than that of the footplate of the stapes (increasing the force per unit area).
- Movement of the stapes (toward the vestibule) sets up a pressure wave in the perilymph. This wave passes from the vestibule into the scala vestibuli, and travels through it to the apex of the cochlea. At this point (called the **helicotrema**), the scala vestibuli is continuous with the scala tympani. The pressure wave passes into the scala tympani and again traverses the whole length of the cochlea to end by causing an outward bulging of the secondary tympanic membrane.
- In this way, vibrations are set up in the perilymph and through it in the basilar membrane. Movements of the basilar membrane produce forces that result in friction between the "hairs" of hair cells against the membrana tectoria. This friction leads to bending of the "hairs". This bending generates nerve impulses that travel through the cochlear nerve to the brain.
- The presence of efferent terminals on the hair cells probably controls the afferent impulses reaching the brain. It can also lead to sharpening of impulses emanating from particular segments of the spiral organ by suppressing impulses from adjoining areas.
- It has to be remembered that the transverse length of the basilar membrane is not equal in different parts of the cochlear canal. The membrane is shortest in the basal turn of the cochlea, and longest in the apical turn (quite contrary to what one might expect). Different segments of the membrane vibrate most strongly in response to different frequencies of sound thus, providing a mechanism for differentiation of sound frequencies. Low frequency sounds are detected by hair cells in the organ of Corti lying near the apex of the cochlea, while high frequency sounds are detected by hair cells placed near the base of the cochlea. The intensity of sound depends on the amplitude of vibration.

Added Information

Hair cells

With the EM, the "hairs" of hair cells are seen to be similar to microvilli. Each hair has a covering of plasma membrane within which there is a core of microfilaments. Each hair is cylindrical over most of its length, but it is much narrowed at its base. The hair can, therefore, bend easily at this site. The hair on each hair cell is arranged in a definite manner. When viewed from "above", they are seen to be arranged in the form of the letter "V" or "U". Each limb of the "V" has three rows of hairs. The hairs in the three rows are of unequal height being tallest in the "outer" row, intermediate in the middle row, and shortest in the "inner" row. The "V" formed by the hairs of various hair cells are all in alignment, the apex of the "V" pointing toward the "outer" wall of the cochlear canal. At the point corresponding to the apex of the "V", there is a centriole lying just under the apical cell membrane, but a true kinocilium is not present (unlike hair cells of ampullary crests).

The earlier description applies to both inner and outer hair cells.

The direction of the "V" is of functional importance. Like hair cells of the maculae and cristae, those of the cochlea are polarized. Bending of stereocilia toward the apex of the "V" causes depolarization, while the reverse causes hyperpolarization. Ionic gradients associated with depolarization and hyperpolarization are maintained because apices of hair cells and surrounding cells are tightly sealed by occluding junctions.

Planum semilunatum

On each side of each ampullary crest, the epithelium of the semicircular duct shows an area of thickened epithelium that is called the planum semilunatum. The importance of this area is that (among other cells) it contains certain dark cells that have an ultrastructure similar to cells (elsewhere in the body) that are specialized for ionic transport. The cells bear microvilli and have deep infoldings of their basal plasma membrane. The areas between the folds are occupied by elongated mitochondria (compare with structure of cells of the distal convoluted tubules of the kidney). The dark cells are believed to control the ionic content of the endolymph. Similar cells are also present elsewhere in the membranous labyrinth. The planum semilunatum may secrete endolymph.

APPLIED HISTOLOGY

- **Grafts in rhinoplasty**: The conchal cartilage is frequently used to correct depressed nasal bridge. The composite grafts of the skin and cartilage can be used for repair of defects of ala of nose.

- **Grafts in tympanoplasty**: Tragal and conchal cartilage and perichondrium and fat from lobule are often used during tympanoplasty operations.
- **Fissures of Santorini**: Transverse slits in the floor of cartilaginous EAC called "fissures of Santorini" provide passages for infections and neoplasms to and from the surrounding soft tissue (especially parotid gland). The parotid and mastoid infections can manifest in the EAC.
- **Hair follicles** are present only in the outer cartilaginous canal and, therefore, furuncles (staphylococcal infection of hair follicles) are seen only in the cartilaginous EAC.
- Foreign body impacted medial to bony isthmus of EAC is difficult to remove.
- **Foramen of Huschke**: In children and occasionally in adults, anteroinferior bony EAC may have a deficiency that is called foramen of Huschke. Foramen of Huschke permits spread of infections to and from EAC and parotid.

Note: The skin of EAC has a unique self-cleansing mechanism. This migratory process continues from the medial to lateral side. The sloughed epithelium is extruded out as a component of cerumen.

MULTIPLE CHOICE QUESTIONS

1. Outer epithelial layer of tympanic membrane is lined by this epithelium.
    a. Transitional
    b. Pseudostratified
    c. Stratified squamous keratinized
    d. Stratified squamous nonkeratinized
2. All are parts of membranous labyrinth, *except*:
    a. Vestibule
    b. Saccule
    c. Semicircular duct
    d. Cochlear duct
3. Cochlea is a tube that is coiled on itself for:
    a. One and three-fourth
    b. Two and three-fourth
    c. Three and three-fourth
    d. Four and three-fourth
4. Organ of Corti is located on this membrane
    a. Vestibular
    b. Basilar
    c. Tympanic
    d. Otolithic

Answers
1. c   2. a   3. b   4. b

Index

Page numbers followed by *f* refer to figure, *fc* refer to flowchart, and *t* refer to table.

A

Abortions 164
Acetylcholine receptors 97*f*
Achalasia 209
Achlorhydria 209
Achondroplasia 65
Acid hydrolase enzymes 14
Acidophil 291
    cells, types of 291
Acinar glands 38
Acini
    structure of 41
    types of 41*f*
Acinus 214
Acne vulgaris 150
Acoustic meatus, external 325, 326
Acromegaly 305
Acrosome reaction 260
Actin 87, 88
    filament 89*f*
Actinin 89
Active transport 8
Acute respiratory distress syndrome 176
Addison's disease 306
Adenocarcinoma 42
Adenohypophysis 291
Adenoma 42
Adenomyosis 288
Adenosine triphosphate 13, 89
Adhesion spots 9
Adhesive belts 100
Adhesive junctions 9
Adhesive strips 10
Adipocytes 46
Adipose tissue 44, 46, 53, 56
    cell 57*f*
    section 47
Adrenocorticotropin 291
Advanced bell stage 186
Adventitia 171, 190, 191, 219, 235, 282
Afferent fibers 121
    entering cerebellar cortex 250
Agranular cortex 247
Air passages, common features of 166
Albinism 150
Albuminuria 238
    causes of 238
Aldehyde fuchsin 51
Aldosterone 300
Alimentary canal 177
Allocortex 243
Alpha cells 221, 291
Alpha efferents 91
Alveolar ducts 171
Alveolar epithelial cells 174

Alveolar glands 38
Alveolar sacs 171
Alveolar wall, structure of 172
Alveoli 171, 172, 284, 287
Alveolus 174*f*
Amacrine cells 317
Amacrine neurons 322
    connections of 323*f*
Ameloblasts 186
Amine precursor uptake and decarboxylation 40
Amino acid derivatives 289
Ampulla 262, 276, 332
Ampullary crest 332, 335
    functioning of 335
    structure of 335*f*
Amyloid bodies 265
Amyloidosis 112
Anal canal 190, 208
    interior of 208*f*
Anal columns 208
Anal sinus 208
Anal sphincter, internal 190, 208
Anal valves 208
Anchoring junctions 9
Anchoring villi 162, 162*f*
Androgen binding protein 255
Angioma 138
Angiotensin 233
    converting enzyme 130
Angiotensinogen 233
Ansa nephroni 230
Antibodies 100
Antigen 100
    presenting cells 105
Anti-Müllerian hormone 255
Antrum 273
Apical foramen, primary 187
Apocrine 37, 38, 284
Appendices epiploicae 205
Appendicitis, acute 209
APUD cell system 305
Areola 284, 287
Areolae
    primary 76
    secondary 76
Areolar tissue 52
    loose 45*f*, 52
Argentaffin cells 40, 196, 203*f*, 209
Argentophil fibers 51
Argyophil cells 40
Arrector pili muscles 94, 147
Arterioles 129, 132, 132*f*
    afferent 233
    efferent 234

Arteriovenous anastomoses 137, 137*f*
Artery 129, 132
    arcuate 233
    elastic 130-132, 132*t*
    interlobar 233
    large-sized 130
    medium-sized 132, 133
    structure of 130
    within kidney, arrangement of 233*f*
Asthma 176
Astrocytes 16, 116, 117*f*
    fibrous 116
Atherosclerotic lesions 138
Atretic follicles 275
Atrium 171
Auditory canal, external 325
Auditory tube 327
Auerbach's plexus 190
Auricle 325
Autoimmune diseases 112
Autonomic ganglia 126, 126*f*, 127
Autonomic nervous system 113
Axoaxonal synapse 124, 124*f*
Axodendritic synapse 124, 124*f*
Axoneme 18, 34
Axons 115, 116, 116*t*
    hillock 115
    on basis of length of 120
    unmyelinated 119
Axoplasmic flow 116
Axosomatic synapse 124, 124*f*

B

Bacteria 103
Balt 109
Barrett's esophagus 209
Basal body 34
Basal cells 167, 168, 175, 261
    carcinoma 151
Basal folds 36
Basal granule 34
Basal lamina 32, 129, 130, 311
Basement membrane 31*f*, 32, 52, 229*f*
    functions of 33
Basilar membrane 328
Basket cells 153, 244*f*, 247, 250
Basolateral folds 20
Basophil cells 291
    types of 291
Bell stage, early 185, 186*f*
Beta cells 222, 291
Bile 217
    canaliculus 217*f*
    capillaries 215*f*
Biliary apparatus, extrahepatic 217

Biliary duct system 215
Bipolar cells 315
Bipolar neurons 120, 120f, 321
    firing of 322, 323fc
Birbeck bodies 144
Blastomeres 161
Blood 44
    monocyte of 109
    placental barrier 162
    pressure 130
    retinal barrier 317
    testis barrier 255
    thymic barrier 108
    thymus barrier 106
    vessels 91, 96
        basic structure of 129
        innervation of 135
B-lymphocytes 48, 100
    circulation of 100f
Body 150
    tube 1
Bone 44, 52, 67
    cells 67f, 68, 68f
        mature 67
    classification of 71
    deformans 81
    formation of 75
    forming cells 67
    gross appearance of 71
    lamellae 71f
    lining cells 69
    marrow 72, 98, 108, 109
    matrix 69
    membranes 69
    of vault of skull, growth of 78
    osteoblast rimming surface of 68f
    structure 70f, 71
    tissue, composition of 67
    woven 75
Bony cochlea 328
Bony labyrinth 327, 328, 328f
Bony lamellae 76f
Bowman's capsule 227
Bowman's membrane 309
Brain sand 302
Breast
    carcinoma of 288
    human female 287f
Bright's disease 238
Brodmann's areas 247
Bronchial tree 171f
Bronchioles 171
Bronchitis, chronic 176
Brown adipose tissue 56
    cell 57f
Brush border 20, 27, 35
Brush cells 168, 174
Bud stage 185, 186f

C

Calcification 65
    zone of 81
Calcination 71
Calcitonin 296

Calcium
    dependent 9
    independent 9
Calix 335
Canal of Schlemm 308
Canal of Volkmann 72
Canalicular surface 215
Canaliculate lamellar bodies 302
Canaliculi 71
Cancellous bone 72, 74, 76
    structure of 72f
Cap stage 185, 186f
Capillary 129, 133
    lamina 311
    structure of 134
    types of 134
Capsule 39, 102, 103, 221
Cardiospasm 209
Cardiovascular system 129
Carotid body 304
    cells of 304
    functions of 305
    nerve supply of 305
    structure of 304f
Cartilage 44, 52, 60, 168, 172
    bones 75
    cells 61
    components of 60
    elastic 60, 61, 63, 66, 168
    epiphyseal 78
    fibers of 61
    forming tumors 65
    general features of 60
    growth of 60, 65
        zone of 80
    hyaline 60-62, 66, 168
    transformation, zone of 81
    types of 59, 61
    zone of
        proliferating 80
        resting 80
Cartilaginous model, establishment of 80f
Cartwheel appearance 49
Castle, intrinsic factor of 196
Cataract 324
C-cells 296
Celiac sprue 209
Cells 5, 12f, 44, 60, 150
    adhesion molecules 9, 9f, 10f, 11f
        types of 9t
    arrangement of 23, 185f
    basal parts of 153
    body 113, 115, 316
        toward 116
    capsular 116
    components of 5
    drinking 8
    eating 8
    elongated 183f
    flask-shaped 167
    from adrenal
        cortex, ultrastructure of 302f
        medulla, ultrastructure of 302f
    from striated duct, electron microscopic
        structure of 159f

    highly phagocytic 111
    horizontal 316, 316f
    intercalated 232
    intermediate 203
    junctions 9
        classification of 9
    lining distal convoluted tubule,
        ultrastructure of 232f
    lining proximal convoluted tubule,
        ultrastructure of 230f
    membrane 5, 7f, 8f
        carbohydrates of 7
        functions of 8
        lipids in 5
        outer aspect of 7f
        protein in 7
        significance of proteins of 7
        trilaminar structure of 6f
    morphology 23
    nest 61
    number of 37
    organelles 11
    power house of 13
    staining of 21
    structure of 5, 111
    surface, projections from 18, 33
    system 290
    types of 144, 172f, 175
    undifferentiated 203
Cells of Cajal 245
    horizontal 244, 244f
Cells of Clara 172
Cells of Claudius 333
Cells of Hensen 333
Cells of Martinotti 244, 244f
Cells of Merkel 144
Cells of Müller 317
Cells of Polkissen 233
Cells of Sertoli 255
Cementocytes 180
Cementum 180
Central nervous system 110, 113, 240
Centrioles 16
Centroacinar cells 221
Centrosome 16
Centrotubule 89
Cerebellar
    ataxia 251
    cortex 240, 247, 248, 249f
    cortex, structure of 247
    glomeruli 250
    glomeruli, structure of 250f
    islands 250
    nuclei 247, 247f
Cerebellum, cells of 249
Cerebral cortex 240, 243, 244f, 246
    lamina of 244, 245f
    neurons in 244
Cerebrospinal fluid 118
Cervix 281
Chalazion 324
Cheilitis 185
Chemical nature 49, 51
Chemical synapses 124
    classification of 124f

Index

structure of typical 128f
types of 124f
Chief cells 196, 298
Cholecystectomy 223
Cholelithiasis 223
Cholesterol 130
Chondroblastoma 65
Chondroblasts 61, 76
Chondrocytes 60, 61
Chondrogenic layer 60
    inner 60
Chondroitin sulfate 52
Chondrosarcoma 65
Chorion 161
    frondosum 161
    laeve 161
Chorionic plate 161
Chorionic villi 162
Choroid 307, 311
Choroidal epithelial cells 118
Choroidal stroma 311
Choroidocapillaris 311
Chromatin 17
    fiber, structure of 18f
    nature of 17
Chromatophores 46
Chromophil cells 291
Chromophobe cells 291
Chromosomes 18
Chyle 99
Chylomicrons 99
Chylopericardium 111
Chyloperitoneum 111
Chylothorax 111
Chyluria 111
Chyme 191
Cilia 18, 19f, 27f, 33, 34, 35, 35t
    abnormalities of 36
    functions of 19
Ciliaris muscle 311
Ciliary body 307, 311
Ciliary glands 149, 320
Ciliary processes 312
Ciliated cells 167, 168, 276
Ciliated columnar epithelium 27, 28
Cilium 19f, 34f, 316
Circular layer, inner layer of 190
Circumvallate papillae 181
Cisternae, central layers of 14
Clasmatocytes 47
Clear cells 148, 232
Clitoris 282
Closed-face nuclei 17
Cochlea 327-329
    aqueduct of 330
    duct of 330
Cochlear canal, structure of 330f
Collagen 49
    fibers 49, 49t, 50f, 60, 69
    types of 59t
Collecting duct 225f, 232
Collecting tubule 225, 232
Colloid 296
Colon 188, 204, 206, 209
    segment of 205f

Colostrum 284
Columnar cells
    absorptive 202
    basal layer of 31f
Columnar epithelial cells 28
Columnar epithelium 24, 25, 27f, 28
    lining small intestine 203f
    simple 24, 25, 26f, 27, 193
    stratified 31
Communicating junctions 9, 11, 12f
Compact bone 71, 72f, 74, 76
    longitudinal section of 70f, 74
    transverse section 73
Compound tubuloalveolar
    glands 189
    mucous glands 191
    serous gland 219
Concentric lamellae 71
Condenser 2
Cone
    horizontal neuron, connections of 323f
    pedicles 316, 316
Conjunctiva 320
Conjunctival fornix 320
Conjunctival sac 320
Connecting tubule 232
Connective tissue 44, 52, 57, 87f, 174, 262
    basic components of 45fc
    classification of 44
    components of 44
        loose 50f
    diseases of 59
    fibers of 49, 50f
    framework, structure 103
    functions of 56
    histiocytes of 109
    intercellular ground substance of 51
    loose 44, 52
    macrophage cells of 109
    sheath 147
    subendocardial layer of 137
    typical 52
Connexons 11
Conus medullaris 241
Cord and clump type 40
Cornea 307, 308, 310, 323
    junction of 308f
    nutrition of 309
    transparency of 309
Corneal abrasion 324
Corneal epithelium, anterior 309
Corneal neovascularization 324
Corneal opacity 323
Corneal stroma 309
Corneal ulcer 323
Corneoscleral junction 308
Corona radiata 273
Corpora amylacea 265
Corpora arenacea 302
Corpora atretica 275
Corpora cavernosa 265, 282
Corpus albicans 275
Corpus hemorrhagicum 274
Corpus luteum 274, 274f
Corpus spongiosum 265

Cortex 102, 224, 225, 270
Corti, spiral organ of 332, 333
Cortical arches 225
Cortical glomeruli 234
Cortical lobules 225
    concept of 234f
Cortical structure, variations in 247
Corticotropes 291
Cortisol 300
Cortisone 300
Cotyledons, components of 162f
Cretinism 306
Cristae 13
    ampullae 332
Crohn's disease 209
Crown 179
Crypts 202
Crystals, needle-shaped 69
Cuboidal epithelium 24
    simple 24, 26, 26f
    stratified 31
Cumulus oophorus 273
Cupula 335
Cushing's disease 306
Cystitis 238
Cytocrine 37
Cytokeratin 16
Cytokines 100
Cytoplasm 5, 114
Cytoskeleton 15
Cytosol 5, 12

D

Dark cells 148, 232, 330, 331
Dartos muscle 94
Decalcification 70
Decidua 160
    basalis 161
Deep fascia 53
Defense mechanisms, participation in 111
Dehydroepiandrosterone 300
Delta basophils 291
Delta cells 222
Dendrites 115, 116, 116t
Dendritic cells 144
Dendritic processes 144f
Dendroaxonic synapse 124
Dendrodendritic synapse 124
Dense connective tissue 52
    irregular 44, 53, 55
    regular 44, 52, 54
Dense lymphoid tissue 98, 99
Dental caries 185
Dentate nucleus 247
Dentin 180
    types of 180
Dentinal sheath 180
Deoxycorticosterone 300
Deoxyribonucleic acid 13, 17, 18, 18f
Dermal papillae 142, 142f
Dermatan sulfate 52
Dermis 142, 145
    papillary layer 145
    reticular layer 145
Descemet's membrane 309

Desmin 89, 96
Desmosome 9
   electron microscopy appearance of 10f
   structure of 10f
Detrusor muscle 235
Diabetes insipidus 306
Diaphysis 78
Digestive system 177, 188
Dihydrocortisone 300
Dilator pupillae 312
Distal convoluted tubule 230
Domain 52
Duchenne muscular dystrophy 97
Duct of Bellini 225, 232
Ducts 148
   branching of 38
   intercalated 153, 221
   interlobular 153, 221
   intralobar 153
   intralobular 221
   system 39, 153, 221, 285
Ductules, efferent 257
Ductus deferens 253, 262, 263
Duodenal papilla 219f
Duodenum 188, 189, 197, 198, 198t, 199
   part of 190
Dust cells 111, 174
Dyads 93
Dysfunctional uterine bleeding 287

E

Ear
   external 325
   main parts of 326f
   middle 325, 327
Ehlers-Danlos syndrome 59
Elastase 51
Elastic lamina
   external 129, 131
   internal 129, 130
Elastin 51
Electrical synapses 124
Electron microscopy 5, 11f
   high magnifications of 6f
   scanning 19f
Ellipsoid 316
Embryonic connective tissue 44
Enamel 179
   dentin, structure of 180f
   lamellae 180
   organ 185
   spindles 180
   structure of 180f
   tufts 180
Enchondroma 65
Endocardium 24, 137
Endocervix 281
Endochondral ossification 75, 76, 77f
   secondary centers of 78
Endocrine
   cells 196, 203, 209
      distribution of 290
      groups of 290
      in gut, types of 210t
      isolated 290

   functions 303
   gland 37, 39, 40, 290
   pancreas 221
   system 289
Endocytic vesicle 8
Endocytosis 8, 8f
Endolymph 330
Endolymphatic sac 330
Endolysosome 15
Endometriosis 287
Endometrium 276
   thickness of 278, 281f
Endomysium 84, 86
Endoneurium 121
Endoplasmic reticulum 12, 41
Endorphins 294
Endosomes 15
Endosteum 70
   functions of 70
Endothelial cells 106
   basal lamina of 106
Endothelial venules, high 103
Endothelin 130
Endothelium 24, 129, 130, 309
   functions of 130
Entamoeba histolytica 222
Enterochromaffin cells 204, 209
Enterocytes 202
Eosinophil 48, 48f
Ependymal cells 118
Epicardium 137
Epidermal papillae 142, 142f
Epidermal proliferation units 150
Epidermal ridges 142f
Epidermis 10f, 142
   cells of 144
   layer of 142, 143f
Epididymis 253, 260, 261
   duct of 261
Epiglottis 168
Epilemmal junctions 153
Epimysium 85, 86
Epineurium 121
Epiphyseal plate 78, 80
   structure of 81f
Epiphysis 78
   cerebri 302
   fusion of 81
Episclera 308
Epithelia 23, 35
   classification of 23, 24fc
   functions 23
   stratified 23
   unilayered 23
Epithelial cells 35
   renewal of 35
   shape of 35
Epithelial diaphragm 187
Epithelial layer, outer 327
Epithelial lining 202
Epithelial tissue, general features of 23
Epitheliocytes 106
   basal lamina of 106
Epithelioid cells 111
Epithelioreticular cells 106

Epithelium 23, 208
   lining 172, 276, 278
      intestines 42
      renal tubules 21f
   simple 23
   stratified 29
Epitheloid 49
Erythrocytes, abnormal 112
Esophagus 188-192, 208, 223
   part of 190
Estrogens 281
Euchromatic nucleus 17f
Euchromatin 17
Eukaryotic cell 6f
Eustachian tube 327
Excretion 160
Excretory ducts 287
Exocrine 40
   gland 37, 39
      classification of 37
      structural organization of 40f
   pancreas 219
Exocytic vesicles 8
Exocytosis 8
   stages in 8f
Exostoses 70
External piles 209
Extracellular molecules, absorption of 8f
Extraglomerular mesangial cells 233
Extrahepatic ducts 211, 219
Eye piece 1
Eyeball 308f
   layer of 311f
Eyelids 319, 320f, 324

F

Fabricus, bursa of 100
F-actin 88
Fallopian tube 276, 277, 287
Fascia adherens 10
Fasciculi 121, 240
Fast twitch fibers 89
Fastigial nucleus 247
Fat cells 45, 46, 47f, 53f
Fenestra cochleae 328
Fenestrated capillary, structure of 134f
Fetal
   connective tissue 44
   cotyledons, ramifications of 162f
Fibers 60, 69
   efferent 121, 251
   elastic 49, 49t, 50f, 51, 51f, 60
   intrafusal 91
   of Tomes 180
   within lens, arrangement of 319f
Fibrillin 51
Fibrils, arrangement of 260f
Fibroadenoma 288
Fibroblast 45
   structure of 46f
Fibrocartilage 60, 63, 64, 66
Fibromuscular
   coat 219
   lamina 32

Index

stroma 265
tube 189
Fibrous coat, outer 307
Fibrous layer 60
   middle 327
   outer 60
Filiform
   papillae 181
Filtration slits 227, 229*f*
Filum terminale 241
Fimbriae 276
Finger-like processes 191
First meiotic division 258
First polar body 272
Fissure 247
   anterior median 243
Fissures of Santorini 337
Flagella 20, 34
Floating villi 162, 162*f*
Fluids
   inner ear 330
   mosaic model 5
Focal spots 10
Focus knobs 2
Folia 247
Foliate papillae 183
Follicle 295
   primary 272, 273*f*
   secondary 273
   stimulating hormone 257*f*, 281, 291
Follicular cells 272, 296
Follicular type 40
Foramen cecum 181
Foramen of Huschke 337
Fordyce's granules 185
Free macrophages 45
Fungiform 183*f*
   papillae 181
Funiculi 240
Funiculus
   anterior 243
   anterolateral 243
   posterior 243
Fusiform 96
   cells 244*f*
Fusogenic proteins 8*f*

G

G-actin, globular molecules of 89*f*
Galea capitis 259
Gallbladder 211, 217, 218, 223
   microscopic structure 217
Gallstones 223
Gamma-efferents 91
Ganglia 124
Ganglion cell 322, 323*f*
   diffuse 322
   layer of 317
Gap junctions 9, 11
Gastric
   glands 38, 42, 193
   pits 193
   ulcer 209
Gastrin 196

Gastritis 209
Gastroenteropancreatic endocrine system 209
Gastrointestinal tract 177
   enteroendocrine cells of 37
   general plan of 188, 189
Gaucher's disease 112
General connective tissue 44
Genital ducts 252
Genitalia, female external 282
Germ cell 255, 255*f*
   tumors 268
Germinal center 102
Germinal layer 143
Germinative matrix 146
Germinative zone 143
Giant cells 47
   foreign body 49, 111
Gigantism 305
Glabrous skin 139
Gland 23, 37, 189
   adrenal 300
   anterior lingual 183
   cardiac 197
   ceruminous 149
   characteristic features 37
   classification of 37, 38*fc*
   development of 40, 40*f*
   ductless 37, 290
   externally secreting 37
   intermediate submucous 265
   internally secreting 37
   interstitial 275
   intestinal 202
   lacrimal 321, 321*f*
   lactating 284
   mixed 38
   multicellular 37, 39*f*
   outer 265
   secretory elements of 39*f*
   types of 38*f*
Glands of Brunner 198
Glands of Krause 321
Glands of Moll 320
Glands of Wolfring 320
Glands of Zeis 320
Glandular elements, structure of 284
Glandular tissue 284
   arrangement of 267*f*
Glans penis 265
Glassy membrane 147
Glial fibrillary acidic protein 16
Gliocytes, capsular 116
Gliosis 117
Gliosomes 116
Glisson's capsule 212
Globose nucleus 247
Glomerular basement membrane 229
Glomerular capsule 227
Glomerular filtration barrier 229
Glomeruli, efferent arterioles of 234*f*
Glomerulonephritis 238
Glomerulus 227, 251
Glomus 137, 137*f*, 138
   cells 304
   tumor 138

Glossitis, atrophic 185
Glucagon 219
Glucose, storage of 211
Glycocalyx 7, 35, 202
Glycolipid and glycoprotein molecules 7*f*
Glycoprotein 196
   structural 52
Glycosaminoglycans 52, 61
   types of 52*t*
Goblet cells 25, 27*f*, 28, 42, 167, 202, 203*f*
Golgi apparatus 13, 14, 284
Golgi cells 247, 250
Golgi complex 13, 14, 215, 262
   role of 14*f*
   structure of 14*f*
Golgi hydrolase vesicles 15
Gonadotrophs 291
Gonadotropin-releasing hormone 281
Graafian follicle 273
Granular cortex 247
Granular layer 249
   inner 245
   outer 245
Granular layer of Tomes 180
Granule 48
   cells 244, 247, 250
   small 168
Granulosa cells 272, 274
Graves' disease 306
Gravid uterus, wall of 160
Gravis 96
Gray matter 240, 241
Ground substance 51, 61, 69
Growth, interstitial 60, 65
Guanosine triphosphate 13
Gustatory cells 183
Gustatory pore 183
Gut, layer of 189*f*

H

Haemophilus influenzae 176
Hair 145
   cell 333, 335, 336
      inner 333, 334, 334*f*, 334*t*
      outer 333, 334, 334*f*, 334*t*
   follicle 145, 146, 146*f*, 148, 178, 337
      structure of 146
   papilla 145
   parts of 145
   shaft, structure of 145
Hairy skin 139, 140
Hand lens, use of 1
Hassall's corpuscles 106
Haversian canal 71, 72*f*
Haversian system 71, 72, 72*f*, 74
   atrophic 74, 77
   typical 74, 77
Hearing, mechanism of 336
Heart 137
   failure cells 174
Helicotrema 336
Hemangioma 138
Hematopoietic tissue 72
Hemidesmosomes 10

Hemolymphatic tissue 44
Hemorrhoids 209
Henle's layer 146
Heparan sulfate 52
Heparin 52
Hepatic coma 223
Hepatic lobules 212, 214f
Hepatic sinusoids 212
Hepatobiliary system 211
Hepatocyte 215
    cells surface of 215f
Hepatopancreatic duct 219
Herring bodies 294
Hertwig's epithelial root sheath 186
Heterochromatic nucleus 17f
Heterochromatin 17
Heterocrine 152
Hilum 225
Hilus cells 272
Histaminocytes 47
Histiocyte 47, 47f
Histone 17
    complex forming nucleosome core, composition of 18f
Hodgkin's disease 112
Hofbauer cell 49
Holocrine 37, 38f
Homocrine 152
Hordeolum, external 324
Hormones 39, 278, 289
    antidiuretic 294
    control of secretion of 295
    corticotropic 291
    formation of 298fc
    inhibin 257
    luteinizing 257, 281, 291
    production 160
Horn, anterior 241
Houstra coli 205
Huxley's layer 146
Hyaline membrane disease 176
Hyaloplasm 5, 12
Hyaluronic acid 52
Hydronephrosis 238
Hydroxylysine 50
Hydroxyproline 50
Hyperparathyroidism 306
    primary 306
    secondary 306
Hyperplasia 281
Hypertension 138, 238
Hyperthyroidism 306
Hypertrophy 281
    benign prostatic 268
Hypolemmal junctions 153
Hypoparathyroidism 306
Hypophysis cerebri 290, 292, 294f
    blood supply of 294
    pars posterior of 295f
    subdivisions of 290f
Hypothalamo-hypophyseal portal system 295, 295f
Hypothalamus 295f
Hypothyroidism 306

I

Ileum 188, 197, 198, 198t, 201
Immotile cilia syndrome 21, 36, 176
Immune
    responses, role in 111
    system 100
Immunity
    cellular 100
    humoral 100
Immunoglobulins 100
Immunoregulation, disorders of 112
Infections 112
Infundibulum 276, 290
Inner band of Baillarger 245
Insulin 219
Intercalated disc 93
    electron microscopic structure of part of 93f
Intercellular secretory canaliculi 41
Intercellular substance 69
Interlobular arteries 233
Intermediate filaments 15, 16
    functions of 16
Internal ear 325, 327
    basic structure of 328f
Internode 119
Interstitial cell of Leydig 257
Interstitial cells 303
    stimulating hormone 257f, 291
Intervillous space 162, 162f
Intestinal absorptive cells 20f
Intestine 188, 204, 205, 205t
Intramembranous ossification 75, 76f, 78
Iodine, activation of 298
Ions, inorganic 69
Iris 307, 312
Islets of Langerhans 221
Isogenous cell groups 61
Isthmus 276, 327

J

Jejunum 188, 197, 198, 198t, 200
Joint, ligaments of 53
Junctional complex 10f
Junctional tubule 232
Juxtaglomerular apparatus 232
Juxtaglomerular cells 233
    functions of 233
Juxtamedullary glomeruli 234
Juxtamedullary nephrons 227

K

Kartagener's syndrome 36
Keratan sulfate 52
Keratin 31
    precursor of 143
Keratinization, zone of 144
Keratinized stratified squamous epithelium 31
Keratinocytes 144
Keratitis 323
Keratoconus 324
Keratohyalin 143

Kidney 224, 225f, 226
    floating 56
    macroscopic structure 224
    proximal convoluted tubules of 24
Kinetic balance 333
Kinetosome 34
Kinocilia 20, 34
Koilonychia 151
Krebs cycle 13
Kulchitsky cells 168
Kupffer cell 49, 212, 217

L

Labia
    majora 282
    minora 282
Labyrinth 327
Lacis cells 233
Lactiferous
    duct 284, 285
    sinus 284, 285
Lactogenic hormone 291
Lacunae 61, 71
Lamellae 71
    constitute bone 71f
    interstitial 71
Lamellar bone 75
Lamina 314
    cribrosa 308
    densa 32, 229
    fusca 308, 311
    lucida 32
    propria 167, 175, 189, 197, 204, 208, 235, 276
    rara interna 229
    stroma 276
Langerhans
    bodies 144
    cell 49
    dendritic cells of 144
Laryngitis
    acute 176
    chronic 176
Larynx 167
    anterior view of 168f
    cartilage of 167
Lateral funiculus 243
Lateral gray column 243
Leishmaniasis 112
Lemmocytes 116
Lemnisci 240
Lens 307, 317, 324
    capsule 319
    epithelium 319
    fibers 319
    objective 1
Leukocytes 45, 48
Light microscope, parts of 1
Light source 2
Limbus lamina spiralis 332
Limiting membrane, outer 314
Linea gravidarum 151
Lines of Retzius 179

Index

Lingual tonsil 109, 181
Lip 177, 178f, 185
    longitudinal section through 178
Lipoblasts 53
Lipofuscin 257
Lipoprotein, low-density 130
Liquor folliculi 273
Littoral cells 110
Littre's glands 238
Liver 211, 213, 216, 222
    blood supply of 211
    cells of 215, 215f
    cirrhosis of 112
    lobule 212
        classical 212, 212f
    macroscopic structure of 212
Lobar arteries 233
Lobar bronchi 171
Lobe 225
    posterior 291
Lobular bronchiole 171
Lobule 284
    classical 212
Long bone, growth of 79
Loop of Henle 230
Lung 171, 173
Lunule of nail 150f
Lutein 274
Lymph 98, 99
    capillaries 99
    vessels, larger 99
Lymph node 100-103, 111
    blood supply of 102
    structure of 102f
Lymphadenitis 112
Lymphangitis 111
    acute 111
    chronic 111
Lymphatic capillaries 99
Lymphatic duct, right 98
Lymphatic follicles 102
Lymphatic nodules 102
Lymphatic vessels 98, 99
Lymphedema 111
Lymph node 98
Lymphoblasts 102
Lymphocytes 48, 48f, 100
    functions of 100
Lymphohematogenous malignancies 112
Lymphoid organ
    discrete 99
    primary 98, 108
    secondary 98
Lymphoid system 98
Lymphoid tissue 98
    bronchial-associated 99
    diffuse 98, 99
    gut-associated 99
Lymphokines 100
Lysosomal glycogen storage disease 21
Lysosome 14, 15f, 215
    primary 15
    secondary 15
    types of 15fc

M

M cells 204
Macrophage 57, 108, 110
    cells 47, 47f, 211
    fixed 45
Macula 332
    adherens 9
    communicans 11
    densa 233
Malaria 112
Male genital system, control of 257fc
Male reproductive system 252, 253f
Malpighian bodies 105
Malpighian corpuscle 225
Malpighian layer 143
Malt 99, 108
Mammary gland 284-286, 288
    active 284
    lactating 287t
Mammotropin 291
Marfan's syndrome 59
Marrow cavity 72, 79
Masson's trichrome 49
Mast cells 45, 47, 47f
Masticatory mucosa 185
Mastocytes 47
Maternal cotyledons 160, 161f
Matrix 13, 51
    capsular 61, 65
    extracellular 60, 130
    intercellular 60
    unterstitial 61
    vesicles 68
Maturation 260
Mediastinum testis 253
Medulla 102, 145, 224, 270
Medullary rays 225
Meibomian glands 320
Meiotic division, second 258
Meissner's plexus 190, 204
Melanocyte 144, 144f
    stimulating hormone 294
Melanoma, malignant 151
Melanophores 46
Melatonin 303
Membrana granulosa 273
Membrana tectoria 333
Membrane
    bones 75
    internal limiting 317
    of Bruch 311
    outer 13
    proteins 7f
    ruffled 69
    T-system of 89
Membranous labyrinth 327, 330, 332f
    parts of 331f
Menstrual cycle 278
    endometrial changes in 278
    stages of 281f
Merocrine 37, 38f, 285
Mesangium 227, 229f
Mesaxon 118

Mesenchymal cells 46f, 165
    undifferentiated 46
Mesenchymal condensation 75
Mesenchyme 44
Mesothelium 24, 190
Metaphysis 81
Metastatic splenic tumors 112
Microcirculatory unit 138
Microfilaments 15
Microglia 49, 118
Microglial cells 110, 117f
Microscope 1, 1f
    compound 2f
    dark-field 3
    electron 3, 24, 115f, 260f
    fluorescence 3
    interference 3
    types of 3
Microscopy, principle of 2
Microtubules 15, 16f
Microvilli 20, 20f, 27, 33, 35, 35t, 189
Midget ganglion cells 322
Milky spots 111
Mitochondria 13
Mitochondrial cytopathy syndromes 21
Mitochondrion, structure of 13f
Mittleschiebe 88
Monoblasts 109
Monocyte 45, 48
    phagocyte system 109
Mononuclear phagocyte system 47, 109, 217
    cells of 109
    functions of 111
Monosomes 13
Montgomery, tubercles of 287
Mossy fibers 250
Motor endplate 91
Motor fibers 121
Motor neuron 120
    disease 251
    single 91f
Motor unit 91
Muciphages 205
Mucocutaneous junction 177
Mucoepidermoid carcinoma 42
Mucoid connective tissue 44, 165
Mucoid tissue 57, 58f
Mucosa 168, 189, 191, 208
    lining 185
    specialized 185
Mucosa-associated lymphoid tissue 98, 99, 108
    in alimentary system 109
    in respiratory system 109
Mucosal layer, inner 327
Mucous 21, 153
    acini 41, 41f, 41t
    cells 21, 41, 152, 153, 154f, 168
    gland 37
        inner 265
    layer, lamina propria of 235
    membrane 181, 189, 193, 198, 204, 208, 235, 238, 262, 276, 282
    neck cells 196
    secreting Goblet cells 193, 202
    structure of 205f

Müller's cells 317
Müller's muscle 94
Müllerian inhibitory substance 255
Multiadhesive glycoproteins 52, 61
Multilamellar bodies 174
Multilaminar primary follicle 273
Multilayered epithelia 23
Multilocular adipose tissue 56, 57*f*
Multipolar neurons 120, 120*f*
Multivesicular bodies 15, 15*f*
Muscle 262
    bundle 84*f*
    cardiac 84, 91, 92, 96, 96*t*
    coat 235, 238, 282
    dystrophy 96
    fiber 83, 84*f*
        layer contains striated 190
        number of 91*f*
        white 90, 90*t*
    hypertrophy 97
    involuntary 84
    plain 93
    spindles 91
    tendon of 53
    tissue 83
    triad 89
Muscular arterioles 132
Muscular artery 132, 132*t*, 133
Muscular coat 235
Muscular tissue 83
    types of 83
Muscular venules 135
Muscularis externa 189-191, 197, 204, 205, 208
Muscularis mucosae 189, 190, 197, 204
Myasthenia 96
    gravis 96, 97*f*, 112
Myelin sheath 118, 118*f*, 119
    formation of 118, 119*f*
    functions of 119
    of axon, segment of 117*f*
    short segment of 119*f*
Myelinated axons 118
Myelinated nerves 120
Myenteric plexus 190
    of Auerbach 190
Myocardium 137
Myocytes 83
    cardiac 93
Myoepithelial cells 96, 148, 153
Myoepitheliocytes 96
Myofibril 84
    contracts 88*f*
    structure of 87
Myofilaments 87
    in sarcomere, arrangement of 88*f*
    structure of 87
Myoglobin 89
Myomesin 89
Myometrium 278
Myosin 87, 88*f*
    filament 88, 88*f*
    molecule, structure of 88*f*
Myxedema 306

N

Nail 149
    bed 150
    growth of 150
    parts of 150*f*
Nasal cavities 166
Natural killer cells 48
Neocortex, structure of 244
Neonatal line 180
Nephron 225
    parts of 225*f*
Nephrotic syndrome 238
Nerve
    fibers 115
        myelinated 120*t*
        unmyelinated 120*t*
    plexuses 190
    tracts 115
    unmyelinated 120
Nervi vasorum 130
Nervous system 113
    anatomical classification of 114*fc*
    classification of 241*fc*
Nervous tissue 113
    tumors of 126
Nervus conarii 303
Neurilemma 119
Neurilemmal sheath 119
Neurites 115
    ischemic 126
Neuroeffector junctions 153
Neuroendocrine system 290
    diffuse 40, 305
Neuroendocrine transducers 295
Neuroepithelial cells 183
Neurofibrils 114, 115*f*
Neurofilament protein 16
Neuroglia 113, 116
    form cell 244*f*
    found, types of 117*fc*
Neuroglial cells 116, 118
Neurohypophysis 291, 294
Neuron 113, 114*f*
    arrangement of 249*f*
    horizontal 322
    morphological classification of 120*t*
    structure of 113, 115*f*
    types of 120
Neurovascular hilus 91
Nexins 11
Niemann-Pick's disease 112
Nipple 284, 287
Nissl bodies 114
Nissl granules 116
Nissl substance 114, 114*f*
Nodes of Ranvier 119
Nodules
    primary 102
    secondary 102
Nonciliated columnar cells 167
Non-Hodgkin's lymphomas 112
Nonpolar end 5
Nonstriated muscle 83

Normal transmission 97*f*
Nuclear envelope 17
Nuclear lamina 17
Nuclear layer
    external 314
    internal 315
Nuclear membrane 17
Nuclear pores 17
Nucleoli 17, 18
    pars chromosoma of 18
Nucleolus, electron microscopy structure of 18*f*
Nucleoplasm 17
Nucleosome 17
    core 18
Nucleus 5, 16, 240
    emboliform 247
Nutrition 135, 160
Nutritional lobule 214

O

Ocular conjunctiva 320
Oddi, sphincter of 219, 219*f*
Odontoblasts 180, 186
Olfactory cells 175
Olfactory cilia 20, 34
Olfactory epithelium 167, 175, 175*f*
Olfactory mucosa 167, 175*f*
Oligodendrocyte 117, 117*f*, 118
Onychia 150
Oocyte
    primary 272
    secondary 272
Oogenesis 272
    stages of 272*fc*
Oogonia 272
Open-face nuclei 17
Oppositional growth 60, 65
Optic cup 312
Optic nerve 121, 123
    fibers, layer of 317
Optic stalk 312
Optic vesicle 312
Oral cavity 177
    proper 177
Oral mucosa 185
Organ of Corti
    cell in 333*f*
    structure of 331*f*
Organelles 5
Organic ground substance, mixture of 69
Organic matrix 69
Organization 84
Organs 290
Ossification 65, 75
    centers of 78
    primary center of 78, 80*f*
Osteitis deformans 81
Osteoarthritis 65
Osteoblast 67, 67*f*, 68, 68*f*, 75
Osteocalcin 69
Osteocartilaginous exostoses 65
Osteochondromas 65

Index

Osteoclast 49, 67f, 68, 68f
   multinucleated 68f
Osteocyte 67, 67f, 68, 68f, 71f
Osteogenesis imperfecta 59
Osteogenetic layer 70
Osteoid 69, 75
   collagen 69
Osteoma 81
Osteonectin 69
Osteons
   primary 74, 77
   secondary 74, 77
Osteopetrosis 81
Osteoprogenitor cells 68
Osteosarcoma 81
Otolithic membrane 332
Otoscopy 327
Ovarian cycle 275
Ovarian follicle 270, 272, 274f
   fate of 275, 275f
   formation of 272
   mature 273f
Ovarian tumors 287
Ovary 269, 271, 274f, 287
   histological structure of 270f
Oviducts 276
Ovula nabothi 281
Ovulation 273
   pain 287
   time of 274f
Ovum
   fate of 274
   mature 272
   structure of 274f
Oxyntic cell 196
   electron microscope structure of 196f
Oxyphil cells 300
Oxytocin 294

P

Paget's disease 81
Palatine tonsil 109, 110
   coronal section of 109f
Palms 144
Palpebral conjunctiva 320
Pancreas 42, 211, 219, 220, 222, 222t, 223
   types of 210t
Pancreatic acini 221
   accessory 221
   main 221
Pancreatic islets 221
Pancreatic serous acinus 221f
Pancreatitis
   acute 223
   chronic 223
Paneth cells 202, 203, 203f
Panniculus adiposus 53
Papillae 181, 183f
Papillary plexus 145
Para-aortic bodies 303
Paracrine glands 37
Parafollicular cells 296
Parafollicular zone 108
Paraganglia 303
Parasympathetic nervous systems 113

Parathormone 299
Parathyroid
   gland 298, 299, 306
   hormone 299
Parenchyma 39, 103, 152, 212
Parietal cells 196
Parkinson's disease 251
Paronychia 150
Parotid gland 155
   pancreas 38
Parotid salivary gland 154
Pars amorpha 18
Pars anterior 291, 293
Pars distalis 291
Pars filamentosa 18
Pars granulosa 18
Pars intermedia 294, 294f
Pars nervosa 294
Pars tuberalis 291, 293
Passive transport 8
Pecten 208
Peduncles 240
Peg cells 276
Penicilli 103
Penis 265
   transverse section of 267f
Peptic cells 196
Peptides, small 289
Perforating fibers of Sharpey 70
Periarterial lymphatic sheath 105
Perichondrium 60
Perichoroidal space 308
Pericytes 134, 135
Perilymph 330
Perilymphatic cells 330
Perimetrium 281
Perimysium 84, 86
Perinephric fat 53
Perineurium 121
Perinuclear space 17
Periodic acid-Schiff
   method 32
   stain 48
Periodontal ligament 179
Periodontal membrane 180
Periosteal bud 76
Periosteal collar 78, 80f
Periosteum 69
   functions of 70
Peripheral nerves 115, 120, 122
   basic anatomy of 121f
   microscopic structure of 121
Peripheral nervous system 113, 117fc
Peristalsis 190
Peritoneum 219
Peritubular dentin 180
Perivascular connective tissue 106
Peroxisomes 15
Peyer's patch 98, 204
Phagocytosis 8
Phagolysosomes 15, 15f
Phalangeal cells 333, 334
Pharyngeal tonsil 109
Pharynx 167
Phosphatidylcholine 7f

Phospholipid molecule, structure of 7f
Physiological syncytium 93
Pia mater, modification of 241
Pigment cell 45, 46, 46f
   layer 312, 313
Pillar cell 333
Pineal body 303f
Pineal gland 302
   cyclic activity of 303
Pinealocytes 302
Pinna 325, 326
Pinocytosis 8
Pituicytes 294
Pituitary gland 290, 305
Placenta 160, 163
   accreta 164
   components of 160, 162f
   early 162
   fetal surfaces of 161f
   formation of 161
   functions 160
   increta 164
   maternal surfaces of 161f
   percreta 164
   synthesizes 160
   term 162
Placental abnormalities, structural 164
Placental circulation and barrier 162
Placental insufficiency 164
Planum semilunatum 336
Plaques, atheromatous 138
Plasma cell 45, 48, 48f, 57, 103, 204
   membrane 5
      structure of 5
Plasmakinin 153
Plasmatocytes 48
Pleomorphic adenoma 42, 159
Pleura 174
Plexiform cells, internal 317, 322
Plexiform layer 245
   external 315
   internal 317
Plica circularis 189, 198
Pneumocytes 174, 174f
Pneumonia, bacterial 176
Podocytes 227, 229f
Polar body, second 272
Polar end 5
Polycystic ovarian disease 287
Polygonal cells 31f
Polyribosomes 13
Polysomes 13
Pore complex 17
Portal acini 214
   concept of 214f
Portal canal 212
Portal hypertension 223
Portal lobules 214f
Portal triad 212, 214f
Portal vein obstruction 112
Portio vaginalis 281
Postcapillary venules 135
Postmenstrual phase 278
Precapillary sphincter 133, 137, 138

Pregnancy
   corpus luteum of 275
   ectopic tubal 287
   test 287
   tumor 185
Prickle cells 143
Primordial follicle 272, 273f
Principal bronchi 171
Principal cells 232, 261, 262, 298
Principal respiratory organs 171
Prisms 179
Progesterone 281
Prognathism 305
Prolactin 291
Proliferative phase 278t
Promonocytes 109
Prostaglandins 265
Prostate 265, 266, 267f
   carcinoma of 268
   gland, lobes of 267f
Protein 289
   intermediate 9
   link 9
   microtubule-associated 15, 116
   tubulin 15
Proteoglycans 52
Protofilaments 15
Protoplasm 5
Protoplasmic astrocytes 117
Proximal convoluted tubule 229, 230
Pseudostratified ciliated columnar epithelium 29
Pseudostratified columnar epithelium 19f, 29f
Pseudostratified epithelium 28
Psoriasis 150
Ptyalism 42
Pulmonary surfactant 174
Pulp 179, 180
   canal 179
   cavity 179
   white 103
Pulpitis 185
Pupil 312
Purkinje cell 247, 249
   layer 249
Pyloric glands 197
Pyloric sphincter 190
Pyogenic granuloma 185
Pyramidal cell 244, 244f
Pyramidal layer, outer 245

R

Ramus chorii 162f
Rapid transport 116
Receptor cells 183
Receptors 8
Rectum 208, 209
Red marrow 72
Red muscle fiber 90, 90t
Red pulp 103, 105
Renal blood vessels 233
Renal columns 225
   consists of 225
Renal corpuscle 225, 227
   basic structure of 227f

Renal cortex 228
   deeper parts of 234f
   superficial of 234f
Renal interstitium 234
Renal medulla 231
Renal pelvis 225
Renal pyramids 224
Renal sinus 225
Renal tubule 35, 225, 229
Renin 233
Reproductive system, female 269, 270f
Resident cells 44
Resorption bays 68
Respiratory bronchioles 171
Respiratory mucosa 167
Respiratory part of nasal mucosa, structure of 167f
Respiratory system 166
   types of cells of 174fc
Rete cutaneum 145
Rete ridge system 178
Rete subpapillare 145
Rete testis 253
   structure of 257
Reticular cells 45, 57
Reticular fibers 49, 50, 50f, 51f, 60
Reticular lamina 32, 333, 335, 334
Reticular plexus 145
Reticular tissue 57
Retina 307, 312, 313f, 321, 324
   basic structure of 313
   ciliary part of 312
   different parts of 323f
   iridial part of 312
   layer of 313f
   nervous layer of 312
   pigment cell of 314f
Retinal detachment 324
Retinitis pigmentosa 324
Retinoblastoma 324
Rheumatoid arthritis 112
Rhinoplasty 336
Rhodopsin 314
Ribonucleic acid 12
Ribosomes 12, 13
Rod and cone 314
   cells, ultrastructure of 314
   density of 321
   layer of 314
   main parts of 315f
Rod bipolar cells, terminals of 316f
Rod cell 333
   structure of 315f
Rod ganglion cells 322
Rod spherule 316
   synapsing 316f
Rokitansky-Aschoff sinuses 219
Root 150, 179
   formation 187
Root sheath
   inner 146
   outer 146
Russell's bodies 49
Rympanoplasty 337

S

Saccular glands 38
Salivary gland 37, 42, 152, 154f, 177
   cells of 154
   innervation of 153
   major 152, 159
   minor 152
   serous cell in 154f
   tumors of 42, 159
Salivary tumor, mixed 42
Saltatory conduction 119
Sarcolemma 84, 87
Sarcoplasm 84
Sarcoplasmic reticulum 89, 90f
Satellite cells 116, 118
Scala tympani 328
Scala vestibuli 328, 330f
Schwann cell 116, 118, 119, 119f, 120f
   sheath 119
Sclera 307
   junction of 308f
Scleral spur 308
Sclerous connective tissue 67
Sebaceous gland 42, 147, 147f, 148
Sebum 147
Secretion
   mode of 37
   nature of 37
   site of 37
Secretory cells 221, 276
Secretory component 153
Secretory function 189
Secretory part 152
Secretory phase 278t
Secretory unit 287
   shape of 38
Secretory vacuoles, formation of 14f
Section across eyeball 308f
Segmental bronchi 171
Sella turcica 290
Semicircular canals 327, 328, 328f
Seminal vesicle 262, 264
Seminiferous tubules 253
   general structure of 253
   walls of 258f
Sensory 126t
   ganglia 124-126
   neuroepithelium 332
   neuron 120
Seromucous cells 42, 153
Serosa 197, 204, 205, 208, 219
Serous 41t
   acini 41, 153
   cell 21, 41, 152, 153
   coat 103
   demilunes 153
   gland 37
   layer 189, 235
   pericardium, visceral layer of 137
   salivary gland 222, 222t
Sertoli cells, cytoplasm of 258
Serum amylase 223
Sex glands, accessory 252
Sialadenitis 42
Sialorrhea 42

Index

Sickle cell disease 112
Signet ring appearance 53
Sinus venosus sclerae 308
Sinusoid, structure of 135*f*
Sinusoidal surface 215
Sinusoids 129
Skeletal muscle 83, 84, 91, 96, 96*t*
    contraction of 89, 94
    fibers, types of 89
    innervation of 91
    lymphatic of 91
    proteins in 89
    structure of 84*f*
    transverse section of 86, 87*f*
    tumors 96
Skin 52
    appendages of 145
    blood supply of 145
    dermis of 53, 55
    functions 139
    nerve supply of 145
    thick 139, 139*t*, 141
    thin 139, 139*t*, 140, 142*f*
    types of 139
Skull bones, growth of 79*f*
Slit diaphragm 227
Slow transport 116
Small intestine 189, 197, 205, 205*t*, 209
    basic structure of 198*f*
    cells of 202, 202*f*
    structure 198
Smooth muscle 83, 93-96, 96*t*
    cells 94f, 130
        aggregations of 94
    layer 168, 172
Somatodendritic synapse 124
Somatosomatic synapse 124
Space of Disse 217
Special senses
    ear 325
    eye 307
Spermatocytes
    primary 258
    secondary 258
Spermatogenesis 257, 258*f*, 258*fc*
    stages of 257, 259*fc*
Spermatogenic cells 253, 255
Spermatogonia 257
Spermatozoa 252
    capacitation of 260
    maturation of 260
Spermatozoon 260*f*
    structure of 260*f*
        mature 259
Spermiogenesis 258, 259
Spherocytosis 112
Sphincter 96, 190
    ampullae 219
    choledochus 219
    muscle, internal 235
    pancreaticus 219
    pupillae 312
    vesicae 235
Spinal cord 240, 241*f*, 242
    cross-section of 243*t*

Spine 143
    typical 143*f*
Spiral artery 278
Spiral ganglion 331
Spiral lamina 328
Spiral ligament 331
Spiral limbus 332
Spiral prominence 331
Spiral sheath 260
Spiral sulcus
    internal 332
    outer 331
Spleen 98, 103, 104, 112
Splenectomy 105
Splenic circulation 105*f*
Splenic cords 105
Splenic sinusoids 105
Splenic tumors, primary 112
Splenic vein obstruction 112
Splenomegaly 112
    causes of 112
Spongiocytes 300
Spongy bone 71, 72
Squamous cell carcinoma 151
Squamous epithelium 24
    simple 24, 24*f*, 25
    stratified 29, 30, 31*f*, 177, 181, 183*f*
Squamous metaplasia 36
Squamous nonkeratinized epithelium,
    stratified 178, 191
Stave cells 103
Stellate cell 244*f*, 247
    inner 250
    outer 250
Stellate neurons 244
Stem cells 46, 108, 197
    adult 45
    intermediate 144
Stem villus 162
Stereocilia 21, 33, 36
Steroids 289
Stigma 273
Stomach 188, 191, 209
    anatomical regions of 191*f*
    basic structure of mucous membrane of
        193*f*
    functions 193
    fundus 188, 194
    microscopic features 193
    pylorus 188, 195
    region of 193*t*
Storage diseases 112
Storage vesicles 14
Stratum basale 143
Stratum corneum 144
Stratum epithelial
    granulosum 146
    pallidum 146
Stratum germinativum 143
Stratum granulosum 143
Stratum intermedium 186
Stratum lucidum 143, 144
Stratum spinosum 143
    cells of 143*f*
Stria vascularis 330, 331

Striate cortex 247
Striated border 20, 27, 202
    appearance 35
Striated ducts 153
Striated muscle 83
    ultrastructure of 85
Stroma 39, 152, 212, 278, 287
Stye 324
Subcapsular sinus 102
Subcutis 142
Subendothelial connective tissue 129, 130
Sublingual salivary gland 158, 159
Submandibular gland 154, 156, 157
Submucosa 168, 189-191, 197, 204, 205, 208, 238
    glands in 172
Submucosal plexus of Meissner 190
Submucous layer 235
Sulcus terminalis 181
Supercoiling 17
Supporting cells 183, 335
    of Sertoli 253
Suprachoroid lamina 308, 311
Supranuclear granules 203*f*
Suprarenal cortex 300
Suprarenal gland 300, 301, 306
Suprarenal medulla 302
Suspensory ligaments 284
Sustentacular cells 175, 183, 255, 255*f*, 335
Sweat gland 38, 42, 147, 149*f*
    atrophic 149
    parts of typical 149*f*
    typical 147
Synapse 116, 124
Synaptic transmission, mechanism of 128*f*
Synaptic zone, inner 317
Systemic lupus erythematosus 112

T

Taenia coli 190, 205
Tanycytes 118, 295
Tarsal gland 42, 320
Tarsal plate 320
Tarsus 320
Taste bud 183, 183f, 185*f*
Tay-Sachs disease 21
Teeth 177, 179
Tendon, transverse section through 53*f*
Terminal arterioles 132
Terminal bronchioles 171
Terminal buds 302
Terminal web 202
Tertiary hyperparathyroidism 306
Testicular tumors 268
Testis 252, 254, 256
    basic structure of 253*f*
    general structure of 252
Testosterone 252
Thalassemias 112
Theca externa 273
Theca interna 273
Thoracic duct 98
Thoroughfare channels 137
Thymic humoral factor 108
Thymic nurse cells 106

Thymocytes 106, 108
Thymopoietin 108
Thymosin
    alpha-1 108
    beta-4 108
Thymulin 108
Thymus 98, 106, 107, 112
    functions of 108
    lymphocytes of 108
Thyroglobulin, synthesis of 298
Thyroid
    follicles, appearance of 296f
    gland 295, 297, 298fc, 306
        follicular cell of 296f
    hormone, synthesis of 298
Thyrotropes 291
Thyrotropic hormone 291
Thyrotropin 291
Tight junctions, functions of 11
Tissue
    elastic 57
    plasminogen activator 130
    processing 3
T-lymphocytes 48, 49, 100
    circulation of 99f
Tomes process 186
Tongue 177, 181, 182f, 185
    and palate, minor salivary glands of 42
    bald 185
    dorsal surface of 181f
    fissured 185
    geographic 185
    glossitis 185
    hairy 185
    mucous glands of 183
    serous glands of 183
Tonsil 98
Tonsillar crypts 109
Tonsillectomy 112
Tonsillitis 112
Tonsils 109, 112
Tooth 185
    development, stages in 185, 186f
    part of 180f
Trabeculae 103
Trachea 168, 170
Transitional epithelium 31, 32, 33f, 35, 235
Transitional zone 208
Transmembrane proteins 7
Triads 316
Trichohyaline granules 146
Trophoblast 161
Tropocollagen 49
Tropoelastin 51
Tropomyosin 88
Troponin 88, 94
Truncus chorii 162, 162f
Trypsin-like substances 260
Tubal tonsils 109
Tubular glands 38
Tubules 16f
Tubuli recti 253

Tubuloalveolar glands, branched 152
Tumor 36, 151
    chondroblastic 65
Tunica adventitia 129, 131, 132
Tunica albuginea 252, 270
Tunica intima 129, 132
Tunica media 129, 130, 132
Tunica vaginalis 252
Tunica vasculosa 252, 253
Tympani 330f
Tympanic cavity 327
Tympanic lip 332
Tympanic membrane 327
    secondary 328
Tympanum 327
Typical long bone
    development of 78
    formation of 80f

U

Ulcerative colitis 209
Ultraviolet microscope 3
Umbilical arteries 165
Umbilical cord 160, 161f, 164, 165f
    microscopic section of 164
Umbrella cells 235
Unicellular gland 37, 39f
Unicellular goblet cells 37
Unilaminar primary follicle 272
Unilocular adipose tissue 57f
Unipolar neurons 120, 120f
Ureter 234, 236
Ureterocele 238
Urethra 238
    female 238
Urethral sphincter, external 238
Urinary bladder 94, 235, 237
Urinary pole 227
Urinary space 227
Urinary system 224
    functions 224, 238
Urothelium 32
Uterine glands 278, 281f
Uterine part 276
Uterine tubes 276
Uterus 276, 279, 280, 287
    living ligature of 281
    wall of 161f
Utricle 330
Uvea 309

V

Vacuoplasm 5, 12
Vagina 282, 283, 288
Vaginitis 288
Vallate papilla 184f
van Gieson method 49
Varicose veins 138
Vas deferens 94
Vasa recta
    ascending 234
    descending 234

Vasa vasorum 135
Vascular coat 309
Vascular lamina 311
Vascular pole 227
Vasopressin 294
Vasorum 130
Vein 129, 134
    arcuate 234
    interlobar 234
    interlobular 234
    large-sized 136
    valves of 135
Ventral horn 241
Ventral white commissure 243
Venule 132f, 129, 135
Verhoeff's method 51
Vermiform appendix 98, 188, 205, 207
Vermilion 178
Vestibular lip 332
Vestibule 167, 282, 327
Villi 189, 198, 202
Vimentin 16
Visual organs, accessory 319
Vitiligo 150
Vocal folds 167
Volkmann's canal 72f
Voluntary muscle 83
von Kupffer cells 110
von Willebrand factor 130

W

Waldeyer's ring 109
Weibel-Palade bodies 130
Wharton's jelly 164
White fibrocartilage 63
White line of Hilton 208
White matter 240, 243
Wilson's disease 324
Wolff's law 81

X

Xerostomia 42

Y

Yellow marrow 72

Z

Zollinger-Ellison syndrome 209
Zona arcuata 330
Zona fasciculata 300
Zona glomerulosa 300
Zona pectinata 330
Zona pellucida 273
Zona reaction 260
Zona reticularis 300
Zonula adherens 10
Zonula occludens 11, 11f
Zwischenschiebe 88
Zymogen cells 196, 203